Complications of Urogynecology and Reconstructive Pelvic Surgery

Howard B. Goldman
Jacqueline Zillioux
Editors

Complications of Urogynecology and Reconstructive Pelvic Surgery

Third Edition

Springer

Editors
Howard B. Goldman
Glickman Urological & Kidney Institute
Cleveland Clinic
Cleveland, OH, USA

Jacqueline Zillioux
Department of Urology
University of Virginia Health
Charlottesville, VA, USA

ISBN 978-3-032-00338-6 ISBN 978-3-032-00339-3 (eBook)
https://doi.org/10.1007/978-3-032-00339-3

This Springer imprint is published by the registered company Springer Nature Switzerland AG
The registered company address is: Gewerbestrasse 11, 6330 Cham, Switzerland

With deep appreciation to all of my former and current fellows, residents, and visiting observers.
I hope you have learned as much from me as I have learned from you.

Howard B. Goldman, M.D., F.A.C.S

To my husband Alan, whose support and love are my bedrock.

Jacqueline. Zillioux, M.D.

Forewords from the Second Edition

First Foreword

This second edition of Dr. Howard Goldman's *Complications of Female Incontinence and Pelvic Reconstructive Surgery* updates the outstanding first edition which included a multinational authorship related to those issues of quality and safety that are pertinent to female pelvic surgical reconstruction. The second edition updates the first edition by including discussions related to specific procedures, but also more global issues related to surgical reconstruction and risks thereof associated. The first chapter of the book summarizes taxonomic classifications for complications both generally and specifically. The next two chapters—Patient Consent and Perception of Complications and Medical Malpractice—define the importance of the engaged and informed patient and the issues surrounding the importance of obtaining appropriate informed consent from the standpoint of avoiding medical–legal concerns. The last general chapter deals with Medical and Other Types of Complications Related to Pelvic Surgery (and in fact inherent to all surgeries). Following these first four chapters, there then follow chapters on various prolapse repair concerns followed by incontinence concerns and finally specific issues related to management of other lower urinary tract symptom complexes and/or anatomic abnormalities.

It is abundantly clear that surgery is only one aspect of approaching complex female disorders. There is an extremely important presurgical time frame which not only involves the subjective and objective estimation of the patient's condition, bother, and ongoing life burden but also involves the objectification of those symptoms through appropriate, focused, and informed testing which will help the surgeon in his or her preplanning for the surgical procedure. There has been a great deal of discussion and research into the value of certain types of testing modalities (i.e., urodynamics). It is incumbent upon the surgeon, for the unique patient, to make the appropriate choice of objective testing. The wary surgeon is cautioned that operating for symptoms only is fraught with the potential of not completely understanding what is causing those symptoms and complicating the initial symptoms with secondary symptoms arising from surgical intervention. Preoperative preparation, education, and realistic expectation setting are critical for not only the perioperative time frame but also the chronic postoperative time frame where the patient experiences (we hope) some resolution or improvement of their symptoms. Part of urologic pelvic reconstruction is the acknowledgement that rarely is success equivalent to cure but rather remediation and improvement. The successful surgeon is one who counsels his or her patient that they are embarking upon a journey together which hopefully will result in overall improvement, but that the surgeon will stand by their patient regardless of outcome for purposes of helping chronically manage any persistent and/or new conditions that may arise as a direct result of treatment for the initial inciting condition.

This book is a very important contribution and should be used by all who venture into the world of pelvic reconstruction for purposes not only of self-education and edification but also of guidance given the authorities who are listed in this book and their expertise in the various areas of concern.

This text should serve as a fundamental reference book for not only those in training but also those who have mature careers who are looking for a rapid update on specific issues related to female incontinence and pelvic reconstructive surgery and complications resulting therefrom. I personally find this book an outstanding resource. I hope that you will too.

Department of Urology
Vanderbilt University Medical Center
Vanderbilt University Hospital
Nashville, TN, USA

Roger R. Dmochowski

Second Foreword

Female Pelvic Medicine and Reconstructive Surgery (FPMRS) has made significant strides in the last decade, including official subspecialty designation by the American Board of Medical Specialties and an ever expanding armamentarium for treating women with urinary incontinence, pelvic organ prolapse, and other pelvic floor disorders. As pelvic reconstructive surgeons, our goal is to perform safe and effective procedures that improve the quality of lives of women suffering from these disorders. Avoiding and, when necessary, effectively managing perioperative complications are essential goals, particularly in this era of Quality and Safety. The FDA's 2011 public health notification on transvaginal mesh and the resultant media and medico-legal storm has heightened patients' awareness of the potential for surgical complications and made comprehensive knowledge of informed consent, patient selection, and avoiding, recognizing and managing mesh-related complications all the more important. No one understands this better than Howard Goldman, M.D., Vice Chair of Quality and Patient Safety for the Glickman Urologic Institute at the Cleveland Clinic and internationally recognized expert on pelvic surgical complications. In the first edition of *Complications of Female Incontinence and Pelvic Reconstructive Surgery*, Dr. Goldman brought together highly experienced pelvic reconstructive surgeons to share their expertise on the prevention, recognition, and management of a broad spectrum of surgical complications. In this second edition, this novel and highly valuable resource has been expanded significantly to include new chapters exploring the medico-legal implications of surgical complications as well as the informed consent process and patient perception of complications. Additionally, the coverage of sling complications has been vastly expanded and includes separate chapters on complications from midurethral, transobturator, fascial, and single-incision slings and retropubic procedures.

In my opinion, *Complications of Female Incontinence and Pelvic Reconstructive Surgery, Second Edition*, is an essential text that should be on the bookshelves of all FPMRS specialists. It provides practical, real-world advice that should improve your ability to provide high-quality care to your patients.

Department of Obstetrics
Gynecology and Women's Health Institute
Cleveland Clinic
Cleveland, OH, USA

Matthew D. Barber

Prefaces from the First Edition

I am honored and pleased to write a preface for the textbook on Complications of Female Incontinence and Pelvic Reconstructive Surgery. At a time when the subspecialty of female pelvic medicine and reconstructive surgery is in its infancy, I feel having such a resource available to pelvic surgeons is extremely beneficial. Dr. Goldman has invited internationally respected contributors to provide their experience and expertise regarding the avoidance and management of surgical complications related to a variety of female pelvic floor surgeries. As the majority of the surgeries we perform on our female patients are done for quality of life symptoms, it has become apparent that we need to do a better job reporting and managing the untoward outcomes that can sometimes occur after these interventions. This book brings these potential complications to the forefront.

It will be of great use for both general urologists and gynecologists who perform pelvic floor surgeries as well as current and future specialists in female pelvic medicine and reconstructive surgery.

Cincinnati, OH, USA — Mickey Karram

Surgery for incontinence, pelvic organ prolapse, and other disorders of the female pelvic floor has evolved in the past two decades as the specialty of Female Pelvic Medicine and Reconstructive Surgery has incorporated expertise from the fields of urology, gynecology, and colorectal surgery. Today, more surgeons are better equipped to treat disorders of the female pelvic floor than ever before. Unfortunately complications of surgery, whether intraoperative or postoperative, are inevitable even for the most experienced and highly skilled surgeon. Whether it is an unexpected finding in the operating room or an undesirable outcome of surgery, the Female Pelvic Surgeon must be equipped to prevent and manage a variety of complications.

While there are several excellent texts devoted to indications for surgery and the technical aspects of surgical procedures "Complications of Female Incontinence and Pelvic Reconstructive Surgery" fills a need by providing readers with a comprehensive review of the prevention and management of common and not so common complications of female pelvic surgery. Dr. Howard Goldman has assembled a group of highly experienced authors from all three disciplines of Female Pelvic Medicine and Reconstructive Surgery. These authors offer in-depth descriptions of three critical areas: prevention, evaluation, and management of complications. They present practical information and surgical tips based on years of experience and a thorough review of the relevant literature. In addition, a look at the table of contents shows that complications from all types of reconstructive procedures are covered.

I believe that "Complications of Female Incontinence and Pelvic Reconstructive Surgery" will be a great complement to the libraries of those of us who treat female pelvic disorders. Whether one is just starting a career or is highly experienced, this book is a welcome addition.

New York City, NY, USA Victor W. Nitti

Current Edition [3rd Edition]

First Foreword

A renowned surgeon in Abraham Verghese's "The Covenant of Water" remarked to a junior colleague who saved a postoperative catastrophe through diligent awareness, preparation, and attentiveness: "Good surgeons can do any operation. Great surgeons take care of their own complications."

Experts from Urology and Urogynecology have joined forces under the editorial guidance of Drs. Howard Goldman and Jacqueline Zillioux to produce an updated third edition of *Complications of Female Incontinence and Pelvic Reconstructive Surgery* that provides detailed and pragmatic guidance to surgeons committed to complication prevention, diagnosis, and management. As the field of Urogynecology and Reconstructive Pelvic Surgery rests on restoring quality of life, complications that induce suffering are particularly hard for patients and their doctors to endure. Fortunately, procedures in our field are not commonly associated with severe adverse events. This results, however, in many surgeons not having experiential training in how to manage a particular problem. Coalescing evidence-based strategies with expert opinion for the evaluation and management of complications associated with the full breadth of female urology and urogynecology procedures in one textbook is a valuable resource for patient care. It is also an excellent physician resource for board preparation and review.

Since the previous edition of this textbook was published in 2017, practice patterns have evolved with a focus on harm reduction. Procedures such as urethral bulking, single-incision slings, vaginal laser, and hysteropexy have increased in popularity, largely due to lower risks. However, as our patients live longer and get sicker, more challenging interventions and repeat operations are often needed, often with compounded risk. This expanded and updated textbook, arranged primarily by surgical procedure (anterior and posterior compartment repair, uterosacral and sacrospinous ligament fixation, sacrocolpopexy, colpocleisis, colposuspension, fascial slings, synthetic slings, female urethral reconstruction, urethral diverticulectomy, fistula repair, anal sphincteroplasty, cosmetic gynecology, urethral bulking, sacral neuromodulation, intravesical botulinum toxin injection, and flaps) has the addition of the following new chapters: hysteropexy, mesh products, vaginal laser treatments, autologous graft harvest, gender-affirming surgery, and prolapse after cystectomy. This third edition serves as a resource to all pelvic surgeons for mundane to complex complication scenarios.

Department of Urology
Wake Forest School of Medicine
Winston Salem, NC, USA
Catherine A. Matthews

Second Foreword

A foreword is supposed to reflect a personal introduction to a book, written especially for the readers, and is supposed to whet their appetite for proceeding.

To paraphrase a line in the movie Forrest Gump, "it happens." Despite our very well-planned and well-executed efforts to surgically correct or improve a situation, adverse events do occur. Some of these are predictable and have been discussed with the patient beforehand, but some are not very predictable and have not been mentioned, or perhaps they have been, but were described as "very rare." Generally, in a global textbook of a medical discipline, the subject of complications is relegated to the end of a chapter discussing surgical correction. Often, these discussions do not yield as much information as desired by the individual under whose direction the complication has occurred. Thus, the great value of a textbook such as this which deals only with this side of a surgical discipline, in this case the surgical subspecialty of Urogynecology and Pelvic Reconstructive Surgery (URPS).

This is the third edition of this book, and so it has demonstrated "staying power" to the publisher and to the segment of surgeons who practice in these areas. Howard Goldman, a true expert in all areas encompassed by URPS, has added a co-editor for this addition, Jacqueline Zillioux, a rising young expert, and they have again recruited a roster of recognized superstars in these fields as contributors. All chapters have been extensively updated (the last edition was published in 2017), and totally new chapters have been added on hysteropexy, mesh products, vaginal laser treatment, autologous graft harvest, gender affirming surgery, and prolapse occurrence after female cystectomy. New authors have been chosen for the chapters on sacral neuromodulation and on mesh-related pain. All surgeons who practice in the area of URPS, whether fellowship trained or not, will want this book on their shelves or computers, and it will prove to be an essential resource for residents and fellows in these areas as well. The book provides succinct but complete information from patient consent guidelines and how to reduce malpractice risks and how to recognize and correct virtually all adverse events related to the Surgery of Female Incontinence and Pelvic Reconstruction. In my opinion, it represents a most valuable and up-to-date contribution to our field.

Alan J. Wein

Professor of Urology, Director of Business
Development and Mentoring
Desai-Sethi Institute of Urology
University of Miami Miller School of Medicine
Miami, FL, USA

Emeritus Professor, Chief and Program
Director of Urology
University of Pennsylvania Perelman School of Medicine
Philadelphia, PA, USA

Contents

Contributors

Shree Agrawal-Patel Glickman Urological & Kidney Institute, Cleveland Clinic, Cleveland, OH, USA

Emma Bacharach Department of Urology, Medical University of South Carolina, Charleston, SC, USA

Bethany Bandi Department of Urology, Cleveland Clinic Foundation, Cleveland, OH, USA

Matthew D. Barber Department of Obstetrics and Gynecology, Duke University Medical Center, Durham, NC, USA

Lisa M. Barrett Law Department, Cleveland Clinic, Beachwood, OH, USA

Dina A. Bastawros Urogynecology and Reconstructive Pelvic Surgery, Novant Health Pelvic Health Center, Winston-salem, NC, USA

Jerry G. Blaivas Icahn School of Medicine at Mount Sinai Hospital, Department of Urology, New York, NY, USA

Elizabeth Timbrook Brown MedStar Health Department of Urology, MedStar Georgetown University Hospital, Washington, DC, USA

Benjamin Brucker Department of Urology, New York University Langone Medical Center, New York, NY, USA

Kristina A. Burger Urogynecology and Reconstructive Pelvic Surgery, Atrium Health Wake Forest Baptist, Charlotte, NC, USA

Courtney Capella Department of Urology, Thomas Jefferson University, Philadelphia, PA, USA

Laura A. Chang-Kit Encore Urology, Naples, FL, USA

J. Quentin Clemens Department of Urology, University of Michigan, Ann Arbor, MI, USA

Rachel Cline LSU Health Shreveport School of Medicine, Shreveport, LA, USA

Joshua A. Cohn Division of Urology, Fox Chase Cancer Center, Philadelphia, PA, USA

Lindsey Cox Department of Urology, Medical University of South Carolina, Charleston, SC, USA

Maria D'Amico Department of Urology, Thomas Jefferson University, Philadelphia, PA, USA

Ava A. Delu Department of Urology, University of Arizona College of Medicine, Tucson, AZ, USA

Roger R. Dmochowski Department of Urologic Surgery, Vanderbilt University Medical Center, Nashville, TN, USA

Matthew J. Donnelly Office of Professional Staff Affairs, Cleveland Clinic, Cleveland, OH, USA

Erin Dougher Urogynecology, Baylor Scott White, Austin, Texas, USA

Alice Drain Department of Urology, Rutgers University, Robert Wood Johnson Barnabas Health Medical Group, New Brunswick, NJ, USA

Rahul Dutta Fellow Urogynecology and Pelvic Reconstructive Surgery, Departments of Urology and Obstetrics and Gynecology, David Geffen School of Medicine at the University of California, Los Angeles, CA, USA

Amr El Haraki Urogynecology and Reconstructive Pelvic Surgery, Wake Forest School of Medicine, Winston Salem, NC, USA

Michele Fascelli Department of Urology, Cleveland Clinic Foundation, Cleveland, OH, USA

Danni Feng The Arthur Smith Institute for Urology, Lenox Hill Hospital, Hofstra Northwell School of Medicine, Northwell Health System, New York, NY, USA

Farzeen Firoozi The Arthur Smith Institute for Urology, Lenox Hill Hospital, Hofstra Northwell School of Medicine, Northwell Health System, New York, NY, USA

Joel T. Funk Department of Urology, University of Arizona College of Medicine, Tucson, AZ, USA

Natalie Gaines Amarillo Urology Associates, Amarillo, TX, USA

Alienor S. Gilchrist Department of Urology, Piedmont Hospital, Stockbridge, GA, USA

David A. Ginsberg Department of Urology, Keck School of Medicine of USC, USC Institute of Urology, Los Angeles, CA, USA

Mitchell G. Goldenberg Department of Urology, Keck School of Medicine of USC, USC Institute of Urology, Los Angeles, CA, USA

Howard B. Goldman Glickman Urological & Kidney Institute, Cleveland Clinic, Cleveland, OH, USA

Alex Gomelsky Department of Urology, Lousiana State University Health—Shreveport, Shreveport, LA, USA
Department of Urology, University of Florida School of Medicine, Gainesville, FL, USA

Sonia Guérin University of Texas Southwestern Medical Center, Dallas, TX, USA

Priyanka Gupta Department of Urology, University of Michigan, Ann Arbor, MI, USA

Brooke Gurland Department of Surgery, Stanford Pelvic Health Center, Stanford, CA, USA

Barry Hallner Jr Department of Obstetrics and Gynecology, Louisiana State University Health Sciences Center, New Orleans, LA, USA
Urogynecology, Womans Hospital, Baton Rouge, Louisiana, USA

Lacey Hart Department of Urology, University of Arizona College of Medicine, Tucson, AZ, USA

Hashim Hashim Bristol Urological Institute, Southmead Hospital, Bristol, UK

Camryn Hawkins Northeast Ohio Medical University, Rootstown, OH, USA

Sender Herschorn Division of Urology, Sunnybrook Health Science Centre, Toronto, ON, Canada

Michael Ingber Rutgers New Jersey Medical School, Newark, NJ, USA
Department of Urology, Atlantic Health System, Morristown Medical Center, Morristown, NJ, USA

Mickey Karram Division of Urogynecology and Pelvic Reconstructive Surgery, The Christ Hospital, University of Cincinnati, Cincinnati, OH, USA
Department of Obstetrics/Gynecology, University of Cincinnati, Cincinnati, OH, USA

Melissa R. Kaufman Department of Urology, Vanderbilt University Medical Center, Nashville, TN, USA

Michael J. Kennelly Urogynecology and Reconstructive Pelvic Surgery, Atrium Health Wake Forest Baptist, Charlotte, NC, USA

Ashley B. King Woodlands Medical Specialist, Department of Urology, Center for Female Pelvic Medicine and Reconstructive Surgery, Pensacola, FL, USA

Rachel Kopkin Department of Urology and Gynecology, Stanford University, Stanford, CA, USA

Michelle Koski Department of Urology, Kaiser Permanente Medical Center, San Marcos, CA, USA

Dominic Lee Department of Urology, ST George Hospital, Kogarah, NSW, Australia

Jennifer Lee Department of Urology, Kaiser Permanente Los Angeles Medical Center, Los Angeles, CA, USA

Marcelo Mass Lindenbaum Glickman Urological Institute, Cleveland Clinic Foundation, Cleveland, OH, USA

Brian J. Linder Department of Urology, Mayo Clinic, Rochester, MN, USA

Austin J. Martin Department of Urology, Mayo Clinic, Rochester, MN, USA

Catherine A. Matthews Urogynecology and Reconstructive Pelvic Surgery, Wake Forest School of Medicine, Winston Salem, NC, USA

Courtenay K. Moore The Ohio State University, Columbus, OH, USA

Elizabeth R. Mueller Professor Emeritus, Urogynecology and Reconstructive Pelvic Surgery, Loyola University Chicago Stritch School of Medicine, Maywood, IL, USA

Alana Murphy Department of Urology, Thomas Jefferson University, Philadelphia, PA, USA

Victor W. Nitti Shlomo Raz Chair in Urology, Division of URPS, David Geffen School of Medicine at the University of California Los Angeles, Los Angeles, CA, USA

Bahrom Ostad Department of Urology, University of Virginia Health, Charlottesville, VA, USA

Natalie Pace Department of Urologic Surgery, Vanderbilt University Medical Center, Nashville, TN, USA

Dominique Malacarne Pape Department of Obstetrics, Gynecology and Urology, New York Medical College, Valhalla, NY, USA

Javier Pizarro-Berdichevsky Centro de Innovación en Piso Pélvico, Sótero del Rio Hospital, Santiago, Chile
Corporación de Innovación en Piso Pélvico, Santiago, Chile
Gynecology Department, Pontificia Universidad Católica de Chile, Santiago, Chile

Mikolaj Przydacz Department of Urology, Jagiellonian University Medical College, Krakow, Poland
Glickman Urological Institute, Cleveland Clinic, Cleveland, OH, USA

Rajveer S. Purohit Icahn School of Medicine at Mount Sinai Hospital, Department of Urology, New York, NY, USA

Karla Rebullar Department of Urologic Surgery, Vanderbilt University Medical Center, Nashville, TN, USA

William Stuart Reynolds Department of Urologic Surgery, Vanderbilt University Medical Center, Nashville, TN, USA

Paholo Barboglio Romo Department of Urology, University of Michigan, Ann Arbor, MI, USA

Nirit Rosenblum Department of Urology, NYU Langone Medical Center, New York, NY, USA

Elizabeth A. Rourke Department of Urologic Surgery, Louisiana State University Health Science Center, New Orleans, LA, USA

Eric S. Rovner Department of Urology, Medical University of South Carolina, Charleston, SC, USA

Kamran P. Sajadi Department of Urology, Oregon Health and Science University, CH10U, Portland, OR, USA

Dora Jericevic Schwartz Department of Urology, NYU Langone Medical Center, New York, NY, USA

Steven W. Siegel Centers for Continence Care and Female Urology, Metro Urology, Woodbury, MN, USA

Larry T. Sirls Corewell Health William Beaumont University Hospital, Bloomfield Hills, MI, USA

Ellen R. Solomon Urogynecology and Pelvic Surgery, Baystate Medical Center, Springfield, MA, USA

Brandee Spitnale Department of Urology, University of Michigan, Ann Arbor, MI, USA

Noah Stern Department of Surgery Division of Urology, North York General Hospital, Toronto, ON, Canada

Lauren Stewart Department of Urology, NYU Langone Medical Center, New York, NY, USA

Christopher F. Tenggardjaja Bernard J Tyson School of Medicine, Department of Urology, Kaiser Permanente Los Angeles Medical Center, Los Angeles, CA, USA

Laura Thomas Bristol Urological Institute, Southmead Hospital, Bristol, UK

Camille Torres Crane Center for Transgender Surgery, Austin, USA

Christian O. Twiss Department of Urology, University of Arizona College of Medicine, Tucson, AZ, USA

Tyler Trump Center for Urogynecology and Reconstructive Pelvic Surgery, Glickman Urological Institute, Cleveland Clinic, Cleveland, OH, USA

Sandip P. Vasavada Glickman Urological & Kidney Institute, Cleveland Clinic, Cleveland, OH, USA

Lauren Wilson Department of General Surgery, Dartmouth Hitchcock Medical Center, Lebanon, NH, USA

Jack Christian Winters Department of Urology, Louisiana State University Health Sciences Center, New Orleans, LA, USA
Urogynecology, Womans Hospital, Baton Rouge, Louisiana, USA

Katherine L. Woodburn Department of Urology, Wake Forest School of Medicine, Winston Salem, NC, USA

Menaka Yadav Urogynecology and Reconstructive Pelvic Surgery, Loyola University Chicago Stritch School of Medicine, Maywood, IL, USA

Yu Zheng Department of Urology, Brigham and Women's Hospital, Boston, MA, USA

Jacqueline Zillioux Department of Urology, University of Virginia Health, Charlottesville, VA, USA

Philippe E. Zimmern University of Texas Southwestern Medical Center, Dallas, TX, USA

Dani Zoorob Division of Urogynecology and Pelvic Reconstructive Surgery, Department of Obstetrics and Gynecology, Louisiana State University Health Sciences Center in Shreveport, Shreveport, LA, USA

Taxonomy of Complications of Pelvic Floor Surgery

1

Karla Rebullar, Joshua A. Cohn, Alex Gomelsky, Laura A. Chang-Kit, and Roger R. Dmochowski

Introduction

The etymology of the word "taxonomy" is from the Greek *taxis*, meaning orderly arrangement, and *nomos*, meaning law. Stedman's Medical Dictionary defines "taxonomy" as the systemic classification of living things or organisms; however, more recently, the term has come to mean any specialized method of classifying objects or events. The aim of taxonomic classification of surgical complications is to permit comparison of adverse outcomes and assist in risk stratification. In this chapter, we review the existing broader surgical classification systems that may be applicable to female pelvic medicine as well as those systems specifically developed for female reconstructive procedures.

K. Rebullar · R. R. Dmochowski (✉)
Department of Urologic Surgery, Vanderbilt University Medical Center, Nashville, TN, USA
e-mail: karla.rebullar@vumc.org; roger.dmochowski@vumc.org

J. A. Cohn
Division of Urology, Fox Chase Cancer Center, Philadelphia, PA, USA

A. Gomelsky
Department of Urology, Lousiana State University Health—Shreveport, Shreveport, LA, USA
e-mail: alexander.gomelsky@lsuhs.edu

L. A. Chang-Kit
Encore Urology, Naples, FL, USA
e-mail: lchangkit@encoreurology.com

The Need for Taxonomy of Complications

Complications are an unfortunate but inevitable aspect of patient care and surgery, in particular. Complications are usually multifactorial and can accompany even the most minor, least invasive, and routine procedures. The tracking and reporting of surgical complications are essential to identifying areas for quality improvement. Historically, reporting of complications has been inconsistent, and, therefore, outcomes are difficult to compare. Martin and colleagues developed a list of ten critical elements of accurate and comprehensive reporting of surgical complications [1]. These criteria included: (1) providing the methods for data accrual, (2) duration of follow-up, (3) outpatient information, (4) definition of complications, (5) mortality rate and cause of death, (6) morbidity rate and total complications, (7) procedure-specific complications, (8) severity grade, (9) length-of-stay data, and (10) risk factors included in the analysis. The authors found that of 119 articles published between 1975 and 2001 reporting data on 22,530 patients who had undergone pancreatectomy, esophagectomy, and hepatectomy, none reported all ten criteria, and only 2% reported nine out of ten. The most frequently omitted criteria were outpatient information (22%), definitions of complications (34%), risk factors included in the analysis (29%), and severity grade (20%). Similarly, Donat and

H. B. Goldman, J. Zillioux (eds.), *Complications of Urogynecology and Reconstructive Pelvic Surgery*, https://doi.org/10.1007/978-3-032-00339-3_1

colleagues found that only 2% of 109 studies between 1995 and 2005 encompassing 150,000 patients following urologic oncology procedures met nine or more of the ten criteria [2]. Seventy-nine percent failed to report definitions for complications, 67% complication severity, 63% outpatient data, 59% comorbidities, and 56% duration of reporting period. Both studies highlighted the need to develop standardized systems for reporting complications and disseminate these systems.

Reporting of complications in female pelvic reconstruction suffers from similar challenges. Depending on the type of procedure and definition of complication, the prevalence of complications in reconstructive pelvic surgery varies significantly. For example, a meta-analysis [3] of randomized controlled trials (RCTs) for midurethral sling (MUS) reported rates of bladder penetration of 0–24%, hematoma formation 0–16.1%, bladder erosion 0–13.1%, and vaginal extrusion 0–5.9%. Postoperative storage and voiding lower urinary tract symptoms (LUTS) were reported in 0–41.3% and 0–55.1% of women, respectively. Furthermore, many of the RCTs did not report any data on the abovementioned complications. In a meta-analysis of RCTs in the treatment of pelvic organ prolapse (POP), Maher and coworkers [4] similarly reported that only 16 out of 56 (29%) RCTs evaluating 5954 women reported data on the impact of surgery on bladder outcomes.

The reporting of complications in surgery and in female reconstructive surgery may be inconsistent for several reasons. First, a complication by one surgeon's consideration may not be seen as one by another surgeon and therefore may not be consistently reported. Second, specific abnormal cutoff values for measures such as estimated blood loss and postvoid residual volume (PVR) are not universally agreed upon, complicating the reporting of outcomes such as hemorrhage and urinary retention, respectively. Third, prior studies had primarily focused on outcomes such as anatomic success in pelvic organ prolapse (POP) repair or resolution of incontinence in MUS placement, failing to note other potential sequelae of surgery, such as voiding dysfunction or dyspareunia, which may have a significant impact on quality of life (QoL).

Reasons for underreporting may include lack of centralized registries for reporting complications, disincentives to report such as professional embarrassment or retribution, the cumbersome nature of reporting complications in a busy clinical practice, or complications occurring remote from surgery of which the provider may not be aware. The ideal classification and reporting method would mitigate any of these potential reasons, resulting in increased reporting of complications and greater opportunity for quality improvement.

Existing Complication Classification Systems

In 1992, Clavien and coworkers [5] proposed a classification system for surgical complications that would in conjunction with subsequent work by Dindo and colleagues [6] develop into the predominant classification scheme for reporting adverse outcomes. Clavien and colleagues distinguished between three types of negative outcomes: complications, failure to cure, or sequelae [5]. Complications were defined as any deviation from the normal postoperative course, which also included asymptomatic complications such as arrhythmias and atelectasis. A sequela was defined as an "after effect" of surgery that was inherent to the procedure. Failure to achieve a cure meant that the original purpose of the surgery was not achieved, even if the surgery had been executed properly and without complications. What has come to be known as the Clavien–Dindo classification of complications considers only complications and not treatment failures or sequelae.

The Clavien–Dindo classification system consists of five grades [6]. Grade I complications include any deviation from the normal postoperative course without the need for any pharmacological treatment or surgical, endoscopic, or radiological intervention. Grade I therapeutic regimens include replacement of electrolytes, physiotherapy, and medications such as antiemetics, antipyretics, analgesics, and diuretics. Wound infections that are opened at the bedside also fall into this grade. Grade II complications require pharmacological treatment with medications other than those allowed for grade I complications. Transfusion of blood products and total parenteral nutrition constitute grade II complications. Grade III complications require surgical, endoscopic, or radiological intervention. This category is subdivided into IIIa (not under general anesthesia) and IIIb (under general anesthesia). Grade IV complications are life-threatening and require intermediate or intensive care management. Central nervous system complications such as brain hemorrhage, ischemic stroke, and subarachnoid bleeding are included in this category, while transient ischemic attacks are not. Category IV is subdivided into IVa (single-organ dysfunction, with or without dialysis) and IVb (multiorgan dysfunction). The death of a patient is a grade V complication. The suffix "d" (for "disability") is added to the respective grade of complication if the patient suffers from a complication at the time of discharge. This label indicates the need for follow-up to fully evaluate and grade the complication.

In essence, the grading of complications using the modified Clavien system is related to the intensity of the treatment directed at correcting the complication [6]. The intent is a link between the severity of the complication and its associated morbidity. Dindo and colleagues validated the modified Clavien classification in 6336 patients undergoing elective surgery in their institution over a 10-year period. Adjusting for surgical complexity, the authors found that the Clavien grade of complications significantly correlated with the duration of the hospital stay, a surrogate marker of outcome. A strong correlation was also observed between the complexity of surgery (and assumed higher complication rates) and the frequency and severity of complications. Furthermore, over 90% of surgeons in an international survey conducted by the authors found the classification system to be simple, reproducible, and logical, and reported that they would support the introduction of the classification system into their clinical practice. The modified Clavien system has now become the most widely used complication classification system across surgical disciplines [7], including urology [8].

In 2011, a classification of complications directly related to the insertion of prostheses (meshes, implants, tapes) or grafts in female pelvic floor surgery was introduced [9]. Following this initial joint effort of the International Urogynecological Association (IUGA) and International Continence Society (ICS), classification systems were published in 2012 for complications related to native tissue female pelvic floor [10] and POP repair [11].

The 2011 prostheses complication report specifically combined the input of members of the Standardization and Terminology Committees of the IUGA and the ICS and a Joint IUGA/ICS Working Group on Complications Terminology and was assisted at intervals by many expert external referees [9]. An extensive process of 11 rounds of internal and external review took place with exhaustive examination of each aspect of the terminology and classification. The decision-making process was conducted by collective opinion (consensus). The classification of each complication is broken down into three parts: category (C), time (T), and site (S). The category (C) is stratified by location of compromise (vagina, urinary tract, bowel or rectum, skin or musculoskeletal system, and hematoma or systemic compromise) and symptom severity (asymptomatic, symptomatic, presence of infection, and abscess formation). The timing of complication (T) is subdivided into four groups (intraoperative to 48 h, 48 h to 2 months, 2–12 months, and >12 months), while the site of complication (S) includes vagina (at or away from the suture line), due to trocar passage, other skin or musculoskeletal site, and intra-abdominal location. A patient may have more than one complication, and the most severe endpoint and corresponding time point are chosen for each. Additionally, grades of pain may be assigned as a subclassification of the complication category. The subjective presence of pain by the patient only may be graded from "a" to "e" (asymptomatic or no pain to spontaneous pain). Each complication is assigned a category time site (CTS) code consisting of three or four letters and four numerals and should theoretically encompass all conceivable scenarios for describing operative complications and healing abnormalities. There is notably no classification of functional issues or urinary tract infection (UTI).

The 2012 IUGA/ICS Joint Terminology and Classification of the Complications Related to Native Tissue Female Pelvic Floor Surgery was written by the same lead author as the 2011 joint report and proposed a slightly modified CTS system [10]. The CTS system for native tissue repair is virtually identical on its surface to the system developed for insertion of prostheses. However, because there is no mesh, tape, or other implant in native tissue repair, the definitions for "exposure" and "extrusion" are applied to permanent suture material "visualized through separated vaginal epithelium" and "protruding into the vaginal cavity," respectively. In addition, the terms "granulation" (i.e., "fleshy connective tissue projections on the surface of a wound, ulcer, or inflamed tissue surface") and "ulcer" (i.e., "lesion through the skin or a mucous membrane resulting from loss of tissue, usually with inflammation") were added to the terminology. As with the earlier proposal for classification of implant complications, functional issues and UTIs were omitted from the classification system. A subsequent joint IUGA/ICS report [11] proposed that Clavien–Dindo grade and functional outcomes such as postoperative pain, LUTS, bowel dysfunction, sexual dysfunction, other de novo symptoms, and backache should be reported along with the CTS classification.

Developed in 2013, the Comprehensive Complication Index (CCI), is an alternative system of the Clavien–Dindo that aggregates all patient complications on a continuous scale [12]. Whereas the Clavien–Dindo selects only the single most severe complication, the CCI aims to consider all complications and their respective severity. The overall morbidity is reflected on a scale from 0 (no complication) to 100 (death). The complex CCI formula is outside the scope of this book chapter; however, a calculator is readily available online [13] for clinicians to access (https://www.cci-calculator.com).

Despite the reproducibility and wide acceptance of the Clavien–Dindo system (even with the modification provided by the CCI), the system is not designed to include reporting of intraoperative complications. Recognizing this limitation, the European Association of Urology (EAU) published a classification of intraoperative events in 2020 [14]. They aimed to develop a "simple, systematic, objective, and reproducible" grading system for intraoperative complications. The EAU ad hoc Complications Guidelines Panel developed the grading system using two rounds of expert consensus (≥70% agreement) followed by validation in hypothetical clinical scenarios to test clinical performance. The proposed EAUiaiC (EAU intraoperative adverse incident classification) system comprises eight adverse incidence grades: Grade 0 (no deviation and no consequence to the patient), Grade 1 (requires change in planned intraoperative steps but addressed in a controlled manner with no long-term side effects), Grade 2 (may have short-/long-term side effects), Grade 3 (life-threatening but not requiring tissue/organ removal), Grade 4A (requires tissue/organ removal), Grade 4B (unable to complete procedure as planned) to grade 5B (wrong surgery site or intraoperative death) [14].

To date, there have been no updates to the IUGA/ICS Classification system discussed above, and many recent studies [15, 16] continue to report their complications using either the CTS classification or the Clavien–Dindo.

The Challenge of Implementing a Classification System of Complications

Inherent to the definition of taxonomy is that the classification system should reduce complexity by presenting a logical and hierarchical representation of categories. The classification should likewise provide a means for organizing and accessing vast quantities of data in an intuitive and streamlined manner. Perhaps owing to the complexity of female pelvic reconstruction and any associated standardized schema, the adoption of classification systems in female pelvic surgery has historically lagged.

The most prominent example is the Pelvic Organ Prolapse Quantification (POP-Q) system. While classification systems for pelvic organ support have existed since the 1800s, no system has gained widespread acceptance. In 1996, Bump and colleagues [17] introduced POP-Q, the first and only classification system to be recognized by the ICS, the American Urogynecologic Society (AUGS), and the Society of Gynecologic Surgeons (SGS). Despite extensive study and reportedly excellent inter- and intra-observer reliability [18, 19], 8 years after its introduction, only 40% of members of the ICS and AUGS reported using POP-Q in clinical practice [18]. Some of the reported reasons for not consistently employing the POP-Q were that the system is too confusing and overly time-consuming and that colleagues are not using it. While some of these reasons are not supported by the literature [16], it suggests that even the most rigorous and well-conceived classification systems may not achieve widespread use owing to concerns regarding simplicity of use, established practice patterns, and unfamiliarity. Nevertheless, with the passage of time and persistence from relevant professional organizations, use of the POP-Q system has increased, with 76% of respondents reporting using the system routinely in a survey published in 2011 [21]. The 2016 IUGA/ICS Joint Report on the Terminology for Female Pelvic Organ Prolapse is the most recent example of attempts to simplify the POP-Q system, improve education, and ultimately increase its routine use [20].

The IUGA/ICS classification system for complications related to prosthetic and native tissue repair pelvic floor surgery is likely to face even greater challenges to widespread adoption. While comprehensive, the CTS system may be cumbersome to use and does not immediately appear to reduce the complexity of organizing complications. Furthermore, the CTS classification does not account for the presence of de novo or worsening storage or voiding LUTS commonly associated with surgery for stress urinary incontinence and POP. Multiple studies have reported significant challenges with retrospective coding of complications and poor interobserver reliability with all of the CTS components. Approximately one-third of mesh erosions were reported as unclassifiable [23, 24], and interobserver reliability was observed to be as low as 14.3% for category (C), 28.6% for timing (T), and 0% for site (S) [25]. Furthermore, CTS classification was not found to correlate with patient outcomes or need for further intervention [24], an important benefit of the widely used modified Clavien–Dindo classification system [6]. For proponents of the IUGA/ICS system, these issues may not be insurmountable but will require a widespread increase in knowledge of the system and its application. Haylen and Maher [26] have suggested that "record issues" rather than the classification system were responsible for poor interobserver reliability in one study and suggested that with improved data and appropriate application of the system, interobserver reliability may have been as high as 87% [23]. More recently, Haylen and coworkers [22] reported markedly improved confidence and ability in scoring all three CTS components following a formal 15-minute instructional lecture with eight clinical case examples [27]. In 2015, the first study [28] reporting mesh complications via the IUGA/ICS classification system (and not aiming to evaluate the system itself) was published, although one of the authors on this retrospective study contributed to the IUGA/ICS joint document detailing the system. Challenges certainly remain in the application of the CTS system, and questions continue to exist regarding its applicability and utility.

Despite its merits, the modified Clavien–Dindo classification, while simpler to integrate, appears to be constructed for grading surgical procedures with a significant prevalence of postoperative intervention, reoperation, and morbidity. It can certainly be argued that because reconstructive pelvic surgery is often performed in otherwise healthy individuals, it is associated with a lower prevalence of "traditional" morbidity. Thus, the modified Clavien–Dindo classification may not be sensitive enough to classify the complications typically associated with reconstructive pelvic surgery. Additionally, unlike the CTS or EAUiaic system, the Clavien–Dindo classification does not take into account intraoperative complications. Thus, intraoperative events such as iatrogenic injuries to the urinary tract, bowels, or vessels would not be reported via the Clavien–Dindo classification, unless they had subsequent postoperative sequelae (such as blood transfusion, take-back into the operating room, etc.)

Complications in urologic pelvic surgery may be classified as general or specific, by their temporal relationship to the surgery itself and by their relationship to a technique or specific material used in the procedure. These are summarized in Table 1.1. Taking into account these complications, a modification of the Clavien classification could combine the benefits of the well-regarded Clavien system with the specificity to pelvic surgery of the IUGA/ICS joint classification system (Table 1.2).

Using Table 1.2 as a guide, an even further step can be taken and use the CCI calculator [13] to take into consideration all the complications that occurred. For example, a patient who underwent a pubovaginal sling insertion that suffers postoperatively from de novo LUTS (IIb), received antibiotics for incisional wound infection (IIa), and a DVT (IVa), will typically only be classified as having a Grade IVa complication, essentially dismissing the two other complications the patient had. With the CCI, all complications will be aggregated into a score, and for this patient is 51.7 (versus a 42.4 if only the DVT was accounted for).

Despite the depth and breadth of the aforementioned classification systems, none take into account patient perception of severity. In 2022, Pizzoferrato and colleagues published the results of their survey among 529 women who underwent pelvic floor repair surgery [29]. Each participant was asked to rate their perception of complication severity, and their responses were compared to the Clavien–Dindo classification. Interestingly, only 52% of the women's classification was concordant with clavien dindo (CD). Self-catheterization, long-term medication use, and severe persistent pain were perceived as more serious than CD classification or the surgeon's perceptions.

Table 1.1 Common complications in reconstructive pelvic surgery

Time	General	Specific	Reoperation
Perioperative	Acute bleeding		Hematoma drainage
	Transfusion		
	Organ injury		Repair organ injury
	Pneumonia, atelectasis		
	Ileus		
	Arrhythmia, MI, CVA, PE, DVT, death		
Postoperative <30 days	MI, CVA, PE, DVT, death	UTI	I&D wound
	Incisional pain	Wound infection	Sling revision
	Pelvic pain	AUR	
	PSBO	Leg pain	
		Storage LUTS	
		Voiding LUTS	
		Extrusion	Sling/mesh revision
		Erosion into GU tract	
Postoperative >30 days	Incisional pain	Storage LUTS	Sling/mesh revision
	Pelvic pain	Voiding LUTS	
		Dyspareunia	
		Extrusion	
		Erosion into GU tract	
		Leg pain	

MI myocardial infarction, *CVA* cerebrovascular accident, *PE* pulmonary embolism, *DVT* deep vein thrombosis, *UTI* urinary tract infection, *I&D* incision and drainage, *AUR* acute urinary retention, *PSBO* partial small bowel obstruction, *LUTS* lower urinary tract symptoms, *GU* genitourinary

Table 1.2 Proposed reconstructive pelvic surgery modification of the Clavien system

Grade	Description	Examples
I	Deviation from normal course (no need for additional intervention)	Trocar bladder puncture, replaced; no formal repair
		Perioperative antipyretics
		Postoperative pelvic floor exercises
IIa	Pharmacological intervention (other than for Grade I)	Antibiotics for UTI or wound infection; antimuscarinics
		Transfusion of blood products
		Analgesics for incisional, pelvic, or leg pain
IIb	Short- or long-term complication, no operative intervention	De novo or worsened storage LUTS
		De novo or worsened voiding LUTS
		Incisional, pelvic, or leg pain
III	Operative intervention required	
	IIIa: Postoperative, office	Incision and drainage wound infection; partial excision of extruded sling/mesh
	IIIb: Intraoperative/immediately postoperative	Repair organ injury (bladder, ureter, colorectal, vascular); endovascular embolization for bleeding
	IIIc: Postoperative, operating room	Sling/mesh incision/revision/excision; urethrolysis; laparotomy for small bowel obstruction; SNM
IV	Life-threatening event	
	IVa: Single-organ dysfunction	DVT, PE, MI, CVA/CNS, admission to ICU
	IVb: Multiorgan dysfunction	
V	Death	

UTI urinary tract infection, *LUTS* lower urinary tract symptoms, *DVT* deep vein thrombosis, *PE* pulmonary embolism, *MI* myocardial infarction, *CVA* cerebrovascular accident, *CNS* central nervous system event, *ICU* intensive care unit, *SNM* sacral neuromodulation

Conclusions

A practical taxonomic classification of complications in reconstructive pelvic surgery would be a valuable instrument for reporting outcome measures and quality indicators. While both the modified Clavien and the IUGA/ICS classification systems contain valuable components, at present, a single, comprehensive, user-friendly, and widely accepted system does not exist. The determination of an optimal classification system that incorporates both intraoperative and postoperative events would further increase quality and transparency, and lead to an improved ability of surgeons to learn from each other's experiences and compare and share data.

Although less objective, integrating a validated complication severity classification that takes into account patient perception of complications may be beneficial to improve our understanding of patient expectations and the ramifications these complications have on their daily lives.

References

1. Martin RCG, Brennan MF, Jaques DP. Quality of complication reporting in the surgical literature. Ann Surg. 2002;235:803–13.
2. Donat SM. Standards for surgical complication reporting in urologic oncology: time for a change. Urology. 2007;69:221–5.
3. Novara G, Galfano A, Boscolo-Berto R, Secco S, Cavalleri S, Ficarra V, et al. Complication rates of tension-free midurethral slings in the treatment of female stress urinary incontinence: a systematic review and meta-analysis of randomized controlled trials comparing tension-free midurethral tapes to other surgical procedures and different devices. Eur Urol. 2008;53:288–308.
4. Maher C, Feiner B, Baessler K, Schmid C. Surgical management of pelvic organ prolapse in women. Cochrane Database Syst Rev. 2013;4:CD004014.
5. Clavien PA, Sanabria JR, Strasberg SM. Proposed classification of complications of surgery with examples of utility in cholecystectomy. Surgery. 1992;111:518–26.
6. Dindo D, Demartines N, Clavien P-A. Classification of surgical complications: a new proposal with evaluation in a cohort of 6336 patients and results of a survey. Ann Surg. 2004;240:205–13.

7. Clavien PA, Barkun J, de Oliveira ML, Vauthey JN, Dindo D, Schulick RD, et al. The Clavien–Dindo classification of surgical complications: five-year experience. Ann Surg. 2009;250:187–96.
8. Yoon PD, Chalasani V, Woo HH. Use of Clavien–Dindo classification in reporting and grading complications after urological surgical procedures: analysis of 2010 to 2012. J Urol. 2013;190:1271–4.
9. Haylen BT, Freeman RM, Swift SE, Cosson M, Davila GW, Deprest J, et al. An International Urogynecological Association (IUGA)/International Continence Society (ICS) joint terminology and classification of the complications related directly to the insertion of prostheses (meshes, implants, tapes) and grafts in female pelvic floor surgery. Neurourol Urodyn. 2011;30:2–12.
10. Haylen BT, Freeman RM, Lee J, Swift SE, Cosson M, Deprest J, et al. International Urogynecological Association (IUGA)/International Continence Society (ICS) joint terminology and classification of the complications related to native tissue female pelvic floor surgery. Neurourol Urodyn. 2012;31:406–14.
11. Toozs-Hobson P, Freeman R, Barber M, Maher C, Haylen B, Athanasiou S, et al. An International Urogynecological Association (IUGA)/International Continence Society (ICS) joint report on the terminology for reporting outcomes of surgical procedures for pelvic organ prolapse. Neurourol Urodyn. 2012;31:415–21.
12. Slankamenac K, Graf R, Barkun J, Puhan MA, Clavien PA. The comprehensive complication index: a novel continuous scale to measure surgical morbidity. Ann Surg. 2013;258(1):1–7. https://doi.org/10.1097/SLA.0b013e318296c732.
13. University of Zurich. CCI Calculator. n.d. https://www.cci-calculator.com/cciCalculator.
14. Biyani CS, Pecanka J, Rouprêt M, Jensen JB, Mitropoulos D. Intraoperative adverse incident classification (EAUiaiC) by the European Association of Urology ad hoc complications guidelines panel. Eur Urol. 2020;77(5):601–10. https://doi.org/10.1016/j.eururo.2019.11.015.
15. van Zanten F, van Iersel JJ, Hartog FE, et al. Mesh exposure after robot-assisted laparoscopic pelvic floor surgery: a prospective cohort study. J Minim Invasive Gynecol. 2019;26(4):636–42. https://doi.org/10.1016/j.jmig.2018.06.015.
16. Rac G, Greiman A, Rabley A, et al. Analysis of complications of pelvic mesh excision surgery using the Clavien-Dindo classification system. J Urol. 2017;198(3):638–43. https://doi.org/10.1016/j.juro.2017.04.078.
17. Bump RC, Mattiasson A, Bø K, Brubaker LP, DeLancey JO, Klarskov P, et al. The standardization of terminology of female pelvic organ prolapse and pelvic floor dysfunction. Am J Obstet Gynecol. 1996;175:10–7.
18. Hall AF, Theofrastous JP, Cundiff GW, Harris RL, Hamilton LF, Swift SE, et al. Interobserver and intraobserver reliability of the proposed International Continence Society, Society of Gynecologic Surgeons, and American Urogynecologic Society pelvic organ prolapse classification system. Am J Obstet Gynecol. 1996;175:1467–70. discussion 1470–1
19. Kobak WH, Rosenberger K, Walters MD. Interobserver variation in the assessment of pelvic organ prolapse. Int Urogynecol J Pelvic Floor Dysfunct. 1996;7:121–4.
20. Auwad W, Freeman RM, Swift S. Is the pelvic organ prolapse quantification system (POPQ) being used? A survey of members of the International Continence Society (ICS) and the American Urogynecologic Society (AUGS). Int Urogynecol J Pelvic Floor Dysfunct. 2004;15:324–7.
21. Pham T, Burgart A, Kenton K, Mueller ER, Brubaker L. Current use of pelvic organ prolapse quantification by AUGS and ICS members. Female Pelvic Med Reconstr Surg. 2011;17:67–9.
22. Haylen BT, Maher CF, Barber MD, Camargo S, Dandolu V, Digesu A, et al. An International Urogynecological Association (IUGA)/International Continence Society (ICS) joint report on the terminology for female pelvic organ prolapse (POP). Int Urogynecol J. 2016;27:165–94.
23. Tunitsky E, Abbott S, Barber MD. Interrater reliability of the International Continence Society and International Urogynecological Association (ICS/IUGA) classification system for mesh-related complications. Am J Obstet Gynecol. 2012;206(442):e1–6.
24. Batalden RP, Weinstein MM, Foust-Wright C, Alperin M, Wakamatsu MM, Pulliam SJ. Clinical application of IUGA/ICS classification system for mesh erosion. Neurourol Urodyn. 2016;35(5):589–94.
25. Gowda M, Kit LC, Stuart Reynolds W, Wang L, Dmochowski RR, Kaufman MR. Interobserver variability when employing the IUGA/ICS classification system for complications related to prostheses and grafts in female pelvic floor surgery. Int Urogynecol J. 2013;24:1671–8.
26. Haylen BT, Maher C, Deprest J. IUGA/ICS terminology and classification of complications of prosthesis and graft insertion—rereading will revalidate. Am J Obstet Gynecol. 2013;208:e15.
27. Haylen BT, Lee J, Maher C, Deprest J, Freeman R. Optimizing study design for interobserver reliability: IUGA-ICS classification of complications of prostheses and graft insertion. Int Urogynecol J. 2014;25:751–4.
28. Miklos JR, Chinthakanan O, Moore RD, Mitchell GK, Favors S, Karp DR, et al. The IUGA/ICS classification of synthetic mesh complications in female pelvic floor reconstructive surgery: a multicenter study. Int Urogynecol J. 2016;27(6):933–8.
29. Pizzoferrato AC, Ragot S, Vérité L, Naiditch N, Fritel X. How women perceive severity of complications after pelvic floor repair? J Clin Med. 2022;11(13):3796. https://doi.org/10.3390/jcm11133796.

2 Patient Consent and Patient Perception of Complications

Jennifer Lee and Christopher F. Tenggardjaja

History of Informed Consent

The informed consent process that we have today is born through the medicolegal affairs of the twentieth century. While most of us can recall the dictum of "primum non nocere" or above all first do no harm, most physicians would probably be astonished to know that Hippocratic teaching also includes provisions from withholding the necessary details of treatment from the patient, "concealing most things from the patient … revealing nothing of the patient's future or present condition" [1, 2]. This recalls the time paternalism was the dominant model of practicing medicine, whereby physicians knew best. Early medicine often depended on withholding information from patients. Treatment prior to the turn of the nineteenth century was based on anecdotal and sometimes even baseless evidence. It was not until the late twentieth century that evidence-based medicine was conceived and became popularized [3, 4]. As treatment options and knowledge flourished with the scientific method and rigorous study design, our model for healthcare delivery has also evolved into one of shared decision-making. Shared decision-making though is not to be confused with overwhelming patients with information and then letting them choose among the myriad options [2]. After all, patients depend on physicians to be their fiduciary in such matters to guide them through treatment options. As a result, the informed consent process has evolved in regard to what a physician is expected to disclose.

Unfortunately, the topic of informed consent cannot be broached without referring to the medicolegal affairs that have framed the discussion. Multiple landmark cases have molded what constitutes our modern-day informed consent. The *four* most discussed cases are *Schloendorff v. The Society of New York Hospital* (1914), *Salgo v. Leland Stanford Jr. University Board of Trustees* (1957), *Cobbs v. Grant (1972)*, and *Canterbury v. Spence* (1972). In the case of Mary Schloendorff, the patient consented to an "ether exam" but subsequently underwent a hysterectomy for a fibroid tumor. The patient sued the hospital because she had not consented to surgery. The defendant's claim was that the surgery was done on part of beneficence of the patient [5]. Judge Cardozo's opinion on the case stated "Every human being of adult years and sound mind has a right to determine what shall be done with his own body; and a surgeon who performs an operation without his patient's consent, commits an assault, for which

J. Lee
Department of Urology, Kaiser Permanente Los Angeles Medical Center, Los Angeles, CA, USA
e-mail: Jennifer.x12.lee@kp.org

C. F. Tenggardjaja (✉)
Bernard J Tyson School of Medicine, Department of Urology, Kaiser Permanente Los Angeles Medical Center, Los Angeles, CA, USA
e-mail: Christopher.tenggardjaja@kp.org

H. B. Goldman, J. Zillioux (eds.), *Complications of Urogynecology and Reconstructive Pelvic Surgery*, https://doi.org/10.1007/978-3-032-00339-3_2

he is liable in damages" [6]. The decision ruled in favor of the defendant (the hospital) not being liable for the negligence of its physicians, who were independent contractors of the hospital. More importantly, patient autonomy was reaffirmed, and most of us are familiar with the lack of consent equaling assault and battery.

The Salgo case involved the use of sodium urokon dye for an aortogram, with the complication of permanent paralysis afterward. Although a rare complication inherent with the procedure, it was not disclosed prior. Justice Bray wrote "that the patient's mental and emotional condition is important and in certain cases may be crucial, and that in discussing the element of risk a certain amount of discretion must be employed consistent with the full disclosure of facts necessary to an informed consent" [7]. Katz points out the contradiction within this legal statement of discretion and full disclosure [2]. Indeed, this first mention of informed consent was born of the idea that a physician should be required to fully disclose the discretionary risks to a patient for a certain procedure. Given this apparent contradiction, it is little wonder that we have so many models of informed consent.

In *Cobbs v. Grant*, the plaintiff had a duodenal ulcer for which he underwent surgical intervention that was complicated by a splenic injury requiring a subsequent surgery to remove his spleen. The plaintiff alleged there was negligence in performing the surgery and that the defendant had failed to obtain his informed consent, as he had not disclosed the risk of splenic injury, a rare complication. Although an expert witness, who was another physician, testified that it was not standard practice to discuss the complication of splenic injury, the court initially ruled in favor of the plaintiff. The court stated that "A physician's duty to disclose is not governed by the standard of practice in the community; rather, it is a duty imposed by law. A physician violates his duty to his patient and subjects himself to liability if he withholds any facts which are necessary to form the basis of an intelligent consent by the patient to the proposed treatment" [8]. The ruling made it clear that the standard of disclosure should be centered around what a patient, not a physician would need in order to make a treatment decision.

Lastly, in *Canterbury v. Spence*, the "reasonable patient" model of disclosure was born. The plaintiff underwent spine surgery for a ruptured disc with postoperative disability with mobility, urinary incontinence, and bowel problems [9]. It was alleged that the neurosurgeon did not mention the small risk of serious disability. In this regard, the physician should discuss and disclose information based on what a reasonable person would need to know in order to make an informed decision. This contrasts with the "professional model" in which a physician should discuss and disclose information based on what other colleagues would disclose in similar circumstances (Table 2.1) [5, 10].

Although these and many other legal cases highlight the need for good documentation, informed consent is not only based on legal safeguards but also on ethical principles. Childers and colleagues suggest three main components for ethical informed consent, consisting of

Table 2.1 Models of informed consent

Model	Definition and problems
Professional model	Disclosure and discussion based on what other physicians would disclose in similar circumstances
	Problem: Promotes generalizations and diminishes the importance of individual patient values and interests
Reasonable model	Disclosure and discussion based on what a reasonable patient would want to know
	Problem: What is reasonable to one patient may be unreasonable to the next
Subjective model	Disclosure and discussion based solely on specific interests, values, and life plan of patient
	Problem: Difficult to know every important detail of patient's life; cumbersome to implement consistently
Balanced model: reasonable and subjective	Disclosure and discussion based on the most important and relevant interests, values, and goals of the patient, as identified by both patient and physician

disclosure, patient understanding, and patient decision-making. Disclosure encompasses the patient and physician discussion regarding the details of a treatment or procedure, the indicated need, and the attendant risks [10]. As discussed earlier, several models of disclosing risk to a patient exist, from the professional model to the reasonable model and some amalgam in between. Patient understanding is gauged by the physician and through communication to assess comprehension [11, 12]. Lastly, patient decision-making and incorporating the capacity of the patient to make decisions along with their values and preferences [10]. Indeed, the Declaration of Helsinki and the Nuremburg Trials demonstrate that informed consent is an ethical standard in allowing patients with capacity to make informed decisions about their own care instead of having treatments imposed upon them. This capacity to give consent is based on the ethical principle of patient autonomy. While physicians may scoff at the idea that patients know how best to be autonomous in their decision, we have an obligation to be open about the risks, benefits, and alternatives of a procedure and guide them in their decision-making process [13–15]. At the heart of shared decision-making, physicians serve as facilitators of care who disclose information about treatment options but take into account their patient's preferences to help them come to a conclusion. The decision algorithm for pelvic organ prolapse surgery illustrates this concept. Although quite a prevalent condition, the majority of women with prolapse are not symptomatic [16]. Therefore, for a symptomatic patient, no single treatment option serves to be the "right one." Instead, the female pelvic medicine reconstructive surgeon elicits a history to further elucidate her preferences as to whether a reconstructive versus obliterative surgery might serve her better. And again (based on what the patient's beliefs and preferences are), the reconstructive treatment algorithm further branches out into uterine sparing versus nonuterine sparing and discusses different surgical approaches. Gone are the days of paternalistic surgeon privilege when a one-size-fit-all approach was administered to every patient without any input. What has emerged is an emphasis on shared decision-making that has led to more informed and involved patients, which has led to higher patient satisfaction [17]. This evolution reflects the myriad surgical options we have and also the evidence that one approach is not necessarily superior to another. What is inherent to this shared decision-making model is the physician–patient relationship and the trust and communication that it is built upon.

Informed Consent in URPS

Given the different treatment options for disease processes in urogynecology and reconstructive pelvic Surgery (URPS), it is important for the physician to foster a relationship with the patient. When surgical treatment options are presented, this decision is impacted by the physician–patient relationship. Multiple papers have evaluated the role of the physician's relationship in impacting patient care [18–20]. Nowhere is that more true than during procedures that *affect* quality of life. With these elective procedures, it is important that communication be transparent and deliberate [11]. Tamblyn and colleagues found a significant correlation between low clinical skills examination scores (based on physician communication) and the prediction of likely complaints against physicians in Ontario and Quebec [20]. The difficulty in establishing this relationship and communicating effectively manifests in today's medical environment. Quality patient encounters can be hampered by time constraints of the modern doctor's visit. But, we should consider that given the time to talk, most patients speak for 2 min or less while most physicians interrupt within the first 22 s [21, 22]! While quality of care can be determined by patient-driven opinion-dominated metrics, it becomes increasingly more important for the physician to communicate effectively during the limited time with the patient. Studies have demonstrated that patients respond positively to the doctor who addresses their questions and needs [23–26]. Simple portions of the interview, such as allowing the patient uninterrupted time to address their concerns, asking for additional questions, and demonstrating empathy improve the physician–patient relationship. All of this trust built during the relationship culminates in the shared formulation of a treatment plan. Often, the treatment plan involves shared decision-making on a therapeutic intervention. Intervention takes many forms in female pelvic medicine and reconstructive surgery. A prime example of this is the treatment of idiopathic overactive bladder. Surgery is just one option among many including behavioral modification and medications. Often, education and behavioral modification are all that are needed to make a meaningful impact on one's quality of life. Discussion with a patient regarding caffeine intake reduction and fluid intake modification can make a therapeutic difference without surgical intervention. Regardless of the treatment plan, shared decision-making between patient and physician is paramount, which is evident in the most recent idiopathic overactive bladder guidelines published by the American Urological Association and Society of Urodynamics, Female Pelvic Medicine and Urogenital Reconstruction. The current guidelines have done away with the concept of step therapy. No longer are there "first, second, and third-line therapies" in the treatment of idiopathic overactive bladder, which resulted in a physician-guided treatment algorithm [27]. This dramatic shift to shared decision-making has been imminent with studies demonstrating that shared decision-making improves patient-reported outcomes in patients with lung cancer, colorectal cancer, and when managing cardiovascular risk factors in patients [28,29]. This approach involves education regarding the diagnosis, discussion of treatment options, including the option of no treatment, open dialog between the physician and patient, and lastly mutual decision-making on the treatment option that should be pursued. Numerous studies have demonstrated that information presented in multiple modalities can serve to enhance the patient's knowledge and satisfaction with the shared decision-making experience [30]. Long gone are the paternalistic doctoring models where only one decision was the correct decision. Today's medicine involves taking into account patient's and family's preferences and wishes. Part of the difficulty with informed consent is based on how much risk to divulge to the patient. There is a fine line between giving enough information so the patient can make an informed decision versus overburdening a patient with superfluous details. Already presented with the *Canterbury v. Spence* case was the model of the reasonable patient. But rather than placing all decisions in a rigid matrix, a combined approach taking into account patient preferences and values in addition to what a reasonable patient would want to know is probably the best method of informed consent. In this regard, the surgeon would discuss the risks of a surgery that a reasonable patient would want to know and also include any additional risks, however low risk they may be, that may be in accordance with a patient's values. Framed in this context of overactive bladder treatment, a patient may best be served by sacral neuromodulation for overactive bladder if the risk of urinary retention with another treatment is unacceptable to the patient. This model can only be utilized if a physician has spent time elucidating the patient's preferences and goals through building the physician–patient relationship.

Another difficulty regarding informed consent is the realization that this process happens before any paperwork is signed for surgery. Informed consent, as it applies to surgical procedures, is typically the piece of paper or document in the medical record that has the patient's signature. In reality, the signature documents that the discussion took place prior between the physician and patient. *It does not replace this discussion*. And it is during this discussion that the physician has the ability to impact the patient's perception of any outcome of a surgery. The informed consent should take place in a non-hurried setting where the physician has a chance to explain the procedure, the patient has the chance to ask questions, and the physician has a chance to answer these questions and check for comprehension and understanding [12]. The documentation itself should not be trivialized because it serves as an objective part of the medical record. Components that should be included in any documentation include a description of the procedure in understandable terms, details of the risks/benefits documentation that the risks/benefits and alternatives were discussed including the option of no surgical intervention, and then an attestation that the patient had a chance to ask questions [10, 11]. With most shared decision in URPS cases, we enjoy the luxury of discussing treatment options in our office without the emergent need for an operation. For more complex decisions regarding surgical treatment options, it would serve us well to educate our patients so that they can be an integral part of the shared decision-making process and be diligent about all steps of the informed consent process. An example of this can be found in the subtleties of informed consent in any procedure using synthetic mesh, as well as in gender-affirming surgeries.

Informed Consent and Patient Perception in the Realm of Mesh

Patients need to be able to comprehend the treatment options at hand and informed consent needs the understanding of both parties to proceed. The physician shouldGender-affirming care clearly highlights use empathy to try and understand the patient's preferences, while the patient needs to be able to understand the risks/benefits and alternatives to any procedure. Unfortunately, with all the litigation surrounding mesh-based prolapse repair, patient education between fact and fiction can often be difficult. Multiple studies have demonstrated that patients are misinformed regarding the use of synthetic mesh in prolapse repair, and also the litigation involving the use of synthetic mesh. Unfortunately, patients are also deriving most of their information from sources other than their physicians, demonstrating a need for increased patient education [31, 32]. Pelvic organ prolapse and incontinence are difficult concepts for the patient to clearly understand and recall at baseline [33]. Given the difficulty in understanding this subject, jargon should be kept to a minimum. Language should not be condescending, and the risks and benefits of a procedure should be explained in a simple and concise manner. Regarding procedures, the more information afforded to the patient the better. Given the misconception about synthetic mesh, informational tools such as Frequently Asked Questions (FAQs) from American Urogynecologic Society (AUGS) and Society of Urodynamics, Female Pelvic Medicine, and Urogenital Reconstruction (SUFU) can be used for further patient education. The joint FAQ on mesh mid-urethral slings for stress urinary incontinence highlights the important role of professional societies to also provide information to help patients make informed decisions [34]. These tools serve as an adjunct to informed consent and are not meant to replace discussion between physician and patient but rather to reinforce patient knowledge. The International Urogynecological Association published a consensus paper with a sample consent for use with transvaginal prolapse surgery repair [11]. Again, it should be noted that such an extensive consent serves a twofold purpose, as evidence that a shared decision-making process took place and that informed consent was obtained. Studies have demonstrated that patients better understand informed consent when given information in multiple modalities [30, 35]. This agrees with principles in learning and teaching that not only auditory processing but also visual processing matter as well to enhance comprehension [36]. Interestingly, it is assumed that patients will be able to read their after-visit summary for further information and instructions regarding a procedure. But it should be noted that patient's preferences for receiving information should be ascertained prior to ending a visit because some patients may be illidiopathic overactiveiterate and too ashamed to mention this when receiving their after-visit summary [33, 37, 38]. While many of these considerations are assumed during an office visit or during a process such as informed consent, all of these must be considered to ensure that the patient has all the tools available to be involved in the shared decision-making process.

Informed Consent with Gender-Affirming Surgery

Gender-affirming care clearly highlights the importance of informed patients actively participating in decision-making. Although the first documented gender-affirming surgery was in the early twentieth century, it has not been until the last few decades that gender-affirming surgeries have become more prevalent. This relatively new field in pelvic reconstructive surgery has reaffirmed the importance of shared decision-makingwith involved and educated patients, where the physician–patient relationship is paramount.

Gender-affirming medical care has been largely guided by the Standards of Care (SOC) published by the World Professional Association for Transgender Health (WPATH). While the SOC was established to assist health professionals with a framework for caring for transgender and gender diverse (TGD) individuals, there have been concerns that it has led to more nuanced "requirements" for gender-affirming surgeries than for any other surgical procedure [39]. Many of the guidelines in the previous versions of the SOC placed a burden on individuals who desired gender-affirming surgeries. These individuals were required to get a letter of referral from a mental health care professional demonstrating a return to a paternalistic model of medicine, as patients needed to be considered "eligible" to undergo a procedure [40]. There have been many studies looking at the timeliness of gender-affirming care and patient satisfaction when comparing the WPATH model requiring a formal mental health assessment to an informed consent model, which emphasizes shared decision-making. These studies have demonstrated that relying on the principles of informed consent, in particular having an open discussion about treatment options and confirming the patient's understanding of the risks and benefits of each leads to high patient satisfaction and fewer medical assessments before receiving gender-affirming care than those patients who received care under the WPATH model [41, 42]. The most recently published SOC version 8 has eliminated the need for letters specifically from mental health care professionals and has placed an emphasis on more individualized assessments in the hopes of eliminating barriers to care and strengthening patient autonomy [43]. In particular, there is a need in recognizing the diverse community of TGD individuals and that the various gender-affirming surgeries may be categorized along a spectrum that may or may not align with the patient's goals. For example, a patient's main goal for a gender-affirming surgery may be to have successful penetrative intercourse, or it may be to stand for micturition. This deep understanding can only be obtained by having a trusting physician–patient relationship.

In addition to the physician–patient relationship,surgeons must have a close working relationship with other health care professionals. Gender-affirming care that can eventually include a gender-affirming surgery is a process that involves an interdisciplinary team. Informed consent for these medical and surgical treatments often starts well before an individual decides to pursue surgery. Information is obtained through various channels and often before the individual meets with the surgeon. Given only the recent emergence of research on gender-affirming surgeries, care should be taken to ensure that patients are not misinformed. Informed consent for gender-affirming surgeries is no different than any other urogynecology and reconstructive pelvic surgery procedure in that there should be a strong emphasis on shared decision-making driven by physicians providing the appropriate amount of information that takes into account patient preferences.

Conclusion

Informed consent refers to the process by which the physician and patient agree to a plan formulated concerning the patient's care. There are two key components to informed consent—one, that the physician informs and discloses information to the patient, and two, that the patient consents to this formulated plan of care. The heart of informed consent lies within the shared decision-making between the physician and the patient. Informed consent has both a medicolegal and ethical basis. In URPS, shared decision-making should take place between the physician and patient with clear communication and established rapport to come to a decision that is both acceptable to everyone in regards to treatment outcomes and also the patient's preferences. To that extent, multiple modalities provided by professional societies should be used, such as published FAQ's and other resources. These can be used to clearly communicate and inform patients so that shared decision-making becomes the cornerstone of any treatment plan, and expectations regarding benefits and complications are clearly understood.

References

1. Hippocrates Z. Decorum. Cambridge: Harvard University Press; 1967.
2. Katz J. Reflections on informed consent: 40 years after its birth. J Am Coll Surg. 1998;186(4):466–74.
3. Eddy DM. Practice policies: where do they come from? JAMA. 1990;263(9):1265, 9, 72 passim.
4. Evidence-Based Medicine Working Group. Evidence-based medicine. A new approach to teaching the practice of medicine. JAMA. 1992;268(17):2420–5.
5. Dolgin JL. The legal development of the informed consent doctrine: past and present. Camb Q Healthc Ethics. 2010;19(1):97–109.
6. Schloendorff v. The Society of New York Hospital; 1914.
7. Salgo v. Leland Stanford Jr. University Board of Trustees; 1957.
8. Cobbs v. Grant, Court of Appeal, First District, Division 4, California. https://caselaw.findlaw.com/court/ca-court-of-appeal/1827202.html.
9. Canterbury v. Spence, 464 F.2d 772; 1972.
10. Childers R, Lipsett PA, Pawlik TM. Informed consent and the surgeon. J Am Coll Surg. 2009;208(4):627–34.
11. Miller D, Milani AL, Sutherland SE, Navin B, Rogers RG. Informed surgical consent for a mesh/graft-augmented vaginal repair of pelvic organ prolapse. Consensus of the 2nd IUGA grafts roundtable: optimizing safety and appropriateness of graft use in transvaginal pelvic reconstructive surgery. Int Urogynecol J. 2012;23(Suppl 1):S33–42.
12. Schenker Y, Meisel A. Informed consent in clinical care: practical considerations in the effort to achieve ethical goals. JAMA 2011;305(11):1130–1.
13. Will JF. A brief historical and theoretical perspective on patient autonomy and medical decision making: part I: the beneficence model. Chest. 2011;139(3):669–73.
14. Will JF. A brief historical and theoretical perspective on patient autonomy and medical decision making: part II: the autonomy model. Chest. 2011;139(6):1491–7.
15. Stain SC. Informed surgical consent. J Am Coll Surg. 2016;222(4):717–8.
16. Barber MD, Maher C. Epidemiology and outcome assessment of pelvic organ prolapse. Int Urogynecol J. 2013;24(11):1783–90.
17. Siebinga VY, Driever EM, Stiggelbout AM, Brand PLP. Shared decision making, patient-centered communication and patient satisfaction – a cross-sectional analysis. Patient Educ Couns. 2022;105(7):2145–50.
18. Hickson GB, Clayton EW, Githens PB, Sloan FA. Factors that prompted families to file medical malpractice claims following perinatal injuries. JAMA. 1992;267(10):1359–63.
19. Beckman HB, Markakis KM, Suchman AL, Frankel RM. The doctor–patient relationship and malpractice. Lessons from plaintiff depositions. Arch Intern Med. 1994;154(12):1365–70.
20. Tamblyn R, Abrahamowicz M, Dauphinee D, Wenghofer E, Jacques A, Klass D, et al. Physician scores on a national clinical skills examination as predictors of complaints to medical regulatory authorities. JAMA. 2007;298(9):993–1001.
21. Langewitz W, Denz M, Keller A, Kiss A, Ruttimann S, Wossmer B. Spontaneous talking time at start of consultation in outpatient clinic: cohort study. BMJ. 2002;325(7366):682–3.
22. Rhoades DR, McFarland KF, Finch WH, Johnson AO. Speaking and interruptions during primary care office visits. Fam Med. 2001;33(7):528–32.
23. Hojat M, Louis DZ, Markham FW, Wender R, Rabinowitz C, Gonnella JS. Physicians' empathy and clinical outcomes for diabetic patients. Acad Med. 2011;86(3):359–64.
24. Street RL Jr, Makoul G, Arora NK, Epstein RM. How does communication heal? Pathways linking clinician–patient communication to health outcomes. Patient Educ Couns. 2009;74(3):295–301.
25. Neuwirth ZE. Physician empathy—should we care? Lancet. 1997;350(9078):606.
26. Kim SS, Kaplowitz S, Johnston MV. The effects of physician empathy on patient satisfaction and compliance. Eval Health Prof. 2004;27(3):237–51.
27. Cameron AP, Chung DE, Dielubanza EJ, Enemchukwu E, Ginsberg DA, Helfand BT, et al. The AUA/SUFU guideline on the diagnosis and treatment of idiopathic overactive bladder. J Urol. 2024;212(1):11–20.
28. Kehl KL, Landrum MB, Arora NK, Ganz PA, van Ryn M, Mack JW, et al. Association of actual and preferred decision roles with patient-reported quality of care: shared decision making in cancer care. JAMA Oncol. 2015;1(1):50–8.
29. Elias S, Chen Y, Liu X, Slone S, Turkson-Ocran R, Ogungbe B, et al. Shared decision-making in cardiovascular risk factor management: a systematic review and meta-analysis. JAMA Netw Open. 2024;7(3):e243779.
30. Kinnersley P, Phillips K, Savage K, Kelly MJ, Farrell E, Morgan B, et al. Interventions to promote informed consent for patients undergoing surgical and other invasive healthcare procedures. Cochrane Database Syst Rev. 2013;7:CD009445.
31. Tenggardjaja CF, Moore CK, Vasavada SP, Li J, Goldman HB. Evaluation of patients' perceptions of

mesh usage in female pelvic medicine and reconstructive surgery. Urology. 2015;85(2):326–31.
32. Koski ME, Chamberlain J, Rosoff J, Vaughan T, Kaufman MR, Winters JC, et al. Patient perception of transvaginal mesh and the media. Urology. 2014;84(3):575–82.
33. Anger JT, Lee UJ, Mittal BM, Pollard ME, Tarnay CM, Maliski S, et al. Health literacy and disease understanding among aging women with pelvic floor disorders. Female Pelvic Med Reconstr Surg. 2012;18(6):340–3.
34. Frequently asked questions by providers mid-urethral slings for stress urinary incontinence. In: AUGS/SUFU, editor. 2014.
35. Schenker Y, Fernandez A, Sudore R, Schillinger D. Interventions to improve patient comprehension in informed consent for medical and surgical procedures: a systematic review. Med Decis Mak. 2011;31(1):151–73.
36. Davis TC, Crouch MA, Wills G, Miller S, Abdehou DM. The gap between patient reading comprehension and the readability of patient education materials. J Fam Pract. 1990;31(5):533–8.
37. Reagan KM, O'Sullivan DM, Harvey DP, Lasala CA. Readability of patient information pamphlets in urogynecology. Female Pelvic Med Reconstr Surg. 2015;21(2):63–5.
38. Easton P, Entwistle VA, Williams B. Health in the 'hidden population' of people with low literacy. A systematic review of the literature. BMC Public Health. 2010;10:459.
39. Chiang T, Bachmann GA. The informed consent model is adequate for gender-affirming treatment; issues related with mental health assessment in the United States. J Sex Med. 2023;20(5):584–7.
40. Cavanaugh T, Hopwood R, Lambert C. Informed Consent in the Medical Care of Transgender and Gender-Nonconforming Patients. AMA J Ethics. 2016;18(11):1147–55.
41. Solanki P, Colon-Cabrera D, Barton C, Locke P, Cheung AS, Spanos C, et al. Gender-affirming hormone therapy for the trans, gender diverse, and nonbinary community: coordinating world professional association for transgender health and informed consent models of care. Transgend Health. 2023;8(2):137–48.
42. Spanos C, Grace JA, Leemaqz SY, Brownhill A, Cundill P, Locke P, et al. The informed consent model of care for accessing gender-affirming hormone therapy is associated with high patient satisfaction. J Sex Med. 2020;18(1):201–8.
43. Coleman E, Radix AE, Bouman WP, Brown GR, de Vries ALC, Deutsch MB, et al. Standards of care for the health of transgender and gender diverse people, Version 8. Int J Transgender Health. 2023;sup1:S1–S259.

Medical Malpractice: Analysis of Factors Driving Litigation and Insight into Reducing Risk

3

Lisa M. Barrett and Matthew J. Donnelly

Most physicians have heard the saying: "It is not if you get sued, but when you get sued." Furthermore, if a physician gets sued early enough in their career, there is also the chance that that physician may get sued a second and third time before retirement. Moreover, physicians in certain specialties are more likely to get sued than their counterparts in other specialties.

A study published by the American Medical Association finds that roughly 38% of urologists, 62% of OB/gynecologists, and 59% of general surgeons responding to the survey report being sued for medical malpractice during the course of their career [1]. The same study finds that after the age of 55, the likelihood of a surgeon (of any surgical specialty) being named in a medical practice lawsuit increases by 50% [1]. Urology is considered a moderate to high-risk specialty [2].

L. M. Barrett
Law Department, Cleveland Clinic, Beachwood, OH, USA
e-mail: barretl@ccf.org

M. J. Donnelly (✉)
Office of Professional Staff Affairs, Cleveland Clinic, Cleveland, OH, USA
e-mail: donnelm1@ccf.org

Medical Malpractice Defined and Explained

There is often confusion about what legally constitutes medical malpractice or medical negligence. While the exact definition may differ from state to state, it is generally understood as a physician's deviation from the accepted standard of care when rendering medical services to a patient, thereby causing harm to the patient. In order to successfully prosecute a claim for medical malpractice, a claimant must prove four elements. These elements are as follows: (1) the medical professional owed a duty to the patient; (2) the medical professional breached that duty; (3) the breach of the duty proximately caused injury to the patient; and (4) damages caused by the alleged injury.

Proving that the medical professional owed a duty to the patient is the easiest hurdle to overcome. Once the physician–patient relationship is established, the physician owes a duty of reasonable care to the patient. Usually, the most contentious point in medical malpractice litigation comes when the claimant attempts to prove the second legal requirement. Once duty is established, the claimant then must prove that the physician breached that duty by failing to meet the acceptable standard of medical care. In order to do this, a claimant must show that the physician failed to act as a reasonably prudent physician would under the same or similar circumstances.

H. B. Goldman, J. Zillioux (eds.), *Complications of Urogynecology and Reconstructive Pelvic Surgery*, https://doi.org/10.1007/978-3-032-00339-3_3

In order to prove or defend this element, the vast majority of the time the parties will retain the services of expert witnesses. Expert witnesses are necessary in medical negligence lawsuits because the jury in such cases is overwhelmingly staffed with laypeople with little to no medical knowledge. Expert witnesses who opine on the standard of care are generally of the same specialty as the medical provider(s) accused of negligence.

The third element, causation, is also a hotly contested issue in medical negligence trials. In order for a plaintiff to meet their burden for this element, they must prove that the breach of the aforementioned duty was a proximate cause of the claimed injury. Interestingly, even if a jury finds that the physician breached the standard of care, it can find that the breach did not proximately cause the claimant's injuries and therefore still render a verdict for the physician. In some instances, medical providers even admit their negligence, but defend the entire case on causation. A simple illustration of this type of defense can be found in the following failure-to-diagnose scenario. Suppose a physician identifies a lesion on the patient's kidney following a CT scan but fails to act upon that finding. Approximately three months later, a different physician identifies the lesion and diagnoses the patient with renal cell carcinoma. The first physician was certainly negligent for failing to diagnose and treat the lesion, but that breach of the standard of care caused no harm to the patient, as this patient was correctly diagnosed and treated only three months later. In this scenario, if the jury finds that the three-month delay caused no injury to the patient, the jury should find in favor of the first physician based on that physician's causation defense.

The final element in a medical negligence claim is damages. Damages come in three general forms—economic, noneconomic, and punitive. Economic damages may include past and future medical bills, past and future lost wages, and other quantifiable monetary damages. Noneconomic damages include pain and suffering, mental anguish, and loss of consortium. While rarely sought, punitive damages are another remedy available to claimants that are designed to punish a defendant for willful, wanton, or malicious conduct. They are also designed to deter future misconduct. Importantly, punitive damages are usually not covered by insurance. Expert witnesses such as economists, vocational specialists, and life care planners are used by parties to show potential damages.

The plaintiff has the burden of proof in medical malpractice cases. In other words, the plaintiff has the burden to prove that medical malpractice occurred. The physician does not have to prove that it did not. The plaintiff must prove that it was "more likely than not" that malpractice occurred. This burden applied in civil cases is called "by a preponderance of the evidence" as opposed to the better-known and heightened criminal burden of "beyond a reasonable doubt."

In order for a claimant to bring a lawful claim of medical negligence, they must do so within a certain amount of time under the law. This time limitation is known as the statute of limitations, and it varies greatly from state to state. There may also be differences in the amount of time a claimant can bring a negligence claim as opposed to a wrongful death claim. For example, in Ohio a claimant has one year from the accrual of the alleged negligence to bring a claim for medical malpractice, [3] yet there is a two year timeframe in which to bring a claim for wrongful death arising out of the alleged malpractice [4]. The medical malpractice statute of limitations can be tolled due to a patient being a minor or of unsound mind [5].

Malpractice Claim Frequency and Severity Trends

Recent data from the National Practitioner's Databank shows stable trends in claim frequency, but significant increases in claim severity [6]. The frequency of all paid claims is down since 2001 and has leveled off since 2012. However, claims with a value of $500,000 or more have remained steady, yet are much less frequent than claims with a lesser value (Fig. 3.1). This illustrates that the more frivolous or lesser value cases are being brought less often while the meritori-

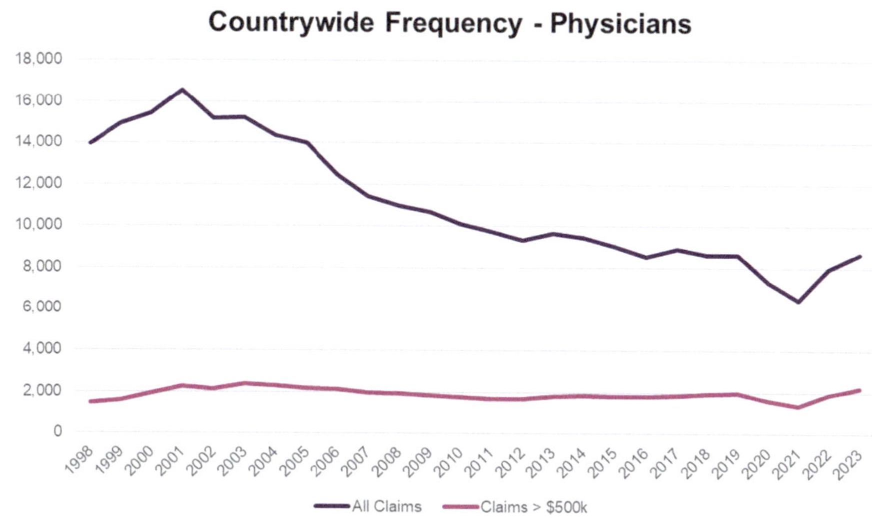

Fig. 3.1 Countrywide frequency, physicians. (Source: National Practitioner Data Bank. http://www.npdb.hrsa.gov/)

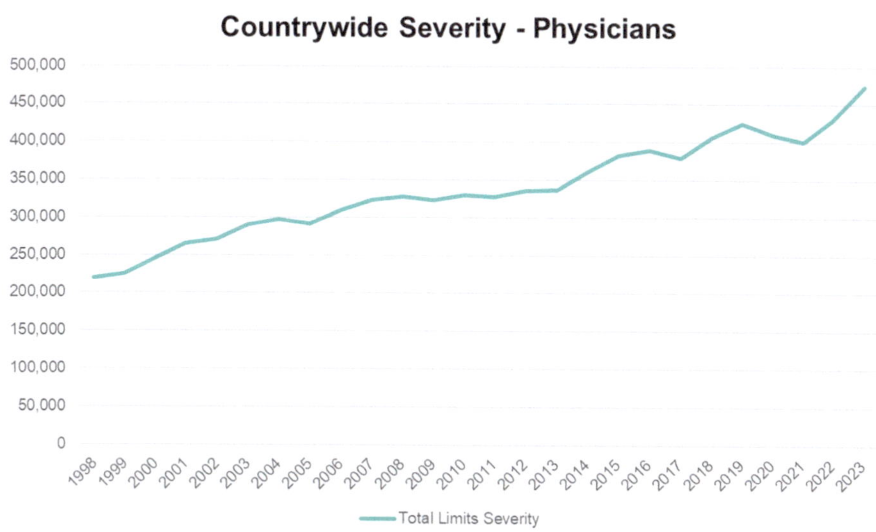

Fig. 3.2 Countrywide severity, physicians. Annual severity trend since 2004: +2.3%. (Source: National Practitioner Data Bank. http://www.npdb.hrsa.gov/)

ous claims are still brought at the same rate. Accordingly, one can hypothesize that while tort reform has had an effect on these lesser value cases, it has had relatively little impact on the frequency of valid claims.

With respect to severity, the country has seen a substantial uptick over the past ten years (Fig. 3.2). Between 2014 and 2020, the average physician indemnity payout has increased by 42% [7]. There are several reasons for this increase. The general cost of prosecuting and defending these cases has grown over time with increases in expert witness and attorney's fees. In some specialties like neurosurgery, expert witnesses are charging over $1500 an hour. Obviously, the wages of injured or deceased patients have increased over this period of time, making the value of corresponding loss of future wage claims increase. Moreover, as the cost of healthcare has increased, so has the cost of life care plans that provide future care for disabled claimants. However, the largest driver for this shift is due to social inflation. Social inflation is defined as the rise of the loss costs to cover medical malpractice claims above the rate of general economic inflation [8].

There are several contributors to social inflation in the arena of medical malpractice, but two factors are most concerning. First is the emergence of third-party funding in the capital market for plaintiff's attorneys. This results in higher settlement costs as the sole intent of the third-party funder is profit, and settlement proceeds must be used to pay back any funding, resulting in the plaintiff receiving a small portion of any resolution [9]. Second, post-COVID juror attitudes (anti-corporate, distrust of science) are more susceptible to the inflammatory narratives used by the plaintiff's attorneys to evoke anger, resulting in enormous jury verdicts [10].

There are steps that we can use to help mitigate this concerning trend. Proactive risk management, quality, and patient safety programs ensure that better care is being delivered. Furthermore, increased focus on the patient experience and caregiver engagement has led to a better physician–patient relationship and overall experience of both the patient and caregiver. Continued advancements in these fields should lead to even more favorable outcomes—in patient care and litigation—in the future.

Why Patients Sue

Patients sue their physician or healthcare provider for a myriad of reasons. There certainly are instances where the care rendered was substandard and a suit is brought to compensate the patient for the harm done. More often, however, there are other factors that influence a claimant's decision to bring a lawsuit. Physicians with a history of litigation share a number of the following patient complaints: failure to listen to their patients; failure to return telephone calls; rudeness; and a lack of respect [11]. It has been suggested that physicians who are at high risk for litigation should better understand environmental and behavioral risk factors that contribute to their risk [11].

Communication

Communication, or lack thereof, is the most common theme found in medical malpractice litigation. George Bernard Shaw once famously said, "The single biggest problem in communication is the illusion that it has taken place." Proper communication is necessary among all participants in a patient's care, including the patient. Obviously, physicians must communicate adequately with their patients in order for the patients to make informed decisions about their healthcare. Proper communication is not only necessary prior to a treatment or procedure, but is just as important during and after the treatment process. Communication among caregivers is also vital to the proper management of a patient. This includes physician-to-physician, physician-to-nurse, and shift-to-shift communications. Oral and written communications are equally important and must be given their proper attention pursuant to the circumstances. Discussions with a patient's family members, especially at the time of discharge, also have an impact on whether poor communication influences a patient's decision to sue.

A recent study by CRICO Strategies directly linked patient deaths to poor communication. The study analyzed over 23,000 medical malpractice claims and suits and found that at least one specific breakdown in communication that contributed to patient harm was present in almost one-third of the cases [12]. Twenty-seven percent of those cases involved surgery [12]. An in-depth review of more than 7500 surgery-related cases revealed that 26% involve significant communication errors [12].

The breakdown between the inpatient and ambulatory settings was fairly even at 44% and 48%, respectively [12]. There was also a fairly even distribution of cases where the breakdown of communication was between two or more healthcare providers or between the providers and their patients [12] (Table 3.1).

Table 3.1 Communication breakdowns

Miscommunication between two or more healthcare providers	Miscommunication between providers and patients	Miscommunications that fall into both categories
57%	55%	12%

Source: Malpractice Risks in Communication Failures 2015 Annual Benchmarking Report [12]

The opportunity for communication errors in surgical cases can occur before, during, and after the surgery. Prior to surgery, failing to properly educate the patient on the procedure's risks, benefits, alternative treatments, and potential outcomes—better known as the informed consent process—is one allegation that occurs frequently in medical malpractice suits. The potential for communication miscues during a surgical procedure is endless. Such errors can occur in writing—whether failing to follow written surgical protocols or clearly documenting in the medical record. Verbal mishaps are also of great potential, ranging from miscommunication concerning instruments and equipment to failing to communicate the patient's status. Finally, postoperative communications can occur in a myriad of ways between caregivers, between caregivers and the patient (and/or family members), and in the written medical chart.

Perceived Arrogance or Lack of Caring

Patients are more likely to sue arrogant and less caring physicians than they are to sue kind and compassionate physicians. The decision to sue one's physician is usually a very personal and difficult decision to make—especially when that physician is well-liked by the patient. When the physician is arrogant, or seems not to care about the patient, the consideration of the personal relationship between the patient and physician is less of a factor. When it is considered, however, and the relationship is viewed in a negative light, it can become a catalyst to sue. In one survey of over 225 patients who sued their physician, a number of respondents stated that in addition to the injury, the lack of sympathy and poor communication that occurred subsequent to the incident was influential in the decision to sue [13].

In the eyes of the patient, the arrogant and dismissive physician does not have time for the patient. The patient is of the mindset that the physician did not carefully discuss the risks, benefits, and alternatives to the treatment, did not allow the patient to ask meaningful questions, and provided an overall negative experience. When a complication occurs, the patient often refers back to the interactions with the physician and concludes that the physician did not care about the patient, had no interest in learning about the patient's unique circumstances, and therefore the surgical technique must have been careless and hurried. Arrogance and the lack of caring during postoperative visits solidify these thoughts and push the patient even further in the direction of suing the physician.

In contrast, a physician who has compassion and takes time to communicate with the patient establishes a much better rapport and level of trust. The patient does not feel like they are "just another number" and has a better understanding of the treatment in question. The patient also feels that they and the physician are on the same team and that they are going through the treatment process together.

Unexpected Outcome

At the outset, it is important to recognize that patients seek medical attention to find a cure. Sometimes this expectation is warranted, sometimes it is not. It is also important to recognize that when patients seek assistance from institutions or physicians with certain name recognition or reputations, they believe they will be cured. In fact, they may have been to several previous physicians who praised these healthcare providers and advised them that only a select number of physicians can solve their problem. The patients sometimes pay large sums of money and travel long distances to seek this treatment. Certainly, after all of this trouble, they expect to be cured. If they are not, or if a complication occurs, they believe the physician must have done something incorrectly.

Scenarios like the aforementioned play out in the minds of patients throughout this country every day. One manner in which to prevent the patient from immediately accusing a physician of negligence upon the occurrence of a complication is to properly and thoroughly educate that patient. Patients have high expectations, and rightfully so, but they also need to understand that complications do occur in the absence of negligence. Patients must understand the risks, benefits, and alternatives to a procedure or surgery. They must understand that the possible outcomes can range from death (in some cases) to complete cure and all potentials in between. When these factors are communicated to the patient, an unexpected outcome should not come as a complete surprise. Setting these expectations should immediately lessen the knee-jerk reaction that negligence occurred. Involving the patient's family members (when appropriate) in the informed consent process is also prudent. Obviously, documenting that the informed consent process took place is necessary and will greatly assist in the defense of medical negligence allegations.

Significant Damages

Every so often, a patient or family will experience damages or a loss so significant that they feel that a lawsuit is the only option. Significant complications and death can devastate a family emotionally and financially. Even when no negligence has occurred, it is this devastation that leaves the patient or family feeling as if litigation is the only option. Such instances include the incapacitation or death of a family's main breadwinner. The shock of the loss is overwhelming. Next come questions about how the family will survive financially and how it will pay for future expenses such as mortgages, college educations, and retirement. Patients and families are left to believe that absent a large settlement or verdict resulting from litigation, they are forever financially doomed. Hopefully, such scenarios are few and far between for patients, their families, and physicians, but they do exist.

Patients/Families Need Answers

Many plaintiffs' lawyers have said that their clients turned to litigation because the hospital or physicians would not answer their questions. When complications or unexpected outcomes occur, patients and family members desire to understand how and why. When they do not receive the answers they seek, or when they feel that hospitals and physicians are hiding evidence, they believe they have no choice but to turn to litigation. Transparency with patients and family members can avoid the need to turn to litigation to seek answers.

To Prevent a Similar Event from Happening Again

A number of patients cite the desire to prevent similar incidents of perceived or actual malpractice from happening again [13]. Injuries due to adverse outcomes or medical negligence can have devastating long-term effects. This can create a patient's desire to prevent future similar outcomes. When a patient feels that there is a lack of cooperation from a physician or hospital system, litigation may be the only avenue to effect change. Accordingly, it behooves healthcare providers to investigate adverse outcomes, either through peer review or other protected mechanisms. Under the proper circumstances, quality and process improvements may be shared with the patient without breaching legal protections provided to the peer review process. These discussions can demonstrate to patients that processes have been put in place to prevent a similar occurrence from happening again in the future, which should lessen the chance of litigation.

Types of Patients That Sue

Wealthy

It is a misconception that low-income patients are more likely to sue their physicians than their more well-off counterparts [14]. Wealthy patients are likely to sue a physician when things go wrong for a number of reasons. Wealthy patients are usually well educated and have researched their medical condition and physician. They have high expectations and view unexpected outcomes with skepticism. In addition, economic damages such as past and future lost wages are greater for wealthy patients, and therefore the potential settlement or verdict range is much higher than it is for middle-class or poor patients. As a practical matter, a wealthy patient's economic damage claim is much more attractive to a plaintiff's attorney than a lower value claim.

Patients with Medical or Legal Connections

Patients with medical or legal connections are more likely to sue because they use those resources when contemplating legal action. Having a physician or attorney as a family member or neighbor makes it easy for the patient to call on that expertise. That physician or attorney may then direct the patient to additional contacts that will further facilitate the investigation into the care in question. Patients without such contacts may find it too burdensome or expensive to seek such guidance on complicated issues such as medical care, whereas the patient with medical or legal connections has free access to medical and legal opinions.

Demanding, Hard-to-Satisfy Patients

Physicians often recognize a future problem when they encounter a patient that demands certain medications, a certain procedure, or is overall difficult to satisfy. These types of patients should raise red flags immediately and should be treated with extra attention. When dealing with a demanding or hard-to-satisfy patient, a physician may need to spend additional time communicating with the patient and documenting those communications. In addition, the physician must not get "pushed around" by the patient or talked into prescribing unnecessary medication or performing an unwarranted procedure. It is important to stick to sound medical decision-making and thoroughly document the rationale for doing so. If such measures are taken, the physician will be well protected against the allegations of this troublesome patient.

Patients That Have Sued Other Physicians

This may seem obvious, but patients who have sued their past physicians are not averse to suing their present or future physicians. However, just because a patient has been involved in prior litigation does not mean that a physician should refuse to see that patient. The patient may have had completely valid reasons for the prior suit, or certain unknown circumstances could have prompted the litigation. Accordingly, prior litigation does not automatically mean that the patient is overly litigious or likely to sue. Prior litigation is reason to be cautious, and additional communication and medical record documentation is advised.

Causes of Action in Surgical Cases

Medical malpractice lawsuits against any surgeon generally involve claims that include failure to diagnose, surgical technique, informed consent, and failure to monitor. However, some variations of these general causes of action appear more frequently in urologic surgery cases. The causes of action most often filed against a urologic surgeon include improper performance of a procedure, error in diagnosis, failure to recognize a complication, failure to supervise or monitor a case, failure to create a proper follow-up plan, and failure to perform a proper preoperative workup of the patient [2, 15].

The failure to recognize a surgical complication is a popular claim against surgeons. Failure to recognize postoperative bleeding is a common postoperative complication. It is important to recognize that this allegation implicates several members of the team that care for the postoperative patient, including the surgeon, trainees, anesthesia, and nursing staff. It is frequently claimed that the patient's lab results, blood pressure, and clinical picture revealed an internal bleed that went unnoticed and unacted upon by the team. A similar allegation involves failing to recognize injury to adjacent structures, organs, or nerves.

Every so often, a patient will experience a complication which leads the patient to believe that the attending surgeon allowed trainees to perform the procedure or surgery without proper supervision. This is especially true in cases where the attending surgeon is "world-renowned" and the patient has the mistaken belief that complications are impossible in this surgeon's hands. Accordingly, when an adverse outcome presents itself, the patient believes that the only possible manner in which such an outcome can occur is if the attending surgeon allowed unsupervised trainees to perform the surgery. It is important to educate the patient on the various roles of the team members and that the attending surgeon may not be the only individual performing portions of the surgery.

One type of claim criticizes the activities of the surgeon even before the surgery begins. A number of intraoperative and postoperative adverse events can be traced to the preoperative workup of the patient. When an expert witness is reviewing a patient's medical chart who experienced an adverse event in the surgical setting, the patient's preoperative records are well studied. On certain occasions the expert will criticize the preoperative workup for a number of reasons. First, the expert may find that the surgeon failed to obtain a complete history and physical. It may also be alleged that the surgeon failed to order appropriate testing such as cardiac clearance, or performed inappropriate or inadequate testing. This is especially true in cases where the patient suffered a respiratory or cardiac event during or subsequent to the operation in question. When arriving at preoperative testing decisions, it is advised to properly document the decision-making process. To that end, the previously mentioned lack of informed consent claim is also a presurgical issue that is often the subject of litigation.

Surgical Mesh Litigation

A major source of litigation indirectly involving pelvic floor surgeons is the product liability lawsuits filed against the manufacturers of surgical mesh used to treat Pelvic Organ Prolapse (POP) and Stress Urinary Incontinence (SUI). Fortunately, surgeons do not usually get sued in ordinary product liability cases, but the lessons learned from the tens of thousands of cases filed against the surgical mesh manufacturers serve as valuable reminders to those operating in this space.

It is well documented that as early as 2008 the US Food and Drug Administration (FDA) issued a Public Health Notification about adverse events relating to urogynecologic use of surgical mesh to treat POP and SUI [16]. The FDA updated this communication in 2011 and warned surgeons that complications from surgical mesh used to repair POP include vaginal mesh erosion, pain, infection, urinary problems, and bleeding [17]. The FDA also warned that organ perforation due to surgical instruments was a more frequently reported complication [17]. Of note, the 2011 update dealt only with complications of transvaginal placement for POP.

Importantly, the FDA's 2011 communications on the subject cautioned that the agency's five year review of relevant literature revealed that "transvaginally placed mesh in POP repair does NOT conclusively improve clinical outcomes over traditional non-mesh repair" [18]. Furthermore, before recommending the placement of surgical mesh, a surgeon should consider the following:

- Nonsurgical alternatives
- Non-mesh surgery
- Abdominal placement of mesh
- Transvaginal placement of mesh when no preferable alternatives exist [13]

When recommending mesh surgery to patients, surgeons must ensure that their patients understand the permanency of mesh and the significant complications that could materialize. It may also be useful to provide patients with outcomes data or literature on these complications.

In addition to making recommendations to surgeons, the FDA also issued recommendations to patients [17, 18]. Accordingly, urogynecologic surgeons may experience more detailed and advanced questioning from patients. Likewise, the increased media attention and attorney advertisements concerning surgical mesh litigation are likely to further educate the public on the risks of surgical mesh.

As with any surgical procedure, the decision to proceed with abdominally or transvaginally placed surgical mesh should be one made with careful deliberation and in consultation with the patient. Documentation of this decision-making and consultation process is an absolutely necessary practice to undertake. This topic is still on the radar of the FDA. Physicians should remain vigilant for any recommendations or considerations coming out of the agency as it continues to monitor the effectiveness of SUI, recently completing a literature review of 30 randomized controlled clinic trials [19].

Conclusion

Certainly, providing a higher quality of care with better outcomes lessens a physician's chances of being sued. But as discussed in this chapter, care, treatment, and outcomes are not the only factors that influence a patient's decision to sue. Recognizing other dynamics such as communication style and setting expectations can certainly change a patient's outlook on the entire medical treatment process. If physicians can combine enhanced surgical technique with proper communication while recognizing what types of patients are more likely to sue when something goes wrong, the physician should be successful in implementing a proactive approach to avoid litigation while rendering appropriate care to the patient.

References

1. Guardado JR. Policy research perspectivies, medical liability claim frequency among US physicians, 2023 Report.
2. Sherer BA, Coogan CL. The current state of medical malpractice in urology. Urology. 2015;86(1):2–9.
3. Ohio Rev Code. 2023;§ 2305.113((A)(1)).
4. Ohio Rev Code. 2023;§ 2125.02((D) (1)).
5. Ohio Rev Code. 2001;§ 2305.16.
6. NPDB. National Practitioner Data Bank. Available at: http://www.npdb.hrsa.gov/, 07/15/2024.
7. White RE. Social inflation drives up malpractice payouts—and insurance rates. Med Econ, May 18, 2023.
8. Insurance Information Institute. What can we do about social inflation? August 18, 2022.
9. Insurance Information Institute. How legal system abuse drives social inflation. July 17, 2022.
10. The Doctors Company. Social inflation and loss development Report January 23, 2023.
11. Hickson GB, Federspiel CF, Pichert JW, Miller CS, Gauld-Jaeger J, Bost P. Patient complaints and malpractice risk. JAMA. 2002;287(22):2951–7.
12. CRICO Strategies. Malpractice risks in communication failures 2015 Annual Benchmarking Report 2015.
13. Vincent C, Young M, Phillips A. Why do people sue doctors? A study of patients and relatives taking legal action. Lancet. 1994;343(8913):1609–13.
14. McClellan FM, White AA, Jimenez RL, Fahmy S. Do poor people sue doctors more frequently? Confronting unconscious bias and the role of cultural competency. Clin Orthop Relat Res. 2012;470(5):1393–7.
15. Badger WJ, Moran ME, Abraham C, Yarlagadda B, Perrotti M. Missed diagnoses by urologists resulting in malpractice payment. J Urol. 2007;178(6):2537–9.
16. U.S. Food and Drug Administration. FDA Public Health Notification: Serious Complications Associated with Transvaginal Placement of Surgical Mesh in Repair of Pelvic Organ Prolapse and Stress Urinary Incontinence. October 20, 2008:1–3.
17. U.S. Food and Drug Administration. Update on Serious Complications Associated with Transvaginal Placement of Surgical Mesh for Pelvic Organ Prolapse: FDA Safety. Communication July 13. 2011:1–6.

18. U.S. Food and Drug Administration, CDRH: Center for Devices and Radiological Health. Urogynecologic Surgical Mesh: Update on the Safety and Effectiveness of Transvaginal Placement for Pelvic Organ Prolapse. July 2011:1–15.
19. U.S. Food and Drug Administration. Stress urinary incontinence: surgical mesh considerations and recommendations. April 11, 2024.

General Complications of Pelvic Reconstructive Surgery

4

Ellen R. Solomon and Matthew D. Barber

Assessing Perioperative Risk

Before a patient undergoes pelvic reconstructive surgery, the risk of potential complications should be carefully assessed and addressed with the patient. Complications may occur during or after the procedure and it is imperative to recognize high-risk patients and minimize risk from surgery before a patient is brought to the operating room. The lifetime risk of a woman undergoing prolapse or incontinence surgery by the age of 85 is 19% [1, 2]. The prevalence of perioperative complications among women undergoing reconstructive pelvic surgery has been reported to be as high as 33% [3]. There are a multitude of factors which are found to increase perioperative risk. A large retrospective cohort study including 1,931 women who had undergone prolapse surgery found an overall complication rate of 14.9% [4]. The complications identified included infection, bleeding, surgical injuries, pulmonary, and cardiovascular morbidity. These complications were associated with medical comorbidities (odds ratio 11.2) and concomitant hysterectomy (odds ratio 1.5). Risk factors for complications after pelvic reconstructive surgery are listed in Table 4.1.

Obesity is an increasingly important risk factor for perioperative complications. The prevalence of obesity continues to rise in industrialized countries [5]. With obesity, there is an increase in comorbid conditions, including the incidence of cardiac disease, type II diabetes, hypertension, stroke, sleep apnea, and some cancers [6]. One study of obese and overweight women found that obese women had significantly increased estimated blood loss and operative time [7]. In a retrospective cohort study from 2007, obese patients who underwent vaginal surgery were matched to patients who were of normal weight, and perioperative comorbidities and complications were analyzed. This study found that there was no difference in perioperative complications between obese and nonobese patients; however, there was

Table 4.1 General risk factors of pelvic reconstructive surgery

Risk factors
Age
Central nervous system disease
Coronary heart disease
Diabetes
Frailty
Hypertension
Obesity
Peripheral artery disease
Pulmonary disease

E. R. Solomon
Urogynecology and Pelvic Surgery, Baystate Medical Center, Springfield, MA, USA
e-mail: ellen.solomonmd@baystatehealth.org

M. D. Barber (✉)
Department of Obstetrics and Gynecology, Duke University Medical Center, Durham, NC, USA
e-mail: matthew.barber@duke.edu

H. B. Goldman, J. Zillioux (eds.), *Complications of Urogynecology and Reconstructive Pelvic Surgery*, https://doi.org/10.1007/978-3-032-00339-3_4

a higher rate of surgical site infection in the obese population [8].

In obese women undergoing hysterectomy, the abdominal approach results in significantly higher rates of wound infection than those receiving a vaginal hysterectomy [9]. In a recent systematic review, it was found that compared with vaginal and laparoscopic hysterectomy, patients with a Body Mass Index (BMI) over 35 who underwent abdominal hysterectomy had more postoperative complications and longer hospitalizations [10]. Overall, vaginal surgery appears to be a safer approach for obese women [11]. It is important to assess BMI when planning the route of surgery and to consider the increased risks with this population. In a large retrospective cohort study performed in Sweden, it was found that women who had a BMI ≤25were more likely to have increased blood loss, and longer duration of surgery, and women with a BMI ≥35 were more likely to have postoperative infections [12]. Furthermore, in an extremely large retrospective study where data was abstracted from the American College of Surgeons National Safety and Quality Improvement Project registry, 55,409 women who underwent hysterectomy for benign conditions were studied and it was found that patients with BMIs 40 or higher had five times the odds of wound dehiscence, five times the odds of wound infection, and 89% higher odds of sepsis compared to women with normal BMIs under 25 [13]. Furthermore, in a large retrospective study of over 18,800 women undergoing hysterectomy for benign conditions, the rates of total abdominal hysterectomy increased from 45.7% in patients with ideal body weight to 62% in morbidly obese patients, which has higher morbidity than laparoscopic and vaginal approaches [14].

Age is also an important factor to consider when assessing perioperative risk. The median age of patients who undergo pelvic reconstructive surgery is 61.5 years [15]. Increasing age corresponds with increasing medical comorbidities, including chronic illness, hypertension, coronary heart disease, diabetes, pulmonary disease, and central nervous system disease [16]. A retrospective cohort study of 264,340 women undergoing pelvic surgery found that increasing age is associated with higher mortality risks and higher complication risks. Specifically, elderly women (>age 80) were found to have an increased risk of perioperative complications compared with younger women [17]. In this same study, elderly women who underwent obliterative procedures (e.g., colpocleisis) had a lower risk of complications compared to patients who underwent reconstructive procedures for prolapse. In a prospective study of 2-year postoperative survival, survival was worse among 80-year-olds who experienced a postoperative complication [18]. In a retrospective chart review of patients ≥75-years old, 25.8% of patients had significant perioperative complications, including significant blood loss, pulmonary edema, and congestive heart failure. Independent risk factors that were predictive of perioperative complications in this patient population included length of surgery, coronary artery disease, and peripheral vascular disease [19]. In a retrospective cohort study including 508 women undergoing urogynecologic surgery, women who were older than age 65 had an increased risk of postoperative complications on the Dindo-Clavien scale when compared to women who were younger than age 65 [20]. When choosing to perform a prolapse or incontinence procedure on an elderly patient, it is important to review the patient's comorbidities.

Frailty, the accumulation of age-related physical and cognitive deficits, is a well-established risk factor for perioperative complications. A recent large (n = 107,890) retrospective cohort study of Medicare beneficiaries (women ≥65 years old) undergoing prolapse surgery found that moderately to severely frail women had a sevenfold increased risk of prolonged hospital stay (≥3 days) or UTI and threefold greater risk of 30-day complication compared to non-frail women [21]. Recognizing that frailty and advanced age are not synonymous, a novel surgical risk calculator incorporating frailty was also recently developed for older patients undergoing prolapse and stress urinary incontinence surgery to help individualize counseling [22].

Cardiac risk factors also impact postoperative morbidity in pelvic surgery. In a retrospective cohort study by Heisler et al. [23], perioperative complications were increased in patients with a history of myocardial infarction or congestive heart failure, perioperative hemoglobin decrease greater than 3.1 g/dL, preoperative hemoglobin less than 12.0 g/L, or history of prior thrombosis. In a retrospective analysis of cardiac comorbidities in pelvic surgery by Schakelford et al. [24], hypertension and ischemic heart disease were statistically significant risk factors for perioperative cardiac morbidity. It is important to ensure that a patient's cardiac status is optimized prior to proceeding with surgery [25]. In a retrospective cohort study of 4,315 patients undergoing elective major noncardiac surgery, predictors of major cardiac complications included high-risk types of surgeries, history of ischemic heart disease, history of congestive heart failure, history of cerebrovascular disease, preoperative treatment with insulin, and a serum creatinine of ≥2.0 mg/dL [26]. To further decrease cardiac morbidity in patients undergoing surgery, it has also been shown that continuing beta blockers in the perioperative period in patients with chronic beta blockade will decrease cardiovascular mortality [27]. Additionally, it has been recently determined via a retrospective cohort study of patients undergoing pelvic reconstructive surgery that the rate of mortality, cardiac arrest, myocardial infarction, and acute ischemic stroke was 4.8 per 1000 surgeries. Risk factors according to this study included major preexisting cardiac conditions, diabetes, neurologic disease, or coagulopathy [28]. Consultation with the patient's primary care physician or cardiologist prior to surgery is often warranted in patients with cardiac disease.

In conclusion, when considering pelvic reconstructive surgery, it is important to examine and evaluate the whole patient, including their medical comorbidities, in order to appropriately assess their perioperative risk. This knowledge will help determine whether or not surgery is appropriate and, when appropriate, what route of surgery and procedure may be best for the individual patient. In high-risk patients, the vaginal route is often the lowest risk approach. In elderly patients no longer interested in sexual activity, obliterative procedures should be considered because of their quick surgical times and low risk of complications relative to reconstructive procedures.

Venous Thromboembolism

Deep venous thrombosis (DVT) and pulmonary embolism (PE), jointly referred to as venous thromboembolism (VTE), are among the leading causes of preventable perioperative morbidity and mortality. In the perioperative period, the risk of death after VTE is approximately 3–4% [29]. During surgery, the combination of epithelial damage, venous stasis, and hypercoagulability, collectively referred to as Virchow's triad, increases the risk of any patient undergoing surgery. Many pelvic reconstructive surgeries require the dorsal lithotomy position and steep Trendelenberg, positions that exacerbate the risk of venous stasis. The postoperative risk of VTE may be elevated up to 1 year after the initial procedure has been performed, but is highest in the immediate perioperative period [30].

The risk of VTE has been well studied in the general surgery, urology, and gynecologic oncology populations. Recently, there have been large studies that have addressed this issue in the population of patients who undergo pelvic reconstructive surgery. In a large cohort study by Montoya et al., it was found that the risk of VTE in this patient population that used intermittent pneumatic compression devices as the main form of postoperative thromboprophylaxis was 0.25% [31]. This is similar to a smaller study by Solomon et al. where the risk of VTE was 0.3% [32]. In a large systematic review by Rahn et al. it was found that intermittent pneumatic compression devices provide sufficient prophylaxis for most patients undergoing pelvic reconstructive surgery [33]. Risk factors that the authors determined should have additional chemoprophylaxis with intermittent compression devices were patients with two out of the three risk factors assessed: age over 60, history of cancer, or history of past VTE.

In another retrospective cohort study of 1,356 patients undergoing sling and/or prolapse procedures, the rate of VTE was 0.9% in women who had a sling alone and 2.2% in women who had concomitant prolapse surgery (*P* = 0.05) [34]. While this study gives rise to concern of concomitant procedures, it remains unclear if any of the patients received thromboprophylaxis during this study, and therefore it is difficult to assess actual patient risk. In a retrospective review by Nick et al. [35], the incidence of DVT was assessed among patients who underwent laparoscopic gynecologic surgery and was found to be 0.7% in this population. Overall, it seems that the risk is below 1% in the population undergoing these procedures.

A number of risk factors for VTE have been suggested for women undergoing pelvic surgery. In a retrospective review of 1232 patients who underwent surgery for gynecologic conditions in Japan, it was found that malignancy, history of VTE, age greater than 50, and allergic-immunologic disease were all statistically significant risk factors for VTE [36]. However, this study only found three episodes of VTE in patients with benign disease, making it significantly underpowered for this patient group. In a questionnaire study by Lindqvist et al. [37] that included 40,000 women, it was found that moderate drinkers and women who engaged in strenuous exercise most days were at half the risk of VTE compared to women who were heavy smokers and led sedentary lifestyles (increased risk of 30%).

In a retrospective review of gynecologic surgery patients, 1862 patients were given VTE prophylaxis with intermittent compression devices alone, and the incidence of VTE was 1.3%. The risk factors associated with VTE were diagnosis of cancer, age over 60, and anesthesia over 3 h. Patients with two or three of these variables had a 3.2% incidence of developing VTE vs. 0.6% in patients with zero or one risk factor [38].

The question of which thromboprophylactic modality is best in the perioperative period is difficult to answer for women undergoing pelvic reconstructive surgery. As mentioned previously, in the study by Montoya et al. [31], the rate of VTE among patients who underwent pelvic reconstructive surgery was 0.25% where the only thromboprophylaxis used was sequential compression devices placed during the perioperative period. The American College of Obstetricians and Gynecologists [39] follows the recommendations provided by the American College of Chest Physicians from the Seventh ACCP Conference on Antithrombotic and Thrombolytic Therapy, published in 2004. The ACCP has since updated its recommendations for prophylaxis in all surgical patients. (Table 4.2) Furthermore, they recommend chemothromboprophylaxis in patients who are moderate and high risk. Most female pelvic reconstructive surgery patients fall into the "high" risk category. Therefore, it is now recommended that most patients in our population should receive chemothromboprophylaxis [40]. However, the rate of thromboprophylaxis is below 1.5% in our population, and it could be argued that our patients fall into the very low risk category, where no specific recommendations for prophylaxis are made.

It is essential to be able to recognize the symptoms of VTE in the postoperative patient. While many patients who have VTE may be asymptomatic, the symptoms of dyspnea, orthopnea, hemoptysis, calf pain, complaints of calf swelling, chest pain, and tachypnea may signify a thrombotic event [41]. The physical signs that suggest VTE include hypotension, tachycardia, crackles, decreased breath sounds, lower extremity edema, tenderness in the lower extremities, and hypoxia [42]. Although the signs and symptoms of VTE are well known, it is difficult to rule out VTE by clinical diagnosis alone. A systematic review evaluating the d-dimer test used in combination with clinical probability to rule out VTE found that the d-dimer test is a safe and relatively reliable first-line test to use. After a 3-month follow-up, only 0.46% of patients were later diagnosed with PE [43]. However, d-dimer test is not useful in pregnant patients, the elderly, and hospitalized patients due to decreased specificity [44].

Compression ultrasonography is a noninvasive, easy, and cost-effective procedure for the diagnosis of DVT in the lower extremities. The sensitivity and specificity for detecting DVT using compression ultrasonography in symptomatic patients are 89% and 96%, respectively,

Table 4.2 American College of Chest Physicians risk for venous thromboembolism in patients undergoing surgery

Level of risk	Definition	Recommended prevention strategy
Very low	<0.5% risk of VTE (Most outpatient or same-day surgery)	No specific recommendations
Low	Minor surgery (1.5% risk)(e.g., spinal surgery for nonmalignant disease)	Mechanical prophylaxis, preferably with SCDs
Moderate	Major surgery includes most general, open gynecologic and urologic cases (3% risk) (Gynecologic non-cancer surgery, cardiac surgery, thoracic surgery, and spinal surgery for malignant disease)	LMWH, LDUH, plus mechanical thromboprophylaxis with ES or SCDs
High	Major surgery, or patients with additional VTE risk factors (6% risk) (bariatric surgery, Gynecologic cancer surgery, craniotomy, traumatic brain injury, spinal cord injury)	LMWH or LDUH, plus mechanical prophylaxis; use mechanical prophylaxis until bleeding risk diminishes
High-risk cancer surgery		LMWH or LDUH plus mechanical prophylaxis and extended-duration prophylaxis with LMWH post-discharge.
High risk, LDUH and LMWH contraindicated or not available		Fondaparinux or low-dose aspirin (160 mg); mechanical prophylaxis with SCDs, ES, or both.

Modified with permission from Gould et al. [38]
Bid twice daily, *LDUH* low-dose unfractionated heparin, *LMWH* low-molecular-weight heparin, *tid* three times daily, *VTE* venous thromboembolic events, *SCDs* sequential compression devices, *ES* elastic stockings

although the sensitivity is decreased in patients with calf DVT or asymptomatic patients [45]. Compression ultrasonography may also be used in conjunction with other diagnostic tests if PE is suspected [46]. If compression ultrasound is negative but the patient remains symptomatic, venography may be used to further rule out DVT [47].

Indicated imaging for patients presenting with signs and symptoms of PE include ventilation perfusion scanning (V/Q), computed tomography (CT) pulmonary angiography, and spiral CT of the chest. The V/Q scan was the imaging modality of choice for decades; however, due to the lack of ease of use and potential for indeterminate testing, CT has become the modality of choice [48]. CT angiography has a specificity of 96% as well as 83% sensitivity [41]. This has become the gold standard for PE diagnosis. CT looking for PE may vary across centers due to the type of CT used and the radiologist's ability to make the diagnosis.

It is important to start anticoagulation immediately once VTE has been diagnosed; furthermore, if there is high suspicion for PE, anticoagulation may be started even before the diagnosis is confirmed. According to the 2021 second update of the American College of Chest Physicians (CHEST) Guideline and Expert Panel on Antithrombotic Therapy for VTE Disease, clinically stable patients with surgery-provoked PE can be treated on an outpatient basis with close follow-up for 3-months with a direct-acting oral anticoagulant (i.e., apixaban, dabigatran, edoxaban, and rivaroxaban) [49]. Direct-acting oral anticoagulants are now strongly recommended in most scenarios over vitamin K antagonist (i.e., warfarin) due to more favorable safety profiles without the need for monitoring or titration. Acute PE with hypotension should be considered for thrombolysis. If the patient has contraindications to anticoagulation therapy, an inferior vena cava (IVC) filter can be considered.

Pulmonary Complications

Postoperative pulmonary complications are a frequent cause of morbidity and mortality. Postoperative pneumonia, atelectasis, pneumothorax, and respiratory failure are postoperative complications that increase length of stay and are more common than postoperative cardiac complications [50]. The incidence of postoperative pulmonary complications in gynecologic patients has been reported to be between 1.22 and 2.16% [51]. There are multiple risk factors that may increase pulmonary complications in the postoperative surgical patient. In a prospective randomized trial of patients who underwent non-thoracic surgery, on multivariate analysis, four risk factors for postoperative pulmonary complications were age greater than 65, positive "cough test," perioperative nasogastric tube, and duration of anesthesia (procedures lasting longer than 2.5 h) [52]. A retrospective review of patients undergoing gynecologic laparoscopy found that operative time greater than 200 min and age greater than 65 contributed to hypercarbia. Predictors of the development of pneumothorax included pneumoperitoneum, CO_2 pressure greater than 50 mmHg, and operative time greater than 200 min [53].

In a retrospective review of 3226 patients who underwent hysterectomy for benign conditions, it was found that the overall incidence of pulmonary complications in the benign gynecologic patient population was extremely low, −0.3% (95% CI, 0.17–0.57%) [54].

Surgical approach is also a contributing factor to the development of a postoperative ulmonary complication. A study of patients undergoing abdominal surgery found that age greater than 60, smoking history within the past 8 weeks, body mass index greater than or equal to 27, history of cancer, and incision site in the upper abdomen or both upper/lower abdominal incisions were identified as independent risk factors for postoperative pulmonary complications [55].

In a prospective randomized control trial involving 994 patients by Xue et al. [56], patients were divided into three groups (1) elective superficial plastic surgery, (2) upper abdominal surgery, and (3) thoracoabdominal surgery. It was found that the incidence of hypoxemia in the postoperative period was closely related to the operative site, where upper abdominal and thoracoabdominal sites gave the greatest risk. When evaluating this study, patients undergoing pelvic reconstructive surgery would most likely fall into the low-risk category, similar to elective superficial plastic surgery, with a low risk of hypoxemia in the postoperative period.

Another risk factor associated with postoperative pulmonary complications is smoking. In a prospective cohort study of patients referred for non-thoracic surgery, the risk for postoperative pulmonary complications was increased by age of greater than 65 years or more and smoking of 40 pack-years or more [51]. In a retrospective review performed on 635,265 patients from the American College of Surgeons National Surgical Quality Improvement Program database, current smokers had increased odds of postoperative pneumonia and unplanned intubation [57]. Pulmonary complications significantly decrease after 8 weeks of smoking cessation [58]. Chronic obstructive pulmonary disease (COPD) patients are at increased risk of having postoperative pulmonary complications. Preoperative pulmonary function tests may help to identify patients with increased pulmonary risk [59]. Patients with COPD were found to be 300–700 times more likely to have a postoperative pulmonary complication in a prospective cohort study [51]. Nasogastric intubation instead of oro-gastric intubation increases the risk of pneumonia in this patient population as well [60].

Sleep apnea is an additional risk factor for postoperative pulmonary complications. Obstructive sleep apnea is defined as partial or complete obstruction of the upper airway during sleep [61]. The prevalence of sleep apnea is around 5% [62]. In an additional study evaluating the prevalence of sleep apnea in the general surgery population, 22% of surgical patients were found to have obstructive sleep apnea [63]. Therefore, we can hypothesize that obstructive sleep apnea is a prevalent and important risk factor for postoperative pulmonary complications in our population as well. In a retrospective cohort study of orthopedic and general surgery patients by Memtsoudis et al. [64], 51,509 patients with sleep apnea who underwent general surgery procedures were assessed for postoperative pulmonary complications. It was found that patients with sleep apnea developed pulmonary complications more frequently than their matched controls. Due to relaxation of the pharyngeal muscles from anesthetic agents, sedatives, and opioids, patients with obstructive sleep apnea may have increased airway collapse in the postoperative period [65]. The supine position that occurs during surgery and in the postoperative period may worsen obstructive sleep apnea [66]. Anesthesia may also blunt the hypercapnic and hypoxic respiratory drive as well as the arousal response. In a study performed by Bolden et al. [67], the frequency of postoperative hypoxemia was measured in OSA patients in the postoperative period, where 16% of the patients studied found multiple measured postoperative desaturations.

To avoid hypoxemia in OSA patients, it is necessary to encourage patients to bring in their home continuous positive airway pressure (CPAP) machines or to order home CPAP settings for the hospital machines. Careful evaluation of the patient is essential to preventing postoperative complications. If a patient is suspected to have OSA but has not been diagnosed, it is useful to place the patient under continuous pulse oxygen saturation monitoring for the first 24 h after surgery [61].

Atelectasis and hypoxemia are common after surgery, especially surgeries that involve the abdomen or thorax. Early on, atelectasis may result from soft tissue edema in the upper pharynx due to intubation and tongue manipulation. Later, especially in patients who have undergone abdominal surgery, there is decreased ability to take in deep breaths or cough due to postoperative pain. Postoperative patients have decreased functional residual capacity [68]. These factors lead to hypoventilation. Diagnosis of atelectasis may be made clinically and/or via imaging tests. Atelectasis may present as postoperative fever, decreased breath sounds at the lung bases, and can be found on chest X-ray or CT.

Pre- and postoperative incentive spirometry is the most common prevention and treatment intervention for atelectasis. Incentive spirometry used in the perioperative period enhances postoperative functional residual capacity and reminds patients to continue to take in large breaths. If a patient becomes hypoxic from atelectasis, bronchoscopy may be performed to remove secretions from the airway [69]. CPAP can be used in the postoperative period and has also been shown to decrease intubation in patients who are at high risk of hypoxemia from atelectasis after abdominal surgery [70].

Postoperative pneumonia is a common postoperative pulmonary complication. Hospital-acquired pneumonia refers to pneumonia that develops after 48 h in the hospital. Diagnosing postoperative pneumonia can be difficult. Infiltrates from atelectasis, pulmonary edema, and acute lung injury can all look identical to pneumonia on chest X-ray. Diagnosis should be suspected if the patient has new-onset fever, purulent sputum, leukocytosis, hypoxemia, and infiltrate on chest X-ray (American Thoracic Society, 2002) [71]. In a prospective case series of patients presenting with postoperative pneumonia within 14 days of surgery, 61% of patients developed pneumonia within the first 5 days postoperatively. The most common etiologic agents were *Staphylococcus aureus*, *Streptococci*, and *Enterobacter* [72].

Treatment of postoperative pneumonia should begin with broad-spectrum antibiotics given the polymicrobial nature of hospital-acquired pneumonia. Recommendations by the American Thoracic Society and the Infectious Disease Society of America include coverage for aerobic bacteria as well as anaerobic coverage. Most hospitals have guidelines for treating hospital-acquired pneumonia based on regional microbial infections.

Urinary Tract Infection

Urinary tract infections (UTIs) are one of the most common infections seen in the postoperative period. The incidence of UTIs rises with increasing age. Eighty percent of UTIs are caused by bladder instrumentation, with catheter-associated UTI (CAUTI) being most common [73]. The rate of bacteriuria after undergoing an anti-incontinence procedure has been estimated to be between 17% and 85% [74]. Reconstructive pelvic surgery almost always involves bladder instrumentation via cystoscopy and/or catheter placement, thereby increasing the risk of UTI in these patients. Additional risk factors for UTI include inefficient bladder emptying, pelvic relaxation, neurogenic bladder, asymptomatic bacteruria, decreased ability to get to the toilet, nosocomial infections, physiologic changes, and sexual intercourse, all seen commonly in the reconstructive pelvic surgery population [75]. Development of a fever in the postoperative period after female pelvic reconstruction should warrant a urinary tract evaluation; however, it is rare that a lower UTI causes fever in itself.

There have been multiple trials evaluating the risk of UTI after urogynecological procedures, including the SISTEr trial of Burch vs autologous sling for treatment of stress urinary incontinence, where the reported rate of UTI was 48% in the sling cohort and 32% in the Burch cohort during the first 24 months of follow-up [76]. In the TOMUS trial, retropubic midurethral slings were associated with significantly more UTIs than transobturator slings in the first 6 weeks after surgery (13% vs 8%, $p = 0.3$) and after 24 months of follow-up (21% vs 13%, $p = 0.02$) [77]. In a case-control study of women undergoing surgery for stress urinary incontinence and/or pelvic organ prolapse, 9% of women developed UTI, and the risk of UTI was significantly increased by previous history of chronic or multiple UTIs, prolonged duration of catheterization, and increased distance between the urethra and anus [78].

Signs and symptoms of UTI in women are varied. Common cystitis symptoms include frequency, urgency, nocturia, dysuria, suprapubic discomfort, hematuria, and occasional mild incontinence. Fever, chills, general malaise, and costovertebral angle tenderness are associated with upper UTI [74]. There are multiple ways to diagnose UTI. Urine dipstick testing can detect the presence of leukocytes, bacteria, nitrates, and red blood cells. It also measures glucose, protein, ketones, blood, and bilirubin. In the office, the dipstick test can be used as a rapid diagnostic test. It can measure leukoesterase, nitrates, hematuria, and pyuria. In the setting of leukocytosis, and/or nitrites and hematuria, the sensitivity to detect UTI is 75%, but the specificity is 66% with a positive predictive value of 81% and a negative predictive value of 57% [79]. The most important predictor of UTI measured by microscopy is leukocytosis; however, leukocytosis alone is not sufficient to diagnose UTI [80]. The gold standard to diagnosing UTI is a urine culture. The traditional diagnosis of UTI by culture is greater than 100,000 colony-forming units/mL (CFU); however, many women may have asymptomatic bacteruria. In a study performed by Schiotz [81], 193 women who underwent gynecologic surgery and had a Foley catheter for 24 h were assessed for bacteruria; 40.9% of patients had asymptomatic bacteruria, while only 8.3% of patients actually developed UTI. In contrast, those with fewer than 100,000 CFU but symptoms of UTI can also be appropriately diagnosed as having a UTI.

The most common pathogen causing complicated and uncomplicated UTI is *E. coli*. The definition of complicated UTI is associated with a condition that increases the risk of acquiring an infection or failing first-line treatment. Many patients with pelvic floor disorders with UTI may fit into the complicated category because they are status/post-catheterization and procedures [82]. Other uropathogens include *Klebsiella*, *Pseudomonas*, *Enterobacter*, *Enterococcus*, and *Candida*. The initial therapy for treatment of UTI traditionally has been Trimethoprim-Sulfamethoxazole (TMP-SMX) if the resistance in the population is less than 20%. However, due to empiric treatment of UTIs in the past, resistance to TMP-SMX and amoxicillin is high and has been reported to be up to 54% for TMP-SMX and 46% for penicillins. Nitrofurantoin has been well studied and is an additional agent used frequently to treat UTIs. It is a cost-effective agent that may be used in the setting of fluoroquinolone and TMP-SMX resistance [83]. *When treating a postoperative reconstructive patient, it is important to evaluate the antimicrobiogram in the specific hospital setting and to prescribe accordingly.*

It is clear that patients who undergo female pelvic reconstructive procedures require antibiotic prophylaxis at the time of the procedure [84]. The American Urologic Association Best Practice Guidelines [85, 83] recommend antibiotic prophylaxis for vaginal surgery to prevent both postoperative UTI and postoperative pelvic infection (Table 4.3). A prospective randomized trial by Ingber et al. [86] found that patients who were given single-dose antibiotic therapy for midurethral slings had a low rate of postoperative UTI (5.9%). Clinical trials have been mixed about whether multiple doses of antibiotics in the perioperative period decrease UTI rates beyond single-dose therapy, although most recent guidance suggests a single dose [85, 87]. What is also unclear is the need for prophylactic antibiotics beyond the perioperative period in patients who will require prolonged catheterization. In a randomized, double-blind controlled trial by Rogers et al. [84], 449 patients who underwent pelvic organ prolapse and/or stress urinary incontinence surgery and had suprapubic catheters placed were given either placebo or nitrofurantoin monohydrate daily while the catheter was in place to assess the rate of UTI. The study found that there was a significant decrease in positive urine cultures, as well as symptomatic UTIs at suprapubic catheter removal with nitrofurantoin prophylaxis; however, there was no difference in symptomatic UTIs at the 6–8 week postoperative visit. A similar trial evaluating nitrofurantoin daily prophylaxis in patients with prolonged transurethral catheterization after pelvic reconstructive surgery found that daily nitrofurantoin during catheterization did not reduce the risk of postoperative UTI [88].

Surgical Site Infections

Infection complicating pelvic surgery can occur in three different settings (1) fever of unknown origin, (2) operative site infection, and (3) infection remote from surgery. The pathological source of most surgical site infections is bacteria located on the skin or in the vagina. Skin flora is usually aerobic Gram-positive *cocci*, but may include Gram-negative, anaerobic, and/or fecal flora if incisions are made near the perineum and groin [88]. Pelvic reconstructive surgery almost always involves the vagina and perineum and therefore places all of our patients at increased risk for surgical site infections. Other patient comorbidities that may increase the risk of surgical site infections include advanced age, obesity, medical conditions, cancer, smoking, malnutrition, and immunosuppressant use [89, 90]. Other risk factors for surgical site infection include poor hemostasis, length of stay, length of operative time, and tissue trauma. Specific risk factors for obese patients include increased bacterial growth on skin, decreased vascularity in the subcutaneous tissue, increased tension on wound closure due to increased intra-abdominal pressure, decreased tissue concentrations of prophylactic antibiotics, and a higher prevalence of diabetes with poor glucose control and longer operating time [91]. In a retrospective chart review of patients who underwent midline abdominal incisions, patients with increased subcutaneous fat were 1.7 times more likely to develop a superficial incisional infection [92]. In a prospective study of 5279 patients who underwent hysterectomy, it was found that obese patients who underwent abdominal hysterectomy

Table 4.3 American Urological Association recommended antimicrobial prophylaxis for urologic procedures

Procedures	Organisms	Antimicrobials of choice	Alternative antimicrobials	Duration of therapy
Vaginal surgery and/or slings	*E. coli*, *Proteus* sp., *Klebsiella* sp., *Enterococcus*, skin flora, and Group B *Strep.*	First/second-generation cephalosporin (*note that 2nd generation provides better anaerobic coverage, but cefazolin is equivalent in sling procedures*)	Ampicillin/sulbactam Aztreonam and metronidazole Aztreonam and clindamycin Clindamycin	Single dose

Modified from AUA Best Practice Guidelines [83]

were five times more likely to have wound infection. The route of surgery was an additional risk factor for infection, with the highest risk in patients who underwent abdominal hysterectomy. Patients who underwent laparoscopic or vaginal hysterectomy were more likely to have remote pelvic infections compared with abdominal hysterectomy [90]. In a large retrospective study of over 22,000 patients undergoing hysterectomy, the rate of surgical site infection overall was 2.04% and it was found that β-lactams given prior to incision were associated with the lowest rate of surgical site infections [93]. It is therefore advised that patients with penicillin allergies should be questioned on their reaction thoroughly and may necessitate penicillin allergy testing prior to surgery to avoid alternate antibiotics if possible. In another large retrospective study of over 55,000 patients undergoing hysterectomy, it was found that compared with those of normal BMI, women with BMIs 40 or higher had five times the odds of wound dehiscence, five times the odds of wound infection, and 89% higher odds of sepsis [13]. Women should be counseled about these findings prior to undergoing hysterectomy.

Use of synthetic mesh may be an additional risk factor for surgical site infection. There have been multiple case studies describing mesh infection. In one retrospective case study of patients who had undergone abdominal sacrocolpopexy, 27% of patients who underwent hysterectomy at the time of sacrocolpopexy became infected, requiring mesh removal vs. 1.3% of patients in the same study that had undergone sacrocolpopexy alone [94]. In an additional case series of 19 women who had undergone intravaginal slingplasty with synthetic mesh, six women had infected mesh that had to be removed [95]. In randomized trials comparing native tissue vaginal repair to transvaginal mesh placement using wide-pore [96] polypropylene, the risk of infection appears to be low in some trials and elevated in others [97]; however, many of these studies are small and are not adequately powered to detect differences in infectious morbidity.

Diagnosis of surgical site infection includes pain and tenderness at the operative site and fever. Fever is defined as a temperature of greater than 38 °C on two or more occasions occurring at least 4 h apart [98]. Skin erythema, induration, and/or drainage of purulent or serosanguinous fluid may be visualized on examination. On pelvic exam, there may be pelvic, vaginal cuff, or parametrial tenderness. There may be a leukocytosis on complete blood count [99]. If pelvic abscess is suspected, ultrasound, CT scan, or Magnetic Resonance Imaging (MRI) may be used for diagnosis. Ultrasound is a cost-effective way to image a patient with a suspected abscess. The sensitivity and specificity of pelvic ultrasound to look for pelvic abscess are 81% and 91%, respectively [99]. CT may be used to diagnose pelvic abscess when the diagnosis by ultrasound is equivocal. However, CT increases exposure to ionizing radiation, which may be problematic in younger patients.

Patients with superficial wound cellulitis may be treated with oral therapy. If there is evidence of a wound seroma or hematoma, a small portion of the wound may be opened and/or evacuated. It is important to probe the wound to ensure the fascia is intact [100]. It may be necessary to remove staples and sutures in the infected area. Admission is recommended if a patient is febrile, has signs of peritonitis, has failed oral agents, has evidence of a pelvic or intra-abdominal abscess, is unable to tolerate oral intake, or has laboratory evidence of sepsis [97]. Patients requiring admission should receive broad-spectrum parenteral antibiotics. Pelvic abscess may need drainage via opening of the vaginal cuff, CT, or ultrasound-guided drainage [101]. A vaginal cuff abscess may necessitate opening part of or, in some cases, the entire cuff to allow for sufficient drainage. If mesh has been placed, it may need to be removed if directly involved with the infection in order to achieve adequate resolution.

Prevention of wound infection is paramount to the practice of reconstructive pelvic surgery. Good surgical technique, hemostasis, and gentle tissue handling may decrease the risk of infection [99]. There have been multiple studies that suggest perioperative cleansing of the vagina with saline increases the infection rate [102, 103]. Currently, there is no evidence to suggest that

Table 4.4 Recommended antibiotic prophylaxis by the American College of Obstetrics and Gynecology

Procedures	Antibiotic	Dose (single dose)
Hysterectomy, female pelvic reconstructive procedures, procedures involving mesh	Cefazolin *Or for patients with PCN allergies*: Clindamycin *or* Metronidazole *plus* Gentamicin *or* Azetronam	2 g IV (or 3 g if weighs >120 kg) 900 mg or 500 mg IV 5 mg/kg or 2 g IV

Modified from Ref. [89]
IV intravenously, *g* grams, *mg* milligrams

cleansing the vagina with any preparation reduces postoperative infection. However, in a retrospective cohort trial of 669 patients who underwent sacral nerve modulation therapy, it was found that chlorhexidine washing prior to the procedure may decrease rates of surgical site infections in this population [102].

The use of prophylactic antibiotics is an imperative strategy for lowering surgical site infections. Antibiotics should be given within 30 min of incision time to allow for the minimal inhibitory concentrations (MIC) of the drug to be in the skin and tissues at the time of incision. It is important to note that some drugs such as vancomycin, metronidazole, and fluconazole require longer infusion times ranging from 30 min to 2 h. Recommendations for prophylactic antibiotic regimens from the AUA and ACOG are listed in Tables 4.3 and 4.4. Cefazolin is most commonly used in pelvic surgery because of its broad antimicrobial spectrum [89]. Patients who are morbidly obese with a BMI greater than 35 should receive increased dosing of antibiotics [90]. Procedures lasting longer than 3 h and blood loss greater than 1500 cc require redosing of antibiotics.

Nerve Injury

Intraoperative nerve injury is a preventable iatrogenic complication. Injury to nerves in the upper and lower extremities, while uncommon, may occur during laparotomy, robotic, laparoscopic, and vaginal procedures. In a prospective cohort study of women who underwent elective gynecologic surgery, the overall incidence of postoperative neuropathy was 1.8% [104]. Brachial plexus injury has a reported incidence of 0.16% [105]. Risk factors for developing nerve injuries during surgery include increased operating room time, patient positioning, and history of smoking [106]. Stretching or direct compression of the nerve results in ischemia, and when prolonged, necrosis can develop [107]. With muscle relaxants given during anesthesia, patients are unable to reposition themselves from nonphysiologic positions, and the risk of nerve damage increases. With nerve compression, blood flow to the nerve is decreased; therefore, operating room time is a critical factor for nerve injury. The longer a patient is incorrectly positioned, the worse the nerve injury. With the development of robotic surgery, it has been theorized that brachial plexus injuries may become more common [108]. Most robotic procedures require steep Trendelenberg positioning, and depending on the operator, may require longer operating room times. Other risk factors include a history of diabetes, alcoholism, and history of herpes zoster [109].

Nerve injuries to the upper extremity mostly occur from overstretching or compression of the brachial plexus or the ulnar nerve. Brachial plexus injury may result in both sensory and/or motor injury. Risk factors for brachial plexus injury includes Trendelenberg positioning, longer operating room time, use of shoulder braces, abduction of the arm ≥90°, and unequal shoulder support [104]. Patients with brachial plexus injury may present with numbness of the first, second, and third digits and the radial side of the fourth digit. Patients may experience motor deficits that involve the shoulder, wrist, arm, and hand. In severe cases, patients may experience Erb's palsy or Klumpke's paralysis [107]. Patients with ulnar nerve injury may present with sensory loss of the lateral hand, with loss of sensation in the fourth and fifth digits.

Management of brachial plexus injury includes physical therapy, analgesics, nonsteroidal anti-inflammatory medications, physical therapy, and neuroleptic medications. Prevention of brachial plexus injury includes utilizing the minimum amount of Trendelenberg positioning, decreasing operating room times as much as possible, avoiding abduction or extension of the upper extremities, and avoiding shoulder braces [107]. For robotic and laparoscopic surgeries, we recommend padding and tucking the patient's arms to her sides, using a "thumbs up" hand position with the patient's palms facing her thighs to avoid overabduction. To avoid sliding down the operating room table while in Trendelenberg, placing the patient on an egg crate mattress that is taped to the operating room table and then padding the patient's chest with additional foam and taping the foam down to the operating room table can be helpful (Fig. 4.1).

Common lower extremity nerve injuries associated with female pelvic reconstructive medicine include femoral, lateral femoral cutaneous, obturator, sciatic, and common peroneal nerve injuries. Risk factors for lower extremity nerve injuries include ill positioning of the lower extremities using stirrups, lithotomy position, slender patients, smokers, Trendelenberg position, and operating room time greater than 4 h [110]. In laparoscopic and vaginal surgeries, the femoral nerve may be injured due to the stretch encountered from the lithotomy position. The lateral cutaneous femoral nerve is one of the most common nerves injured from the lithotomy position, and injury is caused by compression and

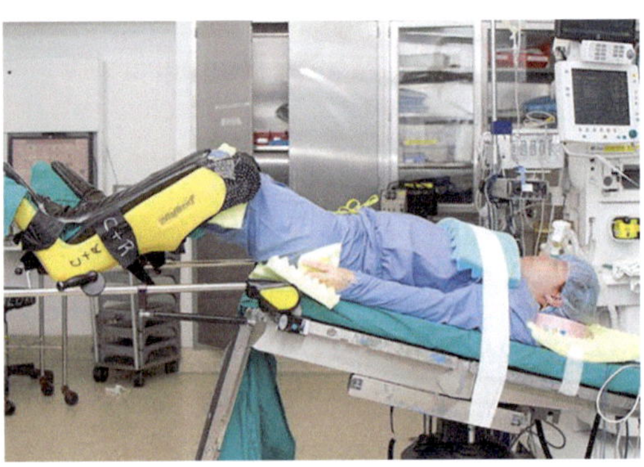

Fig. 4.1 Appropriate positioning of patients for laparoscopic or robotic pelvic reconstructive procedures with padding and taping to prevent neurologic injury

stretching under the inguinal ligament, most likely from prolonged flexion of the lower extremities. The obturator nerve may be injured from prolonged flexion of the legs in the lithotomy position. Sciatic nerve injury is less common in the dorsal lithotomy position; however, it may be caused by overflexion of the hip with abduction and external rotation. The common peroneal nerve can be injured via direct pressure on the nerve when legs are touching the pole of the candy cane stirrups—boot stirrups may aid in decreasing the risk of injury to this nerve [109].

To prevent lower extremity neuropathies caused by female pelvic reconstructive surgery, it is necessary to utilize the correct positioning of the lower extremities. Whenever possible, avoid candy cane stirrups as they offer little support and may cause undue hip abduction and external rotation. When positioning the lower extremities in boot stirrups, make sure the heel of the patient's foot fits directly into the boot. Padding the lateral aspect of the knee avoids injury to the peroneal nerve. When placing a patient in high lithotomy, the knee should be flexed 90–120°, hip flexion should be less than 60°, and abduction of the thighs should be no greater than 90° (Figs. 4.2 and 4.3). Nerve injuries from reconstructive pelvic surgery are minimized when the patient's extremities are positioned correctly.

Injury to the pudendal and other pelvic nerves may occur during specific pelvic reconstructive procedures. In the Optimal trial which randomized 374 women with apical vaginal prolapse to either sacrospinous ligament fixation or uterosacral vault suspension neurologic pain requiring intervention (medications, trigger point injections, or suture release) occurred more frequently after sacrospinous ligament fixation (6.9% vs. 12.4%) and persisted to 4–6 weeks after surgery more often (0.5% vs 4.3%) [110]. In the TOMUS trial, neurologic complications were noted more frequently in slings performed via the transobturator approach than the retropubic approach (9.7% vs. 5.0%, $p = 0.04$); however, most of these were minor and represented transient inner thigh numbness and weakness that resolved by 6 weeks

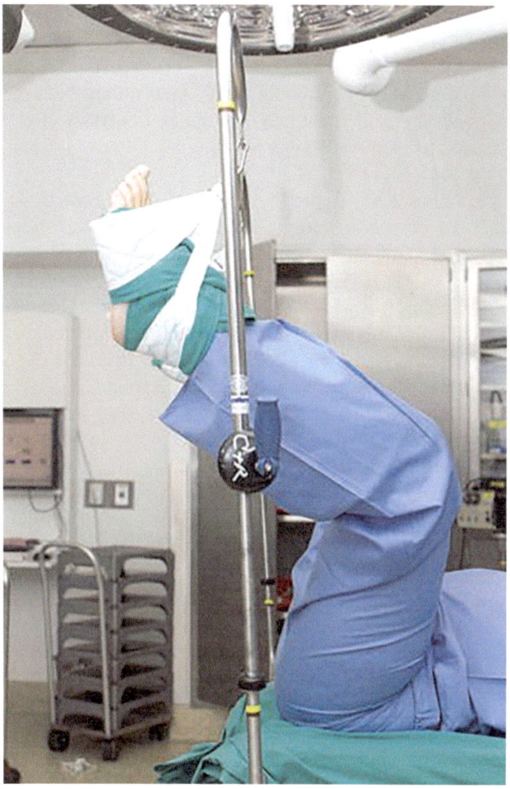

Fig. 4.2 Appropriate positioning of the lower extremities for dorsal lithotomy position using candy cane stirrups

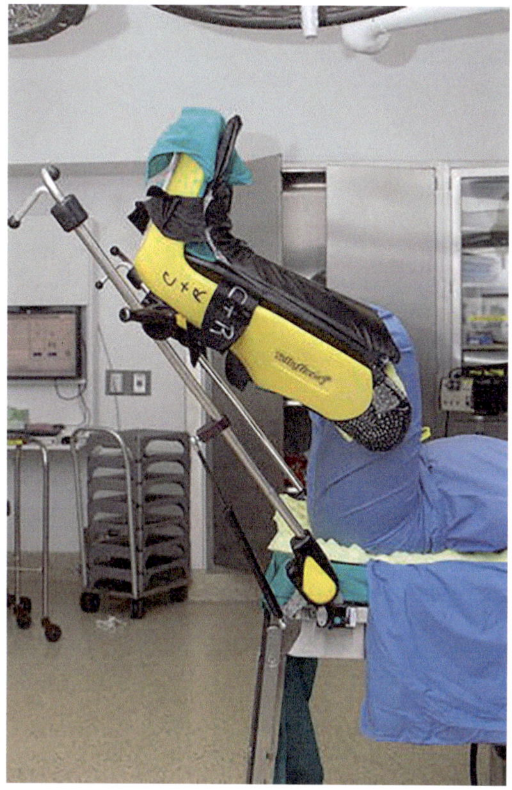

Fig. 4.3 Appropriate positioning of the lower extremities for dorsal lithotomy position using Boot stirrups

[77]. Of note, four patients (0.7%) had persistent postoperative neurologic symptoms at 24 months after surgery without any difference between the transobturator and retropubic approaches.

Diagnosis of postoperative neuropathy should include a thorough musculoskeletal and neurological exam (Table 4.5). The patient may also experience pain, numbness, and tingling in the dermatomes of the nerve routes. Electromyography (EMG) and MRI are procedures that may further aid in diagnosis. Treatment includes oral analgesics, nonsteroidal anti-inflammatory medications, low-dose antidepressants, neurologic medications including gabapentin and pregabalin, and physical therapy,

Table 4.5 Motor and sensory defects associated with lower extremity neuropathy

Nerve	Motor function	Sensation
Femoral	Hip flexion and knee extension	Anterior and medial thigh, medial calf
Lateral femoral cutaneous	N/A	Anterior and lateral thigh
Sciatic	Foot dorsiflexion and eversion	Foot, toes
Obturator	Thigh adduction and internal rotation	Medial aspect of the thigh
Common peroneal	Foot dorsiflexion and eversion	N/A

N/A not applicable

especially for prolonged neuropathies. Surgery and steroid injections may be used for severe cases [109].

References

1. Smith FJ, Holman CD, Moorin RE, Tsokos N. Lifetime risk of undergoing surgery for pelvic organ prolapse. Obstet Gynecol. 2010;116(5):1096–100.
2. Maher C, Feiner B, Baessler K, Schmid C. Surgical management of pelvic organ prolapse in women. Cochrane Database Syst Rev. 2013;4:CD004014.
3. Lambrou NC, Buller JL, Thompson JR, Cundiff GW, Chou B, Montz FJ. Prevalence of perioperative complications among women undergoing reconstructive pelvic surgery. Am J Obstet Gynecol. 2000;183:1355–60.
4. Handa VL, Harvey L, Cundiff GW, Kjerulff KH. Perioperative complications of surgery for genital prolapse: does concomitant anti-incontinence surgery increase complications? Adult Urol. 2004;65:483–7.
5. National Task Force on the Prevention and Treatment of Obesity. Overweight, obesity, and health risk. Arch Intern Med. 2000;160:898–904.
6. Must A, Spandano J, Coakley EH, Field AE, Colditz G, Dietz WH. The disease burden associated with overweight and obesity. JAMA. 1999;282:1523–9.
7. Rogers RG, Lebkuchner U, Kammerer-Doak DN, Thompson PK, Walters MD, Nygaard IE. Obesity and retropubic surgery for stress incontinence: is there really an increased risk of intraoperative complications? Am J Obstet Gynecol. 2006;195:1794–8.
8. Chen CCG, Collins SA, Rodgers AK, Paraiso MFR, Walters MD, Barber MD. Perioperative complications in obese women vs normal-weight women who undergo vaginal surgery. Am J Obstet Gynecol. 2007;197(98):e1–8.
9. Pitkin RM. Vaginal hysterectomy in obese women. Obstet Gynecol. 1977;49:567–9.
10. Blikkendaal MD, Schepers EM, van Zwet EW, Twijnstra AR, Jansen FW. Hysterectomy in very obese and morbidly obese patients: a systematic review with cumulative analysis of comparative studies. Arch Gynecol Obstet. 2015;292(4):723–38.
11. Isik-Akbay EF, Harmanli OH, Panganamamula UR, Akbay M, Gaughan J, Chatwani AJ. Hysterectomy in obese women: a comparison of abdominal and vaginal routes. Obstet Gynecol. 2004;104:710–4.
12. Bohlin KS, Ankardal M, Stjerndahl JH, Lindkvist H, Milsom I. Influence of the modifiable life-style factors body mass index and smoking on the outcome of hysterectomy. Acta Obstet Gynecol Scand. 2016;95(1):65–73.
13. Shah DK, Vitonis AF, Missmer SA. Association of body mass index and morbidity after abdominal, vaginal, and laparoscopic hysterectomy. Obstet Gynecol. 2015;125(3):589–98.
14. Mikhail E, Miladinovic B, Velanovich V, Finan MA, Hart S, Imudia AN. Association between obesity and the trends of routes of hysterectomy performed for benign indications. Obstet Gynecol. 2015;125(4):912–8.
15. Luber KM, Boero S, Choe JY. The demographics of pelvic floor disorders: current observations and future projections. Am J Obstet Gynecol. 2001;184:1496–503.
16. Toglia MR, Nolan TE. Morbidity and mortality rates of elective gynecologic surgery in the elderly woman. Am J Obstet Gynecol. 2003;189:1584–9.
17. Sung VW, Weitzen S, Sokol ER, Rardin CR, Myers DL. Effect of patient age on increasing morbidity and mortality following urogynecologic surgery. Am J Obstet Gynecol. 2006;194:1411–7.
18. Kawalpreet M, Bacchetti P, Leung JM. Prognostic significance of postoperative in-hospital complications in elderly patients. I. Long term survival. Anesth Analg. 2003;96:583–9.
19. Stepp KJ, Barber MD, Yoo EH, Whiteside JL, Paraiso MFR, Walters MD. Incidence of perioperative complications of urogynecologic surgery in elderly women. Am J Obstet Gynecol. 2005;192:1630–6.
20. Bretschneider CE, Robinson B, Geller EJ, Wu JM. The effect of age on postoperative morbidity in women undergoing urogynecologic surgery. Female Pelvic Med Reconstr Surg. 2015;21(4):236–40.
21. Reddy R, Zhao S, Boscardin WJ, Nik-Ahd F, Van Kuiken M, Suskind AM. The role of frailty on surgical outcomes following pelvic organ prolapse surgery in medicare beneficiaries: a national study. Urology. 2022;168:96–103. https://doi.org/10.1016/j.urology.2022.06.031.
22. Nik-Ahd F, Zhao S, Wang L, Boscardin WJ, Covinsky K, Suskind AM. UroARC: a novel surgical risk calculator for older adults undergoing pelvic organ prolapse and stress urinary incontinence surgery. Neurourol Urodyn. 2025;44(1):143–52. https://doi.org/10.1002/nau.25573.
23. Heisler CA, Aletti GD, Weaver AL, Melton LJ, Cliby WA, Gebhart JB. Improving quality of care: development of a risk-adjusted perioperative morbidity model for vaginal hysterectomy. Am J Obstet Gynecol. 2010;202(137):e1–5.
24. Schakelford DP, Hoffman MK, Kramer PR, Davies MF, Kaminiski PF. Evaluation of peroperative cardiac risk index values in patients undergoing vaginal surgery. Am J Obstet Gynecol. 1995;173:80–4.
25. Potyk D, Raudaskoski P. Peroperative cardiac evaluation for elective non cardiac surgery. Arch Fam Med. 1998;7:164–73.
26. Lee TH, Marcantonio ER, Mangione CM, Thomas EJ, Polanczyk CA, Cook EF, et al. Derivation and prospective validation of a simple index for prediction of cardiac risk of major noncardiac surgery. Circulation. 1999;100:1043–9.

27. Shammash JB, Trost JC, Gold JM, Berlin JA, Golden MA, Kimmel SE. Perioperative beta-blocker withdrawal and mortality in vascular surgical patients. Am Heart J. 2001;141:148–53.
28. Roberts K, Slopnick E, Chapman G, Mangel J, Sheyn D. Adverse cardiovascular events associated with female pelvic reconstructive surgery. Female Pelvic Med Reconstr Surg. 2021;27(4):230–7.
29. Colwell CW, Collis DK, Paulson R, McCutchen JW, Bigler GT, Lutz S, et al. Comparison of enoxaparin and warfarin for the prevention of venous thromboembolic disease after total hip arthroplasty. J Bone Joint Surg Am. 1999;81:932–9.
30. Sweetland S, Green J, Liu B, et al. Duration and magnitude of the postoperative risk of venous thromboembolism in middle aged women: prospective cohort study. BMJ. 2009;339:1–8.
31. Montoya TI, Leclaire EL, Oakley SH, Crane AK, Mcpencow A, Cichowski S, Rahn DD, Fellows' Pelvic Research Network of the Society of Gynecologic Surgeons. Venous thromboembolism in women undergoing pelvic reconstructive surgery with mechanical prophylaxis alone. Int Urogynecol J. 2014;25(7):921–6.
32. Solomon ER, Frick AC, Paraiso MFR, Barber MD. Risk of deep venous thrombosis and pulmonary embolism in urogynecologic surgical patients. Am J Obstet Gynecol. 2010;203(510):e1–4.
33. Rahn DD, Mamik MM, Sanses TV, Matteson KA, Aschkenazi SO, Washington BB, Steinberg AC, Harvie HS, Lukban JC, Uhlig K, Balk EM, Sung VW, Society of Gynecologic Surgeons Systematic Review Group. Venous thromboembolism prophylaxis in gynecologic surgery: a systematic review. Obstet Gynecol. 2011;118(5):1111–25.
34. Anger JT, Weingberg AE, Gore JL, Wang Q, Pashos MJ, Leonardi LV, et al. Thromboembolic complications of sling surgery for stress urinary incontinence among female Medicare beneficiaries. Urology. 2009;74:1223–6.
35. Nick AM, Schmeler KM, Frumovitz MM, Soliman PT, Spannuth WA, Burzawa JK, et al. Risk of thromboembolic disease in patients undergoing laparoscopic gynecologic surgery. Obstet Gynecol. 2010;116(4):956–61.
36. Suzuki N, Yoshioka N, et al. Risk factors for perioperative venous thromboembolism: a retrospective study in Japanese women with gynecologic diseases. Thromb J. 2010;8:1–9.
37. Lindqvist PG, Epstein E, Olsson H. The relationship between lifestyle factors and venous thromboembolism among women: a report from the MISS study. Br J Haematol. 2008;114:234–40.
38. Clarke-Pearson DL, Dodge RK, Synan I, McClelland RC, Maxwell GL. Venous thromboembolism prophylaxis: patients at high risk to fail intermittent pneumatic compression. Obstet Gynecol. 2003;101(1):157–63.
39. ACOG Committee on Practice Bulletins No. 84: prevention of deep vein thrombosis and pulmonary embolism. Obstet Gynecol. 2007;110(2 Pt 1):429–40.
40. Gould MK, Garcia DA, Wren SM, Karanicolas PJ, Arcelus JI, Heit JA, Samama CM, American College of Chest Physicians. Prevention of VTE in nonorthopedic surgical patients: antithrombotic therapy and prevention of thrombosis, 9th ed: American College of Chest Physicians Evidence-Based Clinical Practice Guidelines. Chest. 2012;141(2 Suppl):e227S–77S.
41. Okadome M, Saito T, et al. Postoperative pulmonary embolism including asymptomatic cases in gynecologic oncology. Int J Gynecol Cancer. 2010;20:655–63.
42. Stein PD, Beemath A, Matta F, et al. Clinical characteristics of patients with acute pulmonary embolism: data from PIOPED II. Am J Med. 2007;120:871–9.
43. Cate-Hoek AJT, Prins MH. Management studies using a combination of D-dimer test results and clinical probability to rule out venous thromboembolism: a systematic review. J Thromb Haemost. 2005;3:2465–70.
44. Agnelli G, Becattini C. Acute pulmonary embolism. N Engl J Med. 2010;363:266–74.
45. Qaseem A, Snow V, et al. Current diagnosis of venous thromboembolism in primary care: a clinical practice guideline from the American Academy of Family Physicians and the American College of Physicians. Ann Intern Med. 2007;146:454–8.
46. Moores LK, King CS, Holley AB. Current approach to the diagnosis of acute nonmassive pulmonary embolism. Chest. 2011;140:509–18.
47. Krivak TC, Zorn KK. Venous thromboembolism in obstetrics and gynecology. Obstet Gynecol. 2007;109:761–77.
48. Desciak MC, Martin DE. Perioperative pulmonary embolism: diagnosis and anesthetic management. J Clin Anesth. 2011;23:153–65.
49. Stevens SM, Woller SC, Kreuziger LB, et al. Antithrombotic therapy for VTE disease: second update of the CHEST Guideline and Expert Panel Report. Chest. 2021;160(6):e545–608. https://doi.org/10.1016/j.chest.2021.07.055. [published correction appears in Chest. 2022 Jul;162(1):269. doi: 10.1016/j.chest.2022.05.028]
50. Lawrence VA, Hilsenbeck SG, Mulrow CD, Dhanda R, Sapp J, Page CP. Incidence and hospital stay for cardiac and pulmonary complications after abdominal surgery. J Gen Intern Med. 1995;10:671–8.
51. Pappachen S, Smith PR, Shah S, Brito V, Bader F, Koury B. Postoperative pulmonary complications after gynecologic surgery. Int J Obstet Gynecol. 2006;93:74–6.
52. McAlister FA, Bertsch K, Man J, Bradley J, Jacka M. Incidence of and risk factors for pulmonary complications after nonthoracic surgery. Am J Respir Crit Care Med. 2005;171:514–7.
53. Murdock CM, Wolff AJ, Van Geem T. Risk factors for hypercarbia, subcutaneous emphysema, pneu-

mothorax and pneumomediastinum during laparoscopy. Obstet Gynecol. 2000;95:704–9.
54. Solomon ER, Muffly TM, Barber MD. Common postoperative pulmonary complications after hysterectomy for benign indications. Am J Obstet Gynecol. 2013 Jan;208(1):54.e1–5.
55. Brooks-Brunn JA. Predictors of postoperative pulmonary complications following abdominal surgery. Chest. 1997;111:564–71.
56. Xue FS, Li BW, Zhang GS, Liao X, Zhang YM, Liu JH, et al. The influence of surgical sites on early postoperative hypoxemia in adults undergoing elective surgery. Anesth Analg. 1999;88:213–9.
57. Turan A, Mascha EJ, Roberman D, Turner PL, You J, Kurz A, et al. Smoking and perioperative outcomes. Anesthesiology. 2011;114(4):837–46.
58. Warner MA, Divertie MB, Tinker JH. Preoperative cessation of smoking and pulmonary complications in coronary artery bypass patients. Anesthesiology. 1984;60(4):380–3.
59. Doyle RL. Assessing and modifying the risk of postoperative pulmonary complications. Chest. 1999;115:77S–81.
60. Ephgrave KS, Kleiman-Wexler R, Pfaller M, Booth B, Werkmeister L, Young S. Postoperative pneumonia: a prospective study of risk factors and morbidity. Surgery. 1993;114:815–21.
61. Adesanya AO, Lee W, Greilich NB, Joshi GP. Perioperative management of obstructive sleep apnea. Chest. 2010;138:1489–98.
62. Young T, Peppard PE, Gottlieb DJ. Epidemiology of obstructive sleep apnea. A population health perspective. Am J Respir Crit Care Med. 2002;165:1217–39.
63. Hwang D, Shakir N, Limann B, Sison C, Kaira S, Shulman L, et al. Association of sleep-disordered breathing with postoperative complications. Chest. 2008;133:1128–34.
64. Memtsoudis S, Liu SS, Ma Y, Chiu YL, Walz JM, Gaber-Baylis BA, et al. Perioperative pulmonary outcomes in patients with sleep apnea after noncardiac surgery. Anesth Analg. 2011;112:113–21.
65. Bolden N, Smith CE, Auckley D. Avoiding adverse outcomes in patients with obstructive sleep apnea (OSA): development and implementation of a perioperative OSA protocol. J Clin Anesth. 2009;21:286–93.
66. Johnson MM, Conde MV. In: Maneker S, editor. Overview of the management of postoperative pulmonary complications. Waltham: UpToDate; 2011.
67. Bolden N, Smith CE, Auckley D, Maraski J, Ramachangdra A. Perioperative complications during use of an obstructive sleep apnea protocol following surgery and anesthesia. Int Anesth Res Soc. 2007;105:1869–70.
68. Wahba RM. Airway closure and intraoperative hypoxaemia: twenty-five years later. Can J Anaesth. 1996;43:1144–9.
69. Barrett CR. Flexible fiberoptic bronchoscopy in the critically ill patient, methodology and indications. Chest. 1978;73:746–9.
70. Squadrone V, Coha M, Cerutti E, et al. Continuous positive airway pressure for treatment of postoperative hypoxemia. JAMA. 2005;293:589–95.
71. American Thoracic Society and the Infectious Diseases Society America. Guidelines for the management of adults with hospital-acquired, ventilator-associated, and healthcare-associated pneumonia. Am J Respir Crit Care Med. 2005;171(4):388–416.
72. Montavers P, Veber B, Auboyer C, Dupont H, Gauzit R, Korinek AM, et al. Diagnostic and therapeutic management of nosocomial pneumonia in surgical patients: results of the Eole study. Crit Care Med. 2002;30:368–75.
73. Lo E, Nocolle L, Classen D, et al. Strategies to prevent catheter-associated urinary tract infections in acute care hospitals. Infect Control Hosp Epidemiol. 2008;29:S41–50.
74. Nygaard IE, Kreder KJ. Complications of incontinence surgery. Int Urogynecol J. 1994;5:353–60.
75. Karram MM, Kleeman SD. Lower urinary tract infection. In: Walters M, Karram MM, editors. Urogynecology and reconstructive pelvic surgery. 3rd ed. Philadelphia: Mosby Elsevier; 2007. p. 413–24.
76. Albo ME, Richter HE, Brubaker L, Norton P, Kraus S, Zimmern PE, et al. Burch colposuspension versus fascial sling to reduce urinary stress incontinence. N Engl J Med. 2007;356:2143–55.
77. Brubaker L, Norton PA, Albo ME, Chai TC, Dandreo KJ, Lloyd KL, Lowder JL, Sirls LT, Lemack GE, Arisco AM, Xu Y, Kusek JW. Urinary incontinence treatment network. Adverse events over two years after retropubic or transobturator midurethral sling surgery: findings from the Trial of Midurethral Slings (TOMUS) study. Am J Obstet Gynecol. 2011;205(5):498.e1–6.
78. Sutkin G, Alperin M, Meyn L, Wiesenfeld HC, Ellison R, Zyczynski HM. Symptomatic urinary tract infections after surgery for prolapse and/or incontinence. Int Urogynecol J. 2010;21:955–61.
79. Little P, Moore MV, Turner S, Rumsby K, Warner G, Lowes JA, et al. Effectiveness of five different approaches in management of urinary tract infection: radomised controlled trial. BMJ. 2010;340:c199.
80. Komoroff AL. Urinalysis and urine culture in women with dysuria. Ann Intern Med. 1986;104:212–8.
81. Schiotz HA. Urinary tract infections and bacteriuria after gynecological surgery: experience with 24-hour Foley catheterization. Int Urogynecol J. 1994;5:345–8.
82. Hooten TM, Stamm WE. Diagnosis and treatment of uncomplicated urinary tract infection. Infect Dis Clin N Am. 1997;11:551–81.
83. Mckinnell JA, Stollenwerk NS, Jung CW, Miller LG. Nitrofurantoin compares favorably to recommended agents as empirical treatment of uncomplicated urinary tract infections in a decision and cost analysis. Mayo Clin Proc. 2011;86(6):480–8.
84. Rogers RG, Kammerer-Doak D, Olsen A, Thompson PK, Walters MD, Lukacz ES, et al. A randomized,

double-blind, placebo-controlled comparison of the effect of nitrofurantoin monohydrate macrocrystals on the development of urinary tract infections after surgery for pelvic organ prolapse and/or stress urinary incontinence with suprapubic catheterization. Am J Obstet Gynecol. 2004;191:182–7.
85. Lightner DJ, Wymer K, Sanchez J, Kavoussi L. Best practice statement on urologic procedures and antimicrobial prophylaxis. J Urol. 2020;203(2):351–6. https://doi.org/10.1097/JU.0000000000000509.
86. Ingber MS, Vasavada SP, Firoozi F, Goldman HB. Incidence of perioperative urinary tract infection after single-dose antibiotic therapy for midurethral slings. Urology. 2010;76:830–4.
87. Andy UU, Harvie HS, Ackenbom MF, Arya LA. Single versus multi-does antibiotic prophylaxis for pelvic organ prolapse surgery with mesh/graft. Eur J Obstet Gynecol. 2014;181:37–40.
88. Deiter AA, Amundsen CL, Edenfield AL, Kawasaki A, Leven PJ, Visco AG, Siddiqui NY. Oral antibiotics to prevent postoperative urinary tract infection: a randomized controlled trial. Obstet Gynecol. 2014;123(1):96–103.
89. ACOG Committee on Practice Bulletins No. 104: antibiotic prophylaxis for gynecologic procedures. Obstet Gynecol. 2009;113(5):1180–9.
90. Walsh C, Scaife C, Hopf H. Prevention and management of surgical site infections in morbidly obese women. Obstet Gynecol. 2009;113:411–5.
91. Boesch CE, Umek W. Effects of wound closure on wound healing in gynecologic surgery. J Reprod Med. 2009;54:139–44.
92. Brummer THI, Jalkanen J, Fraser J, Heikkinine AM, Kauko M, Makinin J, et al. Prevention and management of surgical site infections in morbidly obese women. Hum Reprod. 2011;26:1741–51.
93. Uppal S, Harris J, Al-Niaimi A, Swenson CW, Pearlman MD, Reynolds RK, Kamdar N, Bazzi A, Campbell DA, Morgan DM. Prophylactic antibiotic choice and risk of surgical site infection after hysterectomy. Obstet Gynecol. 2016;127(2):321–9.
94. Mattox TF, Sanford EJ, Varner E. Infected abdominal sacrocolpopexies: diagnosis and treatment. Int Urogynecol J Pelvic Floor Dysfunct. 2004;15:319–23.
95. Baessler K, Hewson AD, Tunn R, Schuessler B, Maher CF. Severe mesh complications following intravaginal slingplasty. Obstet Gynecol. 2005;106:713–6.
96. Hiltunen R, Nieminen K, Takula T, Heiskanen E, Merikari M, Niemi KI, et al. Low-weight polypropylene mesh for anterior vaginal wall prolapse. Obstet Gynecol. 2007;110:455–62.
97. Vakili B, Huynh T, Loesch H, Franco N, Chesson RR. Outcomes of vaginal reconstructive surgery with and without graft material. Am J Obstet Gynecol. 2005;193:2126–32.
98. Lazenby GB, Soper DE. Prevention, diagnosis, and treatment of gynecologic surgical site infections. Obstet Gynecol Clin N Am. 2010;37:379–86.
99. Moir C, Robins ER. Role of ultrasonography, gallium scanning, and computed tomography in the diagnosis of intraabdominal abscess. Am J Surg. 1982;143:582–5.
100. Walters MD, Barber MD. Complications of hysterectomy. In: Karram M, editor. Hysterectomy for benign disease. Philadelphia: Saunders Elsevier; 2010. p. 195–212.
101. Levenson RB, Pearson KM, Saokar A, Lee SI, Mueller PR, Hahn PF. Image-guided drainage of tuboovarian abscesses of gastrointestinal or genitourinary origin: a retrospective analysis. J Vasc Interv Radiol. 2011;22(5):678–86.
102. Kjolhede P, Shefquet H, Lofgren M. Vaginal cleansing and postoperative infectious morbidity in vaginal hysterectomy. A register study from the Swedish National Register for Gynecological Surgery. Acta Obstet Gynecol Scand. 2011;90:63–71.
103. Kjolhede P, Shefqet H, Lofgren M. The influence of preoperative vaginal cleansing on postoperative infectious morbidity in abdominal total hysterectomy for benign indications. Acta Obstet Gynecol. 2009;88:408–16.
104. Bohrer JC, Walters M, Park A, Polston D, Barber MD. Pelvic nerve injury following gynecologic surgery: a prospective cohort study. Am J Obstet Gynecol. 2009;201(531):e1–7.
105. Romanowski L, Reich H, McGlynn F, Adelson MD, Taylor PJ. Brachial plexus neuropathies after advances laparoscopic surgery. Fertil Steril. 1993;60:729–32.
106. Warner MA, Warner DO, Harper CM, Schroeder DR, Maxon PM. Lower extremity neuropathies associated with lithotomy positions. Anesthesiology. 2000;93:938–42.
107. Britt BA, Gordon RA. Peripheral nerve injuries associated with anesthesia. Can Anaesth Soc J. 1964;11:514–36.
108. Shveiky D, Aseff JN, Iglesia CB. Brachial plexus injury after laparoscopic and robotic surgery. J Minim Invasive Gynecol. 2010;17:414–20.
109. Parks BJ. Postoperative peripheral neuropathies. Surgery. 1973;74:348–57.
110. Barnett JC, Hurd WW, Rogers RM, Williams NL, Shapiro SA. Laparoscopic positioning and nerve injuries. J Minim Invasive Gynecol. 2007;14:664–72.

5 Anterior Compartment Repair

Alana Murphy, Maria D'Amico, Courtney Capella, and Courtenay K. Moore

Introduction

The first true surgical anterior colporrhaphy was performed in 1866 by the controversial American gynecologist James Marion Sims [1]. Over the next 50 years, various techniques were used until transvaginal repair of anterior compartment prolapse was popularized by Kelly in the early twentieth century [2]. While this plication technique has generally fallen out of favor for the treatment of stress urinary incontinence (SUI), the same principles are utilized in contemporary anterior compartment repairs.

In addition to a traditional colporrhaphy, the role of various materials to augment anterior compartment repair continues to evolve. While several studies support superior anatomic results with mesh repairs, one must factor in the higher complication rates, the 2016 FDA ruling reclassifying transvaginal mesh kits for pelvic organ prolapse (POP) from a class II (moderate risk) to class III (high risk), and subsequent 2019 ban on all transvaginal mesh products for POP repair. This chapter will focus on complications associated with native tissue anterior repairs. The specific complications associated with the use of mesh in transvaginal surgery will be discussed in detail in another chapter.

Potential anterior compartment repair complications include intraoperative hemorrhage and blood transfusion, genitourinary tract injury, onset of de novo SUI, and postoperative urinary retention. Given the infrequent nature of these complications, there is a paucity of the literature focusing on intraoperative and immediate postoperative complications. In this regard, data on the immediate and shorter term complications must be extracted from studies that focus primarily on long-term anatomical and functional outcomes. Utilization of this data is further complicated by the inclusion of concomitant procedures. Women with high-grade anterior compartment prolapse may require a simultaneous vault procedure to adequately address all aspects of pelvic floor support. While these additional procedures often have complication profiles similar to anterior repairs, the complication rates are often higher. This chapter will focus on the complications and complication rates only for anterior repairs.

A. Murphy (✉) · M. D'Amico · C. Capella
Department of Urology, Thomas Jefferson University, Philadelphia, PA, USA
e-mail: alana.murphy@jefferson.edu; maria.damico@jefferson.edu; courtney.capella@jefferson.edu

C. K. Moore
The Ohio State University, Columbus, OH, USA
e-mail: Courtenay.moore@osumc.edu

H. B. Goldman, J. Zillioux (eds.), *Complications of Urogynecology and Reconstructive Pelvic Surgery*, https://doi.org/10.1007/978-3-032-00339-3_5

Injury to the Lower Urinary Tract

The incidence of lower urinary tract injuries varies based on the type of vaginal surgery, ranging from 0 to 19.5 per 1000 surgeries performed, with injuries occurring more commonly after reconstructive pelvic and incontinence surgery than other gynecological surgeries [3–5]. While injuries are uncommon, the consequences of unrecognized injuries can significantly increase patient morbidity.

Bladder Injuries

Bladder injury at the time of anterior colporrhaphy is very rare. Gilmour et al. conducted a systematic review of the literature from 1966 to 2004 and found that the rate of bladder injuries during urogynecologic surgery, excluding hysterectomies, varied from 12.1/1000 surgeries to 16.3/1000 surgeries when intraoperative cystoscopy was performed [3]. Of those studies that performed intraoperative cystoscopy, 95% of bladder injuries were diagnosed and corrected intraoperatively compared to a 43% detection rate when cystoscopy was not performed, underscoring the importance of intraoperative cystoscopy [4].

While the majority of studies on bladder injuries during urogynecological surgery include multiple concomitant procedures, several report on the rate of bladder injury after anterior colporrhaphy alone. In a study by Kwon et al. of 346 women who underwent traditional anterior colporrhaphy, there were no reported bladder injuries [6].

When comparing the rate of bladder injury between traditional anterior colporrhaphy and transvaginal mesh kits, two randomized controlled studies found there to be no difference in the rate of cystotomy, with Weber et al. reporting no injuries and Hiltunen reporting one in the mesh group [7, 8]. A 2011 randomized controlled study by Altman et al. found there to be a higher rate of cystotomy in the transvaginal mesh group versus traditional anterior colporrhaphy, 3.5% versus 0.5%. However, this did not reach statistical significance ($p = 0.07$) [9].

Immediate recognition of bladder injury during anterior compartment repairs is essential in reducing postoperative morbidity and potential fistula formation. As cited earlier, intraoperative cystoscopy increases the rate of intraoperative diagnosis and repair. If an intraoperative cystotomy is detected, the injury should be closed in two layers with absorbable sutures. Should the injury be missed, depending on the duration of postoperative catheter drainage and the extent of the injury, the patient is at risk for developing a vesicovaginal fistula requiring either prolonged catheter drainage or a vesicovaginal fistula repair.

Ureteral Injuries

Ureteral injuries occur infrequently after routine gynecological procedures (0.5–1.5%), with patients undergoing complex reconstructive procedures for pelvic organ prolapse at an increased risk of ureteral injury [10]. Like bladder injuries, the incidence of ureteral injuries varies depending on the type of urogynecologic surgery, ranging from 2% to 11% [4, 11]. Women with pelvic organ prolapse are at an increased risk of ureteric injury given the anatomic distortion caused by the prolapse itself, with 12–20% of women with symptomatic pelvic organ prolapse having moderate to severe hydronephrosis secondary to chronic obstruction from ureteral kinking [11].

The majority of the studies on ureteral injuries during gynecologic surgery do not separate the rate of injury by procedure. However, a study by Kwon et al. looked at the incidence of ureteral injury after anterior colporrhaphy alone [6]. Of the 346 procedures performed, there were seven reported ureteral injuries (2.0%). There was no comment on the POP-Q staging of the women with ureteral injuries. All injuries were recognized at the time of surgery. Additionally, a retrospective review of 700 patients undergoing anterior vaginal prolapse and/or apical suspension looked at rates of ureteral obstruction with universal cystoscopy [12]. In the anterior colporrhaphy alone cohort, they identified a rate of 0.4% ($n = 574$), which was alleviated by suture removal. In their entire study, they identified a positive predictive value for universal intraoperative cystoscopy of 99.3%.

Intraoperative Diagnosis

If a ureteral injury does occur, the ability to identify the injury at the time of the initial operation is paramount to avoid the permanent damage associated with unrecognized injuries. The single most controllable factor adversely affecting the outcome of ureteral injuries is delayed diagnosis. Studies have shown that intraoperative recognition and repair of ureteral injuries decreases postoperative morbidity, minimizes loss of renal function and need for nephrectomy. Early recognition also decreases the incidence of ureterovaginal fistulas as compared to postoperative diagnosis with delayed repair [13].

If a ureteral injury is suspected during abdominal surgery, direct inspection of the ureter is recommended. However, during vaginal surgery, direct visualization of the ureter is usually not feasible. Therefore, intraoperative cystoscopy has been recommended as a means to identify ureteral injuries during vaginal surgery while obviating the need for an abdominal incision. If efflux is unable to be visualized, adjunctive agents can be used. Historically, intravenous indigo carmine was utilized but it is no longer commercially available since 2014 [14]. Intravenous methylene blue dye has a risk of methemoglobinemia or serotonin syndrome in certain patient populations. Oral phenazopyridine and intravenous sodium fluorescein are additional agents that can be used, although contingent on renal function [14]. By patiently observing and comparing to the opposite ureter, one may detect subtle sluggish flow, which may suggest partial obstruction.

If fluoroscopy is available, another method of assessing ureteral patency is retrograde ureterography. If fluoroscopy is not available, a one-shot excretory urogram can be obtained 10 min after the administration of intravenous contrast material (one mL/pound of body weight). Fluoroscopically, ureteral injuries present as urinary extravasation or high-grade obstruction.

Delayed Diagnosis

Most ureteral injuries are unsuspected and diagnosed postoperatively [15]. In a study by Meirow et al., the mean delay to diagnosis of patients sustaining ureteral injuries after gynecologic surgery was 5.6 days [16]. Undiagnosed ureteral injuries are associated with significant morbidity, the formation of ureterovaginal fistulas, and potential loss of renal function [17]. The majority of patients present with fever, flank pain, continuous incontinence, pyelonephritis, ileus, peritonitis, or anuria. However, 5% of patients remain asymptomatic and are diagnosed at a later date secondary to a nonfunctioning or hydronephrotic kidney [15]. Delayed diagnosis is most often (66–76%) made by CT pyelography, excretory urography, or retrograde ureterography [18].

Immediate Intraoperative Management

The management of ureteral injuries depends on the time of diagnosis, location, nature, and extent of the injury. Injuries recognized intraoperatively must be treated immediately. Inadvertent ligation or kinking of the ureter should be treated by suture removal and repeat cystoscopy to ensure ureteral efflux. Typically, if recognized immediately, ureteric damage is minimal as these injuries include other tissue in the ligature [13]. If the extent of the ureteral injury is in question, at minimum, ureteral stent placement is warranted [13]. For more severe injuries, when ureteral viability is unlikely, exploration and direct visualization of the ureter is recommended [19]. The involved ureter should be primarily repaired or resected, debrided, and re-anastomosed over a stent. If the diagnosis of an intraoperative ureteral injury is made during retrograde ureterography, an attempt at retrograde stent placement should be made.

Delayed Management

The type of repair and the timing of delayed-recognition injury repair are controversial. Postoperatively noted suture entrapment can be managed conservatively with immediate attempt at placement of a double-J ureteral stent or nephrostomy tube drainage if the suture is absorbable [20]. However, placement is only possible in 20–50% of patients [18]. In a study by Ghali, only two of 21 (19%) iatrogenic ureteral injuries identified postoperatively were able to be stented [18]. When stent placement is possible, as many as 73% of patients will not require surgical repair.

If the diagnosis is delayed, the traditional recommendation is that repair of iatrogenic ureteral injuries after urogynecologic surgery should not be undertaken for three to six months [21]. However, more recent studies suggest similar outcomes after immediate and delayed repairs [21]. Given that most injuries after vaginal surgery occur to the distal one-third of the ureter, intervention often involves ureteral reimplantation or ureteroneocystostomy. Ureteroneocystostomy is used to repair distal ureteral injuries close to the bladder or in the intramural tunnel.

Hemorrhage

Hemorrhage is a rare complication of anterior compartment repair. During a traditional suture plication repair, proper dissection between the vaginal epithelium and the underlying vaginal muscularis (or the controversially named pubocervical fascia) will minimize blood loss and reduce the risk of postoperative hemorrhage. Judicious use of electrocautery during the anterior vaginal wall dissection can also be used to maintain hemostasis. A randomized controlled trial (RCT) by Altman and colleagues included 389 women who underwent isolated anterior compartment repair [9]. Women with stage >2 prolapse were randomized to a repair using trocar-guided transvaginal mesh (n = 200) or a traditional colporrhaphy (n = 189). The two treatment groups did not differ significantly in terms of POP-Q stage or previous anterior compartment repairs. The traditional colporrhaphy group had a significantly lower mean estimated blood loss (EBL) (35.4 ± 35.4 mL) compared to the trocar-guided transvaginal mesh group (84.7 ± 163.5 mL, $p < 0.001$). The study reported five cases (1.3%) of clinically significant intraoperative blood loss, with all five patients having undergone trocar-guided transvaginal mesh placement: four patients (1.0%) had an EBL greater than 500 mL and one patient (0.3%) had an EBL greater than 1000 mL and a subsequent retropubic hematoma. The authors did not provide data on transfusion rates. Due to its focus on anterior compartment repairs without concomitant pelvic floor procedures, the Altman study is a valuable addition to the limited body of literature that addresses the complications of isolated anterior compartment repairs.

Studies that included concomitant pelvic floor procedures also provide data regarding the low incidence of hemorrhage associated with anterior compartment repair [8, 22–24]. Weber and colleagues performed the very first randomized study of anterior compartment repairs, comparing standard placation, plication with mesh, and ultra-lateral anterior colporrhaphy [7]. Subjects were excluded if they underwent an anti-incontinence procedure other than a suburethral plication. Subjects undergoing additional procedures for prolapse were included. Of the 109 women undergoing anterior compartment repair with concomitant pelvic floor procedures, one patient (0.9%) in the standard anterior colporrhaphy group required transfusion.

An RCT by Hiltunen and colleagues, comparing anterior colporrhaphy with and without tailored mesh, included 201 women with pelvic organ prolapse [8]. Subjects were excluded from the study if they had gynecologic malignancies, apical prolapse mandating apical fixation, SUI, or if their main symptomatic compartment was the posterior vaginal wall. Women could be included if they underwent concomitant vaginal hysterectomy, reduction of an enterocele, culdoplasty, or posterior colporrhaphy without mesh. Women were randomized to traditional anterior compartment repair (n = 97) or anterior compartment repair reinforced with mesh (n = 104). A total of 29 patients (14%) underwent an isolated anterior compartment repair with no concomitant procedure. There was no difference in rates of previous vaginal surgery or concomitant hysterectomy between groups. All patients had vaginal packing in place for 20 h postoperatively. Although the mean EBL in the traditional repair group (114 ± 109 mL) was less than the mean EBL in the mesh group (190 ± 23 mL), the difference was not statistically significant. There was no statistically significant difference in clinically significant blood loss (EBL >400 mL) between the groups (3.1% vs 9.6%, $p = 0.07$). Two patients in total (1.0%), though not specified in what group, required blood transfusions. In a more recent retrospective cohort study using data from the ACS-NSQIP database between 2010 and 2017, Darvish et al. identified a postoperative transfusion rate of 0.9% (10/1164 patients) for those undergoing anterior colporrhaphy (without graft) [25]. Patients in the study underwent anterior colporrhaphy with or without use of a graft, and with or without concomitant procedures including vaginal hysterectomy, apical suspensions, and slings. Those undergoing posterior colporrhaphy were excluded.

Careful attention should be paid during dissection of the anterior vaginal wall and muscularis to minimize blood loss. Hemostasis can typically be attained using electrocautery. If electrocautery is insufficient, a figure-of-eight stitch with a 2–0 or 3–0 Vicryl suture can be used to over-sew a small vessel. When closing the anterior vaginal wall incision, great care should be taken to achieve a secure closure. A tight closure can provide an additional degree of hemostasis by allowing tamponade within the closed anterior compartment.

The low incidence of clinically significant blood loss affects our routine postoperative care pathway. Given that hemorrhage is a rare complication of anterior compartment repair, our practice is not to obtain routine postoperative lab work. A vaginal pack can be placed at the completion of the anterior compartment repair and removed after one hour in the recovery room. If the patient is admitted for observation, then the vaginal packing can be removed in the early morning of the first postoperative day. Vaginal packs are sometimes used as a means to reduce postoperative hemorrhage, despite the lack of evidence in the literature. An RCT from Thiagamoorthy and colleagues assessed the effect of vaginal packing after a vaginal hysterectomy and/or pelvic floor repair [26]. Women were randomized to receive a vaginal pack ($n = 86$) or no vaginal pack ($n = 87$). A total of five patients were withdrawn from the no packing group due to intraoperative bleeding. The study demonstrated no significant difference in mean postoperative hemoglobin on the first postoperative day (11.75 g/dL vs 11.94 g/dL, $p = 0.061$) and six weeks postoperatively (12.55 g/dL vs 12.49 g/dL, $p = 0.884$) between the packing and the no packing group. Although the packing group had less postoperative hematomas ($n = 4$) compared to the no packing group ($n = 9$), the difference was not significant ($p = 0.098$). Despite the lack of statistical significance, all three clinically significant complications related to bleeding were in the no-packing group. One patient returned to the operating room from the recovery room for hemorrhage and two patients required repeat admission for intravenous antibiotics to treat an infected pelvic hematoma.

A more recent systematic review by Porta-Roda et al. that included 4 clinical trials and 337 participants provided no clear evidence that vaginal packing led to clinically meaningful reductions in adverse effects, including vaginal bleeding, hematoma formation, or postoperative vaginal cuff infection [27].

Hemorrhage recognized in the postoperative setting is rare after an anterior compartment repair. If a patient demonstrates a clinical sign of hemorrhage, such as significant transvaginal bleeding or tachycardia, a vaginal packing should be placed, vital signs closely monitored, and serial hematologic profiles checked until stable values are achieved. As demonstrated in the previously discussed studies, less than 1% of patients will require a transfusion after an anterior compartment repair. In cases of severe hemorrhage that are not responsive to transfusion or are associated with significant hemodynamic instability, angiography with selective embolization should be utilized to control the hemorrhage.

De novo Stress Urinary Incontinence

De novo SUI should be included in the preoperative discussion of potential postoperative complications with greater emphasis in patients with high-grade anterior compartment prolapse. Women with severe anterior compartment prolapse may not experience SUI due to urethral kinking, and SUI may not be detected by the patient or the physician until the prolapse is reduced or surgically repaired [28]. According to the International Continence Society (ICS), SUI with prolapse reduction (or occult SUI) is defined as SUI observed only after the reduction of coexistent prolapse [29]. Once any degree of urethral kinking is relieved with reduction of the anterior compartment prolapse, the mechanism of de novo SUI is likely multifactorial and may include urethral hyper-suspension or intraoperative damage to the sphincter [30]. In addition to intraoperative factors, reduction of anterior compartment prolapse may unmask compromised periurethral support or frank intrinsic sphincter deficiency [31]. In order to minimize the risk of developing de novo SUI, each patient without subjective and/or objective evidence of SUI should be assessed for SUI with prolapse reduction before undergoing anterior compartment repair for high-stage prolapse.

Proper assessment of SUI with prolapse reduction requires adequate reduction of the patient's anterior compartment prolapse. In the office setting, our practice is to perform a stress test after the anterior prolapse is reduced with half of a speculum. If SUI is not demonstrated in the office, the patient is then referred for urodynamic evaluation with prolapse reduction. The most common techniques for prolapse reduction include a vaginal pack, a pessary, and a speculum. No general consensus exists regarding the best method for prolapse reduction. A study conducted by Mattox and Bhatia demonstrated no difference in maximal urethral closure pressure whether a Smith-Hodge pessary, a ring pessary, or half of a Graves speculum was used for prolapse reduction [32]. Visco and colleagues found that rates of SUI with prolapse reduction differed based on the method of prolapse reduction, which included a pessary, manual reduction, a forceps, a swab, and a speculum [33]. When interpreting urodynamic results, it is important to remember that each method of prolapse reduction may partially obstruct the urethra and lead to a false-negative SUI assessment.

A recent meta-analysis by Oliveira and colleagues studied the risk factors for women undergoing surgery for POP. Associations were identified between de novo stress urinary incontinence and occult urinary incontinence ($p = 0.004$), diabetes ($p = 0.005$), and advanced pelvic organ prolapse ($p = 0.01$) [34].

Controversy continues to surround the management of women with either isolated SUI with prolapse reduction or no evidence of subjective or objective SUI with prolapse reduction. Should these women undergo a concomitant anti-incontinence procedure at the time of anterior compartment repair?

A study done by Chaikin and colleagues on 24 stress continent women with stage III or IV POP found 14 patients (58.3%) to have SUI with prolapse reduction on preoperative urodynamics and subsequently underwent pubovaginal sling placement with concomitant anterior compartment repair [35]. The remaining 10 patients (41.7%) had no SUI with prolapse reduction and underwent isolated anterior compartment repair. Two of the patients (14%) in the pubovaginal sling group had persistent postoperative SUI, while no patient in the group without occult SUI developed de novo SUI at a mean follow-up of 44 months.

Liang and colleagues reported on 79 stress continent women with stage III or IV POP [36]. The patients were divided into three treatment groups based on the presence or absence of SUI with prolapse reduction on preoperative urodynamics. In group I, 32 patients with SUI with prolapse reduction underwent total vaginal hysterectomy (TVH), anterior/posterior (AP) repair, and a mid-urethral sling (MUS). In group IIa, 17 patients with SUI with prolapse reduction underwent TVH and AP repair with no anti-incontinence procedure. In group IIb, 30 patients without SUI with prolapse reduction underwent

TVH and AP repair with no anti-incontinence procedure. Postoperatively, group I had three patients (9.4%) with subjective SUI and zero patients with objective SUI. Group IIa had 11 patients (64.7%) with subjective SUI and 9 patients (52.9%) with objective SUI on repeat urodynamics. Group IIb had three patients (10.0%) with subjective SUI and zero patients with objective SUI. The data presented by both Chitin and colleagues and Liang and colleagues suggest that the rate of de novo SUI is low in women with no SUI with prolapse reduction, while women with SUI with prolapse reduction appear to benefit from a concomitant anti-incontinence procedure.

The Colpopexy and Urinary Reduction Efforts (CARE) trial addressed the role of an anti-incontinence procedure at the time of POP repair [37]. A total of 322 women with stage II or greater POP were randomized to abdominal sacrocolpopexy with Burch colposuspension (n = 157) or abdominal sacrocolpopexy alone (control group, n = 165). All women were considered stress continent if they answered "rarely" or "never" to six questions regarding SUI on the Medical, Epidemiological, and Social Aspects of Aging (MESA) questionnaire, irrespective of preoperative urodynamics results. Three months postoperatively, 23.8% of patients in the Burch group and 44.1% of patients in the control group ($p < 0.001$) reported some degree of SUI. When patients with SUI with prolapse reduction were excluded, de novo SUI was reduced from 38.2% to 20.8% in the control group versus the Burch group ($p = 0.007$). A two-year update of the CARE trial reported that the reduction in de novo SUI was durable, with 32.0% of the Burch group and 45.2% of the control group meeting one or more criteria for SUI [38]. The CARE study also supports the utility of preoperative urodynamic testing in reportedly stress continent women as a valuable tool to enhance preoperative counseling and planning. Examination of the preoperative urodynamic results revealed that 3.7% of women demonstrated urodynamic SUI without prolapse reduction, and 6–30% of women demonstrated SUI when their prolapse was reduced (the range of SUI with prolapse reduction rates reflects the use of various methods for reducing prolapse). Regardless of whether or not they underwent Burch colposuspension, patients who demonstrated SUI with prolapse reduction were more likely to have postoperative SUI compared to women without SUI with prolapse reduction (Burch 32% vs 21% [$p = 0.19$], controls 58% vs 38% [$p = 0.04$]) [33]. Widespread application of the lessons learned in the CARE trial is limited by the use of the Burch procedure as the anti-incontinence procedure.

The Outcomes Following Vaginal Prolapse Repair and Midurethral Sling (OPUS) trial randomly assigned women undergoing vaginal correction of stage 2 or higher anterior prolapse without symptoms of stress incontinence to receive either a mid-urethral sling or sham incisions during surgery [39]. At 3 months, the rate of urinary incontinence was 23.6% in the sling group and 49.4% in the sham group ($p < 0.001$). At 12 months, urinary incontinence was present in 27.3% and 43.0% of patients in the sling and sham groups, respectively ($p = 0.002$). The number of patients required to treat with a sling to prevent one case of SUI at 12 months was 6.3. While sling placement at the time of vaginal surgery for stage 2 or higher POP resulted in lower rates of SUI, it did result in a higher adverse events rate (bladder perforations, urinary tract infection, major bleeding, and incomplete emptying).

Our preference is to perform a concomitant anti-incontinence procedure in patients who demonstrate SUI preoperatively on physical exam, during preoperative pessary use, or during UDS. Since an anterior compartment repair alters the axis of the anterior vaginal wall and may affect the urethral axis, our practice is to perform an anti-incontinence procedure after the anterior compartment repair. If de novo SUI occurs in previously stressed continent women after anterior compartment repair, we perform an anti-incontinence procedure at a later date.

Iatrogenic Bladder Outlet Obstruction (BOO)/Urinary Retention

Postoperative voiding dysfunction and urinary retention rates following pelvic reconstructive surgery range from 2.5% to 24% with the vast majority of patients undergoing concomitant anterior, posterior, and apical prolapse repairs [40]. Unlike anti-incontinence procedures, very few studies have examined risk factors for iatrogenic BOO after an isolated anterior colporrhaphy.

Hakvoort et al. conducted a retrospective study looking at predictors of short-term urinary retention, defined as a post-void residual (PVR) urine volume > 200 mL, after vaginal prolapse surgery in 345 women [41]. Patients were excluded if they underwent a colpocleisis, sacrocolpopexy, or had undergone a prior anti-incontinence procedure. Of the 345 patients, transient urinary retention occurred in 100 patients (29%). Catheterization was required after 72 hours in 30 patients (8.7%) and after six days in four patients (1.1%). In this study population, postoperative urinary retention was temporary, with all patients voiding spontaneously with a PVR volume < 200 mL by two months after surgery. Intraoperative blood loss exceeding 100 mL, high-stage anterior prolapse (grade ≥ 3 cystocele), and levator or Kelly plication were independent risk factors for postoperative urinary retention.

Wang et al. conducted a retrospective cohort study of 294 women undergoing POP repair without an anti-incontinence procedure. A total of 49 women (16.7%) failed their postoperative voiding trial. The women who failed postoperative voiding trials were more likely to have undergone an anterior colporrhaphy ($p = 0.001$) and more likely to have had an elevated preoperative PVR volume (≥150 ml) ($p = 0.001$) [42].

Fernandez-Gonzalez et al. randomized patients undergoing anterior colporrhaphy with native tissue, with or without posterior repair, to catheter removal after either 24 h or 48 h postoperatively [43]. They excluded patients with SUI who had undergone concomitant anti-incontinence procedure, those undergoing concomitant apical compartment surgery, and those with voiding dysfunction on preoperative urodynamics. They defined a successful void trial as a PVR <100 ml, and if PVR was less than the volume of micturition, they measured a second PVR. There were 37 patients in the 48-hour protocol and 40 patients in the 24-hour protocol, and they detected no differences in postoperative urinary retention: three patients (8.1%) in the 48-hour group vs one patient (2.5%) in the 24-hour group ($p = 0.346$).

Due to the risk of postoperative voiding dysfunction and urinary retention, all patients undergoing an anterior colporrhaphy should undergo assessment of their voiding function prior to discharge. This voiding assessment is typically a combination of PVR measurement and assessment of a patient's symptoms. If a patient is found to have postoperative urinary retention, mechanical bladder drainage with either an indwelling catheter or intermittent catheterization is required until normal voiding function is achieved. Although there is no robust data to support a postoperative protocol to minimize urinary retention following an anterior colporrhaphy, general recommendations include early ambulation, avoidance or minimization of constipation, and limitation of postoperative narcotic analgesia.

Summary

While complications during anterior compartment repairs are rare, they do occur. Attention to detail and an in-depth knowledge of pelvic anatomy can reduce the risk of complications and potential patient morbidity.

References

1. Lensen EJ, Withagen MR, Kluivers KB, et al. Surgical treatment of pelvic organ prolapse: a historical review with emphasis on the anterior compartment. Int Urogynecol J. 2013;24(10):1593–602.
2. Kelly HA. Incontinence of urine in women. Urol Cutan Rev. 1913;XVII:291–3.

3. Gilmour DT, Das S, Flowerdew G. Rates of urinary tract injury from gynecologic surgery and the role of intraoperative cystoscopy. Obstet Gynecol. 2006;107:1366–72.
4. Barber MD, Visco AG, Weidner AC, et al. Bilateral uterosacral ligament vaginal vault suspension with site-specific endopelvic fascia defect repair for treatment of pelvic organ prolapse. Am J Obstet Gynecol. 2000;183:1402–10; discussion 1410-1.
5. Harris RL, Cundiff GW, Theofrastous JP, et al. The value of intraoperative cystoscopy in urogynecologic and reconstructive pelvic surgery. Am J Obstet Gynecol. 1997;177:1367-9; discussion 1369–71.
6. Kwon CH, Goldberg RP, Koduri S, et al. The use of intraoperative cystoscopy in major vaginal and urogynecologic surgeries. Am J Obstet Gynecol. 2002;187:1466–71; discussion 1471-2.
7. Weber AM, Walters MD, Piedmonte MR, et al. Anterior colporrhaphy: a randomized trial of three surgical techniques. Am J Obstet Gynecol 2001;185:1299–304; discussion 1304-6.
8. Hiltunen R, Nieminen K, Takala T, et al. Low-weight polypropylene mesh for anterior vaginal wall prolapse: a randomized controlled trial. Obstet Gynecol. 2007;110:455–62.
9. Altman D, Vayrynen T, Engh ME, et al. Anterior colporrhaphy versus transvaginal mesh for pelvic-organ prolapse. N Engl J Med. 2011;364:1826–36.
10. Liapis A, Bakas P, Giannopoulos V et al: Ureteral injuries during gynecological surgery. Int Urogynecol J Pelvic Floor Dysfunct. 2001;12:391–3; discussion 394.
11. Handa VL, Maddox MD. Diagnosis of ureteral obstruction during complex urogynecologic surgery. Int Urogynecol J Pelvic Floor Dysfunct. 2001;12:345–8.
12. Gustilo-Ashby AM, Jelovsek JE, Barber MD, et al. The incidence of ureteral obstruction and the value of intraoperative cystoscopy during vaginal surgery for pelvic organ prolapse. Am J Obstet Gynecol. 2006;194(5):1478–85.
13. Brandes S, Coburn M, Armenakas N, et al. Diagnosis and management of ureteric injury: an evidence-based analysis. BJU Int. 2004;94:277–89.
14. Cohen SA, Carberry CL, Smilen SW. American Urogynecologic Society consensus statement: cystoscopy at the time of prolapse repair. Female Pelvic Med Reconstr Surg. 2018;24(4):258–9.
15. Visco AG, Taber KH, Weidner AC, et al. Cost-effectiveness of universal cystoscopy to identify ureteral injury at hysterectomy. Obstet Gynecol. 2001;97:685–92.
16. Meirow D, Moriel EZ, Zilberman M, et al. Evaluation and treatment of iatrogenic ureteral injuries during obstetric and gynecologic operations for nonmalignant conditions. J Am Coll Surg. 1994;178:144–8.
17. Rafique M, Arif MH. Management of iatrogenic ureteric injuries associated with gynecological surgery. Int Urol Nephrol. 2002;34:31–5.
18. Ghali AM, El Malik EM, Ibrahim AI, et al. Ureteric injuries: diagnosis, management, and outcome. J Trauma. 1999;46:150–8.
19. Assimos DG, Patterson LC, Taylor CL. Changing incidence and etiology of iatrogenic ureteral injuries. J Urol. 1994;152:2240–6.
20. Harshman MW, Pollack HM, Banner MP, et al. Conservative management of ureteral obstruction secondary to suture entrapment. J Urol. 1982;127:121–3.
21. Ku JH, Kim ME, Jeon YS, et al. Minimally invasive management of ureteral injuries recognized late after obstetric and gynaecologic surgery. Injury. 2003;34:480–3.
22. Iglesia CB, Sokol AI, Sokol ER, et al. Vaginal mesh for prolapse: a randomized controlled trial. Obstet Gynecol. 2010;116:293–303.
23. Feldner PC Jr, Castro RA, Cipolotti LA, et al. Anterior vaginal wall prolapse: a randomized controlled trial of SIS graft versus traditional colporrhaphy. Int Urogynecol J Pelvic Floor Dysfunct. 2010;21:1057–63.
24. Moore RD, Miklos JR. Vaginal repair of cystocele with anterior wall mesh via transobturator route: efficacy and complications with up to 3-year followup. Adv Urol. 2009;743831.
25. Darvish R, Davenport A, Dao A, et al. Evaluation of 30-day complication rates following vaginal anterior compartment repair with and without graft augmentation in a propensity score matched cohort. World J Urol. 2021;39(6):2191–6.
26. Thiagamoorthy G, Khalil A, Cardozo L, Srikrishna S, Leslie G, Robinson D. The value of vaginal packing in pelvic floor surgery: a randomised double-blind study. Int Urogynecol J. 2014;25(5):585–91.
27. Porta-Roda O, Cornet-Cortada A, Font-Vilamitjana A, Huguet-Galofré E, Lleberia-Juanós J, Solà-Arnau I. Vaginal packing after vaginal hysterectomy: systematic review and recommendations. Int Urogynecol J. 2023;34(4):789–96. https://doi.org/10.1007/s00192-022-05331-1.
28. Bump RC, Fantl JA, Hurt WG. The mechanism of urinary continence in women with severe uterovaginal prolapse: results of barrier studies. Obstet Gynecol. 1988;72:291–5.
29. Haylen BT, de Ridder D, Freeman RM, et al. An International Urogynecological Association (IUGA)/International Continence Society (ICS) joint report on the terminology for female pelvic floor dysfunction. Neurourol Urodyn. 2010;29:4–20.
30. Zivkovic F, Tamussino K, Ralph G, et al. Long-term effects of vaginal dissection on the innervation of the striated urethral sphincter. Obstet Gynecol. 1996;87:257–60.
31. Goepel C, Hefler L, Methfessel HD, et al. Periurethral connective tissue status of postmenopausal women with genital prolapse with and without stress incontinence. Acta Obstet Gynecol Scand. 2003;82:659–64.

32. Mattox TF, Bhatia NN. Urodynamic effects of reducing devices in women with genital prolapse. Int Urogynecol J. 1994;5:283.
33. Visco AG, Brubaker L, Nygaard I, et al. The role of preoperative urodynamic testing in stress-continent women undergoing sacrocolpopexy: the Colpopexy and Urinary Reduction Efforts (CARE) randomized surgical trial. Int Urogynecol J Pelvic Floor Dysfunct. 2008;19:607–14.
34. Oliveira IKB, Calisto SLS, Ferreira CWS, et al. Occult urinary incontinence, diabetes, obesity, prolapse severity, and type of surgical repair as risk factors for de novo stress urinary incontinence in women undergoing surgery repair of pelvic organ prolapse: a systematic review and meta-analysis. Neurourol Urodyn. 2025;44(1):194–206.
35. Chaikin DC, Groutz A, Blaivas JG. Predicting the need for anti-incontinence surgery in continent women undergoing repair of severe urogenital prolapse. J Urol. 2000;163:531–4.
36. Liang CC, Chang YL, Chang SD, Lo TS, Soong YK. Pessary test to predict postoperative urinary incontinence in women undergoing hysterectomy for prolapse. Obstet Gynecol. 2004;104(4):795–800.
37. Brubaker L, Cundiff GW, Fine P, et al. Abdominal sacrocolpopexy with Burch colposuspension to reduce urinary stress incontinence. N Engl J Med. 2006;354:1557–66.
38. Brubaker L, Nygaard I, Richter HE, et al. Two-year outcomes after sacrocolpopexy with and without burch to prevent stress urinary incontinence [published correction appears in Obstet Gynecol. 2016;127(5):968–9. doi: 10.1097/AOG.0000000000001428.]. Obstet Gynecol. 2008;112(1):49–55.
39. Wei JT, Nygaard I, Richter H, et al. A midurethral sling to reduce incontinence after vaginal prolapse repair. NEMJ. 2012;366(25):2358–67.
40. Geller EJ. Prevention and management of postoperative urinary retention after urogynecologic surgery. Int J Women's Health. 2014;6:829–38.
41. Hakvoort RA, Dijkgraaf MG, Burger MP, et al. Predicting short-term urinary retention after vaginal prolapse surgery. Neurourol Urodyn. 2009;28(3):225–8.
42. Wang R, Won S, Haviland MJ, et al. Voiding trial outcome following pelvic floor repair without incontinence procedures. Int Urogynecol J. 2016; Epub ahead of print.
43. Fernandez-Gonzalez S, Martinez Franco E, Martínez-Cumplido R, et al. Reducing postoperative catheterisation after anterior colporrhaphy from 48 to 24 h: a randomised controlled trial. Int Urogynecol J. 2019;30(11):1897–902.

Rectocele Repair

6

Rahul Dutta, Benjamin Brucker, Alice Drain, and Victor W. Nitti

Introduction

Pelvic organ prolapse of the posterior compartment is a herniation of the posterior vaginal wall or anterior rectal wall into the lumen of the vagina. Defects in the posterior compartment may result from nerve (i.e., pudendal nerve) damage or disruption of connective tissue and muscular attachments [1]. Many factors, including childbirth, aging, estrogen deficiency, chronic abdominal straining (usually from constipation [2]), and heavy physical labor, weaken the pelvic floor and its associated support structures. There are also genetic factors that predispose women to this condition. Childbirth, one of the most associated factors contributing to posterior compartment defects, can cause stretching of the prerectal and pararectal fascia with detachment of the prerectal fascia from the perineal body. This allows for the formation of a rectocele in a dose-dependent fashion [3]. In addition, childbirth damages and weakens the levator musculature and its fascia, attenuating the decussating prerectal levator fibers and the attachment of the levator ani to the central tendon of the perineum. The result is a convex sagging of the levator plate with a loss of the normal, horizontal vaginal axis. The vagina becomes rotated downward and posteriorly, no longer providing horizontal support. These anatomic changes allow downward herniation of the pelvic organs along the new vaginal axis.

Posterior compartment prolapse is not uncommon. A cross-sectional study (Women's Health Initiative Hormone Replacement Therapy Clinical Trial) found that 18.6% of 16,616 women with a uterus had a rectocele on a baseline pelvic examination and 18.3% of 10,727 women who had undergone hysterectomy had a rectocele [4]. Rates of anterior prolapse (cystocele) were higher in both groups at 34.3% and 32.9%, respectively. Isolated posterior compartment defects are more uncommon and are seen most often in women after severe posterior tears associated with vaginal delivery or in women who have previously undergone correction of the anterior or apical compartment. More frequently, posterior

R. Dutta
Fellow, Urogynecology and Pelvic Reconstructive Surgery, Departments of Urology and Obstetrics and Gynecology, David Geffen School of Medicine at the University of California, Los Angeles, CA, USA

B. Brucker
Department of Urology, New York University Langone Medical Center, New York, NY, USA

A. Drain
Department of Urology, Rutgers University, Robert Wood Johnson Barnabas Health Medical Group, New Brunswick, NJ, USA

V. W. Nitti (✉)
Shlomo Raz Chair in Urology, Division of URPS, David Geffen School of Medicine at the University of California Los Angeles, Los Angeles, CA, USA
e-mail: VNitti@mednet.ucla.edu

H. B. Goldman, J. Zillioux (eds.), *Complications of Urogynecology and Reconstructive Pelvic Surgery*, https://doi.org/10.1007/978-3-032-00339-3_6

compartment defects are associated with more global pelvic floor dysfunction and vaginal prolapse. Management should also consider the role the posterior plate and the genital hiatus may play in preventing recurrent pelvic organ prolapse and restoring sexual function.

Up to 80% of rectoceles seen on physical examination are asymptomatic [5]. In cases of asymptomatic isolated rectoceles, or small rectoceles, with concomitant anterior and/or apical prolapse, surgical intervention should be approached cautiously because of the potential complications that will be discussed later. However, when rectoceles are symptomatic, surgical correction is an option. Symptoms associated with rectocele include constipation, incomplete rectal emptying, rectal pressure, and vaginal bulge [6]. Some patients will also describe stool being trapped in the rectocele pocket and the need to apply perineal or vaginal pressure (splinting) to facilitate defecation.

Nonsurgical Therapies

Although it is not the intent of this chapter to discuss the evidence behind alternative therapies, these must be considered when trying to avoid surgical complications.

Observation, or watchful waiting, may be appropriate if the patient has little bother or only minor symptoms from her posterior compartment laxity. A support device such as a pessary can also be considered in a woman with symptoms from pelvic organ prolapse. In the authors' experience, posterior compartment prolapse symptoms can be difficult to treat with these devices. However, if the decision is made to trial a pessary, the process of fitting a pessary in a woman with posterior compartment predominant prolapse should not be any more difficult than fitting women with anterior or apical prolapse [7]. If a woman derives symptomatic improvement, she can be taught how to remove and clean the pessary, or it can be changed on a regular basis in a physician's office. In either case, routine examination is necessary to ensure that there is no unwanted irritation or granulation tissue development. Topical vaginal estrogen can also help prevent these pessary-related complications.

Pelvic floor muscle rehabilitation can also be considered as a therapy for posterior compartment prolapse. There is a paucity of data to support its use in preventing progression or improvement of rectocele-specific symptoms. However, rectoceles are often not isolated findings. The pelvic floor disorders that may coexist may be effectively addressed with nonsurgical options. For example, pelvic floor exercises are useful in the treatment of stress urinary incontinence. Women with concomitant disorders of the pelvic floor may favor the nonsurgical route for the treatment of the rectocele because of the improvement in the symptoms of other conditions.

In summary, nonsurgical therapies should be discussed with patients in most cases. Given the favorable side effect profile, there is no great downside to attempting these therapies if a woman so desires. They can be used if they help correct the bothersome symptoms. Nonsurgical options are also important in counseling patients who are poor surgical candidates secondary to medical comorbidities.

Surgical Approaches

Rectocele repairs can be approached via the abdominal, transvaginal, and transanal approaches. Urogynecologists and pelvic reconstructive surgeons most often perform the repair transvaginally [1]. There is no definitive evidence that suggests which surgical approach is best. Based on three randomized controlled trials comparing transvaginal and transanal repair, one analysis concluded that the transvaginal approach has superior subjective and objective outcomes compared to the transanal approach [8]. In contrast, a later literature review comparing the transvaginal to the transanal approach found that there was no significant difference in outcomes [9]. Surgeon's skill, patient's desires, anatomic, and functional outcomes are all important to consider. As importantly, the potential unwanted outcomes, or complications, must be considered. As we are considering potential complications, which vary based on each different surgical approach, some relative indications for the route of repair that is selected should be considered.

The abdominal approach may be indicated in cases where a rectal prolapse is concomitantly noted. The abdominal approach has also become more popular with the widespread use of robotic-assisted laparoscopic surgical platforms. This has led to more publications describing the abdominal approach for rectocele repair [10, 11]. In cases of apical prolapse with a large rectocele, the posterior leaf of the sacrocolpopexy mesh can be extended, even all the way to the perineal body. Patients are often selected for an abdominal repair (i.e., robotic-assisted laparoscopic sacrocolpopexy) because of a predominance of apical descent. This should be remembered when reviewing the literature of nonrandomized patients. The studies may include women with some degree of posterior prolapse, but this is often not the predominant defect.

The vaginal approach may be preferred by some surgeons if other transvaginal procedures are needed during the same procedure (i.e., concomitant vaginal hysterectomy with midurethral sling). Further, if compromised anal sphincter function exists, the surgeon may like to avoid excessive anal dilation from the retractors utilized during the transanal approach to repair this posterior defect. Finally, if the defect is a high rectocele, it may be difficult to repair through a transanal approach [10, 12]. A Cochrane review in 2010 suggested that for posterior vaginal wall prolapse, the vaginal approach was associated with a lower rate of recurrent rectocele or enterocele or both than the transanal approach (RR 0.24, 95% CI 0.09–0.64) [13]. The review noted a higher postoperative narcotic use and blood loss in this vaginal repair group. A randomized trial from 2020 found more improvement in both dyspareunia and constipation with transvaginal approach compared to transperineal. Although there was no difference in complications, hospital stay was shorter in the transvaginal patients [14].

The transanal approach is utilized if there is other perianal or rectal pathology that needs to be treated concurrently such as redundant rectal mucosa and hemorrhoids. A disadvantage of the transanal approach is that the patient is placed in the prone jackknife position, and it can be difficult to perform a simultaneous perineorrhaphy if needed.

In addition to the approach used, there are other questions that remain. Should a surgeon utilize mesh or graft material? Are traditional repairs vs. site-specific repairs more appropriate? This chapter will address some of the more common complications, and in doing so may help answer some of these questions, or at least inspire future investigation into those questions that remain unanswered. Technique selection and operative plan are always the first step to consider when aiming to minimize and manage complications.

Furthermore, recent literature suggests that for both vaginal and abdominal prolapse repairs, decreasing the size of the genital hiatus reduces the risk of prolapse recurrence [15, 16]. Thus, the addition of a perineal repair (or perineorrhaphy), wherein the transverse perineal muscles are plicated at the midline to rebuild the perineal body and narrow the genital hiatus, has become more "standard" when fixing other compartments.

Complications of Posterior Repair

Before detailing the potential complications following rectocele repair, one must consider that rectocele repair is often performed concomitantly with other pelvic organ prolapse and/or urinary incontinence surgery. Thus, there is a limited body of evidence on outcomes and complications following rectocele repair alone, and much of the data comes from studies where multicompartment prolapse is addressed.

Hemorrhage

Excessive bleeding or hemorrhage is a complication of rectocele repair regardless of the surgical approach. The rectovaginal septum and pararectal fascia are rich in blood vessels. In cases where the tissue is "loose or disrupted," as it often is in cases of posterior prolapse, these vessels tend to retract after they are cut, making identification difficult. This complication should be considered during the preoperative evaluation, intraoperatively, and in the postoperative management of patients. Mild blood loss is a relatively unavoidable result when surgical repair is selected. The surgeon's role, however, should be aimed at preventing hemorrhage by attempting to be aware during all phases of patient care.

Preoperative Prevention: Evaluation of Risk Factors and Preoperative Planning of Surgical Approach

Avoidance of excessive bleeding or hemorrhage starts with the preoperative evaluation. A thorough history and physical exam can help identify any bleeding diatheses or hereditary bleeding problems that may require further workup.

Review of patient medication and dietary supplements can identify agents that may contribute to intraoperative and postoperative bleeding. These agents include medications such as aspirin, NSAIDs, clopidogrel, and supplements such as fish oil. Cessation of antiplatelet agents approximately 7 days prior to surgery will reduce the risk of bleeding; however, the surgical team must weigh the risk of bleeding against the potential for adverse outcomes arising from the relative hypercoagulable state that can exist if antiplatelet agents are stopped. Any chronic antithrombotic agent use is associated with a higher risk of multiple complications after prolapse surgery. In a single-institution retrospective review of nearly 400 cases, only four bleeding complications were encountered, all of which were in patients on antithrombotic medication and received a rectocele repair as part of their procedure [17]. Despite this, careful consideration is recommended where there is a question regarding the safety of stopping antiplatelet agents. For example, one study suggests patients are 2.4 times more likely to experience acute coronary syndrome or death during the first 90 days of discontinuing clopidogrel therapy compared to days 91–180 [18]. This is especially important in patients with coronary artery disease, veno-occlusive disease, and a history of cerebral vascular accidents. Care must also be taken with other medications that affect the clotting cascade. Medications such as Coumadin/warfarin, apixaban, or argatroban should prompt consultation to decide on appropriate perioperative management. The risk of bleeding must be weighed against the risk of adverse outcomes resulting from stopping these medications, i.e., thrombocclusion [19, 20].

Preoperative lab tests can help identify patients with bleeding diatheses especially if it is suggested by history. Depending on institutional regulations, surgeon's preference, and patient's history, coagulation studies and platelet counts can be evaluated preoperatively. Other test such as bleeding times and clotting factor levels can be evaluated if indicated.

Physical examination is also important in attempting to avoid surgical bleeding complications. Inspection for prior surgical scars, as well as signs of potential vascular abnormalities, should be routine. This information can aid in the selection of which approach is most appropriate, as well as the need for other preoperative evaluations. For example, vulvar varicosities (though rare) may lead a surgeon to evaluate the patient with imaging to rule out aberrant vasculature or pelvic congestion syndrome. In a patient with abnormal vasculature, blind passage of trocars (i.e., those found in mesh repairs) should be used with extreme caution [21].

Intraoperative Risk: Avoidance and Identification of Hemorrhage

Meticulous surgical techniques should aim to establish excellent intraoperative hemostatic control. This should also reduce the risk of excessive "oozing" in the postoperative period. Obviously, stopping bleeding by controlling injured vessels is preferred over managing bleeding from uncontrolled vessels. Good visualization can help achieve this goal. This is provided by suction, irrigation, lap pads, and lights. Other general intraoperative considerations (use of electrocautery, suturing technique, etc.) will not be discussed in detail here.

Surgeons have various techniques at their disposal to treat patients with rectoceles. Each technique comes with different expected blood loss and may also have different potential sites of hemorrhage. For example, a double-blind, randomized controlled trial, including women with at least stage 2 symptomatic rectocele, that compared native tissue repair to augmenting the native tissue repair with porcine subintestine submucosal (SIS) graft showed that those who received graft had a significantly greater estimated blood loss (125 mL vs. 100 mL, $p = 0.005$) [22]. This difference is not likely to be clinically significant, but it does illustrate a point. We do need to look objectively at new techniques/materials used and the additional surgical time required to ensure that complications (even if rare) do not become more common. This is true even if the alteration to technique (such as in this study) would not seem to impact the complication.

The tactics to avoid or identify hemorrhage also differ depending on the surgical approach to posterior compartment repair. Cadaveric studies examining the vascularity in the paravesical and pararectal space near the sacrospinous ligament found a large amount of collateral blood supply and anastomosis with significant anatomical variation of the vasculature. For a vaginal approach at the sacrospinous ligament, the inferior gluteal artery and its coccygeal branch are the most prominent arteries susceptible to injury, while the hypogastric and pudendal venous plexi have been reported as the most likely venous sources of significant bleeding [23]. Abdominal approaches to the repair of pelvic organ prolapse routinely require dissection and identification of the sacral promontory. The presacral venous plexus that runs on the anterior aspect of the sacrum can result in significant bleeding that can be difficult to control using conventional measures such as suturing, clipping, or electrocautery. Especially when patients are in the lithotomy position, the hydrostatic pressure can increase two to three times that of the inferior vena cava [24]. Intraoperative management of presacral bleeding with the use of hemostatic matrix (FloSeal; Baxter Healthcare Corporation, Fremont, CA) and an absorbable hemostat (Surgicel® Fibrillar; Ethicon, Somerville, NJ) has been advocated by some as first-line treatment for presacral bleeding if it is encountered intraoperatively [25]. More traditionally, things like long periods of compression, sterile thumbtacks, or the use of a fat bolster have been utilized.

In cases where pneumoperitoneum is utilized (i.e., laparoscopy, with or without robotic assistance), some suggest that inspection after intra-abdominal pressure has been decreased to physiologic levels can be performed to identify any bleeding areas that may be masked by the effects of the positive pressure that pneumoperitoneum provides. The converse of this has also been utilized as a way of controlling bleeding in laparoscopic or robotic-assisted laparoscopic cases. For example, temporarily increasing pneumoperitoneum pressures to compress venous structures can provide time for inspection, gathering necessary instruments, or mobilizing surgical staff. High flow surgical units (SurgiQuest, Milford, CT) can be used if bleeding is anticipated or encountered to allow for more aggressive use of suction without losing the intra-abdominal pressure needed to visualize bleeding structures.

Another question regarding technique is whether the use of robotic assistance decreases the risk of bleeding compared to pure laparoscopy. A 2011 study compared the minimally invasive abdominal techniques (pure laparoscopic to robotic-assisted laparoscopic) for the repair of a rectocele. The laparoscopic group had a higher intraoperative blood loss compared to the robotic group (mean, 45 ± 91 mL vs. 6 ± 23 mL; $p = 0.048$); however, this difference may not be clinically significant [10]. A 2014 systematic review to evaluate the role of robotic assistance in laparoscopic rectopexy found that robotic rectopexy had no effect on the recurrence rate of rectal prolapse, but did decrease intraoperative blood loss by a weighted mean difference of −0.44 (95% CI −0.71, −0.16) [11]. A review of the National Surgical Quality Improvement

Program (NSQIP) found a 0.5% rate of blood transfusion following over 3000 cases of laparoscopic or robotic sacrocolpopexy [26]. Devastating complications such as hemorrhage from posterior repair alone are relatively rare, but this makes it harder to look at as an endpoint in small-scale studies. The studies are often underpowered to show differences in these types of complications.

Utilizing the vaginal approach for an isolated posterior prolapse repair does not allow for a substantial space for blood to accumulate without the surgeon being aware. In cases where it is difficult to identify the specific site of bleeding, temporary packing can be very useful. It is recommended to direct a vaginal sponge in a posterior-lateral direction toward the ischial spine for a minimum of 10 min [23]. Packing not only allows the patient's innate clotting cascade to begin to work but also allows the surgical staff to obtain equipment necessary to assist in visualization. Lighted retractors (i.e., Miyazaki retractor) (Fig. 6.1a, b) can be quite useful in vaginal surgery if visualization of bleeding is difficult. As mentioned earlier, hemostatic agents such as FloSeal (Baxter Healthcare Corporation, Fremont, CA) can also be quite effective in vaginal surgery if specific sites of bleeding cannot be identified or traditional methods are unsuccessful at stopping bleeding. If suture ligation (i.e., figure of eight sutures) is needed, utilizing a finger in the rectum may reduce the chance that a hemostatic stitch injures the rectal wall and results in another set of postoperative complications. In most cases, these sutures will be delayed absorbable. In most cases of isolated posterior repair via a vaginal approach, completing the procedure and closing the vaginal wall is the best way to limit blood loss.

Vasoconstrictive agents such as lidocaine with epinephrine or pitressin are used by some surgeons during the vaginal dissection. Vasoconstriction prevents bleeding during the dissection, which can potentially minimize intraoperative blood loss. When the vasoactive substance is mixed with an anesthetic, there may be the additional benefit of reduced postoperative pain. The downside of using vasoconstrictive agents is that bleeding vessels may be "hidden" while the agent is active and become problematic when it wears off postoperatively. The question of distortion of tissue planes is also raised if a site-specific repair is selected. One study from 2015 randomized eighty women undergoing vaginal prolapse repair to receive hydrodissection with an ornipressin solution or normal saline and found significantly reduced blood loss (35 vs 81 mL) with ornipressin use without any cardio-

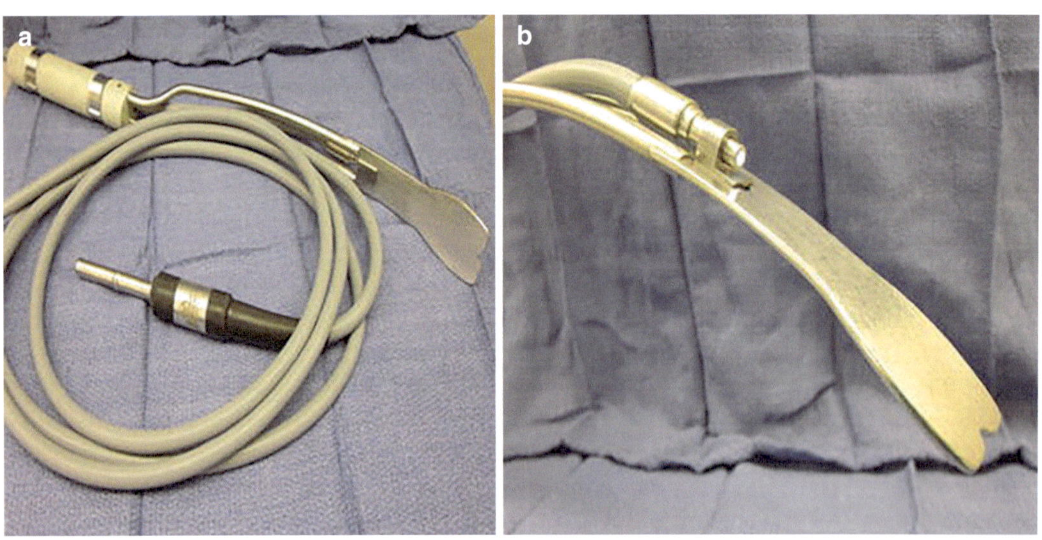

Fig. 6.1 The Miyazaki retractor is shown here (**a**). This retractor has a fiber optic light on the end (**b**) that is useful when the surgeon is working in a narrow space and visualization is poor

vascular complications. Although this was not rectocele repairs specifically and a small blood loss difference that would not be clinically significant in most cases, it is reasonable to expect that the vasoconstrictors may make a real difference in cases where more bleeding is encountered or expected [27].

If extensive dissection is carried out during a vaginal repair or if there is a high suspicion that postoperative bleeding may occur, we recommend placement of vaginal packing while the patient is still anesthetized. This allows for tighter packing with less discomfort to the patient. The packing can be removed the next morning if the patient is staying overnight or in the recovery room prior to discharge, if the patient is set to be discharged the same day. However, it is not necessary in patients where there is not a high concern for postoperative bleeding [28] as packing may increase immediate postoperative pain [29].

If blind passage of trocars or anchoring sutures is selected for a vaginal repair, it is important to have an intimate knowledge of anatomy, appropriately identify landmarks, and maintain a high suspicion of anatomic variations to minimize the risk of vessel injury. A prospective study looking at outcomes with mesh kits reported the adverse outcomes of mesh-augmented vaginal anterior and posterior repairs. They reported excessive bleeding (defined as ≥500 ml) in 5.1% of patients with prolapse treated with mesh kits [30].

Stapled Transanal Rectal Resection (STARR) can be used for the treatment of internal rectal prolapse, as well as rectocele. Postoperative bleeding is not rare following a stapled hemorrhoidopexy and occurs in about 5% of cases [31]. The bleeding usually occurs at the level of the endorectal suture line. After a stapled rectal resection, reinforcing this staple line with a hand-sewn suture has been suggested to decrease this risk of hemorrhage [32]. Careful inspection is important to identify any bleeding vessel after a STARR procedure.

At least one study compared intraoperative blood loss across rectocele repair techniques. There was less intraoperative blood loss in the STARR group compared to blood loss in the group undergoing standard vaginal rectocele repair (STARR, 43 mL; transvaginal rectocele repair, 108 mL; $p = 0.0015$) [33]. However, the study showed a higher complication rate from the transanal resection group (STARR 61.1% vs. transvaginal rectocele repair 18.9%, $p = 0.0001$). Similarly, meta-analysis in a Cochrane Review in 2013 comparing methods of surgical management of pelvic organ prolapse reported that the transanal approach was associated with significantly lower blood loss (a difference of 79 mL, 95% CI 40–119) compared to the transvaginal repair [13]. Obviously, a single outcome, such as intraoperative blood loss, must not be the only driving factor for selecting an appropriate procedure.

Postoperative Evaluation and Management

It is important to identify postoperative hemorrhage in a timely manner because treatment and resuscitation can prevent other unwanted complications. Education and good communication with the recovery room staff are necessary to help identify patients who may require intervention. The standard recovery room protocol in the immediate postoperative period should include monitoring heart rate, blood pressure, urine output, and inspection of surgical incisions or pads. In cases with known bleeding, serial complete blood cell labs with a coagulation panel every 4–6 h is recommended [23].

Patients who are hemodynamically stable but are noted to have excessive oozing from the surgical site should have a vaginal packing placed to help tamponade bleeding vessels and minimize the potential space for blood loss. Aside from packing gauze, other compressive devices utilize balloons (i.e., Foley catheters) to allow for appropriate pressure. These maneuvers are not applicable to abdominal repairs, as the potential space is often too large to contain and cannot be effectively compressed. Surgeons must carefully balance the benefits of improved visualization of bleeding structures with robotics and laparoscopy with the disadvantage of intraperitoneal entry and the resultant potential space for bleeding when deciding on approach. Patients with postoperative hematomas may be monitored expectantly with hemoglobin levels every 6 h and monitoring for signs of infection, or drained.

When conservative measures of fluid resuscitation and packing are not sufficient, more invasive measures may be necessary. This is especially true if a patient becomes hemodynamically unstable. Reexploration allows for identification of bleeding vessels and a tighter closure of the posterior vaginal wall, resulting in better hemostatic control. Reexploration also allows for removal of clot or accumulated blood that, if left in situ, may prolong recovery. This can be effective; however, one must make this decision to reexplore carefully. Bleeding that has slowed from tamponade, whether intrinsic or iatrogenic, now becomes brisker or uncontrolled after clot evacuation relieves pressure on the vessel or vessels. If during an intra-abdominal reexploration the patient becomes increasingly unstable or coagulopathic and the source of bleeding cannot be identified, the surgeon can consider packing the abdomen with surgical laps until resuscitation can be achieved.

Another option for uncontrolled bleeding is the selective embolization of bleeding vessels. Depending on availability and expertise, super selective embolization may be successfully performed [34, 35]. The time required to transfer a patient to an interventional radiology suite must be considered when deciding to utilize embolization.

The use of cross-sectional imaging (i.e., CT scan) before reexploration and/or intravascular intervention can be considered in a hemodynamically stable patient. A flow chart is provided as a reference for clinicians to use if postoperative bleeding is suspected. The assessment and management of bleeding complications from posterior compartment repairs must be managed in an individual manner based on clinical scenario and available resources.

Dyspareunia and Sexual Function

Sexual function is a complex process that involves many organs and structures of the female pelvis. Further, there is an intricate interaction with the central nervous system, hormonal axis, peripheral nerves, and blood vessels. Women with pelvic organ prolapse may present with varying degrees of sexual dysfunction, and the aims of pelvic organ prolapse surgery are to prevent worsening this dysfunction and, hopefully, to restore or improve a woman's sexual function. The effects of pelvic organ prolapse on sexual function are varied and difficult to study. Although prolapse may not directly be associated with dyspareunia, comorbid urinary incontinence, poor patient body image, and the effects on partner experience may affect libido and sexual satisfaction. Fortunately, most women report an improvement in sexual function following surgery for prolapse [36]. There is overall conflicting evidence whether rectocele specifically is a contributor to dyspareunia and sexual dysfunction, which may owe to the heterogeneity of techniques and definitions of repair [36]. Although some recent larger retrospective studies report no association between rectocele repair and dyspareunia and sexual dysfunction [37], surgeons must carefully consider preoperative sexual function and operative technique when approaching the posterior compartment. If there is no dysfunction to start and a woman desires to continue being sexually active, the surgeon should strive to avoid creating a problem. Despite the best efforts, painful intercourse, or dyspareunia, is a potential complication of any pelvic organ prolapse repair, and this section will focus on this potential outcome from posterior prolapse repair.

Preoperative: Evaluation and Counseling

It is very important when taking a history preoperatively to assess if a patient is sexually active, plans on becoming active, and what her current sexual function is. Dyspareunia is reported as a presenting symptom in 29% of women undergoing rectocele repair [38]. Further, dyspareunia is a known potential complication of posterior compartment repair, so the above must be openly discussed preoperatively. There are numerous questionnaires that can be utilized to objectively classify a woman's sexual function both pre- and postoperatively. For example, the Sexual History Form and the Female Sexual Function Index are validated measures [39, 40]. Some questionnaires are for general sexual function, and others have been validated specifically in the pelvic organ prolapse population. This preoperative assessment is important to help counsel the patient on the appropriate repair. It is also useful so that there is a baseline to compare postoperative outcomes against if results are not satisfactory.

Women with rectoceles can present with other aspects of sexual dysfunction along with dyspareunia. Out of a selective group of 68 women with sexual dysfunction who were undergoing fascial suture rectocele repairs, 85% were noted to have dyspareunia as a presenting symptom [41]. After the repair at six-month follow-up, the patients showed significant improvement for desire ($p > 0.001$), satisfaction ($p > 0.0001$), and pain ($p > 0.0001$). There were no significant changes for arousal ($p = 0.0897$), lubrication ($p = 1$), or orgasm ($p = 0.0893$). Only one patient experienced de novo dyspareunia that was attributed to a postoperative infection resulting in excessive scar tissue of the posterior wall of the vagina. A systematic review by Jha and colleagues of 14 articles that assessed sexual function and dyspareunia before and after anterior and/or posterior prolapse repair with native tissue found significant improvements postoperatively in sexual function and dyspareunia [42]. Unfortunately this analysis included all patients who had prolapse repair regardless of whether anterior, posterior, or combined, and no subanalysis limited to posterior repairs was performed. The authors did note that in studies by Colombo [43], Haase [44], and Dua and colleagues [45], higher rates of dyspareunia were reported in patients who underwent a colpoperineorrhaphy or posterior repair in addition to an anterior repair than in those patients who underwent an isolated anterior repair.

As noted earlier, after prolapse repair, there is often an improvement in many of the sexual function domains; however, some studies suggest that posterior repair may have higher rates of postoperative dyspareunia than repair of other compartments of pelvic organ prolapse. One such study looked at a cohort of women who underwent anti-incontinence surgery and concomitant pelvic organ prolapse repair. They divide these women into two groups for comparison: those who had posterior repair and those who did not have a posterior repair. Although both groups had improvements postoperatively in their Pelvic Organ Prolapse-Urinary incontinence Sexual Function Questionnaire (PISQ) score, the women who did not have posterior repairs were noted to have a lower incidence of dyspareunia than those who had posterior repairs [46]. A systematic review of complications after vaginal prolapse repair found that reported rates of dyspareunia varied widely after prolapse repair surgery. Seventy studies were identified with reports of dyspareunia, with an average rate of 9.1% and a range of 0–66.7%. These studies were not analyzed based on the location of repair; however, five of the papers cited posterior repair as a risk factor for dyspareunia [47]. In a prospective database of 3515 Finnish women who underwent prolapse repair in 2015, having a rectocele repair as part of their surgery was associated with dyspareunia at both 6 months and 5 years after surgery [48].

Intraoperative Considerations: Technique, Mesh, and Surgical Approach

Surgical techniques to decrease the risk of dyspareunia are mostly based on expert opinion, as there are few well-designed, randomized controlled trials to assess the impact of different methods of posterior prolapse repair on sexual function and dyspareunia. In this section, we will consider several technical aspects of posterior repair: approach (transvaginal, transanal, etc.), technique (within the approach itself, such as midline plication and levatorplasty), and the use of mesh augmentation (synthetic or biologic). Sexual function and dyspareunia have not been found to correlate with anatomical success of prolapse repair.

The surgical approach, whether abdominal, vaginal, or transanal, may affect postoperative dyspareunia rates. In a randomized study comparing transanal and transvaginal rectocele repairs, none of the subjects reported de novo dyspareunia, while 27% reported improvement of sexual function, slightly in favor of the transanal repair [49]. Like prior studies, this study also found higher rates of prolapse recurrence with the transanal approach. In the previously mentioned 2020 randomized trial by Balata and colleagues, improvements in sexual quality of life were significantly higher with the transvaginal approach compared to the transperineal. They also found a reduction in dyspareunia with the transvaginal approach and an increase with the transperineal approach, though the difference did not reach statistical significance [14]. Though less common, dyspareunia is also seen with the abdominal approach. Sergent and colleagues found that sacrocolpopexy with polyester mesh had a de novo dyschezia rate of 1.7% and dyspareunia rate of 0.8% [50]. Claerhout and coworkers utilized polypropylene mesh in abdominal repairs and found de novo constipation rates of 5% and de novo dyspareunia of 19% with mesh [51]. A comparison of these few small studies is not meant to replace a large, randomized study (that would be more appropriately powered to show differences in these domains), but rather to illustrate that different mesh types (i.e., polyester vs. propylene) used abdominally may result in different dyspareunia rates.

When considering transvaginal repairs and dyspareunia, one must consider the exact procedures that were performed, as there may be differences between levatorplasty, midline plication (or traditional posterior repair), and site-specific repairs. A 2013 meta-analysis by Karram et al. looked at both anatomic and subjective outcomes. Traditional posterior colporrhaphy with midline plication had a reported mean postoperative dyspareunia rate of 18% (range 5–45%) based on analysis of seven studies with a total of 522 patients, and site-specific repair was found to have an identical mean postoperative dyspareunia rate of 18% (range 7–67%) based on analysis of eight studies with a total of 487 patients [8]. Weaker evidence within this meta-analysis suggested that levatorplasty was associated with more dyspareunia. Numerous other studies have associated levatorplasty with increased dyspareunia. In a prospective study, 93 women who had undergone prolapse repair completed the validated International Consultation on Incontinence modular Questionnaire-Vaginal Symptoms (ICIQ-VS) at 6 and 12 months postoperatively. The study found that the subjective vaginal and sexual matters scores improved less in women who had levator plication sutures during posterior vaginal repair compared to those who did not. Furthermore, the women with levator plication showed a significant increase in postoperative dyspareunia ($p \leq 0.05$) while women who underwent posterior repair only had no change in their incidence of dyspareunia [52]. It is believed that the de novo dyspareunia that occurs with levatorplasty results from pressure atrophy of the included muscle and the subsequent scarring that takes place [53, 54]. This may not be the complete cause, however, as dyspareunia can be associated with posterior colporrhaphy even if there is no concomitant levatorplasty or synthetic material used. Another study compared traditional posterior colporrhaphy to site-specific repairs in a retrospective chart review and again found similar rates of dyspareunia and bowel symptoms, though the site-specific repair had a higher recurrence rate of a symptomatic bulge beyond the hymenal ring (11% vs. 4%, $p = 0.02$) [55]. In 2017 retrospective review of 151 patients who had a repair of their rectovaginal fascia but not a levator plication, patients had significant improvements in sexual function and only a 1.8% rate of de novo dyspareunia was reported with a mean follow-up of 64 months [56].

One study of sexually active women undergoing posterior repair looked at whether vaginal dimensions at the time of surgery predicted dyspareunia and did not find an effect [54]. However, expert opinion suggests avoiding excessive tightening of the posterior vagina during a rectocele repair. Additionally, given that perineorrhaphy is often routinely performed alongside a rectocele repair to improve long-term pelvic organ prolapse recurrence outcomes, the surgeon must take care not to overly narrow the genital hiatus while reconstructing the perineal body. Both a narrow vaginal canal and a genital hiatus can contribute to postoperative dyspareunia. This can also occur with perineorrhaphy alone without concomitant rectocele repair. The surgeon's fingers can be used intraoperatively to calibrate the vagina to an appropriate size. Some advocate calibrating the vagina to 2–3 fingerbreadths, which should prevent anatomic difficulties with vaginal penetration in women who are interested in resuming this type of sexual activity [53].

The surgeon may choose to utilize an absorbable mesh, biologic graft, or permanent mesh. In concordance with the United States Food and Drug Administration's (FDA) decision to prohibit the sale of transvaginally placed synthetic mesh kits for the treatment of pelvic organ prolapse, the authors do not recommend the use of kits in the transvaginal correction of rectocele. Additionally, the joint American Urogynecologic Society (AUGS) and American College of Obstetrics and Gynecology (ACOG) statement on pelvic organ prolapse (revised 2024) recommends against the routine placement of transvaginal mesh (both biologic and synthetic) in the posterior compartment, citing both no improvement in outcomes as well as higher rates of mesh complications [57]. The International Urogynecological Association (IUGA) Grafts Roundtable that convened in 2005 suggested the following patient factors as relative contraindications for the use of biomaterials in pelvic floor reconstructions: pelvic irradiation; severe urogenital atrophy; immunosuppression; active infection; and comorbidities such as poorly controlled diabetes, morbid obesity, and heavy smoking [58], and we would agree with these relative contraindications for the use of biomaterials in posterior repairs.

However, practitioners who do not place transvaginal mesh themselves may encounter patients suffering from postoperative complications of that mesh. The use of mesh to augment posterior repairs is a potential contributor to postoperative dyspareunia. In a systematic review from 2021 of all prolapse repair types, they found that all metrics of sexual function were similar between transvaginally placed mesh and native tissue repairs; however, they found that dyspareunia was higher after transvaginal mesh placement than abdominal sacrocolpopexy. While there was no subgroup analysis for rectocele repairs, this is worth considering when choosing an approach to prolapse repair [59]. It is important to remember that the mesh may contract after it is placed intraoperatively. Mesh has been shown to contract or retract after placement, with some showing up to a 66% decrease in size [60]. To date, there is no clear evidence that this gradual decrease in mesh size is associated with dyspareunia, but it is a potential explanation for those who believe that mesh augmentation of the posterior compartment can worsen sexual outcomes. Mesh should be tailored or placed to avoid excessive tension and accommodate for such potential tightening. If vaginally placed mesh is anchored in structures such as muscle, the presence of a tight mesh band can lead to pulling on these muscle groups that may result in significant discomfort during intercourse. Mesh exposure and extrusion may also cause sexual complications and will be discussed later in this chapter.

Although mostly based on expert opinion, there are a few areas of surgical technique that should be considered when placing mesh posteriorly for surgeons who choose to do so. Appropriate thickness of the vaginal flaps and meticulous closure of any vaginal incisions may reduce mesh-related complications. Care must be used to ensure appropriate placement of mesh so that it does not bunch or roll in the vagina. This can form areas of inflammatory reactions that can be uncomfortable for women and may also be felt by male partners. Another potential cause of dyspareunia is vaginal narrowing. Vaginal narrowing can occur secondary to excessive trimming of the vaginal wall, which also results in tenuous coverage of any foreign material utilized. For abdominally placed mesh, differences in technique, such as the extent of the posterior dissection or the width of the dissection with subsequent mesh fixation, have also been proposed as potential factors that might lead to differences in painful intercourse post-abdominal sacrocolpopexy.

Sexual function outcomes following vaginally placed biologic grafts have also been considered. Studies have been conflicted regarding whether graft augmentation of posterior repair improves anatomic or functional outcomes [61–63]. Therefore, the decision to utilize a graft or mesh should be weighed against the potential risks, including dyspareunia. Paraiso and colleagues compared posterior colporrhaphy, site-specific repair, and site-specific repair with porcine small intestine submucosa graft in a randomized trial [62]. They found no difference in postoperative dyspareunia (PISQ-12 and asking "Do you feel pain during intercourse?"). There were also no differences in quality of life measures or bowel function. Perioperative and postoperative morbidity did not show a difference, albeit the study was underpowered to discern differences in these events. Importantly, however, they reported a lower failure rate with traditional repair techniques compared to the site-specific repair with porcine small intestine submucosa graft for rectoceles. This study suggests that sexual complications do not differ significantly based on repair type, but biologic agents have higher failure rates. A prospective cohort study of 50 women undergoing posterior wall repair and prespinous colpopexy with a biological small intestinal submucosa graft reported statistically significant improvement in vaginal symptoms and sexual matters score at 6-month follow-up [64]. One weakness of this study was that it did not have a control arm, so only limited conclusions can be drawn concerning the use of graft. Of note, this study found that concomitant pelvic surgery did not affect the outcomes of posterior wall repair with prespinous colpopexy and biological graft.

If the surgeon and patient elect to use a permanent mesh, selecting the appropriate type of mesh is an intraoperative decision that can minimize morbidity. Macroporous, monofilament, polypropylene mesh (type 1) has been found to have the most favorable biocompatibility profile of the synthetic meshes that are currently available. The lack of interstices allows native collagen to grow into the material and the large pore size allow for entry of macrophages and the body's other immune mediators [65]. However, several series have found that transvaginal synthetic mesh in the posterior compartment is associated with postoperative dyspareunia, as high as 69% [66, 67]. Additionally, many women experience improvement in dyspareunia following synthetic vaginal mesh removal, lending further credibility that placement of the mesh is a unique risk factor for dyspareunia and sexual dysfunction [68].

Based on the available studies, if a vaginal approach is elected for posterior repair, we would caution against the use of permanent mesh given the high incidence of recurrence, dyspareunia, and mesh complications. Because most studies have found no significant reduction in recurrence rate with a higher complication rate with transvaginally placed mesh, we do not recommend it in routine settings. This is in concordance with most major physician organizations, including IUGA, AUGS, and ACOG. In our practice, we only use biologic grafts when a native tissue repair is impossible, as in the case of a completely obliterated rectovaginal septum. We do not use synthetic transvaginal mesh. We must clarify, however, that this does not mean we recommend against the use of abdominally placed sacrocolpopexy mesh in the posterior vaginal wall, as it is very apparent that mesh complications and dyspareunia are far less common with this approach.

There are other intraoperative techniques to prevent dyspareunia that may not fit neatly into a category. For example, the use of copious irrigation and perioperative antibiotics is something that routinely happens. These are simple methods to reduce the risk of infection. These techniques are included in this section because of the potential complications that infection can carry. An abscess of a local surgical site infection, for example, may result in excessive scarring and inflammation that potentially leads to painful intercourse.

Postoperative Evaluation and Management of Dyspareunia

To identify postoperative dyspareunia, the surgeon should ask specific questions regarding the patient's sexual function. As with preoperative evaluations, standardized questionnaires can be utilized to aid with evaluation. Patient's bother and time from surgery must be considered when discussing potential treatments of this outcome. If a patient elects for therapy for dyspareunia, conservative treatment options exist. Topical lubricants, vaginal estrogen, and even topical local anesthetics have been described to help lessen or alleviate some of the milder symptoms. Systemic or local anxiolytics such as benzodiazepines have also been utilized to help relax pelvic floor muscles. When palpation on physical examination reveals pain at specific trigger points, injections with local anesthetics and/or steroids can be considered.

Physical therapy with the optional use of vaginal dilators is another method that can help address symptoms. Vaginal dilators are thought to improve dyspareunia by stretching the levator ani muscles and softening or preventing scar formation (Fig. 6.2). A randomized controlled trial of sexually active patients with no preoperative dyspareunia undergoing posterior colporrhaphy was done to determine when vaginal dilators could be safely used during the early postoperative period [69]. Patients were randomized to daily vaginal dilator use from postoperative weeks 4–8 or to no dilator use. No difference was found between those using dilators compared to controls regarding de novo dyspareunia rates, Patient Global Impression of Improvement scores, or Pelvic Organ Prolapse/Urinary Incontinence Sexual Function Questionnaire-12 scores. Of note, in contrast to prior studies that reported improvement in dyspareunia with dilator use [22, 62], this study found no change in overall sexual function from baseline at 6 months. The authors attributed this difference to the relatively low dyspareunia rates at baseline and the lack of a standardized definition of dyspareunia across studies.

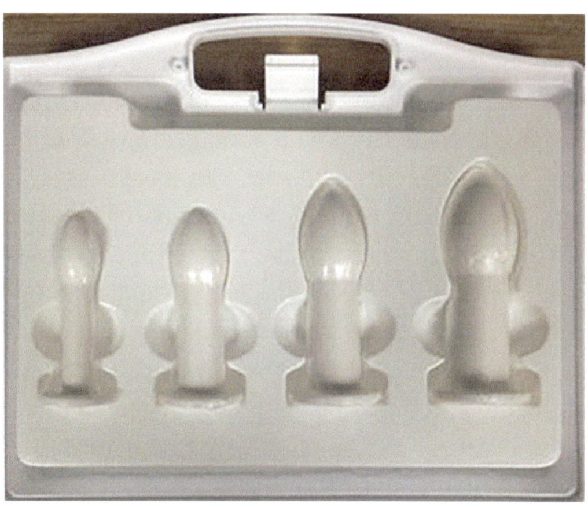

Fig. 6.2 Vaginal dilators come in increasing sizes to allow progressive vaginal dilation. Dilators are thought to improve dyspareunia by stretching the levator ani muscles and softening or preventing scar formation

Careful physical examination is also extremely useful to determine the specific cause of dyspareunia and to identify what will respond best to surgical intervention. Palpation for tight bands of tissue, extrusions, and tender pelvic muscles is an important aspect of the physical exam to identify potential causes of dyspareunia and to direct management of this complication. If a discrete band of tissue is identified on physical exam attached to the vaginal wall and incorporated into the levator ani muscles, operative release of this tissue can help to alleviate symptoms of pain during intercourse. Operative removal of synthetic mesh may be indicated as well, especially if there is tenderness associated with mesh palpation or any mesh exposure [68]. Aside from the release of excessively tight tissue, graft material may be necessary if there is a paucity of local tissue to reconstruct an adequate vaginal lumen. Excessive narrowing of the vaginal introitus or canal may also require surgical intervention.

Other therapies have also been studied for the treatment of dyspareunia. There is level III evidence to support the use of botulinum toxin in the treatment of severe refractory vaginismus. This comes from a study of 24 women where the etiology of vaginismus was not specified in the inclusion criteria. After failing other therapies, these women were injected with 150–400 units of onabotulinum toxin type A in three sites on each side of the puborectalis muscle. After a mean follow-up of 12 months, none of the patients had recurrent vaginismus, and 75% were able to achieve satisfactory intercourse [70]. More specifically, there are case reports describing the use of botulinum toxin in a postoperative patient who experienced de novo dyspareunia and vaginismus [71, 72].

Rectal Injury

Injuring structures that lie adjacent to or in the surgical field is a potential complication of any surgical intervention. The defect that results in a rectocele is a deficiency of tissue or support between the vagina and rectum. The intimate relationship of the rectum to the rectocele defect makes the rectum a potential source for inadvertent injury.

Preoperative Prevention: Imaging, Bowel Preparation, and Estrogen

Preoperative imaging may be useful during surgical planning; however, there is no standardized method for radiographic rectocele evaluation. It has been reported that 80% of colorectal surgeons use defecography before a rectocele repair compared to only 6% of gynecologists [73]. This variance is due in part to a lack of evidence demonstrating superior outcomes associated with the use of preoperative defecography. Defecography provides a two-dimensional view of rectal emptying and is useful to exclude patients with pelvic floor dyssynergia who will not benefit from an operation. The dynamic nature of the test and use of contrast allows for visualization and identification of the rectocele and any adjacent enterocele, sigmoidocele, or intussusception. Knowledge of associated defects theoretically may aid in the avoidance of injury and surgical planning, for example, the addition of a sigmoid resection or sigmoidopexy. A benefit of defecation proctography to dynamic MRI is that it is performed in a position of gravity, which permits study of anatomy and function under conditions that better recreate daily life [74]. However, some studies have shown a lack of utility in obtaining preoperative defecography. In an older study, 74 patients with rectocele and symptoms of obstructed defecation were prospectively enrolled and underwent preoperative defecography in addition to a standardized questionnaire and physical exam [75]. Following a combined transvaginal/transanal rectocele repair, they were again evaluated with defecography, and, at a median follow-up of 58 months, the results of the rectocele repair were independently evaluated. Outcome analysis found that clinical success was not influenced by preoperative size of the rectocele, barium trapping, internal intussusception, rectal evacuation, perineal descent, or radiologic evidence of anismus, leading the authors to question the role of defecography in predicting clinical outcomes. Another study retrospectively looked at 170 patients who had undergone defecography and compared detection of prolapse on clinical and radiographic exam [5]. The authors concluded that most radiographic rectoceles and cystoceles are found on physical exam, while correlation is poor between defecography and physical exam in cases of enteroceles and sigmoidoceles. A more recent study analyzed the correlation between rectocele size on physical examination and defecography presenting to a high-volume pelvic reconstruction clinic and found that although the two were correlated, one did not predict the other, and only physical exam rectocele size was a predictor for surgery [76].

Depending on surgeon's preference, a bowel prep may be used preoperatively for abdominal and transanal posterior repairs. A bowel prep does not necessarily decrease the risk of rectal injury; however, it does decrease the risk of gross contamination if in fact a rectal injury occurs. Some laparoscopic/robotic surgeons have suggested that more complete bowel prep decreases distention secondary to bulky stool or excessive bowel gas that can make dissection more challenging and interfere with visualization. Women with symptomatic rectoceles can have a significant degree of constipation and trapping of stool at baseline. In cases where women have excessive amounts of stool in the rectal vault, intraoperative rectal exam or manipulation can be a more challenging proposition. Patients may benefit from a modified bowel prep. An enema given preoperatively can be an effective way of cleaning out the rectal vault if that is all that is needed preoperatively. Enemas are generally well tolerated and do not dehydrate patients the same way a full bowel prep would.

Preoperative use of estrogen in postmenopausal women can also be considered to thicken the vaginal wall, as this may facilitate dissection. Postmenopausal vaginal atrophy may increase the risk of visceral injury due to difficulty identifying proper planes of dissection and thinning of the vaginal wall. A randomized controlled trial found that preoperative estrogen treatment for 2–12 weeks restored vaginal cytology to the premenopausal state [77]. Vaginal wall thickness was not restored, however. Multivariate analysis has shown that local estrogen therapy has no protective effect on vaginal extrusion or exposure after vaginal mesh surgery or when mesh is used for sacrocolpopexy (level 4) [78]. A double-blind, randomized controlled trial on the role of low-dose estrogens in improving the outcomes of pelvic organ prolapse surgery when used preoperatively reported that epithelial and muscularis thickness was increased 1.8- and 2.7-fold, respectively ($p = 0.002$, $p = 0.088$) by estrogen. The intervention effect was assessed by measuring full-thickness vaginal wall biopsies after 6 weeks of topical estrogen use compared to placebo. In addition to increased wall thickness, the biopsies showed that estrogen use increased the synthesis of mature collagen and decreased degradative enzyme activity. Prior studies had also shown this increase in collagen synthesis with topical estrogen but had not shown a change in the thickness of the vaginal wall. A recent randomized trial aimed to address whether at least 5 weeks of preoperative vaginal estrogen improved surgical success following native tissue apical suspension via a vaginal route. Of the 186 patients who underwent surgery, 65% had a concomitant rectocele repair. Although there was no difference in surgical failure, there was a significant improvement in surgeons' perceived tissue quality at the time of surgery [79]. There are no comparative studies to provide evidence regarding the routine use of local or systemic estrogen therapy before or after prolapse surgery using mesh. None of these studies look specifically at the risk reduction with preoperative estrogen on the relatively rarely reported complication of rectal injury.

Intraoperative Avoidance: Positioning and Risk of Rectal Injury

Patient positioning is important to minimize complications during posterior repair. Digital rectal examinations during transvaginal rectocele repair help to avoid or recognize rectal injury during dissection and or suture/trocar placement, and a draping technique that permits this should be utilized. The finger allows the surgeon to ensure that the rectal wall is not violated. Further, after repair, the surgeon can perform palpation via rectal exam to identify the presence of suture or mesh material that may have been inadvertently placed through the lumen of the rectum. In a retrospective look at rectal injury during vaginal surgery, Hoffman and coworkers found that over an 11-year period they had a 0.7% injury rate utilizing a vaginal approach for a variety of surgical indications including prolapse [71]. After reviewing the cases they felt that prevention of injury required careful sharp dissection, preliminary dissection on either side of the midline, and occasionally the insertion of a finger into the rectum. They suggest that injection of sodium chloride solution or a dilute vasoconstrictor may also facilitate dissection. The authors of this chapter do not routinely utilize this technique during the posterior dissection because of the potential for distortion of the already thin tissue planes.

If an abdominal approach with laparoscopic or robotic assistance is selected, good basic laparoscopic/robotic technique should be observed. These practices include utilizing oral or nasal gastric decompression and placement of a Foley catheter. Use of these measures is aimed at minimizing the risk of injury to hollow viscous organs. We also avoid the use of nitrous oxide to prevent distention of the bowel. Decompression of the bowel and bladder is especially important when gaining access to the abdominal cavity, and thus these measures are not necessarily aimed at reducing rectal injury. However, intraoperatively, they allow for better visualization and can prevent inadvertent injury during dissection.

Historically, mesh prolapse repair kits required placement via blind trocar passage, potentially increasing the risk of rectal injury. In one series of mesh prolapse repair kits with only short-term follow-up, the authors found that they had a 1.1% rectal injury rate [80]. Interestingly, the injured patients sustained the rectal injury during the initial dissection and not from the trocar passage. Both patients had the injury repaired primarily, and one did have a posterior mesh placed while the other was converted to a more traditional colporrhaphy. Injury to the rectum has been noted in another series of patients treated with mesh kits, where rectal injury was not caused by the initial dissection [81]. In this series of 62 patients, one patient (1.6%) had a rectal injury identified postoperatively in week one when a rectoscopy was performed for refractory defecatory pain and revealed an arm of the prolapse repair kit mesh traversing the lumen of the rectum. Today, when mesh is placed vaginally, it is as a freestanding implant rather than with an associated kit with trocars. There are not much data regarding the safety of the placement of mesh after recognizing a rectal injury, but we would recommend against it in most cases.

Patients with pelvic organ prolapse can have a significant posterior defect that the surgeon can attempt to address from the abdominal route, whether open, laparoscopic, or robotic. To achieve this, the dissection is carried down toward the perineal body between the vaginal wall and rectum. In one series of 165 women with vaginal vault prolapse undergoing laparoscopic sacrocolpopexy using a polypropylene mesh, three (2%) sigmoid perforations were noted. These injuries were all in women being treated for rectocele, presumably during the posterior dissection. All injuries were recognized intraoperatively and successfully treated by laparoscopic suture repair [82]. Another series of 124 women undergoing laparoscopic sacrocolpopexy (using multifilament polyethylene terephthalate-polyester) noted two intraoperative rectal injuries (1.6%). One of the rectal injuries was immediately recognized and successfully repaired; the procedure proceeded as planned with uneventful follow-up for this patient. The other intraoperative rectal injury was not recognized, however, and the patient developed a rectovaginal fistula secondary to the occult rectal perforation. This was noted 3 weeks after the surgery, and the fistula was debrided and closed with suture. A transitory colostomy was concomitantly performed. This patient, unfortunately, also developed a lumbosacral spondylodiscitis diagnosed at 4 months and required prolonged antibiotic therapy before complete resolution [50].

Identification of Injury

Regardless of approach, recognition of a rectal injury remains paramount in trying to minimize morbidity to the patient. Ideally, an injury of the rectum is identified intraoperatively to avoid the sequelae of a delayed diagnosis and to potentially allow for correction of the injury, obviating the need for a repeat operation. If an injury is suspected, adequate exposure is needed to investigate the integrity of the rectal wall. Rectal irrigation with saline or betadine may help confirm a small injury. Another technique is to fill the surgical field with irrigation and gently force air into the rectum with a Toomey or bulb syringe. This allows for the identification of bubbles if a full-thickness injury is present.

If an injury is recognized intraoperatively, the surgeon must perform an adequate mobilization of the injured area. The mobilization allows for appropriate exposure so that the injury can be closed in its entirety. Mobilization of the rectum away from other tissue is also usually necessary to allow the surgeon to complete the prolapse repair and is critical to a tension-free repair. After mobilization, a two-layer closure should be performed. The first layer uses delayed absorbable sutures to close the rectal mucosal defect (usually in a running fashion). The second layer is an imbricated seromuscular layer, and a permanent suture or a delayed absorbable suture in a Lembert-type fashion has been utilized. It should be noted that during the dissection required to mobilize the injured bowel, it is often possible to identify additional tissue (fat, fascia) that can be used to cover the two-layered closure.

The final factor to achieve the best possible outcome from an intraoperative repair of a rectal injury is to give patients appropriate postoperative instructions. It is important to ensure that the patient has soft bowel movements. Also, patients should avoid anything per rectum for approximately 6 weeks. Fecal diversion is usually not necessary. Certainly, if the surgeon is unsure of the need for diversion or is not comfortable with the repair, an intraoperative consult can be called.

Delayed Presentation of Unrecognized Rectal Injury

At times, rectal injury may not be recognized until postoperatively. A case report described a patient with ongoing complaints of severe pain radiating down her leg, pelvic pain, dyspareunia, dyschezia, diarrhea, and new-onset fecal incontinence after a vaginal mesh was placed 5 months prior [83]. On physical exam, mesh was palpable at the vaginal apex and traversing the rectal lumen 6 cm from the anal verge. The authors attributed the rectal injury to inadequate medial retraction of the rectum at the time of sacrospinous ligament fixation. A retrospective study of STARR procedures reported a high rate (18%) of postoperative complications [84]. Though these all followed STARR resections and reported complications with this procedure vary greatly across studies [85], approaches to management can be applied to most rectal injuries. One patient presented with sepsis on postoperative day 1 with fever, hypotension, and retroperitoneal air and was treated with antibiotics. Though rare, a high suspicion must be maintained for perforation following posterior repair. In the study, two patients had abscesses at the level of the anastomosis requiring surgical drainage. Drainage should be considered in all patients who present with fluid collections, which may be caused by abscess or hematoma. If infected, the surgical site should be examined for foreign bodies that may serve as a nidus for infection and inflammation. In the STARR review, a granulomatous staple line led to chronic bleeding in eight patients and resolved after their removal. Any infection should be allowed to cool down before further intervention. In severe cases such as rectovaginal fistula, a diverting colostomy may be required. Identification and management of mesh complications and fistula will be discussed further later.

Rectovaginal Fistula

Cases of rectovaginal fistula have been reported with the use of mesh to augment a posterior colporrhaphy and posterior intravaginal slingplasty (Fig. 6.3a, b) [86]. Women with rectovaginal fistula may present with foul-smelling vaginal discharge, systemic signs of infection, and possibly pelvic or perineal adenopathy. A case series of 10 patients who underwent rectovaginal fistula repairs following prolapse repair with mesh highlighted the morbidity of mesh complications in the posterior compartment [87]. Patients underwent a mean of 4.4 surgeries for definitive fistula repair, with 40% requiring bowel diversion. Five of the patients in the series originally underwent a combined anterior and posterior repair, while three had isolated posterior repairs. On average, patients presented 7.1 months following prolapse repair. Fifty percent of the patients had visible mesh on physical exam, and all but two patients had confirmation of mesh extrusion on proctoscopy or colonoscopy. The authors reported that repairs were most successful when all mesh was removed, as noted earlier, for handling cases with intrarectal mesh without frank fistula.

The evaluation of a suspected rectovaginal fistula includes a thorough history, physical examination, imaging, and, if any uncertainty remains, an exam under anesthesia. The elements of history that both increase the likelihood of finding and difficulty in repairing a rectovaginal fistula include a history of multiple surgeries, pelvic radiation, and inflammatory bowel disease. When a fistula is not obvious on awake examination, proctoscopy and thorough vaginal examination with a patient under sedation can assist in identifying the exact location of the fistula and its relationship to the anal sphincter complex. It has become standard of care to obtain preoperative

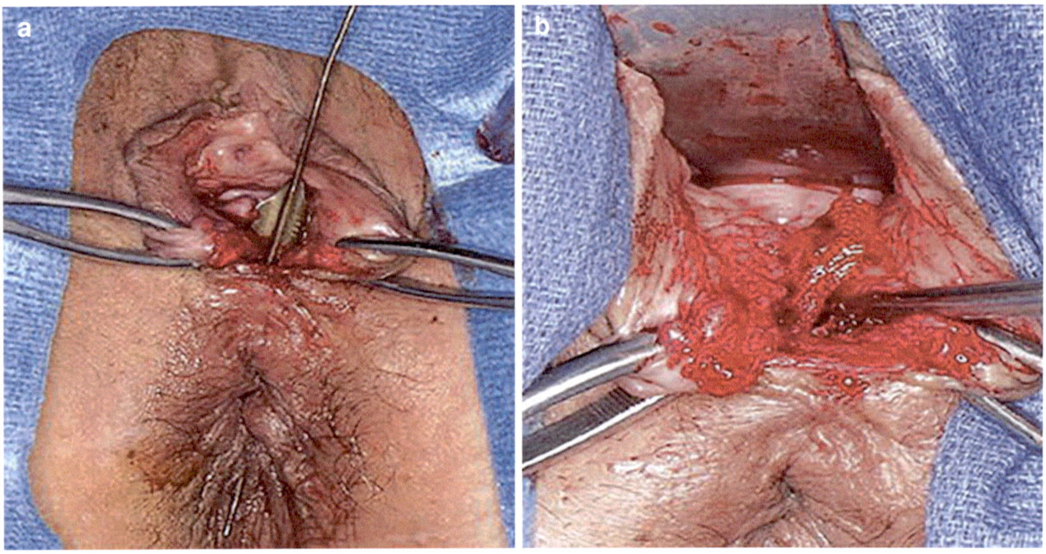

Fig. 6.3 Rectovaginal fistula. (**a**) Rectovaginal fistula demonstrated by a lacrimal duct probe entering the vagina and exiting the anus. (**b**) Posterior intravaginal sling plasty polypropylene mesh protruding through the dissected rectovaginal fistula. (Reproduced with permission from Hilger and Cornella [86])

imaging in cases of suspected rectovaginal fistulas [88]. Anal endosonography and/or MRI are recommended to better define anal fistula anatomy, aid with planning of surgical approach, and to avoid recurrence of disease. Anal endosonography is often preferred because it is a quick exam, well tolerated by patients, and able to accurately identify the internal opening of the fistula and inter- or transsphincteric fistulas; however, it is highly operator dependent. MRI is recommended for evaluation of patients with recurrent fistula or Crohn's disease because it provides superior image quality, especially if an endoluminal coil is utilized in addition to a surface coil. The endoanal coil enhances spatial resolution, which allows the precise size and location of the internal fistula opening to be visualized, provides information about sphincter integrity, and visualization of both ano- and rectovaginal fistulas. The superior utility of MRI was shown in a prospective trial of 104 patients with suspected fistula [89]. Each patient underwent characterization of their fistula by physical exam, endosonography, and MRI, and the results of these three separate modalities were compared to a reference standard. This study found that fistula classification was made correctly 61% of the time by clinical exam, 81% by endosonography, and 97% by MRI. Furthermore, it found that MRI has increased sensitivity for the detection of horseshoe extensions or abscesses. In fistulas that are more proximal or difficult to identify, CT or fluoroscopy with a contrasted enema can help with localization [90].

Repairs of these fistulas are more involved than repairs of straightforward mesh extrusions. It is imperative to identify and deal with the internal fistula opening, which is usually at the dentate line and can be located using palpation and gentle probes. The injection of air, hydrogen peroxide, or methylene blue may further aid in localization. Because of their complexity, it is recommended to involve a colon and rectal specialist as soon as the rectovaginal fistula is suspected. These repairs often require local tissue flaps, and in more complicated cases diverting colostomy may be considered. If a colon and rectal specialist is not present and intraoperative difficulties are encountered, such as unexpected anatomy, compromised anal canal, or failure to locate the internal opening, the procedure may be abandoned and a draining seton may be employed until a specialist is available to perform a sphincter-saving procedure [91].

Other Complications

Immediate Postoperative Complications: Pain, Urinary Retention, Constipation, and Urinary Tract Infections

Postoperative pain, urinary retention, constipation, and urinary tract infections are all common and typically self-limited following rectocele repair. Although these may not be considered true "complications" in urogynecologic surgery and severe by surgeons, they can be significant sources of distress for patients and contribute to healthcare costs by way of emergency department visits and telephone calls.

Pain in the immediate postoperative period following posterior repairs, although expected and not a true complication, can be managed in a multitude of ways. Additionally, minimizing postoperative narcotic burden is paramount in the context of today's opiate crisis. Basic surgical techniques outlined above to prevent intra- and postoperative hemorrhage are imperative in preventing severe postoperative pain, especially since hematoma formation and infection are often the proximate causes for significant pain. Otherwise, in the recent past, a variety of techniques with local anesthetic application have attempted to reduce postoperative pain and narcotic burden.

Most of these recent studies have failed to produce a significant difference in postoperative pain and narcotic burden. When patients were randomized to liposomal bupivacaine or normal saline for posterior repair hydrodissection, there was no difference in pain scores or other postoperative outcomes (including complications) [92]. Similarly, in patients undergoing posterior repair, perineorrhaphy, or colpocleisis who were randomized to placebo or 20 cc of liposomal bupivacaine into the levator muscles, lateral vagina, and/or perineum, there were no reductions in pain or postoperative narcotics [93]. Patients undergoing a vaginal prolapse repair that included a posterior repair who were randomized to muscle block of the iliococcygeus and puborectalis muscles with either 0.5% bupivacaine or normal saline did not have reduced postoperative pain scores or analgesic use [94]. Pudendal block at the time of prolapse repair has mixed results in the literature. In a randomized controlled trial in 2021 of 120 patients (60 per group), pudendal block with liposomal bupivacaine and 0.25% bupivacaine vs 0.25% bupivacaine alone reduced postoperative pain scores and analgesic (but not narcotic) use in patients getting posterior repair alone or in combination with other prolapse repairs. Interestingly, the likelihood of a successful voiding trial was not different between the groups [95]. In another study from 2024, 44 patients undergoing pelvic organ prolapse repair surgery were randomized to a pudendal block with 0.5% bupivacaine or no pudendal block; there was no difference in the primary outcome of opiate use in the first 24 h following surgery. They also found no difference in pain scores in the 24 and 48 h following surgery [96]. A randomized trial from 2005 of 102 patients found similar results [55].

Some authors suggest that pain is the primary contributor to transient postoperative urinary retention, which has been reported at rates higher than 30% following rectocele repair [97]. In a retrospective review of 458 patients, rectocele repair was not an independent risk factor for urinary retention, but worse postoperative pain was [98]. Regardless, surgeons must be aware of the possibility of transient urinary retention following posterior repair or any prolapse repair. It is routine practice within our high-volume division to have every patient complete a voiding trial (either active or passive) prior to discharge following prolapse repair.

Constipation, although common after any surgery, is particularly common after pelvic surgery. It is uniquely distressing to patients and can contribute to postoperative pain. Some suggest it also may contribute to postoperative urinary retention as well, though there is little data to directly support this. A meta-analysis from 2023 synthesizing evidence from four moderate-quality studies suggested that multi-agent laxative regimens were superior to docusate alone or no treatment in the treatment of bothersome postoperative constipation [99]. Additionally, other principles of enhanced recovery after surgery (ERAS) protocols should be adhered to prevent constipation. These include early ambulation as well as clear liquids up to 2 hours prior to surgery [100].

Urinary tract infection is also a potential complication following rectocele repair or any prolapse repair. In a large study of a Swedish registry, 7799 women underwent an isolated rectocele repair. The authors found no difference in the rate of postoperative urinary tract infections following surgery between those who did and did not receive perioperative intravenous antibiotic prophylaxis, which was 11% in both groups [101].

Mesh Extrusion or Exposure

Complications with mesh extrusion or exposure are a concern when mesh is used for vaginal prolapse repairs transvaginally or transabdominally, though the incidence is significantly higher with vaginally placed mesh. In 2011, IUGA and the International Continence Society (ICS) published a joint terminology and classification scheme to standardize nomenclature for complications of prostheses, including mesh [102]. This advocated replacement of the more general term "erosion" with extrusion, defined as the passage gradually out of a body structure or tissue, and exposure, defined as a condition of displaying, revealing, exhibiting, or making accessible. Adoption of this terminology has not been complete, and earlier papers often utilize the older terms, leading to imprecision of reported complications.

Risk factors for mesh exposure are similar whether they occur in the vaginal lumen, where it may be discovered on routine pelvic examinations during follow-up, or in the rectum. A 2011 meta-analysis of prolapse repair data found that most graft "erosions," defined in the analysis as exposed graft material in the vagina or surrounding pelvic organs, occur within 1 year of surgery and should be suggested when patients present with dyspareunia, discharge, and/or vaginal pain [47]. This analysis found rectocele repair at the time of vaginal prolapse repair, increasing age, and concomitant hysterectomy to be risk factors for vaginal graft "erosion." In contrast, a more recent systematic review of risk factors for mesh "erosion" found fewer graft "erosions" with increasing age and identified concomitant hysterectomy to be a potential protective factor [103]. This review also identified greater parity, diabetes mellitus, smoking, premenopausal status, and estrogen replacement therapy as risk factors for mesh "erosions" after urogynecologic surgery. A prospective study looking at outcomes with mesh kits found that the Apogee kit used for posterior repairs had a lower rate of mesh extrusion or exposure than the Perigee kit used for anterior repairs [30]. Like the meta-analysis described earlier, the study identified concomitant hysterectomy as a risk factor for extrusion or exposure along with increased parity, previous native tissue repair, concomitant repair of both compartments, concomitant sling, smoking, and constipation.

Mesh extrusion into the vaginal epithelium can be seen if mesh is used to augment posterior repairs [104]. Care must be used to ensure the appropriate planes of dissection. Improper dissection can potentially lead to a thinned vaginal wall that can increase the chance of mesh extrusions when it is used to cover the mesh. Dwyer and coworkers had a 9% overall extrusion rate noted with the use of monofilament polypropylene mesh placed in the anterior and posterior compartments (and one patient who developed a rectovaginal fistula) [104]. In a long-term retrospective review of patients who underwent both mesh-augmented and native tissue rectocele repair, 13% of women had a vaginal mesh exposure at a mean follow-up of 5.3 years; more than half of those patients were treated for the exposure surgically. Both patient cohorts had similar surgical success rates [105]. Posterior vaginal mesh extrusion is handled in much the same way that any mesh extrusion is handled, as discussed elsewhere in this book. Observation may be warranted if asymptomatic. Topical local estrogen is another conservative approach, and finally, local excision and closure of the vaginal epithelium may be necessary. This may be performed under local anesthesia utilizing an Allis clamp to grasp the exposed mesh prior to sharp excision. In cases of pain secondary to mesh contraction, which may present with prominent bands under the vaginal mucosa, incision may be all that is needed. Lim and coworkers retrospectively noted a 12.9% incidence of vaginal mesh extrusion at 1 year when a Vicryl–Prolene mesh was used with posterior colporrhaphy [66]. The authors noted that all of these extrusions were dealt with easily by trimming the area, without the need for mesh removal, in the outpatient setting. In cases when mesh exposure exceeds 5 mm or is compounded, we recommend performing the excision in the operating room.

Mesh can also extrude into the rectal lumen, where it is less likely to be visualized or palpated during a routine postoperative speculum examination of the vagina. A digital rectal exam should thus be considered part of the postoperative physical exam, especially if a posterior repair was performed. There are case reports and prolapse repair series that describe a small, but real, number of women who develop mesh extrusions, exposure, or misplacements into the rectum recognized postoperatively [106–108]. Successful diagnosis of mesh extrusion into the rectum requires a high index of suspicion. Women may present with rectal bleeding, change in bowel habits, or worsening dyspareunia several months after posterior prolapse repair with mesh. Physical examination is often all that is needed to confirm suspicion of a mesh complication, but more involved testing with a rigid sigmoidoscope may also be necessary. Figure 6.4a, b shows an example of mesh seen by an endoscope in the rectal wall. We know from the trauma literature on penetrating rectal injuries that rigid sigmoidoscopy is much more sensitive than digital rectal exam for uncovering rectal injury. This is a different population with a different mechanism of injury; however, if suspicion is high that a rectal injury occurred (or developed), digital rectal exam alone may not be adequate [109].

For cases of transvaginal excision of synthetic mesh with involvement of the rectum, the basic idea is to remove as much (if not all) of the mesh as possible and to repair any violations of the rectum. Data on surgical techniques and outcomes of mesh excision are limited to small retrospective studies. Based on the extent of the injury and comfort of the surgeon, these procedures can be done in conjunction with a colorec-

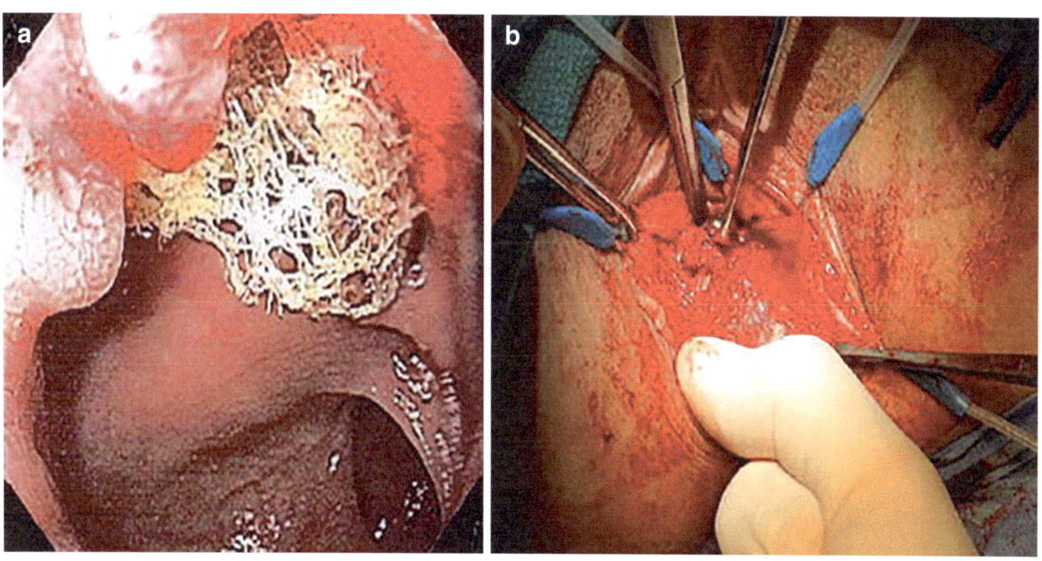

Fig. 6.4 Posterior mesh complication. (**a**) View during a sigmoidoscopy of an eroded (or misplaced) mesh visualized in the lumen of the rectal wall. (**b**) An intraoperative photo of the mesh removal via a transvaginal approach. The surgeon's finger is placed in the rectum to aid in the removal of the mesh. (Reproduced with permission from Hurtado et al. [106])

tal surgeon. A posterior midline vaginal incision is probably most common as it allows for complete exposure. The vaginal epithelium should then be dissected from the fibromuscularis laterally. The mesh should be identified, and it is useful to facilitate the initial dissection by grasping it with an instrument such as an Allis clamp. Ideally, the distal edge of the mesh is now identified and freed sharply. At this point, the mesh should be dissected off the rectovaginal septum in a cephalad direction. The use of a finger in the rectum can help the surgeon appreciate the appropriate depth of dissection as well as the area(s) of rectal violation. Furthermore, the rectal exam can identify the location of the anal sphincter. Awareness of this location allows us to avoid unnecessary sphincter injury. The mesh should be removed laterally to the pelvic sidewalls to as great an extent as possible, assuming this does not worsen the extent of the injury or potentially prevent adequate tissue from being repaired. This is often aided by incising the mesh down the middle, allowing for dissection above and below the synthetic mesh, freeing it completely. In many cases, mesh can become incorporated into the rectal submucosa or placed through the rectal mucosa, and to remove it, it may be necessary to resect a full-thickness portion of the anterior rectal wall. The defect should be closed in at least two layers in a watertight fashion. A proctoscope or other means of irrigating the rectum (i.e., a catheter) should be used to ensure that the closure is adequate. After the mesh removal and defect repair, a rectocele may be present, and this should be closed without synthetic material. The vaginal epithelium is then closed.

Bladder Injury

Bladder injury is an uncommon complication during posterior prolapse repair. A series of patients with mesh prolapse repair kits had a 1.6% intraoperative bladder injury rate [80]. The authors noted that these injuries were secondary to the trocar placement and not dissection. Another series discussed earlier of 124 patients who underwent laparoscopic sacrocolpopexy noted three bladder injuries (2.4%) [82].

If mesh is discovered in the lumen of the bowel or bladder, attempts to treat the mesh complication can be done endoscopically. This is usually done by cutting the exposed mesh and allowing the mucosa or urothelium to heal over the excised arm of the mesh. However, if this is unsuccessful, not possible, or if a more definitive approach is desired, a mesh excision with repair of the adjacent involved organ is warranted. This can be done by a transabdominal or transvaginal approach, depending on the approach of original mesh placement, the site of the mesh complication, the surgeon's skill set, and the potential need for concomitant procedures.

Summary

See Fig. 6.5 for a summary of the main complications of posterior compartment repair.

	Hemorrhage	Dyspareunia	Rectal Injury
Preoperative	Identify bleeding diathesis o Hereditary risk o Medication	Assess Function/Dysfunction o Degree of sexually activity o Future plans for sexual activity o Sexual Function questionnaires	Imaging in select cases o dynamic MRI o defecating proctogram Consider bowel prep (modified or full) Preoperative estrogen
Intraoperative	Maintain proper visualization Awareness of vasculature o Inferior gluteal artery + coccygeal branch, hypogastric and pudental venous plexi- *Vaginal approach* o Presacral venus plexus- *Abdominal approach* Reinforce staple line with hand-sewn suture- *STARR Approach* Utilize compression, packing, hemostatic matrix, absorbable hemostat, pneumoperitoneum	Avoid levator plication if possible Avoid excessive tightening of the posterior vagina and the introitus-calibrate often Consider relative contraindications to mesh use. However if utilizing mesh: o Place without excess tension, bunching or rolling o Accommodate for contracture o Avoid anchoring in muscle o Minimize trimming of vagina Reduce infection with irrigation and perioperative antibiotics	Position patient to permit digital rectal examination Identify injury early if able o Inspect posterior dissection, utilize irrigation and/or air o Palpate via rectal exam for suture or mesh If injury recognized and primary repair viable adhere to basic principles o Mobilize area o Irrigation o Two-layer closure: 1st running delayed absorbable, 2nd imbricating Lembert permanent or delayed absorbable suture
Postoperative	Recovery Room Protocol o HR, BP, UOP, inspection of incision o CBC, coagulation panel q4-6 hrs with known bleed o Vaginal packing If Bleeding Suspected o Hematoma- Hgb q6hrs o Cross-sectional imaging o Reexploration –or– IR Selective Embolization	Use Sexual Function questionnaires to identify dysfunction Conservative Measures o Topical lubricants, vaginal estrogen, topical anesthetics, anxiolyties o Physical therapy, vaginal dilators Interventions o Trigger-point injections o Botulinum toxin for vaginismus o Surgical release of tissue bands o Reconstruction for narrowing	Postoperative instructions o Bowel regimen, soft stool o 6 wks nothing per rectum Delayed Presentation of Injury o Palpate for foreign body(s) o Maintain high suspicion for perforation o Drain abscess or hematoma if found Additional Evaluation of Fistula o Anal endosonography or MRI o Colorectal specialist, draining seton, identify internal opening

This chart contains an assortment of tips and suggestions and is not meant to imply standard of care. Utilizing these thechniques does not in all cases reduce the risk of complications or improve outcome as the data remains limited.

Fig. 6.5 Summary of preoperative, interoperative, and postoperative complications and their management

References

1. Lowenstein L, Meuller ER. Posterior vaginal prolapse repair. In: Graham SDKT, editor. Glenn's urologic surgery. Lippincott Williams and Wilkins; 2010.
2. Sun G, de Haas RJ, Trzpis M, Broens PMA. A possible physiological mechanism of rectocele formation in women. Abdom Radiol. 2023;48(4):1203–14. https://doi.org/10.1007/s00261-023-03807-2.
3. Dietz HP, Gómez M, Atan IK, Ferreira CSW. Association between vaginal parity and rectocele. Int Urogynecol J. 2018;29(10):1479–83. https://doi.org/10.1007/s00192-017-3552-8.
4. Hendrix SL. Pelvic organ prolapse in the Women's Health Initiative: gravity and gravidity. Am J Obstet Gynecol. 2002;186(6):1160–6.
5. Kelvin FM, Maglinte DD, Benson JT. Evacuation proctography (defecography): an aid to the investigation of pelvic floor disorders. Obstet Gynecol. 1994;83(2):307–14.
6. Schwandner T. Transvaginal rectal repair: a new treatment option for symptomatic rectocele? Int J Color Dis. 2009;24(12):1429–34.

7. Clemons JL. Risk factors associated with an unsuccessful pessary fitting trial in women with pelvic organ prolapse. Am J Obstet Gynecol. 2004;190(2):345–50.
8. Karram M, Maher C. Surgery for posterior vaginal wall prolapse. Int Urogynecol J. 2013;24 https://doi.org/10.1007/s00192-013-2174-z.
9. Leanza V, Intagliata E, Leanza G, Cannizzaro MA, Zanghi G, Vecchio R. Surgical repair of rectocele. Comparison of transvaginal and transanal approach and personal technique. G Chir. 2014:34.
10. Wong MT, Meurette G, Rigaud J, Regenet N, Lehur PA. Robotic versus laparoscopic rectopexy for complex rectocele: a prospective comparison of short-term outcomes. Dis Colon Rectum. 2011;54 https://doi.org/10.1007/DCR.0b013e3181f4737e.
11. Rondelli F, Bugiantella W, Villa F. Robot-assisted or conventional laparoscoic rectopexy for rectal prolapse? Systematic review and meta-analysis. Int J Surg. 2014;12 https://doi.org/10.1016/j.ijsu.2014.08.359.
12. Goh JTW, Tjandra JJ, Carey MP. How could management of rectoceles be optimized? ANZ J Surg. 2002;72(12):896–901.
13. Maher C, Feiner B, Baessler K, Schmid C. Surgical management of pelvic organ prolapse in women. In: The Cochrane Collaboration, editor. Cochrane Database of Systematic Reviews. John Wiley & Sons, Ltd; 2013:CD004014.pub5. https://doi.org/10.1002/14651858.CD004014.pub5.
14. Balata M, Elgendy H, Emile SH, Youssef M, Omar W, Khafagy W. Functional outcome and sexual-related quality of life after transperineal versus transvaginal repair of anterior rectocele: a randomized clinical trial. Dis Colon Rectum. 2020;63(4):527. https://doi.org/10.1097/DCR.0000000000001595.
15. Vaughan MH, Siddiqui NY, Newcomb LK, et al. Surgical alteration of genital hiatus size and anatomic failure after vaginal vault suspension. Obstet Gynecol. 2018;131(6):1137–44. https://doi.org/10.1097/AOG.0000000000002593.
16. Bradley MS, Askew AL, Vaughan MH, Kawasaki A, Visco AG. Robotic-assisted sacrocolpopexy: early postoperative outcomes after surgical reduction of enlarged genital hiatus. Am J Obstet Gynecol. 2018;218(5):514.e1–8. https://doi.org/10.1016/j.ajog.2018.01.046.
17. High R, Kavanagh A, Khavari R, Stewart J, Antosh DD. Outcomes in pelvic organ prolapse surgery in women using chronic antithrombotic therapy. Urogynecology. 2017;23(6):372. https://doi.org/10.1097/SPV.0000000000000405.
18. Stephenson JJ. Incidence of death and recurring acute coronary syndrome after stopping clopidogrel therapy in a large commercially-insured population in the US. Curr Med Res Opin:1079–1087.
19. Hall R, Mazer CD. Antiplatelet drugs: a review of their pharmacology and management in the perioperative period. Anesth Analg. 2011;112(2):292–318.
20. Vasudeva P. Antiplatelet drugs and the perioperative period: what every urologist needs to know. Indian J Urol. 2009;25(3):296–301.
21. Trouboul C, et al. Major venous hemorrhagic complication during transvaginal cystocele repair using the transobturator approach. Obstet Gynecol. 2008;111(2):492–5.
22. Sung VW, Rardin CR, Raker CA, Lasala CA, Myers DL. Porcine subintestinal submucosal graft augmentation for rectocele repair: a randomized controlled trial. Obstet Gynecol. 2012;119 https://doi.org/10.1097/AOG.0b013e31823d407e.
23. Pahwa AK, Arya LA, Andy UU. Management of arterial and venous hemorrhage during sacrospinous ligament fixation: cases and review of the literature. Int Urogynecol J. 2016;27 https://doi.org/10.1007/s00192-015-2818-2.
24. Wang QY. New concepts in severe presacral hemorrhage during proctectomy. Arch Surg. 1985;120(9):1013–20.
25. Germanos S. Control of presacral venous bleeding during rectal surgery. Am J Surg. 2010;200(2):33–5.
26. Linder BJ, Occhino JA, Habermann EB, Glasgow AE, Bews KA, Gershman B. A national contemporary analysis of perioperative outcomes of open versus minimally invasive sacrocolpopexy. J Urol. 2018;200(4):862–7. https://doi.org/10.1016/j.juro.2018.03.131.
27. Henn EW, Nondabula T, Juul L. Effect of vaginal infiltration with ornipressin or saline on intraoperative blood loss during vaginal prolapse surgery: a randomised controlled trial. Int Urogynecol J. 2016;27(3):407–12. https://doi.org/10.1007/s00192-015-2821-7.
28. Subramanya J, Curtiss N, Balachandran A, Duckett J. Should we use a vaginal pack to reduce blood loss at the time of prolapse surgery? Eur J Obstet Gynecol Reprod Biol. 2016;206:181–3. https://doi.org/10.1016/j.ejogrb.2016.09.025.
29. Westermann LB, Crisp CC, Oakley SH, et al. To pack or not to pack? A randomized trial of vaginal packing after vaginal reconstructive surgery. Urogynecology. 2016;22(2):111. https://doi.org/10.1097/SPV.0000000000000238.
30. Karmakar D, Hayward L, Smalldridge J, Lin S. Vaginal mesh for prolapse: a long-term prospective study of 218 mesh kits from a single centre. Int Urogynecol J. 2015;26 https://doi.org/10.1007/s00192-015-2658-0.
31. Ravo B. Complications after stapled hemorrhoidectomy: can they be prevented? Tech Coloproctol. 2002;6(2):83–8.
32. Dodi G, Pietroletti R, Milito G, Binda G, Pescatori M. Bleeding, incontinence, pain and constipation after STARR transanal double stapling rectotomy for obstructed defecation. Tech Coloproctol. 2003;7 https://doi.org/10.1007/s10151-003-0026-4.
33. Harris MA, Ferrara A, Gallagher J, DeJesus S, Williamson P, Larach S. Stapled transanal rec-

tal resection vs. transvaginal rectocele repair for treatment of obstructive defecation syndrome. Dis Colon Rectum. 2009;52 https://doi.org/10.1007/DCR.0b013e31819edbb1.
34. Phillips C, Hacking N, Monga A. Super-selective angiographic embolisation of a branch of the anterior pudendal artery for the treatment of intractable post-operative bleeding. Int Urogynecol J. 2006;17(3):299–301.
35. Araco F. Selective embolization of the superior vesical artery for the treatment of a severe retroperitoneal pelvic haemorrhage following Endo-Stitch sacrospinous colpopexy. Int Urogynecol J Pelvic Floor Dysfunct. 2008;19(6):873–5.
36. Fatton B, de Tayrac R, Letouzey V, Huberlant S. Pelvic organ prolapse and sexual function. Nat Rev Urol. 2020;17(7):373–90. https://doi.org/10.1038/s41585-020-0334-8.
37. Lukacz ES, Sridhar A, Chermansky CJ, et al. Sexual activity and dyspareunia 1 year after surgical repair of pelvic organ prolapse. Obstet Gynecol. 2020;136(3):492. https://doi.org/10.1097/AOG.0000000000003992.
38. Richardson ML, Elliot CS, Sokol ER. Posterior compartment prolapse: a urogynecology perspective. Urol Clin North Am. 2012;39 https://doi.org/10.1016/j.ucl.2012.06.005.
39. Rogers RG, Kammerer-Doak D, Villarreal A, Coates K, Qualls C. A new instrument to measure sexual function in women with urinary incontinence or pelvic organ prolapse. Am J Obstet Gynecol. 2001;184 https://doi.org/10.1067/mob.2001.111100.
40. Rosen R. The Female Sexual Function Index (FSFI): a multidimensional self-report instrument for the assessment of female sexual function. J Sex Marital Ther. 2000;26(2):191–208.
41. Brandner S. Sexual function after rectocele repair. J Sex Med. 2011;8(2):583–8.
42. Jha S, Gray T. A systematic review and meta-analysis of the impact of native tissue repair for pelvic organ prolapse on sexual function. Int Urogynecol J. 2015;26 https://doi.org/10.1007/s00192-014-2518-3.
43. Colombo M, Vitobello D, Proietti F, Milani R. Randomised comparison of Burch colposuspension versus anterior colporrhaphy in women with stress urinary incontinence and anterior vaginal wall prolapse. BJOG. 2000;107 https://doi.org/10.1111/j.1471-0528.2000.tb13276.x.
44. Haase P, Skibsted L. Influence of operations for stress incontinence and/or genital descensus on sexual life. Acta Obstet Gynecol Scand. 1988;67 https://doi.org/10.3109/00016348809004283.
45. Dua A, Jha S, Farkas A, Radley S. The effect of prolapse repair on sexual function in women. J Sex Med. 2012;9 https://doi.org/10.1111/j.1743-6109.2012.02660.x.
46. Komesu YM. Posterior repair and sexual function. Am J Obstet Gynecol. 2007;197(1):101 1–6.
47. Abed H, Rahn DD, Lowenstein L. Incidence and management of graft erosion, wound granulation, and dyspareunia following vaginal prolapse repair with graft materials: a systematic review. Int Urogynecol J. 2011;22 https://doi.org/10.1007/s00192-011-1384-5.
48. Wihersaari O, Karjalainen P, Tolppanen AM, Mattsson N, Nieminen K, Jalkanen J. Sexual activity and dyspareunia after pelvic organ prolapse surgery: a 5-year nationwide follow-up study. Eur Urol Open Sci. 2022;45:81–9. https://doi.org/10.1016/j.euros.2022.09.014.
49. Nieminen K. Transanal or vaginal approach to rectocele repair: a prospective, randomized pilot study. Dis Colon Rectum. 2004;47(10):1636–42.
50. Sergent F. Mid-term outcome of laparoscopic sacrocolpopexy with anterior and posterior polyester mesh for treatment of genito-urinary prolapse. Eur J Obstetr Gynecol Reprod Biol.
51. Claerhout F. Medium-term anatomic and functional results of laparoscopic sacrocolpopexy beyond the learning curve. Eur Urol. 2009;55(6):1459–67.
52. Ulrich D, Dwyer P, Rosamilia A, Lim Y, Lee J. The effect of vaginal pelvic organ prolapse surgery on sexual function. Neurourol Urodyn. 2015;34.
53. Pancholy AB, Silva WA, Karram MM. Rectocele-anatomic and functional repair. In: Cardoza L, Staskin D, editors. Textbook of female urology and urogynocology. Informa Heathcare; 2010. p. 799–812.
54. Weber AM, Walters MD, Piedmonte MR. Sexual function and vaginal anatomy in women before and after surgery for pelvic organ prolapse and urinary incontinence. Am J Obstet Gynecol. 2000;182 https://doi.org/10.1067/mob.2000.107436.
55. Abramov Y. Site-specific rectocele repair compared with standard posterior colporrhaphy. Obstet Gynecol. 2005;105(2):314–8.
56. Schiavi MC, D'Oria O, Faiano P, et al. Vaginal native tissue repair for posterior compartment prolapse: long-term analysis of sexual function and quality of life in 151 patients. Urogynecology. 2018;24(6):419. https://doi.org/10.1097/SPV.0000000000000463.
57. Hi TAC, of O and G and the AUSUTPB is updated as. Pelvic organ prolapse. Urogynecology. 2019;25(6):397. https://doi.org/10.1097/SPV.0000000000000794.
58. Sung VW. Graft use in transvaginal pelvic organ prolapse repair: a systematic review. Obstet Gynecol. 2008;112(5):1131–42.
59. Antosh DD, Dieter AA, Balk EM, et al. Sexual function after pelvic organ prolapse surgery: a systematic review comparing different approaches to pelvic floor repair. Am J Obstet Gynecol. 2021;225(5):475.e1–475.e19. https://doi.org/10.1016/j.ajog.2021.05.042.
60. Gauruder-Burmester A. Follow-up after polypropylene mesh repair of anterior and posterior compartments in patients with recurrent

prolapse. Int Urogynecol J Pelvic Floor Dysfunct. 2007;18(9):1059–64.
61. Grimes CL, Tan-Kim J, Whitcomb EL, Lukacz ES, Menefee SA. Long-term outcomes after native tissue vs. biological graft-augmented repair in the posterior compartment. Int Urogynecol J. 2012;23 https://doi.org/10.1007/s00192-011-1607-9.
62. Paraiso MFR. Rectocele repair: a randomized trial of three surgical techniques including graft augmentation. Am J Obstet Gynecol. 2006;195(6):1762–71.
63. Yurteri-Kaplan LA, Gutman RE. The use of biological materials in urogynecologic reconstruction: a systematic review. Plast Reconstr Surg. 2012;130 https://doi.org/10.1097/PRS.0b013e31826154e4.
64. Madhu C, Cooke J, Harber P, Holmes D. Functional outcomes of posterior vaginal wall repair and prespinous colpopexy with biological small intestinal submucosal (SIS) graft. Arch Gynecol Obstet. 2014;290 https://doi.org/10.1007/s00404-014-3254-0.
65. Gomelsky A, Penson DF, Dmochowski RR. Pelvic organ prolapse (POP) surgery: the evidence for the repairs. BJU Int. 2011;107(11):1704–19.
66. Lim Y. A long-term review of posterior colporrhaphy with Vypro 2 mesh. Int Urogynecol J. 2007;18(9):1053–7.
67. Milani R. Functional and anatomical outcome of anterior and posterior vaginal prolapse repair with prolene mesh. BJOG Int J Obstet Gynaecol. 2005;112(1):107–11.
68. Grisales T, Ackerman AL, Rogo-Gupta LJ, Kwan L, Raz S, Rodriguez LV. Improvement in dyspareunia after vaginal mesh removal measured by a validated questionnaire. Int Urogynecol J. 2021;32(11):2937–46. https://doi.org/10.1007/s00192-021-04923-7.
69. Antosh DD, Gutman RE, Park AJ. Vaginal dilators for prevention of dyspareunia after prolapse surgery: a randomized controlled trial. Obstet Gynecol. 2013;121 https://doi.org/10.1097/AOG.0b013e3182932ce2.
70. Ghazizadeh S, Nikzad M. Botulinum toxin in the treatment of refractory vaginismus. Obstet Gynecol. 2004;104(5 Pt 1):922–5.
71. Hoffman MS. Injury of the rectum during vaginal surgery. Am J Obstet Gynecol. 1999;181(2):274–7.
72. Park A, Paraiso MFR. Successful use of botulinum toxin type a in the treatment of refractory postoperative dyspareunia. Obstet Gynecol. 2009;114(2 Pt 2):484–7.
73. Lefevre R, Davila GW. Functional disorders: rectocele. Clin Colon Rectal Surg. 2008;21 https://doi.org/10.1055/s-2008-1075862.
74. Maglinte DD, Bartram C. Dynamic imaging of posterior compartment pelvic floor dysfunction by evacuation proctography: techniques, indications, results and limitations. Eur J Radiol. 2007;61 https://doi.org/10.1016/j.ejrad.2006.07.031.
75. Dam JH, Gosselink MJ. Role of defecography in predicting clinical outcome of rectocele repair. Dis Colon Rectum. 1997;40 https://doi.org/10.1007/BF02054989.
76. Wallace SL, Torosis M, Rogo-Gupta L. Does rectocele on defecography equate to rectocele on physical examination in patients with defecatory symptoms? Urogynecology. 2021;27(1):18. https://doi.org/10.1097/SPV.0000000000000719.
77. Rachaneni S, Latthe P. Role of perioperative low dose vaginal oestrogens in improving the outcomes of pelvic organ prolapse surgery. Med Hypotheses. 2013;81 https://doi.org/10.1016/j.mehy.2013.09.019.
78. Tayrac R, Sentilhes L. Complications of pelvic organ prolapse surgery and methods of prevention. Int Urogynecol J. 2013;24 https://doi.org/10.1007/s00192-013-2177-9.
79. Rahn DD, Richter HE, Sung VW, Pruszynski JE, Hynan LS. Perioperative vaginal estrogen as adjunct to native tissue vaginal apical prolapse repair: a randomized clinical trial. JAMA. 2023;330(7):615–25. https://doi.org/10.1001/jama.2023.12317.
80. Abdel-fattah M, Ramsay I, Scotland Study GW. Retrospective multicentre study of the new minimally invasive mesh repair devices for pelvic organ prolapse. BJOG Int J Obstet Gynaecol. 2008;115(1):22–30.
81. Altman D. Short-term outcome after transvaginal mesh repair of pelvic organ prolapse. Int Urogynecol J. 2008;19(6):787–93.
82. Granese R. Laparoscopic sacrocolpopexy in the treatment of vaginal vault prolapse: 8 years experience. Eur J Obstet Gynecol Reprod Biol. 2009;146(2):227–31.
83. Lang P, Oliphant S, Mizell J, Austin B, Barr S. Rectal perforation at the time of vaginal mesh placement and subsequent abdominal mesh removal. Int Urogynecol J. 2015;26 https://doi.org/10.1007/s00192-015-2683-z.
84. Gagliardi G, Pescatori M, Altomare DF. Results, outcome predictors, and complications after stapled transanal rectal resection for obstructed defecation. Dis Colon Rectum. 2008;51 https://doi.org/10.1007/s10350-007-9096-0.
85. Ripamonti L, Guttadauro A, Lo Bianco G, et al. Stapled Transanal rectal resection (Starr) in the treatment of obstructed defecation: a systematic review. Front Surg. 2022;9 https://doi.org/10.3389/fsurg.2022.790287.
86. Hilger W, Cornella J. Rectovaginal fistula after Posterior Intravaginal Slingplasty and polypropylene mesh augmented rectocele repair. Int Urogynecol J Pelvic Floor Dysfunct. 2006;17(1):89–92.
87. Choi JM, Nguyen V, Khavari R, Reeves K, Snyder M, Fletcher SG. Complex rectovaginal fistulas after pelvic organ prolapse repair with synthetic mesh: a multidisciplinary approach to evaluation and management. Female Pelvic Med Reconstr Surg. 2012;18 https://doi.org/10.1097/SPV.0b013e318270ae15.
88. Israel BL, Gary MC, Shirley WJ, Longo W. Utility of magnetic resonance imaging in anorectal dis-

ease. World J Gastroenterol. 2007;13 https://doi.org/10.3748/wjg.v13.i23.3153.
89. Buchanan G, Halligan S, Bartram CI, Williams AB, Tarroni D, Cohen CRG. Clinical examination, endosonography, and MR imaging in preoperative assessment of fistula in Ano: comparison with outcome-based reference standard. Radiology. 2004;233 https://doi.org/10.1148/radiol.2333031724.
90. Tonolini M. Elucidating vaginal fistulas on CT and MRI. Insights Imaging. 2019;10(1):123. https://doi.org/10.1186/s13244-019-0812-9.
91. Abou-Zeid AA. Anal fistula: intraoperative difficulties and unexpected findings. World J Gastroenterol. 2011;17 https://doi.org/10.3748/wjg.v17.i28.3272.
92. Evans SKL, Abimbola O, Myers EM, Tarr ME. A novel injection technique for extended-release local anesthetic after posterior colporrhaphy and perineorrhaphy: a randomized controlled study. Urogynecology. 2021;27(6):344. https://doi.org/10.1097/SPV.0000000000000855.
93. Jones CL, Gruber DD, Fischer JR, Leonard K, Hernandez SL. Liposomal bupivacaine efficacy for postoperative pain following posterior vaginal surgery: a randomized, double-blind, placebo-controlled trial. Am J Obstet Gynecol. 2018;219(5):500.e1–8. https://doi.org/10.1016/j.ajog.2018.09.029.
94. Kaeser CT, Rothenberger R, Zoorob D, Whiteside JL. Bupivacaine use after posterior Colporrhaphy to reduce postoperative pain: a multicenter, double-blinded, placebo-controlled, randomized clinical trial. Urogynecology. 2022;28(2):72. https://doi.org/10.1097/SPV.0000000000001082.
95. Dengler KL, Craig ER, DiCarlo-Meacham AM, et al. Preoperative pudendal block with liposomal and plain bupivacaine reduces pain associated with posterior colporrhaphy: a double-blinded, randomized controlled trial. Am J Obstet Gynecol. 2021;225(5):556.e1–556.e10. https://doi.org/10.1016/j.ajog.2021.08.034.
96. Torosis M, Fullerton M, Kaefer D, Nitti V, Ackerman AL, Grisales T. Pudendal block at the time of transvaginal prolapse repair: a randomized controlled trial. Urogynecology. 2024;30(8):706. https://doi.org/10.1097/SPV.0000000000001448.
97. Book NM, Novi B, Novi JM, Pulvino JQ. Postoperative voiding dysfunction following posterior colporrhaphy. Urogynecology. 2012;18(1):32. https://doi.org/10.1097/SPV.0b013e31824041a4.
98. Yadav M, Patel K, Turrentine MA, Orejuela F, Jackson E, Kilpatrick C. Postoperative pain and urinary retention after vaginal reconstructive surgery. Urogynecology. 2021;27(3):e497. https://doi.org/10.1097/SPV.0000000000001019.
99. Woodbury CF, Coughlin AC, Dubois B, Romanova A. Prevention of postoperative constipation in urogynecology patients: a systematic review. Urogynecology. 2023;29(2):175. https://doi.org/10.1097/SPV.0000000000001281.
100. Latthe P, Panza J, Marquini GV, et al. AUGS-IUGA joint clinical consensus statement on enhanced recovery after urogynecologic surgery. Urogynecology. 2022;28(11):716. https://doi.org/10.1097/SPV.0000000000001252.
101. Mörlin V, Golmann D, Borgfeldt C, Bergman I. Antibiotic prophylaxis in posterior colporrhaphy does not reduce postoperative infection: a nationwide observational cohort study. Int Urogynecol J. 2023;34(11):2791–7. https://doi.org/10.1007/s00192-023-05617-y.
102. Haylen BT, de Ridder D, Freeman RM, et al. An International Urogynecological Association (IUGA)/International Continence Society (ICS) joint report on the terminology for female pelvic floor dysfunction. Neurourol Urodyn. 2010;29(1):4–20. https://doi.org/10.1002/nau.20798.
103. Deng T, Liao B, Luo D, Shen H, Wang K. Risk factors for mesh erosion after female pelvic floor reconstructive surgery: a systematic review and meta-analysis. BJU Int. 2016:117. https://doi.org/10.1111/bju.13158.
104. Dwyer P, O'Reilly B. Transvaginal repair of anterior and posterior compartment prolapse with Atrium polypropylene mesh. BJOG. 2004;111(8):831–6.
105. Gillor M, Langer S, Dietz HP. Long-term subjective, clinical and sonographic outcomes after native-tissue and mesh-augmented posterior colporrhaphy. Int Urogynecol J. 2019;30(9):1581–5. https://doi.org/10.1007/s00192-019-03921-0.
106. Hurtado E, Bailey HR, Reeves K. Rectal erosion of synthetic mesh used in posterior colporrhaphy requiring surgical removal. Int Urogynecol J Pelvic Floor Dysfunct. 2007;18(12):1499–501.
107. Sullivan ES, Longaker CJ, Lee PY. Total pelvic mesh repair: a ten-year experience. Dis Colon Rectum. 2001;44(6):857–63.
108. Ferry P, Sedille L, Roncheau V. Rectal mesh exposure after laparoscopic sacrocolpopexy. J Minim Invasive Gynecol. 2014:21. https://doi.org/10.1016/j.jmig.2013.09.005.
109. Hargraves MB. Injury location dictates utility of digital rectal examination and rigid sigmoidoscopy in the evaluation of penetrating rectal trauma. Am Surg. 2009;75(11):1069–72.

7 Uterosacral Ligament Suspension

Kamran P. Sajadi and Sandip P. Vasavada

Introduction

Uterosacral ligament vaginal vault suspension (USVVS) is one of the most common native-tissue transvaginal apical suspensions and offers a minimally invasive alternative to sacrocolpopexy in selected patients. Nonetheless, as with any major surgical procedure, there are complications specific to this approach. Complications common among all reconstructive pelvic surgeries—including urinary tract infection, wound infection, venous thrombosis, and position-related neuropraxias—are discussed elsewhere. We focus on major complications related to USVVS including hemorrhage, ureteral injury or obstruction, bowel injury, and peripheral nerve injuries specific to this approach.

Hemorrhage

The incidence of hemorrhage requiring blood transfusion during USVVS is 1.3–1.6% [1, 2]. Prompt attention to bleeding is necessary because this procedure is intraperitoneal, and therefore it can be difficult to control by tamponade alone. When bleeding is encountered during USVVS, it is important to remember that the most common sources may be the uterine vessels if a concomitant vaginal hysterectomy was performed. For this reason, leaving long suture tags on the pedicles for easy retrieval and examination can be invaluable. The distal uterosacral ligament lies close to the uterine vessels, close to the ureter, and is the weakest part of the ligament; and therefore targeting suspension sutures toward the middle or proximal uterosacral ligament is the best approach. Minor to moderate bleeding from the placement of the uterosacral ligament suture can be controlled by applying tension to the suture until the end of the operation, at which point it can be tied down to stop the bleeding. If bleeding is more significant or hematoma starts to form in the adjacent peritoneal tissues, consideration should be given to tying the sutures down. This may then occlude the bleeding point and prevent expansion of a hematoma and control bleeding.

Ureteral Injury and Obstruction

Ureteral obstruction from USVVS usually results from kinking of the ureter during plication of the uterosacral ligament to the vaginal cuff and, less commonly, direct ureteral suture injury. The distal uterosacral ligament is intimately involved

K. P. Sajadi
Department of Urology, Oregon Health and Science University, CH10U, Portland, OR, USA

S. P. Vasavada (✉)
Glickman Urological & Kidney Institute, Cleveland Clinic, Cleveland, OH, USA
e-mail: vasavas@ccf.org

H. B. Goldman, J. Zillioux (eds.), *Complications of Urogynecology and Reconstructive Pelvic Surgery*, https://doi.org/10.1007/978-3-032-00339-3_7

with the cardinal ligament—which contains the uterine vessels—and lies in close proximity to the ureter. Anatomic studies of the ligament demonstrate that the middle and proximal segments may be ideal for use in apical suspension, with the mean ± SD distance from the ureter 0.9 ± 0.4 cm distally, 2.3 ± 0.9 cm in the middle segment, and 4.1 ± 0.6 cm proximally (Fig. 7.1) [3]. Ureteral kinking is minimized by placing sutures from lateral to medial, which is away from the ureter [4]. Patient demographics and the number and type of suture used have not been shown to predict ureteral kinking [1, 5], but the use of a suture placement device may be protective against ureteral obstruction [5]. Obstruction can occur in up to 11% of procedures [6], but the incidence is markedly reduced by performing cystoscopy at the conclusion of the procedure. With intraoperative cystoscopy, the contemporary incidence of intraoperative ureteral kinking is 3.2–4.5% [1, 7], and postoperatively identified (i.e., not detected by intraoperative cystoscopy) ureteral obstruction is 0.5% [1]. Historically, indigo carmine or sodium fluorescein is injected intravenously, and cystoscopy is performed to visualize efflux of dye from each ureter. If a strong ureteral jet is seen from both sides after the vault suspension has been completed, then ureteral obstruction is unlikely. In the United States, indigo carmine has limited availability, but a few alternatives exist [8]. In our experience, methylene blue takes too long to be excreted once administered and has risks of drug interactions with several classes of drugs patients may be taking. Preoperative oral phenazopyridine can be administered; however, this requires preoperative planning. We prefer to use sodium fluorescein (10% solution, 0.25–1 mL IV), which produces rapid excretion of a bright, neon-yellow efflux that is easy to visualize (Fig. 7.2c) [9]. Anecdotally, one should readily visualize the ureteric orifices first before sodium fluorescein administration as the cystoscopic field will quickly become opacified with the neon-yellow

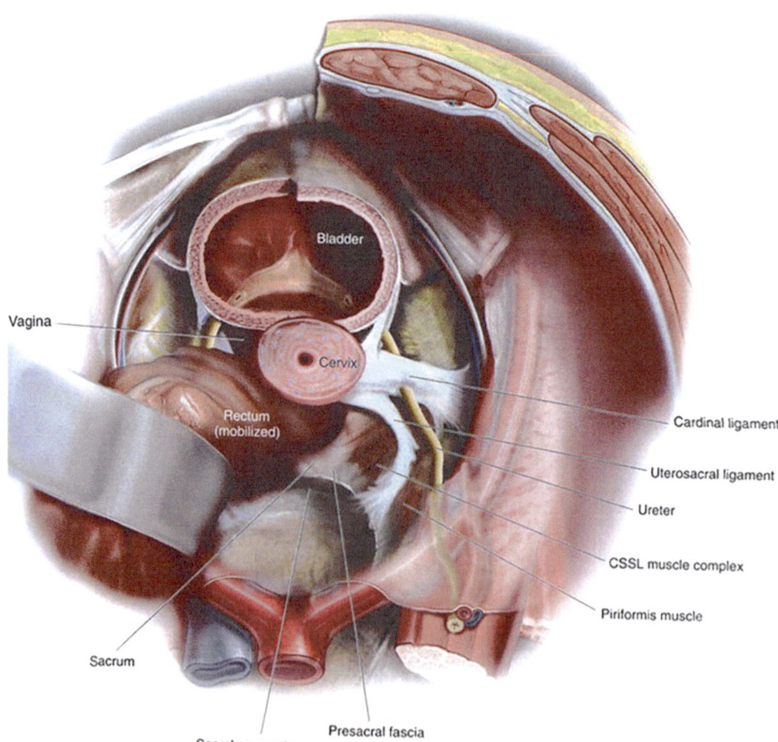

Fig. 7.1 Abdominal view illustrating the relationship between the ureter and the uterosacral ligament. Proceeding cephalad, the uterosacral ligament proceeds medially while the ureter proceeds laterally. Vault suspension to the proximal third and therefore has the lowest rate of ureteral obstruction. (Used with permission of Elsevier from Vaginal Repair of Vaginal Vault Prolapse. In: Baggish MS, Karram MM: Atlas of pelvic anatomy and gynecologic surgery, 3rd ed. Philadelphia: Elsevier Saunders; 2011;709)

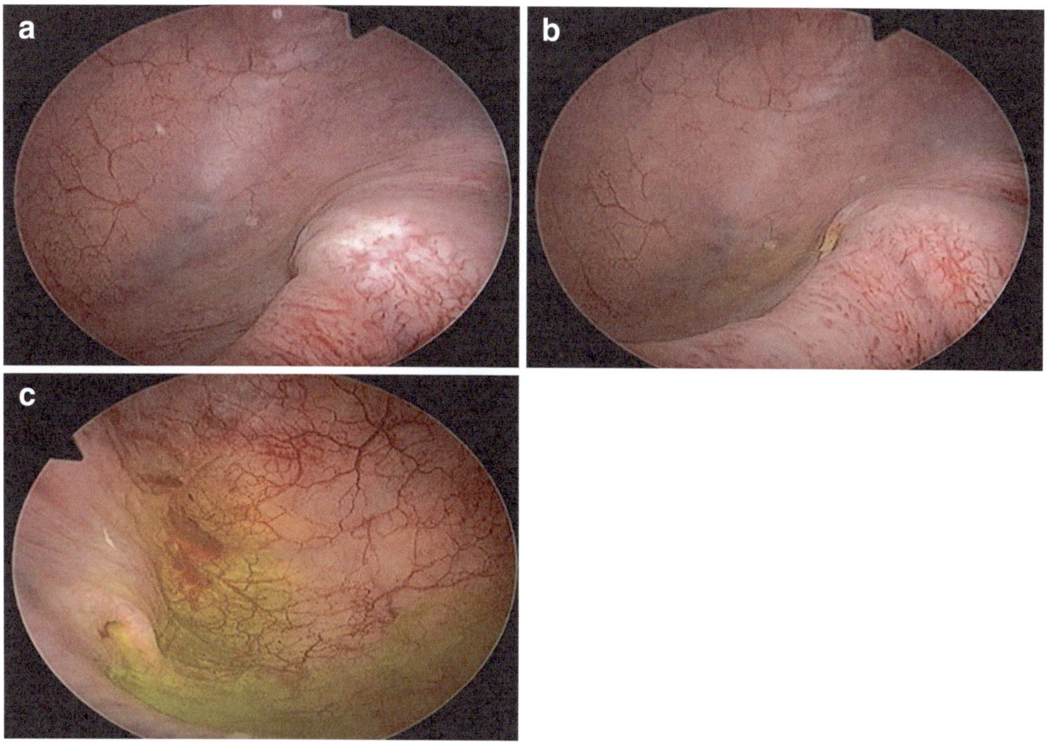

Fig. 7.2 (**a**) Cystoscopic view of the right ureteral orifice. (**b**) Following IV administration of sodium fluorescein, brisk efflux of neon-yellow urine occurs, indicating ureteral patency. (**c**) Within minutes of administration, efflux from the contralateral ureteral begins to discolor the entire bladder contents

efflux and make further identification of the ureteric orifices challenging. A study of hysterectomies showed that cystoscopy is cost-effective when the rate of injury is at least 2% [10], and intraoperative as opposed to postoperative diagnosis of ureteral obstruction substantially reduces morbidity [11]. Indigo carmine dye has recently been reintroduced into the market and many may transition back to it as it has some favorable characteristics including less staining, and more rapid time to efflux [8].

Ureteral Obstruction: Intraoperative Presentation

When there is no efflux from one or both sides, it is important to have a clear plan and algorithm in place for diagnosis and management (Fig. 7.3). First, consider the patient scenario. Reevaluate the patient's history to consider if she has had a prior nephrectomy or ureteral reimplant; in the latter case, the ureter may efflux from a different position. If the patient has had any previous abdominal imaging, it can be helpful in identifying the occasional case of a prior nephrectomy or congenital absence of the ipsilateral kidney.

In addition, confirm the time of administration of sodium fluorescein with the anesthesiologist or nurse, as early delivery may mean that all dye has been excreted. Many different maneuvers have been attempted to promote more rapid excretion of the dye. Most commonly, ensuring adequate hydration by the anesthetist and/or administrating a diuretic such as furosemide may promote more rapid renal excretion of sodium fluoroscein. Resuming a level position or reverse Trendelenburg to encourage gravitational drain-

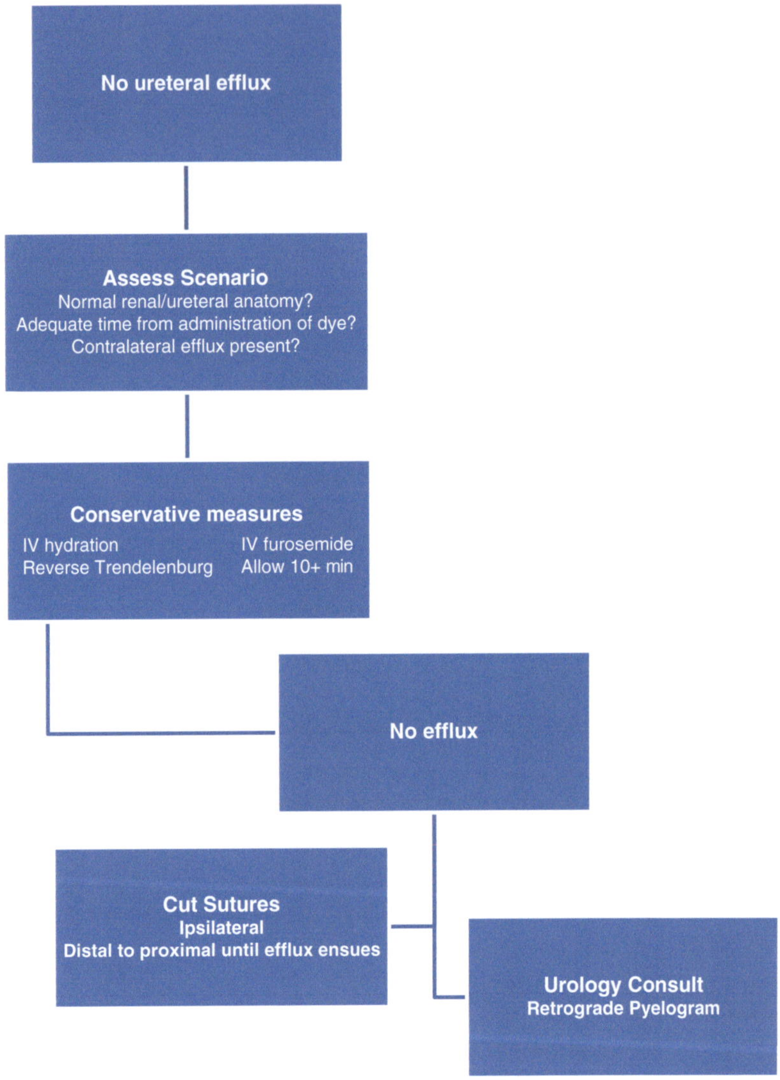

Fig. 7.3 Algorithm for evaluation and management when ureteral efflux is not seen cystoscopically following USVVS

age has also been performed although these reports are anecdotal. Once sufficient time has passed to confirm a lack of excretion from one or both sides, there are a few ways to proceed. One option is to cut the more distal (i.e., more lateral) uterosacral plication suture (the uterosacral ligament is closest to the ureter distally) out of the vaginal cuff, and observe if efflux then occurs. With an assistant, it is possible to cut this suture while the cystoscope is still in place. If this suture was the cause, brisk efflux will usually immediately ensue and most pelvic reconstructive surgeons would not attempt to replace the suture in this situation because replacing or not replacing those sutures does not seem to affect the rate of prolapse recurrence [1]. If efflux does not ensue, remove the remaining sutures on that side, one at a time, proceeding from the most lateral and caudal to the most medial and cranial. It is important to remember, however, that if a concomitant anterior colporrhaphy was performed, that procedure also carries a risk of ureteral obstruction, and it may be prudent to remove those sutures although the rate of ureteral kinking with USVVS is higher than from anterior colporrhaphy [5].

Occasionally, there will still be a lack of efflux even after the removal of all potentially offending sutures. If the patient lacks preoperative upper urinary tract imaging or sufficient historical reason to explain the lack of efflux, urologic consultation is indicated. The most common obstacle to performing retrograde ureterography in such cases is that these patients are often not positioned appropriately on the bed or on an appropriate operative table for pelvic fluoroscopy. Therefore, many urologists will attempt blind passage of a wire or ureteral catheter into the ureter to assure patency. If this is done, a flexible-tipped, soft hydrophilic wire should be used, and even then, there is a risk of converting a ureteral kink or obstruction into a ureteral perforation. Making the extra effort to obtain a C-arm and repositioning the patient can significantly improve patient safety. With retrograde ureteropyelography, the urologist can accurately assess the patency of the ureter and make a decision whether or not a stent should be placed. If there is a suspicion of injury and a stent can be passed, it should be left in place for a minimum of 4–6 weeks [11].

Ureteral Obstruction: Postoperative Presentation

Ureteral injury is a potential complication of uterosacral colpopexy even when intraoperative cystoscopy reveals bilateral ureteral efflux. The so-called delayed obstruction may occur due to excessive scarring between the uterosacral plication and the distal ureter, due to compromise of the ureteral blood supply or perhaps because of inadequate intraoperative examination for efflux. Ureteral obstruction presents in the acute postoperative period with flank pain, nausea, vomiting, and potentially fever. The diagnosis should be confirmed with imaging, and the study of choice in patients with normal renal function is CT Urography (CTU, see Fig. 7.4c). The severity of hydronephrosis, site of ureteral obstruction, presence and location of any extravasation, presence or size of a potential urinoma, and the status of the contralateral kidney can all be assessed with a CTU. Once identified, in the acute postoperative period (up to 7 days), cutting the offending colpopexy sutures may be sufficient to relieve the obstruction. It is usually ideal to perform this in the operating room for several reasons. Aside from patient comfort, under anesthesia cystoscopy and retrograde ureteropyelography can be performed at the same time to confirm patency of the ureter following removal of the suture(s). In addition, given the potential for ureteral edema and the severity of the obstruction, many urologists would choose to place an indwelling ureteral stent after relief of the obstruction. With further delay in presentation or failure to unobstruct in this manner, open abdominal or laparoscopic ureterolysis and reimplant are often necessary, although transvaginal ureterolysis and retrograde stenting has also been reported [12]. In a meta-analysis of USVVS, there was a 1.8%

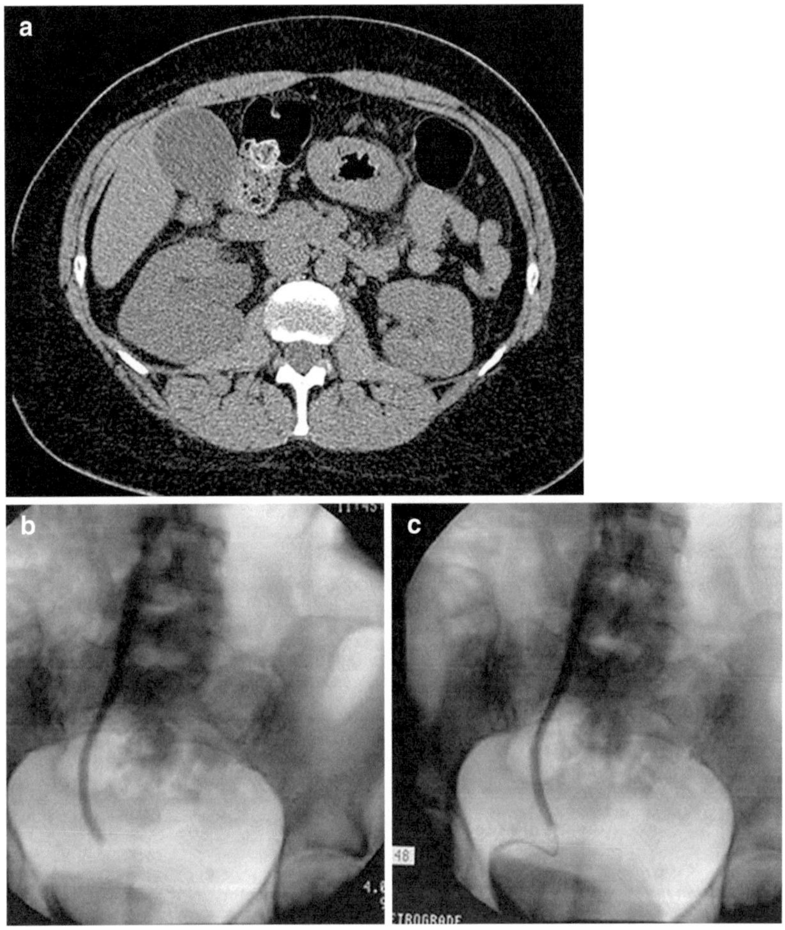

Fig. 7.4 (**a**) A woman with postoperative suspicion of ureteral injury is found to have right hydronephrosis on a CT. (**b**) Right retrograde ureterography demonstrates medial deviation of the distal ureter, and the distal ureter is not opacified. (**c**) A wire was successfully passed, over which a stent was then placed. (Courtesy of Howard Goldman, MD, Cleveland Clinic, OH)

rate of ureteral obstruction, of which 2/3 resolved with suture removal, and the remainder required ureteral reimplantation [2].

Bowel Injury

Despite the intraperitoneal nature of the operation, bowel injury is rare with USVVS and is reported in less than 1% of cases [1, 2]. Small bowel obstruction (SBO) is very rare and was first reported in a series in 2007 [13]. Three patients presented with significant nausea and vomiting on postoperative days 1–14 and were found to have possible SBO [13]. After failing conservative management, all subsequently underwent laparoscopy, and the source of the obstruction was adhesions in two of the patients, and a polypropylene suture in the third. One of the patients required significant adhesiolysis and underwent small bowel resection and enteroenterostomy due to enterotomies during dissection. SBO is more likely with known abdominal and pelvic adhesions or history of endometriosis [1]. Careful attention to surgical technique helps maintain a very low rate of SBO or bowel low. When exposing the uterosacral ligaments, packing of the bowel with tagged, counted laparotomy sponges is usually necessary. The peritoneum should be carefully inspected for abdominal adhesions, the sponges advanced slowly and gently to avoid enterotomies, and gentle retraction on the sponges to minimize trauma. Similarly, these packs should be removed slowly and carefully, and counted, after placing suspension sutures. If performing culdoplasty, care in closing the peritoneum can avoid capturing bowel in the closure and keeping the patient in the Trendelenberg position during this maneuver.

Evisceration

Small bowel evisceration has been reported following vaginal hysterectomy [14, 15]. Evisceration is a surgical emergency, and although some have had success through a transvaginal route alone, usually a transabdominal route is helpful to assess the viability of the small bowel involved [16].

Neurologic and Pain Complications

The intraperitoneal nature of this operation makes direct visualization of retroperitoneal vasculature and nerves difficult, and therefore a thorough anatomic understanding is necessary.

Assessing the position of the ischial spine allows avoidance of the pudendal nerve, which is usually sufficiently far from the uterosacral ligaments [17]. The sacral nerve routes are closer and more susceptible to injury during USVVS. A cadaveric study demonstrated that by tenting the uterosacral ligaments distally and ventrally using an Allis clamp before suture placement, the sacral nerve roots can be avoided [17]. Although tension on the ligament is also distributed to the ureter, this effect is seen most dramatically distally and can be avoided by proximal suture placement [3]. The sacral nerve roots as well as the intrapelvic portion of the sciatic nerve are vulnerable to entrapment during uterosacral suspension, which can explain postoperative pain in some patients [18]. Sensory neuropathies in the S1–S4 distribution have been reported in 1.1–3.8% of patients, but weakness has also been reported [1, 19, 20]. Pain tends to present in the acute postoperative period, in the distribution of the S1 through S4 nerve roots, with a sharp, stabbing pain in the buttock, perineum, and or lower extremity in a dermatomal distribution [19, 21, 22]. Nerve entrapment pain is more common on the right side, which is thought to be due to a predominance of right-handed surgeons, or a relative protective effect of the rectosigmoid junction on the left [17, 19, 21]. Medical management consists of nonsteroidal anti-inflammatories, narcotic pain management, and/or neuromodulating agents such as gabapentin or amitriptyline, and adjuncts can include physical therapy [21]. When conservative measures fail, removal of the ipsilateral sutures is indicated and often causes precipitous relief [21]. Similarly, when pain is severe and abruptly presents upon awakening from surgery or in the recovery room, the sutures on the side of pain should be removed promptly in the operating room [22]. With the appropriate management, neurologic symptoms usually resolve within 12 weeks [1, 19, 21, 22].

Summary

USVVS is a minimally invasive prolapse repair that carries specific risks. Minimize the risk of ureteral kinking by suture placement proximal on the ligament, from lateral to medial, but cystoscopy should be performed regardless to confirm ureteral patency. Less than 2% of cases require blood transfusion, and most minor bleeding resolves with tying suspension sutures. SBO occurs <1% of the time, usually due to adhesive disease. Manual tenting of the ligament can help avoid injury to sacral nerve roots. The incidence of postoperative neuropathies is <4%, and most resolve with conservative measures or suture removal.

References

1. Unger CA, Walters MD, Ridgeway B, Jelovsek JE, Barber MD, Paraiso MF. Incidence of adverse events after uterosacral colpopexy for uterovaginal and posthysterectomy vault prolapse. Am J Obstet Gynecol. 2015;212(5):603.e1–e7.
2. Margulies RU, Rogers MA, Morgan DM. Outcomes of transvaginal uterosacral ligament suspension: systematic review and metaanalysis. Am J Obstet Gynecol. 2010;202(2):124–34.
3. Buller JL, Thompson JR, Cundiff GW, Krueger Sullivan L, Schon Ybarra MA, Bent AE. Uterosacral ligament: description of anatomic relationships to optimize surgical safety. Obstet Gynecol. 2001;97(6):873–9.
4. Wieslander CK, Roshanravan SM, Wai CY, Schaffer JI, Corton MM. Uterosacral ligament suspension sutures: anatomic relationships in unembalmed female cadavers. Am J Obstet Gynecol. 2007;197(6):672.e1–e6.

5. Jackson E, Bilbao JA, Vera RW, Mulla ZD, Mallett VT, Montoya TI. Risk factors for ureteral occlusion during transvaginal uterosacral ligament suspension. Int Urogynecol J. 2015;26(12):1809–14.
6. Gustilo-Ashby AM, Jelovsek JE, Barber MD, Yoo EH, Paraiso MF, Walters MD. The incidence of ureteral obstruction and the value of intraoperative cystoscopy during vaginal surgery for pelvic organ prolapse. Am J Obstet Gynecol. 2006;194(5):1478–85.
7. Barber MD, Brubaker L, Burgio KL, et al. Comparison of 2 transvaginal surgical approaches and perioperative behavioral therapy for apical vaginal prolapse: the OPTIMAL randomized trial. JAMA. 2014;311(10):1023–34.
8. Lepor H, et al. A randomized clinical trial evaluating indigo carmine as a visualization aid for evaluating ureteral patency. Urology. 2024;184:105–11.
9. Doyle PJ, Lipetskaia L, Duecy E, Buchsbaum G, Wood RW. Sodium fluorescein use during intraoperative cystoscopy. Obstet Gynecol. 2015;125(3):548–50.
10. Visco AG, Taber KH, Weidner AC, Barber MD, Myers ER. Cost-effectiveness of universal cystoscopy to identify ureteral injury at hysterectomy. Obstet Gynecol. 2001;97(5 Pt 1):685–92.
11. Kim JH, Moore C, Jones JS, et al. Management of ureteral injuries associated with vaginal surgery for pelvic organ prolapse. Int Urogynecol J Pelvic Floor Dysfunct. 2006;17(5):531–5.
12. Siddighi S, Yandell PM, Karram MM. Delayed presentation of complete ureteral obstruction deligated transvaginally. Int Urogynecol J. 2011;22(2):251–3.
13. Ridgeway B, Barber MD, Walters MD, Paraiso MF. Small bowel obstruction after vaginal vault suspension: a series of three cases. Int Urogynecol J Pelvic Floor Dysfunct. 2007;18(10):1237–41.
14. Patravali N, Kulkarni T. Bowel evisceration through the vaginal vault: a delayed complication following hysterectomy. J Obstet Gynaecol. 2007;27(2):211.
15. Moen MD, Desai M, Sulkowski R. Vaginal evisceration managed by transvaginal bowel resection and vaginal repair. Int Urogynecol J Pelvic Floor Dysfunct. 2003;14(3):218–20.
16. Rollinson D, Brodman ML, Friedman F Jr, Sperling R. Transvaginal small-bowel evisceration: a case report. Mt Sinai J Med. 1995;62(3):235–8.
17. Siddiqui NY, Mitchell TR, Bentley RC, Weidner AC. Neural entrapment during uterosacral ligament suspension: an anatomic study of female cadavers. Obstet Gynecol. 2010;116(3):708–13.
18. Schon Ybarra MA, Gutman RE, Rini D, Handa VL. Etiology of post-uterosacral suspension neuropathies. Int Urogynecol J Pelvic Floor Dysfunct. 2009;20(9):1067–71.
19. Flynn MK, Weidner AC, Amundsen CL. Sensory nerve injury after uterosacral ligament suspension. Am J Obstet Gynecol. 2006;195(6):1869–72.
20. Chung CP, Kuehl TJ, Harris SK, et al. Incidence and risk factors of postoperative urinary tract infection after uterosacral ligament suspension. Int Urogynecol J. 2012;23(7):947–50.
21. Montoya TI, Luebbehusen HI, Schaffer JI, Wai CY, Rahn DD, Corton MM. Sensory neuropathy following suspension of the vaginal apex to the proximal uterosacral ligaments. Int Urogynecol J. 2012;23(12):1735–40.
22. Lowenstein L, Dooley Y, Kenton K, Mueller E, Brubaker L. Neural pain after uterosacral ligament vaginal suspension. Int Urogynecol J Pelvic Floor Dysfunct. 2007;18(1):109–10.

8 Sacrospinous Ligament Fixation

Marcelo Mass Lindenbaum
and Javier Pizarro-Berdichevsky

Introduction

Apical prolapse poses a significant challenge for pelvic reconstructive surgeons. Accurate diagnosis and proper management of apical prolapse are crucial for minimizing the risk of recurrent symptoms in women with multi-compartment prolapse. Abdominal sacrocolpopexy, uterosacral vault suspension, iliococcygeus vault suspension, and sacrospinous ligament fixation (SSLF) are well accepted techniques for the treatment of apical prolapse. Despite the wide availability of traditional and robotic-assisted laparoscopic techniques to minimize the morbidity of transabdominal repair, transvaginal approaches predominate, accounting for 80–90% of pelvic organ prolapse corrective surgeries worldwide [1, 2].

Compared with transabdominal approaches, uterosacral vault suspension, Iliococcygeus fixation, and SSLF are all viable options due to their ease of access, reduced morbidity, recovery times, hospital stay, and suitability for a broader range of ages, health statuses, and surgical histories.

SSLF is a minimally invasive, extraperitoneal technique that can be done with the uterus in situ or post-hysterectomy. Fixation can be performed unilaterally or bilaterally, via either an anterior or posterior approach, with direct suture placement with a curved needle drive, Deschamps needles, Miya hook, Capio, or tackers as Anchorsure, Splentis, among others, at the same time mesh augmentation could be used. The advantages of SSLF include the preservation of vaginal length and width, and the extraperitoneal nature of the procedure minimizes the risk of direct bowel injury and enhances the efficacy of hemostatic maneuvers in the setting of significant bleeding. The main possible disadvantages of this approach include the technical complexity of identifying the anatomical landmarks of the sacrospinous ligament and the posterior deviation of the vaginal axis, which may contribute to the recurrence of anterior prolapse and could be associated with dyspareunia.

The most common practice is to perform a unilateral, right-sided fixation via a posterior approach without mesh. Unilateral fixation offers comparable efficacy to bilateral, and right-sided procedures reduce the risk of indirect bowel injury by alleviating the need to retract the sigmoid colon to visualize the left ligament. The

M. M. Lindenbaum
Glickman Urological Institute, Cleveland Clinic Foundation, Cleveland, OH, USA

J. Pizarro-Berdichevsky (✉)
Centro de Innovación en Piso Pélvico, Sótero del Rio Hospital, Santiago, Chile

Corporación de Innovación en Piso Pélvico, Santiago, Chile

Gynecology Department, Pontificia Universidad Católica de Chile, Santiago, Chile

H. B. Goldman, J. Zillioux (eds.), *Complications of Urogynecology and Reconstructive Pelvic Surgery*, https://doi.org/10.1007/978-3-032-00339-3_8

overall rate of complications associated with SSLF reported in the literature ranges from 2.3 to 16.7% though serious complications comprise only a small fraction of these [2].

Intraoperative and postoperative complications can often be avoided with a thorough understanding of relevant anatomy, meticulous dissection, and suspension suture placement.

Hemorrhage

Because of the anatomic location of the sacrospinous ligament, SSLF poses a greater bleeding risk compared to other transvaginal procedures. The sacrospinous ligament stretches from the ischial spine to the sacrum, forming the inferior border of the greater sciatic foramen. The piriformis muscle, superior and inferior gluteal vessels, and internal pudendal vessels all pass through this foramen. The gluteal vessels and sciatic nerve are near the proximal aspect of the ligament, while the pudendal neurovascular bundle runs immediately inferior and medial to the distal aspect.

Despite the proximity to several major vascular structures, most cases reported in the literature are associated with moderate blood loss. In five randomized controlled trials (RCTs) comparing SSLF with other procedures for vault prolapse, the mean blood loss reported in the literature for SSLF was 59.7–448 mL [2–5]. The reported rate of transfusion is 0.7–3% [2, 5–7], with no statistically significant difference between the type of procedure [2].

A recent meta-analysis compared the rate of hematomas in SSLF compared to other procedures and found no statistically significant differences (RR 0.7 95% CI 0.17, 2.92) [8].

The best first step in mitigating the risk of clinically significant blood loss is establishing the optimal dissection plane, as significant bleeding can occur in the setting of an aberrant dissection plane. Hydrodissection with a vasoconstrictive agent may help delineate the optimal plane between the vaginal epithelium and muscularis, while also offering hemostasis during dissection. This enhances visualization and avoidance of inadvertent injury to adjacent structures. When significant bleeding is noted during dissection, this is often due to the interruption of small venous plexuses in the vagina.

In such cases, vaginal packing should be applied and held in place for 3–5 min for tamponade. The extraperitoneal nature of the dissection should allow for significant slowing of the hemorrhage with this maneuver. Subsequently, the packing can be systematically removed to facilitate cauterization and placement of hemostatic sutures or clips as needed. Correction of the plane of dissection should be undertaken as soon as adequate hemostasis is obtained. Optimization of suspension suture/anchors placement is also imperative to avoid significant bleeding. To avoid vascular injury, suspension sutures/anchors should be placed in the medial aspect of the ligament, approximately 2 cm medial to the ischial spine, at a depth that only includes the ligament, as many vessels run deep to the underlying iliococcygeus muscle. Sutures can be placed either under direct visualization or by palpating the ligament, using a needle driver or a suture passing device (i.e., Capio device, Deschamps ligature carrier, Miya hook ligature carrier, Anchorsure, Splentis, among others). In retrospective and prospective series comparing complications associated with traditional direct vision suspension suture placement vs. placement guided by palpation and use of a suture passing device, there were no statistically significant differences in rates of transfusion or postoperative hematoma [9, 10].

The selection of surgical approach should be guided by the surgeon comfort and experience. When significant bleeding is encountered with suture placement, optimizing visualization is crucial for achieving timely vascular control. Handheld retractors should be used to establish proper exposure of the bleeding vessels and adjacent structures and facilitate precise placement of hemostatic sutures and clips.

It is important to note that the posterior approach could allow for better exposure in this setting than the anterior approach. If visualization remains poor after maximizing exposure with retractors, due to brisk bleeding, firm vaginal packing can be a very effective step to temporarily slow blood loss and allow for gradual inspection of the surgical field. Additionally, application of topical hemostatic agents (i.e., fibrin sealants, thrombin, gel matrix) can also be helpful in establishing hemostasis and improving visualization. Maintaining an open communication with the anesthesia team regarding the magnitude of blood loss is vital to ensure timely laboratory testing and volume resuscitation. If adequate hemostasis cannot be obtained vaginally and major vascular injury is suspected, selective embolization in collaboration with Interventional Radiology should be considered. Vessels can be controlled in this manner without risk to adjacent neural structures.

Urinary Tract Injury

SSLF itself is rarely associated with urinary tract injury; however, the risk is increased when performing a concomitant surgery (i.e., hysterectomy, anterior or posterior repair, mid urethral sling), which is performed in 59–91% of cases [2, 4, 5, 9–11]. In an early systematic review of 17 studies of SSLF outcomes, including 1080 patients, the rate of cystotomy or bladder laceration was 0.3% [6].

Several large contemporary series, describing a variety of approaches, have reported no bladder injury rates unless SSLF is performed with concomitant synthetic mid-urethral sling [5, 9, 11–13]. Ureteral injury is similarly rare. There were no ureteral injuries observed in an RCT of 208 women receiving sacrospinous hysteropexy vs. vaginal hysterectomy with uterosacral ligament fixation [4]. Similarly, no ureteral injuries were observed among 240 women undergoing suspension suture placement under direct visualization or by palpation [9].

Maher et Al.'s Cochrane systematic review and meta-analysis found no difference in ureteric injury rates between uterosacral colpopexy and transvaginal procedures [2].

The anatomical position of the ligament, posterior to the course of the ureter, makes the placement of fixation sutures unlikely to result in ureteral kinking or occlusion. Intuitively, the risk of bladder injury can be minimized with the choice of surgical approach. The anterior approach requires dissection of the ipsilateral paravaginal space as well as mobilization of the bladder away from the vaginal apex conferring the greatest risk of injury. The posterior approach confines dissection to the rectovaginal space and dramatically minimizes the risk of injury. Maintaining the proper plane of dissection can minimize the risk of urinary tract injury with an anterior approach. Excessively deep dissection can result in bleeding and poor visualization, increasing the risk of inadvertent bladder injury.

Cystoscopy is a valuable tool when SSLF is performed via an anterior approach or with multicompartment procedures as it adds minimal morbidity and helps identifying injuries that are unlikely to be apparent without such evaluation.

When ureteral injury or kinking is suspected, a practical and safe approach is to use Indigo Carmine Dye to visualize ureteral patency clearly. A recent phase III RCT studied the use of Indigo Carmine Dye in 96 ureters, comparing a 2.5 mL injection v/s a 5 mL injection and found a median time of 6 min to visualization, with no statistically significant difference between 2.5 and 5 ml injections. The authors also report no adverse events related to Indigo Carmine use [14].

Bladder injuries should be closed in two layers with absorbable sutures. When sluggish or absent ureteral jets are found, removal or revision of sacrospinous fixation sutures is unlikely to be effective. If hysterectomy has been performed, retrograde pyelography or ureteral cannulation with guide wire should be performed. In the setting of concomitant anterior repair, plication sutures should be removed, and the patient reassessed for return of ureteral efflux.

Pain

Pain is one of the most reported complications of SSLF. The reported rate of ipsilateral buttock, perineal, and/or posterior thigh pain is 6–55.4% [4, 11, 13, 15] in the literature. Fortunately, most pain is self-limited and resolves in the early and intermediate postoperative period. Overall, 84–100% of these cases resolved with supportive care and oral analgesia within 6 months of surgery, most within 12 weeks.

Notably, an RCT, that compared intraoperative Bupivacaine injection with placebo, showed no significant difference in patient's perception of postoperative gluteal pain, but patients in the placebo group used significantly more nonsteroidal anti-inflammatory drugs than the treatment group (adjusted OR 1.25; 95% CI, 1.04–1.35; $P = 0.01$) [16]. Nerve block or other injection of analgesic agents or surgery to remove suspension sutures were required in 0–8.7% and 0–13% of cases of pain, respectively [4, 11, 13, 15–18].

There are rare reports of foot drop, most of which resolved spontaneously or with the release of the suspension sutures. Pollack and coworkers reported a case of foot drop that persisted at long-term follow-up despite suspension suture removal [6].

Given the close anatomic relation of the ligament with several neural structures, the prevalence of pain complications comes as no surprise. The risk of damaging the sciatic nerve at the proximal aspect of the ligament and the pudendal nerve in the distal aspect is well known. Reconstructive dogma is that the medial third of the ligament is a virtual "nerve-free zone," and proper suspension suture placement in this region should minimize the risk of neural injury and pain complications.

However, several anatomic and histological studies have shown nerves to the coccygeus and levator ani muscles course over the mid portion of the ligament, nerve fibers run through the substance of the ligament, and that the proximal portion of the pudendal nerve can be near the middle portion of the ligament [19–21]. These findings suggest that even with optimal placement, pain complications remain a salient risk. Be that as it may, careful placement of the suspension suture is the best and most reliable way to avoid pain complications. Completing adequate dissection, confining sutures to the medial third of the ligament approximately 2 cm from the ischial spine, and avoiding incorporation of adjacent soft tissue are vital steps. Pollak and coworkers found that the chosen approach for fixation suture placement, direct visualization vs. palpation, impacts the rate of postoperative pain complications. In a retrospective review of 240 women, placement of sutures in the ligament by palpation and a use of a Deschamps ligature holder resulted in 10% rate of nerve injury compared to none with suture passage under direct visualization or with palpation and utilization of a Miya hook ($p = 0.002$) [9]. However, this finding has not been corroborated to date with an RCT. When significant pain is present after surgery, it is important to recognize symptoms that suggest nerve entrapment. Perineal, vulvar, or gluteal pain that is persistent, unrelieved by pain medication and is worsened with sitting is suggestive of pudendal nerve entrapment.

Posterior leg pain and foot drop are suggestive of sciatic entrapment.

In cases where entrapment is strongly suspected, timely surgical release or revision of ipsilateral suspension sutures should be considered. In all other cases, it is reasonable to pursue a trial of conservative management with medical therapy and/or physical therapy to allow for spontaneous resolution.

Bowel Injury

Compared to uterosacral vault suspension and abdominal sacrocolpopexy, SSLF is associated with a lower risk of visceral injury due to its extraperitoneal location. However, the dissection of the pararectal space utilized to reveal the sacrospinous ligament confers modest risk for rectal injury. Three systematic reviews in the literature report rectal injury rates of 0–1.4% [6, 12, 22]. An RCT of sacrospinous hysteropexy observed no injuries in a cohort of 105 women [4]. Maintaining the proper plane of dissection and avoidance of undue traction on the rectum while exposing the ligament are the two key maneuvers essential for avoiding injury. Hydrodissection helps identify the correct plane between the vaginal epithelium and muscularis and facilitates efficient blunt dissection after initial sharp dissection.

Prior posterior repair may impair the efficiency of hydrodissection, so special attention should be given to reoperative fields. Gentle placement of a gloved finger in the rectum can aid in adherence to the correct plane. Once the plane between the vagina and rectum is fully dissected, the ischial spine is palpated, and the rectum is retracted medially. Retractors used to expose the ligament should be placed with care to avoid undue traction and laceration. Unilateral, right-sided ligament fixation minimizes risk of rectal injury, as it avoids the need to retract the rectosigmoid junction for visualization of the left ligament. When the suspension suture is placed, it is important to avoid inadvertent incorporation of the rectal wall. This is more likely when retraction is insufficient, and sutures are being placed by palpation rather than under direct vision. Careful visual and digital examination should help confirm proper suture placement. Sutures that include rectum should be removed and replaced. Before apical sutures are placed, the rectal wall should be carefully examined to exclude injury. All injuries should be repaired primarily in 2–3 layers of absorbable sutures by the reconstructive surgeon or a general surgery colleague, depending on the surgeon's level of comfort and the degree of injury.

Summary

SSLF is a safe and effective transvaginal approach to apical prolapse. However, the anatomic location of the ligament near numerous vascular and neural structures mandates firm knowledge of pertinent anatomical landmarks and meticulous technique to minimize complications.

Postoperative pain should be an important aspect of the informed consent process.

References

1. Shah AD, Kohli N, Rajan SS, Hoyte L. The age distribution, rates, and types of surgery for pelvic organ prolapse in the USA. Int Urogynecol J Pelvic Floor Dysfunct. 2008;19(3):421–8. https://doi.org/10.1007/s00192-007-0457-y. Epub 2007 Sep 20. PMID: 17882343.
2. Maher C, Yeung E, Haya N, Christmann-Schmid C, Mowat A, Chen Z, Baessler K. Surgery for women with apical vaginal prolapse. Cochrane Database Syst Rev. 2023;7(7):CD012376. https://doi.org/10.1002/14651858.CD012376.pub2. PMID: 37493538; PMCID: PMC10370901.
3. De Gracia S, Fatton B, Cosson M, Campagne-Loiseau S, Ferry P, Lucot JP, Debodinance P, Panel L, Deffieux X, Garbin O, Lamblin G, Carlier-Guérin C, Ramanah R, Fauconnier A, Serrand C, Fritel X, de Tayrac R. Serious complications and recurrence following sacrospinous ligament fixation for the correction of apical prolapse. J Clin Med. 2023;12(2):468. https://doi.org/10.3390/jcm12020468. PMID: 36675397; PMCID: PMC9861510.
4. Detollenaere RJ, den Boon J, Stekelenburg J, IntHout J, Vierhout ME, Kluivers KB, van Eijndhoven HW. Sacrospinous hysteropexy versus vaginal hysterectomy with suspension of the uterosacral ligaments in women with uterine prolapse stage 2 or higher: multicentre randomised non-inferiority trial. BMJ. 2015;351:h3717. https://doi.org/10.1136/bmj.h3717. PMID: 26206451; PMCID: PMC4512203.
5. Barber MD, Brubaker L, Burgio KL, Richter HE, Nygaard I, Weidner AC, Menefee SA, Lukacz ES, Norton P, Schaffer J, Nguyen JN, Borello-France D, Goode PS, Jakus-Waldman S, Spino C, Warren LK, Gantz MG, Meikle SF; Eunice Kennedy Shriver National Institute of Child Health and Human Development Pelvic Floor Disorders Network. Comparison of 2 transvaginal surgical approaches and perioperative behavioral therapy for apical vaginal prolapse: the OPTIMAL randomized trial. JAMA. 2014;311(10):1023–34. https://doi.org/10.1001/jama.2014.1719. Erratum in: JAMA. 2015 Jun 9;313(22):2287. doi: 10.1001/jama.2015.4817. PMID: 24618964; PMCID: PMC4083455.
6. Sze E, Karram MM. Transvaginal repair of vault prolapse: a review. Obstet Gynecol. 1997;89(3):467–75.
7. Solomon ER, St Marie P, Jones KA, Harmanli O. Anterior bilateral sacrospinous ligament fixation: a safe route for apical repair. Female Pelvic Med Reconstr Surg. 2020;26(8):e33–6. https://doi.org/10.1097/SPV.0000000000000857. PMID: 32487884.
8. Xiao X, Yu X, Yin L, Zhang L, Feng D, Zhang L, Gong Z, Zhang Q, Lin Y, He L. Surgical outcomes of sacrospinous hysteropexy and hysteropreservation for pelvic organ prolapse: a systematic review of randomized controlled trials. Front Med (Lausanne). 2024;11:1399247. https://doi.org/10.3389/fmed.2024.1399247. PMID: 39114831; PMCID: PMC11303157.
9. Pollak J, Takacs P, Medina C. Complications of three sacrospinous ligament fixation techniques. Int J Gynaecol Obstet. 2007;99(1):18–22. https://doi.org/10.1016/j.ijgo.2007.04.028. Epub 2007 May 24. PMID: 17531239.
10. Leone Roberti Maggiore U, Alessandri F, Remorgida V, Venturini PL, Ferrero S. Vaginal sacrospinous colpopexy using the Capio suture-capturing device

versus traditional technique: feasibility and outcome. Arch Gynecol Obstet. 2013;287(2):267–74. https://doi.org/10.1007/s00404-012-2540-y. Epub 2012 Sep 2. PMID: 22941353.
11. Lantzsch T, Goepel C, Wolters M, Koelbl H, Methfessel HD. Sacrospinous ligament fixation for vaginal vault prolapse. Arch Gynecol Obstet. 2001;265(1):21–5. https://doi.org/10.1007/s004040000116. PMID: 11327088.
12. Diwadkar GB, Barber MD, Feiner B, Maher C, Jelovsek JE. Complication and reoperation rates after apical vaginal prolapse surgical repair: a systematic review. Obstet Gynecol. 2009;113(2 Pt 1):367–73. https://doi.org/10.1097/AOG.0b013e318195888d. Erratum in: Obstet Gynecol. 2009 Jun;113(6):1377. PMID: 19155908.
13. Maher CF, Murray CJ, Carey MP, Dwyer PL, Ugoni AM. Iliococcygeus or sacrospinous fixation for vaginal vault prolapse. Obstet Gynecol. 2001;98(1):40–4. https://doi.org/10.1016/s0029-7844(01)01378-3. PMID: 11430954.
14. Lepor H, Wiegand L, Patel K, Du W, Gagnon S; 19IC01 investigators. A randomized clinical trial evaluating indigo carmine as a visualization aid for evaluating ureteral patency. Urology. 2024;184:105–11. https://doi.org/10.1016/j.urology.2023.11.005. Epub 2023 Dec 5. PMID: 38061609.
15. Unger CA, Walters MD. Gluteal and posterior thigh pain in the postoperative period and the need for intervention after sacrospinous ligament colpopexy. Female Pelvic Med Reconstr Surg. 2014;20(4):208–11. https://doi.org/10.1097/SPV.0000000000000091. PMID: 24978086.
16. Ferrando CA, Walters MD. A randomized double-blind placebo-controlled trial on the effect of local analgesia on postoperative gluteal pain in patients undergoing sacrospinous ligament colpopexy. Am J Obstet Gynecol. 2018;218(6):599.e1–8. https://doi.org/10.1016/j.ajog.2018.03.033. Epub 2018 Mar 31. PMID: 29614274.
17. Hefni MA, El-Toukhy TA. Long-term outcome of vaginal sacrospinous colpopexy for marked uterovaginal and vault prolapse. Eur J Obstet Gynecol Reprod Biol. 2006;127(2):257–63. https://doi.org/10.1016/j.ejogrb.2005.11.028. Epub 2005 Dec 27. PMID: 16377061.
18. Dietz V, Huisman M, de Jong JM, Heintz PM, van der Vaart CH. Functional outcome after sacrospinous hysteropexy for uterine descensus. Int Urogynecol J Pelvic Floor Dysfunct. 2008;19(6):747–52. https://doi.org/10.1007/s00192-007-0520-8. PMID: 18297228; PMCID: PMC2335287.
19. Roshanravan SM, Wieslander CK, Schaffer JI, Corton MM. Neurovascular anatomy of the sacrospinous ligament region in female cadavers: implications in sacrospinous ligament fixation. Am J Obstet Gynecol. 2007;197(6):660.e1–6. https://doi.org/10.1016/j.ajog.2007.08.061. PMID: 18060971.
20. Wallner C. Buttock pain after sacrospinous hysteropexy. Int Urogynecol J Pelvic Floor Dysfunct. 2008;19(12):1729–30, author reply 1731. https://doi.org/10.1007/s00192-008-0646-3. Epub 2008 Jun 21. PMID: 18568285.
21. Lazarou G, Grigorescu BA, Olson TR, Downie SA, Powers K, Mikhail MS. Anatomic variations of the pelvic floor nerves adjacent to the sacrospinous ligament: a female cadaver study. Int Urogynecol J Pelvic Floor Dysfunct. 2008;19(5):649–54. https://doi.org/10.1007/s00192-007-0494-6. Epub 2007 Nov 24. PMID: 18038107.
22. Chan CYW, Fernandes RA, Yao HH, O'Connell HE, Tse V, Gani J. A systematic review of the surgical management of apical pelvic organ prolapse. Int Urogynecol J. 2023;34(4):825–41. https://doi.org/10.1007/s00192-022-05408-x. Epub 2022 Dec 3. PMID: 36462058.

Abdominal Sacrocolpopexy

9

Michelle Koski, Erin Dougher, Barry Hallner Jr, and Jack Christian Winters

Introduction

With the aging of our population, pelvic organ prolapse is an increasingly common condition that negatively affects patients' quality of life. Vaginal vault prolapse has been reported to occur in as many as 18.2% of all women with prolapse [1], and many would suggest that vaginal vault prolapse is a component of most high-grade anterior compartment descensus. Several repairs exist that reconstitute support to the vaginal vault, and, certainly, there is no single procedure that is optimal for all patients. However, abdominal sacral colpopexy is considered the gold standard approach in patients with recurrent or vault prolapse [2].

M. Koski
Department of Urology, Kaiser Permanente Medical Center, San Marcos, CA, USA

E. Dougher
Urogynecology, Baylor Scott White, Austin, Texas, USA

B. Hallner Jr
Department of Obstetrics and Gynecology, Louisiana State University Health Sciences Center, New Orleans, LA, USA

Urogynecology, Womans Hospital, Baton Rouge, Louisiana, USA

J. C. Winters (✉)
Department of Urology, Louisiana State University Health Sciences Center, New Orleans, LA, USA

Urogynecology, Womans Hospital, Baton Rouge, Louisiana, USA

Abdominal sacral colpopexy (ASC) offers an effective and durable repair for vaginal vault prolapse [3]. It maximizes functional vaginal length and approximates the normal vaginal axis [4]. Patient selection for ASC should be considered for patients with failed prior vaginal repairs, isolated high-grade apical prolapse, patients who desire to maintain sexual function, patients with chronic pain, or when there is concern for chronic intra-abdominal pressure [5, 6]. The procedure may be performed open, laparoscopic, or robotically assisted. There have not been many robust studies to compare the different approaches to ASC. The laparoscopic and robotically assisted route is discussed in a separate chapter. A 2023 Cochrane systematic review and meta-analysis reported similar anatomic outcomes with open versus laparoscopic approaches, although minimally invasive techniques had lower blood loss and shorter length of stay [7]. The review also reported uncertainty in the literature regarding differences in overall complications among the approaches.

In our experience, the key components of the operation include utilization of a lightweight permanent, type I macroporous mesh, secure suture fixation of the graft to the sacral promontory and vaginal cuff (Fig. 9.1), complete enterocele reduction and culdoplasty, and the addition of concomitant anti-incontinence procedures as indicated [5]. We affix the vaginal portion of the graft with multiple sutures to distribute the tension evenly over the vaginal apex (Fig. 9.2) and

H. B. Goldman, J. Zillioux (eds.), *Complications of Urogynecology and Reconstructive Pelvic Surgery*, https://doi.org/10.1007/978-3-032-00339-3_9

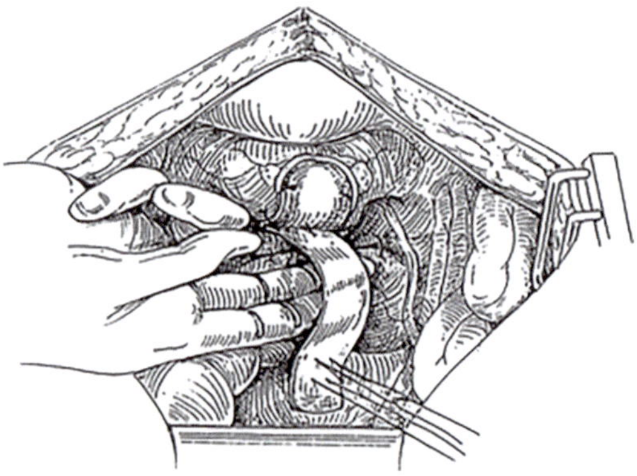

Fig. 9.1 Type 1 macroporous mesh is sutured to the sacral promontory and the vaginal cuff

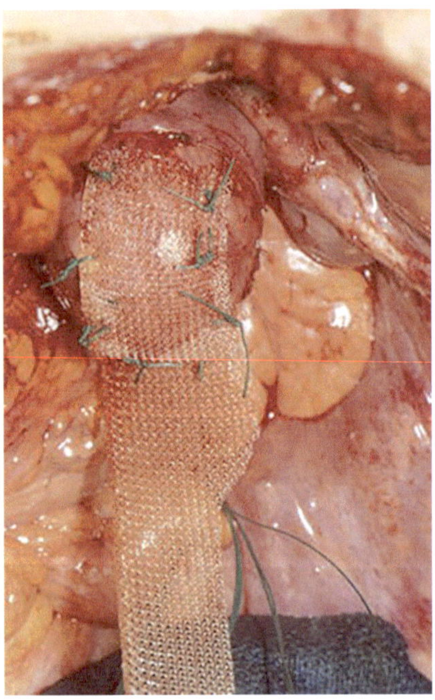

Fig. 9.2 The mesh graft is affixed to the apex of the vagina with multiple sutures for even tension distribution

avoid excessive tension between the apex and sacrum (Fig. 9.3). We routinely close the peritoneum over the mesh. In this chapter, we will address the recognition and management of complications potentially associated with this method of repair.

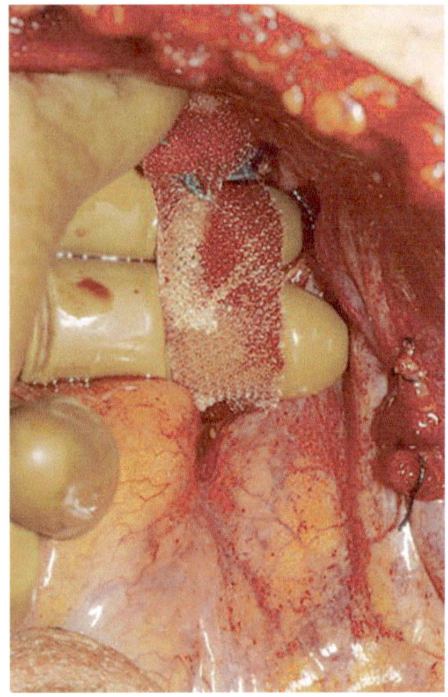

Fig. 9.3 Intraoperative view: graft in final position. A space of two fingerbreadths between the graft and the rectum prevents compression of the rectum under the graft. Incised peritoneum will be closed over graft

Intraoperative Complications

In a large meta-review by Nygaard and colleagues [3], intraoperative complications included hemorrhage or transfusion (0.18–16.9%), cystotomy (0.4–15.8%), enterotomy or proctotomy (0.4–2.5%), and ureteral injury (0.8–1.9%). When compared with the minimally invasive approach, open ASC does involve a longer hospital stay, increased blood loss, and complications associated with those factors [8].

Hemorrhage

Presacral hemorrhage incurred during the dissection of the sacral promontory is one of the most feared complications of ASC, as well as one of the more commonly reported in the literature [3]. Bleeding from the presacral space may be of large volume because the bleeding vessels may retract into the sacrum. Historically, in the 1970s, the operation was described with fixation of the mesh graft to the level of S3–S4 below the sacral promontory in an attempt to create a more natural vaginal axis [9]. After a life-threatening hemorrhage at this site, Sutton advocated for fixation higher on the sacral promontory at the S1–S2 level [10]. This site allows better visualization of the middle sacral artery, and the slight difference in vaginal axis has not resulted in negative outcomes. Careful dissection at the sacral promontory should be used to avoid laceration of the unseen presacral vessels. Excessive blunt dissection should be avoided to prevent shearing of the presacral veins. Monopolar cautery should be used precisely, and diathermy cautery may be helpful as well. If uncontrollable bleeding is incurred, which is not amenable to direct cautery, it may be managed with stainless steel thumbtacks [11], bone wax, or a figure-of-eight stitch [12]. It is important to be aware of the left common iliac vein, as this structure is frequently located more medial than the artery and can be injured during exposure of the promontory.

Cystotomy, Enterotomy, and Ureteral Injury

Injury to the bladder or bowel may occur during dissection or inadvertently. Care should be taken at all points of bladder dissection to maintain a full-thickness dissection and avoid cystotomy. Additionally, we try to avoid excessive cautery in the dissection of the bladder from the vagina. If a bladder injury is detected, it should be closed in two layers with absorbable suture, and an adequately sized urethral catheter should be left for bladder drainage. At this point, it would be at the discretion of the surgeon whether to proceed with mesh attachment to the vaginal apex. Mesh should not be placed adjacent to or in proximity to the cystotomy, as it might predispose to erosion of mesh into the bladder or fistula formation [13]. If vesical injury is missed, patients may present with fever, pain secondary to urinoma or urinary ascites.

Enterotomy with any fecal or enteric soilage precludes the placement of mesh. The bowel injury should be repaired, and the case concluded. If enterotomy is missed, patients with unrecognized bowel injuries often present 1–2 days postoperatively and may lack the typical signs of peritonitis. Patients may present with low-grade fever and leukopenia with a left shift. The clinician should maintain a high index of suspicion and order a computed tomography (CT) scan in these patients.

The ureters should be identified early on in the case to avoid injury from dissection or entrapment, or kinking in the culdoplasty sutures. To ensure patency of the ureter, we perform cystoscopy after the conclusion of the case with D50 for clear visualization of the effluxing urine.

Postoperative Complications

Postoperative complications in a comprehensive review included urinary tract infection (2.5–25.9%), wound infection or separation (0.4–19.8%), ileus (1.1–9.3%), deep venous thrombosis or pulmonary embolism (0.4–5.0%), small bowel obstruction (SBO) (0.6–8.6%), and incisional hernia requiring repair (0.4–15%). Additionally, mesh erosion was noted at an overall rate of 3.4% in the 2178 patients reviewed in this meta-analysis [3].

Vaginal Mesh Erosion

Key signs and symptoms of vaginal mesh erosion include persistent pain, discharge, and occasionally dyspareunia for the woman and/or her partner. Suture erosions are typically asymptomatic [14, 15]. A comprehensive review of ASC quoted an overall mesh erosion rate of 3.4% [3], although rates of erosion quoted in the literature vary [14, 16–18]. While mesh erosions after ASC typically occur 4–24 months after surgery [14, 16], they may also present several years later [19]. Because of this, determining an accurate erosion rate in series is complicated by the length of follow-up. Additionally, mesh type, surgical technique, and modifiable factors may affect the rate of erosion. Predicting mesh erosion can be difficult. Retrospective cohorts have found that mesh exposure is greater in ASC in patients with advanced stage (three or more) prolapse, when performed with concomitant hysterectomy, and patients who have had three or more vaginal procedures [20].

Mesh type appears to affect erosion rates based on the comparison of the literature, although there have been no standardized trials comparing different materials. In the Nygaard meta-analysis, polypropylene carried an erosion rate of 0.5% in comparison to 3.1% for polyethylene terephthalate (Mersilene®; Ethicon/ Johnson & Johnson, Somerville, NJ, USA), 3.4% for polytetrafluoroethylene (Gore-Tex®; W.L. Gore, Flagstaff, AZ, USA), 5.0% for polyethylene (Phillips Sumika, Polypropylene Co., Houston, TX, USA), and 5.5% for Teflon® (E.I. DuPont de Nemours and Co., Wilmington, DE, USA) [3]. No conclusions were made in this review regarding whether certain mesh types predispose to erosion because, in this setting, they could not control for other variables (method of graft placement, concurrent hysterectomy, etc.). However, certainly, particular mesh materials are more at risk for erosion. Govier and colleagues found a 23.8% graft complication rate (mesh erosion or infection) in a retrospective review of 21 patients who underwent ASC using a silicone-coated polyethylene preformed graft [21]. A subanalysis of the Colpopexy and Urinary Reduction Efforts (CARE) study found a nearly fourfold increased risk of mesh erosion if Gore-Tex mesh was used compared to non-Gore-Tex mesh, which reached statistical significance and altered their use of Gore-Tex mesh [17].

Contemporary mesh erosion rates may be lower than those listed in much of ASC literature, as lightweight (25–50 mg/m^2) and ultra-lightweight (<25 mg/m^2) polypropylene meshes are now primarily utilized. A 2022 cross-sectional review of complications reported to the Food and Drug Administration for urogynecologic meshes found that higher weight meshes had higher rates of mesh erosion and pain complication reports. [22]Similarly, a 2023 single-center study comparing two consecutive prospective cohorts of 339 women who underwent laparoscopic sacrocolpopexy with median 93–97 months follow-up found higher rates of mesh-related complication (22.8% vs 7.3%, HR 3.3, 95%CI 1.6–7.1) and reintervention for mesh-complication (18.8% vs 2.1%, HR 4.6, 95%CI 1.9–11.2) with heavier weight vs lighter weight meshes [23]. There were no differences in anatomic success between groups. Furthermore, several recent studies have shown no difference between mesh-related complications or success rates for light vs. ultra-lightweight meshes [24, 25], although one suggested a possible faster time to recurrence with ultra-lightweight mesh [25].

Ongoing concern about synthetic mesh has increased the appeal of biologic materials, but they are not without complications. Allograft fascia lata has been described as a biologic alternative to mesh. Increased risk of abdominal hernias after harvesting of the abdominal fascia has been reported [26]. This material precludes the risk of mesh erosion. However, reports of failures associated with attenuation or absence of the fascia lata graft in reoperation [27, 28], presumably secondary to autolysis, have led to decreased use of this material. A retrospective cohort study comparing polypropylene mesh to Pelvicol® (CR Bard, Murray Hill, NJ, USA) and autologous fascia found a higher rate of failures as well as erosions and other graft-related complications in the Pelvicol group (although it should be noted that Pelvicol was used more frequently in patients undergoing concomitant hysterectomy) [29]. Similar findings of high rates of graft-related complications and unacceptable failure rates were found with porcine grafts [30]. In a randomized trial of 100 women who underwent ASC and were randomized to cadaveric fascia lata vs. polypropylene mesh with a 5-year follow-up, anatomic success was considered greater in the mesh group (93% vs. 62%), and there was no difference in the success of patient symptom improvement (97% vs. 90%) [26]. A recent single-arm trial of total autologous fascia lata sacrocolpopexy reported no treatment failures at median 13-month follow-up.

A modifiable risk factor for erosion after ASC identified by the CARE trial analysis was tobacco use [17]. In their group of 322 patients, smoking was associated with a fivefold increased risk of erosion. A retrospective study of 499 patients undergoing ASC found a nonsignificant trend of smokers requiring more than one surgery for effective treatment of vaginal mesh erosion [31]. The dominant theory is that microvascular vasospasm with associated hypoxia may lead to poor wound healing and vaginal mesh erosion in smokers [19].

Approach and technique affect mesh erosion rates. If a graft or suture is introduced through the vagina in sacral colpoperineopexy, erosion rates are increased. In a retrospective review of 273 patients, there was no statistically significant difference in mesh erosion rates for patients undergoing ASC (3.2%) or purely abdominal sacral colpoperineopexy (4.5%). In patients undergoing sacral colpoperineopexy with vaginal introduction of mesh or sutures, the erosion rates increased to 16% (vaginal placement of sutures) and 40% (vaginal mesh), which maintained statistical significance on multivariate analysis. These patients exhibited a shorter time to mesh erosion as well, with median time to erosion 15.6 months for ASC, 12.4 months for abdominal sacral colpoperineopexy, 9.0 months in the suture group ($P < 0.005$), and 4.1 months in the vaginal mesh group ($P < 0.0001$) [32].

The role of concomitant hysterectomy in mesh erosion after ASC has been debated. In the CARE subanalysis [19], concurrent abdominal hysterectomies were performed in 26% of the patients, who incurred a 14% risk of erosion as compared to 4% in women who had undergone prior hysterectomy. This represented a fivefold increased risk of erosion. Culligan and colleagues found a statistically significant increase in erosion rates in patients undergoing concomitant hysterectomy in a retrospective review of 245 patients (27.3% erosion in those undergoing hysterectomy, 1.3% erosion without hysterectomy) [33]. A retrospective review of 313 patients found a statistically significant fivefold risk of mesh erosion in women on estrogen with concomitant hysterectomy [34]. Of note, they found no significant difference in erosion rates in those undergoing concurrent hysterectomy in the non-estrogen group, or in the overall group as well. These data imply that either estrogen or hysterectomy may increase erosion rates. In our experience, it seems hysterectomy would be the most likely risk factor. In contrast, in a retrospective review of 124 patients undergoing ASC (60 with hysterectomy and 64 without), Brizzolara and Pillai-Allen found a low overall mesh erosion rate of 0.8% and no significant difference in mesh erosions in the hysterectomy group [16]. They attributed their success to the two-layer closure of the cuff, careful handling of tissues, and use of antibiotic irrigation [16]. Based on these findings, if a small vaginal laceration is encountered during colpopexy, we close the laceration in two layers as described in the previous study. In reviewing outcomes of colpopexy following hysterectomy, the significance of the CARE subanalysis, as opposed to retrospective reviews, is that it was prospectively designed to capture complications, including mesh and suture erosions, at regular study intervals in the first 2 years. The CARE trial has since extended its analysis and has found that the complication of mesh extrusion continues long-term up to 10.5% at 7 years [35].

In cases of mesh erosion after combined hysterectomy and ASC, the erosion site is usually at the cuff. This may be secondary to potential vaginal bacterial contamination of the mesh from the opened vagina during hysterectomy. Alternatively, poor healing may occur at the cuff secondary to a devascularizing effect of cuff closure combined with mesh vaginal attachment sutures [19]. Some advocate supracervical hysterectomy as an alternative to total hysterectomy at the time of ASC, with a recent meta-analysis demonstrating lower rates of erosion with supracervical compared to total hysterectomy (0.36^ vs 3.8%, pooled OR 0.26 95% CI 0.18–0.38).

In cases of erosion of Type I mesh (Dacron®; Marlex®; Prolene® [Ethicon, Johnson & Johnson, Somerville, NJ, USA]), treatment with antibiotics and trimming and covering of the mesh is sufficient [15]. Because of the macroporous nature of the mesh, it is expected that macrophages will pass, making complete removal of the graft unnecessary. Additionally, eroded Type III mesh (combinations of multifilament and macroporous components: Teflon, Mersilene) may be treated with partial removal and reclosure of vaginal flaps [15]. However, infected Type II mesh (microporous material: Gore-Tex) must almost always be removed completely, as its microporous nature creates a bacterial sanctuary where access to antibiotics and the immune response is reduced [15, 19].

Conservative therapy with observation and topical estrogen may be initially attempted in small mesh erosions of type I or III mesh (<1 cm). Local excision of mesh is utilized as first-line therapy as well, or in cases of failed conservative therapy. In a series of vaginal erosions of Ethibond® (Ethicon, Somerville, NJ, USA) suture and Marlex and Mersilene mesh, patients presented at an average of 14 months postoperatively (range 4–24). All patients were initially treated with vaginal estrogen and 8 weeks of pelvic rest. Two patients with suture erosions resolved with this regimen, but all five patients with mesh erosion required surgical intervention and were successfully treated with vaginal mesh excision and flap advancement [14]. In another series, local surgical excision of exposed mesh carried a reported efficacy rate of 50% [31]. If the upper portion of the mesh is infected, it must be removed [19]. In the CARE subanalysis, 6% of patients experienced mesh/suture erosion. Most of the women with mesh erosion (13/17) underwent at least one surgery for partial or total mesh removal. Two patients completely resolved, six had persistent problems, and five were lost to follow-up [19]. Of the four women who elected observation, none experienced resolution [19].

Well-circumscribed areas of mesh extrusion may be approached vaginally. We excise only the exposed area with an additional margin of 1–2 cm; not all of the mesh needs to be excised. Surgical exposure of apical mesh extrusions in the post-sacrocolpopexy patient is more challenging than in distal vaginal extrusions. When the apex is well supported, it may be difficult to pull the apex into the forefront of the surgical field. We use a Lone Star® retractor (Cooper Surgical, Trumbull, CT, USA) with sharp hooks placed proximal to the mesh to expose as well as possible. Hydrodissection may be utilized around the area of the extrusion. We grasp the edge of the vaginal margin and dissect laterally between the vaginal margin and the mesh with Metzenbaum scissors to create vaginal flaps that extend about 2 cm circumferentially. If the edge of the mesh is available, we grasp that edge and begin our dissection underneath the mesh. If an edge is not accessible, we incise the mesh and isolate each resultant edge in an Allis clamp. Oftentimes, the mesh will peel off the underlying tissue with a combination of blunt and sharp dissection. We keep the scissor tips pointing toward the mesh. Once the mesh has been separated back to the edges of the initial dissection, we inspect the quality of the edges of our vaginal margins. If there is any question about the quality of the tissue, we will excise or debride the edges. Finally, we re-approximate the vaginal flaps with absorbable suture in a tension-free closure with no mesh under the suture line. Other authors have advocated a partial colpocleisis type approach [31]. If the initial extrusion is extensive or if prior vaginal approaches have failed, an abdominal approach may be attempted. Abdominal excisions are associated with higher blood loss, longer hospitalization, and additional morbidity [31].

In all cases, the approach to extrusions is vaginal unless there is other intra-abdominal pathology warranting correction. In an abdominal approach, extensive scarring and adhesions will be encountered. A full bowel preparation is recommended, and vaginal localization can be assisted with the use of an EEA sizer and or a Lucite vaginal stent. Partial removal of the offending mesh is acceptable unless gross infection is present. The vaginal defect should be repaired in two layers using absorbable sutures. In cases of poor tissue quality, a biologic interposition over the vaginal cuff or omentum may be utilized to assist in cuff healing.

Vaginal Suture Exposure/Erosion

When permanent suture (polytetrafluoroethylene, polypropylene) is used to affix the mesh to the vagina, there is a risk of suture exposure in the vagina. This issue may be asymptomatic or present with similar issues as mesh exposure, with pain, dyspareunia, spotting, or bothersome discharge. A recent randomized controlled trial (RCT) comparing permanent to delayed absorbable sutures for mesh affixation to the vagina during sacrocolpopexy with concomitant hysterectomy had a 2% rate of suture exposure between 3 months and 1 year in the permanent suture group [36]. Similar to mesh exposure/erosion, suture exposure can be managed conservatively with a trial of vaginal estrogen or surgically excised. Depending on patient tolerance and location, this can be attempted in the clinic under local anesthesia. This complication can be avoided by using delayed absorbable sutures instead of permanent sutures. The aforementioned RCT and recent Cochrane review have demonstrated similar anatomic and symptomatic outcomes with delayed absorbable suture compared to permanent, supporting this practice [7, 36].

Erosion of Mesh into the Bladder or Bowel

Patients with mesh erosion into the bladder after ASC may present with hematuria, irritative voiding symptoms, recurrent urinary tract infections, or chronic bladder stones. Diagnosis of this problem hinges on a high index of suspicion and a low threshold to perform cystoscopy. Maintaining a full thickness of the bladder without cystotomy during dissection, or alternatively, minimizing bladder mobilization, may help in avoiding this complication.

Patsner reported a case of erosion of polypropylene mesh and prolene suture into the bladder base, presenting 4 months after ASC, who was treated with open excision after two failed cystoscopic attempts [37]. Shepherd and coworkers performed a retrospective cohort study over 10 years, looking at the mesh/suture erosion rate based on the type of suture. Mesh suture exposure rate was found to vary with the type of suture, 3.7% with Ethibond and 0% with PDS [38]. Yamamoto and coworkers report a vesicovaginal fistula after abdominal hysterectomy and ASC, which occurred adjacent to the edge of the mesh and required abdominal repair [13]. In our experience, we have not had a mesh or suture erosion into the bladder secondary to ASC (Fig. 9.4). To reduce the risk of suture erosion into the bladder, we now use polydioxanone (PDS) suture to fixate the graft to the vagina. Depending on the site of erosion and the amount of mesh, a cystoscopic approach may be attempted. If this fails or is precluded by position or mesh volume, an open cystorrhaphy may be necessary. If the mesh is near the ureteral orifice, the surgeon should consider a retrograde pyelogram or a ureteral stent to delineate the ureter. In a retrospective review of intravesical mesh management cases (from various causes), Frenkl and coworkers concluded that, in their experience, sutures were managed most successfully with endoscopic techniques, where mesh was best managed with cystorrhaphy [39].

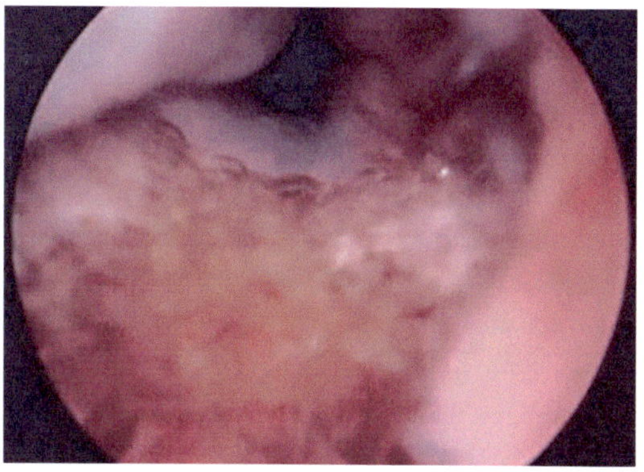

Fig. 9.4 Cystoscopic view of mesh erosion into the bladder

There are a few reported incidences of mesh erosion into the bowel. In a rare report of mesh erosion into the sigmoid colon 8 years after ASC, the patient was noted to have stool in her vagina and was ultimately treated with sigmoid colon resection with a low colorectal reanastamosis and omental J-flap placement [40]. Kenton and coworkers described a Gore-Tex graft erosion into the rectum with spontaneous passage of the graft 7 years post-ASC without fistula formation [41]. Hopkins and Rooney describe a small bowel fistula secondary to adhesion of a loop of terminal ileum to an exposed mesh that had been "minimally retroperitonealized." [42] Based on this, they advocate retroperitonealization of the mesh as a way to prevent adhesion of bowel. Most early descriptions of sacrocolpopexy describe closing the peritoneum over the graft. Other authors question the utility of this step. In a small study of 35 women, three had postoperative bowel obstructions, all resulting from the intestine trapped under the mesh, despite careful retroperitonealization [43]. Due to the low incidence of bowel mesh erosions, it is unlikely that this question will be addressed in a standardized fashion. In order to prevent these complications, we would advise meticulous placement of the mesh with careful attention to ensure an adequate space between the mesh and the sigmoid colon. We routinely close the peritoneum over the mesh.

Ileus and Small Bowel Obstruction

The reported incidence of postoperative ileus is a median 3.6% (range 1.1–9.3%) of patients and reoperation for SBO is a median 1.1% (range 0.6–8.6%) after ASC in the meta-analysis [3]. This review comprised mostly retrospective reports. The findings from a sub-analysis of the CARE trial supported these findings in the framework of a large prospective trial [44]. Of their 322 patients, 5.9% had postoperative gastrointestinal conditions resulting in reoperation, prolonged hospitalization, or readmission. Four patients (1.2%) required reoperation, and all were found to have small bowel entrapment in, or adhesion to, the abdominal wall incision (Fig. 9.5). Overall, the rate of SBO was 1.9–2.5% and the rate of ileus was 2.2–2.8%. Age was found to have a significant association with ileus [44]. A 2014 retrospective cohort of 589 subjects who underwent ASC were found to have a 5% risk of post op ileus/small bowel obstruction; the patients in this group were found to have more previous abdominal surgeries. It is possible that this added risk with an abdominal incision increases the complexity of the case and risk of ileus/SBO [45]. It is worth noting that barbed sutures, popular with minimally invasive approaches due to easier sewing, are associated with increased risk of postoperative SBO related to adhesion to the exposed suture tails/knot [46]. Apart from using non-barbed suture for retroperitonealization, methods to reduce risk include "back-tracking" the suture and trimming flush with the peritoneum.

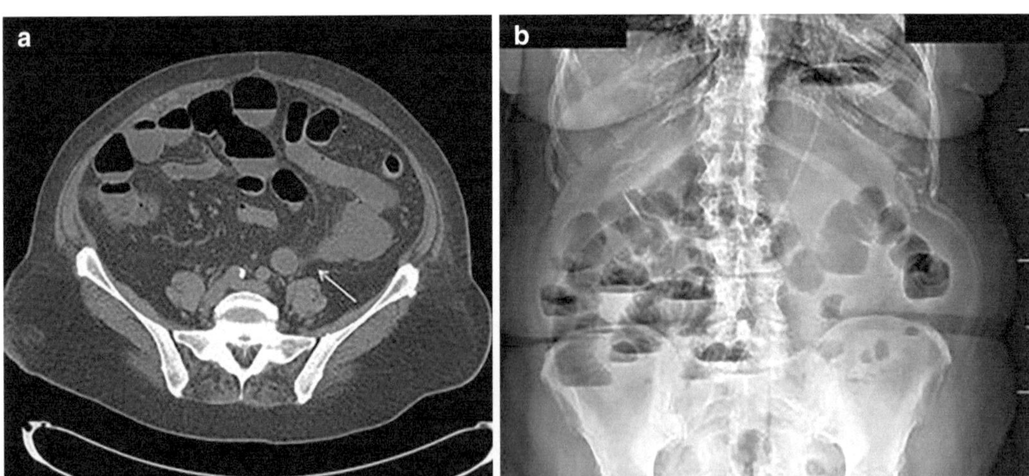

Fig. 9.5 Radiographic images of a patient with partial small bowel obstruction after abdominal sacral colpopexy. The CT scan (*right*) shows distended loops of bowel with a transition point marked with an *arrow*

Recurrence

Recurrent vaginal vault prolapse after ASC with permanent mesh is rare. The extended CARE trial suggested the probability of failure (anatomic or symptomatic) can range from 0.34 to 0.48 up to 7 years after POP repair, with a steadily increasing failure rate after 2 years [35]. Baessler and colleagues proposed that rare cases of symptomatic apical recurrence are usually secondary to detachment of the mesh from the vagina and that separation of the mesh from the sacrum is much less common [15]. If the mesh is still secured to the sacrum, they describe attaching a new mesh to it, which is then sutured to the vagina. They warn against the removal of the original mesh due to the high risk of injury to the ureter and bowel in a potentially difficult dissection. Addison and colleagues reiterate this in their series of recurrences, all resulting from disruption of the mesh from the vaginal apex (one of these cases secondary to a dissection of an enterocele beneath the mesh, causing disruption) [47]. They advocate performing a meticulous culdoplasty with permanent sutures and attachment of the mesh to the vaginal vault with multiple permanent sutures placed through the entire thickness of the vagina over a broad area as methods to help prevent recurrence [47].

Unmasking of Occult Stress Incontinence

We routinely assess for occult stress urinary incontinence (SUI) preoperatively with either urodynamics or cough stress test with the prolapse reduced. Rates of urodynamic SUI with prolapse reduction have been reported, ranging from 25 to 100% in symptomatically continent women using various methods of reduction [48]. Patients undergoing ASC are at significant risk for developing bothersome SUI, even in the absence of preoperative symptoms. In a prospective, controlled trial of 322 previously stress-continent women, 23.8% who underwent Burch colposuspension at the time of ASC showed postoperative SUI compared to 44.1% who underwent ASC alone. Those in the ASC alone group were also more likely to report bothersome SUI symptoms as compared to the Burch group (24.5% vs. 6.1%) [49]. Women who demonstrated preoperative SUI with prolapse reduction were more likely to report postoperative SUI, regardless of concurrent colposuspension (controls 58% vs. 38% ($P = 0.04$) and Burch 32% vs. 21% ($P = 0.19$)) [48]. In this study, the majority of women who did not leak with prolapse reduction did not leak after prolapse surgery (60%). In addition, women who did have a Burch procedure still experienced an approximately 30% rate of recurrent SUI. It is equally important not to over-tension the vagina, as a retrospective cohort analyzed by LeClaire and colleagues found that the abdominal approach and change in point Aa of >3 cm led to increased risk of SUI after sacrocolpopexy [50]. Based on these findings, we use urodynamics to counsel our patients and identify who might best benefit from concurrent anti-incontinence procedures, but we also inform our patients that a negative test does not preclude postoperative incontinence. We prefer to perform midurethral sling concurrently in patients undergoing ASC with symptomatic or occult SUI detected on screening. If women have significant obstructive symptoms on urodynamics with the prolapse reduced, we will perform ASC without a sling. If a woman has no occult SUI or symptoms of SUI, patients choose whether or not to undergo concomitant sling. Our bias is not to place a sling at that time. If patients develop SUI after ASC alone, a midurethral sling or urethral bulking can be performed at a later date with minimal difficulty.

Osteomyelitis and Spondylodiscitis

Osteomyelitis after ASC is rare and is generally heralded by persistent new low back pain. Weidner and colleagues described two cases of lumbosacral osteomyelitis after ASC, both treated successfully and definitively with prolonged parenteral antibiotic therapy guided by aspirated cultures and neither requiring mesh removal [51]. One patient presented with unremitting severe low back pain 5 years after ASC, and the second patient presented 2 months postoperatively. Both sacral fixations were performed with TiCron® (Davis and Geck, Wayne, NJ, USA) suture. Both were diagnosed on MRI, which is the most sensitive method for detecting osteomyelitis and defining the extent of the infection. Plain films and bone scans may be diagnostic, but are less sensitive than MRI. The authors suggest maintaining a higher level of suspicion for osteomyelitis in patients with a history of degenerative disc disease [51], as patients with degenerative disc disease are predisposed to infection due to disruption of the vertebral endplate and neovascularization of disc spaces, which allows bacteria into a normally avascular space [52]. In the rheumatologic literature, Cailleux and colleagues reported on five cases of sacral osteomyelitis after ASC (of a retrospective review of 45 patients with sacral osteomyelitis) [53]. Initial symptoms occurred at an average of 38 days postoperatively. In three of the patients, the same bacterial species was identified in urine cultures 1–4 days postoperatively as in the biopsy of the infected bone.

Since these initial series, there have been more reports, usually in the form of a case report. Nosseir and coworkers reported a case secondary to titanium tacks that resolved with parenteral antibiotics [54]. Muffly and coworkers reported a case of osteomyelitis and infected mesh with a sinus tract after robotic hysterectomy with ASC which required discectomy, sacral debridement, and mesh removal [55]. Another case of sacral osteomyelitis with concomitant mesh erosion and sinus formation required mesh removal and tract resection [56]. Taylor and coworkers described a case that presented with vaginal erosion of mesh and osteomyelitis with progressive neurologic symptoms requiring a decompressive laminectomy [57]. Dalawi reported two cases of pyogenic discitis in patients in which the graft was fixated to the anterior longitudinal ligament; in one patient, stainless steel screws were used, and in the other patient, the graft was fixated with titanium tacks to the ligament [58]. Both patients presented with persistent lower back pain.

We advocate empiric routine preoperative IV antibiotics and meticulous surgical technique with mesh and other permanent implants. We also advocate not using tacks or screws to fixate the graft to the ligament and using new monofilament suture to fixate the graft to the anterior longitudinal ligament that has not been used to fixate the graft to the vagina. It is also likely important to make an effort to just pass the suture through the ligament and not into the actual disc or bone. Patients with degenerative disc disease may be at increased risk of osteomyelitis and should be treated with care as well as a higher index of suspicion postoperatively. MRI should be used to rule out osteomyelitis in the carefully selected patient, and if possible, CT-guided aspiration and culture should be performed to guide antibiotic therapy. Isolated osteomyelitis may respond to prolonged antibiotics alone. In cases that fail antibiotics or in patients with mesh erosion, infection, or sinus tracts, surgery may be required. The surgeon should maintain a low threshold to consult infectious disease, orthopedics, and/or neurosurgery as indicated by the patient's presentation.

Conclusion

Sacrocolpopexy is a well-established standard of care procedure for the surgical correction of vaginal vault prolapse. It has become minimally invasive with the robotic and laparoscopic approach. In many ways, it is now a more comparable alternative to vaginal apical repair operations. Complications occur at a low incidence [3]. For the vast majority of patients, this procedure provides a gratifying outcome, which is durable and anatomic. A thorough knowledge of anatomy, graft biology, and potential complications is optimal in order to assure that this procedure may be performed as safely and efficiently as possible.

References

1. Winters JC, Cespedes RD, Vanlangendonck R. Abdominal sacral colpopexy and abdominal enterocele repair in the management of vaginal vault prolapse. Urology. 2000;56:55–63.
2. Constantini E, et al. Laparoscopic versus abdominal sacrocolpopexy: a randomized controlled trial. J Urol. 2016;196:159–65.
3. Nygaard IE, McCreery R, Brubaker L, et al. Abdominal sacrocolpopexy: a comprehensive review. Obstet Gynecol. 2004;104:805–23.
4. Given FT. Vaginal length and sexual function after colpopexy for complete uterovaginal eversion. Am J Obstet Gynecol. 1993;169:284–7.
5. Winters JC, Delacroix JS. In: Graham SD, Keane TE, editors. Abdominal sacral colpopexy. In Glenn's urologic surgery. Philadelphia: Lippincott Williams & Wilkins; 2010. p. 349–54.
6. Anand M, Weaver A, Fruth B, Gebhart J. Factors influencing selection of vaginal open abdominal, or robotic surgery to treat apical vaginal vault prolapse. Female Pelvic Med Reconstr Surg. 2016;22:236–42.
7. Maher C, et al. Surgery for women with apical vaginal prolapse. Cochrane Database Syst Rev. 2023;2023
8. Pollard ME, Eilber KS, Anger JT. Abdominal approaches to pelvic prolapse repairs. Curr Opin Urol. 2013;23:306–11.
9. Birnbaum SJ. Rational therapy for the prolapsed vagina. Am J Obstet Gynecol. 1973;115:411–9.
10. Sutton GP, Addison WA, Livengood I, C. H, et al. Life-threatening hemorrhage complicating sacral colpopexy. Am J Obstet Gynecol. 1981;140:836–7.
11. Timmons MC, Kohler MF, Addison WA. Thumbtack use for control of presacral bleeding with description of an instrument for thumbtack application. Obstet Gynecol. 1991;78:313–5.
12. Lane FE. Modified technique of sacral colpopexy. Am J Obstet Gynecol. 1982;142:933.
13. Yamamoto Y, Nishimura K, Ueda N, et al. Vesicovaginal fistula caused by abdominal hysterectomy and sacrocolpopexy with polypropylene mesh (GYNEMESH): a case report. Hinyokika Kiyo. 2010;56:517–20.
14. Kohli N, Walsh PM, Roat TW, et al. Mesh erosion after abdominal sacrocolpopexy. Obstet Gynecol. 1998;92:999–1004.
15. Baessler K, Leron E, Stanton SL. In: Stanton SL, Zimmern P, editors. Sacrohysteropexy and sacrocolpopexy. In female pelvic reconstructive surgery. New York: Springer Science; 2002. p. 189–90.
16. Brizzolara S, Pillai-Allen A. Risk of mesh erosion with sacral colpopexy and concurrent hysterectomy. Obstet Gynecol. 2003;102:306–10.
17. Cundiff GW, Varner E, Visco AG, et al. Risk factors for mesh/suture erosion following sacrocolpopexy. Am J Obstet Gynecol. 2008;199(688):e1–688.e5.
18. Nassif J, Yadav GS, Orejuela FJ, Turrentine MA. Rate of mesh erosion after sacrocolpopexy with concurrent supracervical compared with total hysterectomy: a systematic review and meta-analysis. Obstet Gynecol. 2022;140:412–20.
19. Bensinger G, Lind L, Lesser M, et al. Abdominal sacral suspensions: analysis of complications using permanent mesh. Am J Obstet Gynecol. 2005;193:2094–8.
20. Akyol A, Akca A, Ulker V, et al. Additional surgical risk factors and patient characteristics for mesh erosion after abdominal sacrocolpopexy. J Obstet Gynaecol. 2014;40:1368–74.
21. Govier FE, et al. High complication rate identified in sacrocolpopexy patients attributed to silicone mesh. Urology. 2005;65:1099–103.
22. Artsen AM, Sassani JC, Moalli PA, Bradley MS. Complications reported to the food and drug administration: a cross-sectional comparison of urogynecologic meshes. Female Pelvic Med Reconstr Surg. 2022;28 https://doi.org/10.1097/SPV.0000000000001193.
23. Page A-S, et al. Long-term data on graft-related complications after sacrocolpopexy with lightweight compared with heavier-weight mesh. Obstet Gynecol. 2023;141:189–98.
24. Kulkarni M, et al. Outcomes following sacrocolpopexy using ultralight and lightweight mesh. Int Urogynecol J. 2022;33:2475–83.
25. Giugale LE, et al. Assessing pelvic organ prolapse recurrence after minimally invasive sacrocolpopexy: does mesh weight matter? Int Urogynecol J. 2021;32:2195–201.
26. Mueller E. Why complex pelvic organ prolapse should be approached abdominally. Curr Opin Urol. 2013;23:317–22.
27. Fitzgerald MP, Edwards SR, Fenner D. Medium-term follow-up on use of freeze-dried, irradiated donor fascia for sacrocolpopexy and sling procedures. Int Urogynecol J Pelvic Floor Dysfunct. 2004;15:238–42.
28. Fitzgerald MP, Mollenhauer J, Bitterman P, Brubaker L. Functional failure of fascia lata allografts. Am J Obstet Gynecol. 1999;181:1339–46.
29. Quiroz LH, Gutman RE, Shippey S, et al. Abdominal sacrocolpopexy: anatomic outcomes and complications with Pelvicol, autologous, and synthetic graft materials. Am J Obstet Gynecol. 2008;198(557):e1–557.e5.
30. Claerhout F, De Ridder D, Van Beckevoort D, et al. Sacrocolpopexy using xenogenic acellular collagen in patients at increased risk for graft-related complications. Neurourol Urodyn. 2010;29:563–7.
31. Quiroz LH, Gutman RE, Fagan MJ, et al. Partial colpocleisis for the treatment of sacrocolpopexy mesh erosions. Int Urogynecol J Pelvic Floor Dysfunct. 2008;19:261–6.
32. Visco AG, Weidner AC, Barber MD, et al. Vaginal mesh erosion after abdominal sacral colpopexy. Am J Obstet Gynecol. 2001;184:297–302.

33. Culligan PJ, Murphy M, Blackwell L, et al. Long-term success of abdominal sacral colpopexy using synthetic mesh. Am J Obstet Gynecol. 2002;187:1473–82.
34. Wu JM, Wells EC, Hundley AF, et al. Mesh erosion in abdominal sacral colpopexy with and without concomitant hysterectomy. Am J Obstet Gynecol. 2006;194:1418–22.
35. Nygaard I, Brubaker L, Zyczynksi H, et al. Long-term outcomes following abdominal sacrocolpopexy for pelvic organ prolapse. JAMA. 2013;309:2016–24.
36. Matthews CA, et al. Permanent compared with absorbable suture for vaginal mesh fixation during Total hysterectomy and sacrocolpopexy: a randomized controlled trial. Obstet Gynecol. 2020;136:355–64.
37. Patsner B. Mesh erosion into the bladder after abdominal sacral colpopexy. Obstet Gynecol. 2000;95:1029.
38. Shepherd JP, Higdon HL, Stanford EJ, Mattox TF. Effect of suture selection on the rate of suture or mesh erosion and surgery failure in abdominal sacrocolpopexy. Female Pelvic Med Reconstr Surg. 2010;16:229–33.
39. Frenkl TL, Rackely RR, Vasavada SP, et al. Management of iatrogenic foreign bodies of the bladder and urethra following pelvic floor surgery. Neurourol Urodyn. 2008;27:491–5.
40. Rose S, Bunten CE, Geisler JP, et al. Polypropylene mesh erosion into the bowel and vagina after abdominal sacral colpopexy. J Pelvic Med Surgery. 2006;12:45–7.
41. Kenton KS, Woods MP, Brubaker L. Uncomplicated erosion of polytetraflouroethylene grafts into the rectum. Am J Obstet Gynecol. 2002;187:233–4.
42. Hopkins MP, Rooney C. Entero-mesh vaginal fistula secondary to abdominal sacrocolpopexy. Obstet Gynecol. 2004;103:1035–6.
43. Pilsgaard K, Mouritsen L. Follow-up after repair of vaginal vault prolapse with abdominal colposacropexy. Acta Obstet Gynecol Scand. 1999;78:66–70.
44. Whitehead WE, Bradley CS, Brown MB, et al. Gastrointestinal complications following abdominal sacrocolpopexy for advanced pelvic organ prolapse. Am J Obstet Gynecol. 2007;197(78):e1–78.e7.
45. Nosti P, Umoh U, Kane S, et al. Outcomes of abdominal and minimally invasive sacrocolpopexy: a retrospective cohort study. Female Pelvic Med Reconstr Surg. 2014;20:33–7.
46. Stabile G, et al. Case report: bowel occlusion following the use of barbed sutures in abdominal surgery. A Single-Center Experience and Literature Review Front Surg. 2021;8:626505.
47. Addison, W. A., Timmons, M. C., Wall, L. L., et al. Failed abdominal sacral colpopexy: observations and recommendations. Obstet Gynecol 74, 480–483 (1989).
48. Visco AG, Brubaker L, Nygaard I, et al. The role of preoperative urodynamic testing in stress-continent women undergoing sacral colpopexy: the Colpopexy and urinary reduction efforts (CARE) randomized surgical trial. Int Urogynecol J Pelvic Floor Dysfunct. 2008;19:607–14.
49. Brubaker L, Cundiff GW, Fine P, et al. Abdominal sacrocolpopexy with Burch colposuspension to reduce urinary stress incontinence. N Engl J Med. 2006;354:1557–66.
50. Leclaire EL, Mukati M, Juarez D, White D, Quiroz LH. Is de novo stress incontinence after sacrocolpopexy related to anatomical changes and surgical approach? Int Urogynecol J. 2014;25:1201–6.
51. Weidner AC, Cundiff GW, Harris RL, et al. Sacral osteomyelitis: an unusual complication of abdominal sacral colpopexy. Obstet Gynecol. 1997;90:689–91.
52. Cranney A, Feibel R, Toye BW, et al. Osteomyelitis subsequent to abdominal-vaginal sacropexy. J Rheumatol. 1994;21:1769–70.
53. Cailleux N, Daragon A, Laine F, et al. Spondylodiscites infetieuses après cure de prolapses genital: a propos de 5 cas. Journal de Gynecologie Obstetrique et Biologie de la Reproduction. 1991;20:1074–8.
54. Nosseir SB, Kim YH, Lind LR, et al. Sacral osteomyelitis after robotically assisted laparoscopic sacral colpopexy. Obstet Gynecol. 2010;116:513–5.
55. Muffly TM, Diwadkar GB, Paraiso MF. Lumbosacral osteomyelitis after robot-assisted total laparoscopic hysterectomy and sacral colpopexy. Int Urogynecol J Pelvic Floor Dysfunct. 2010;21:1569–71.
56. Hart SR, Weiser EB. Abdominal sacral colpopexy mesh erosion resulting in a sinus tract formation and sacral abscess. Obstet Gynecol. 2004;103:1037–40.
57. Taylor GB, Moore RD, Miklos JR. Osteomyelitis secondary to sacral colpopexy mesh erosion requiring laminectomy. Obstet Gynecol. 2006;107:475–7.
58. Dalwai R, Menon KV, Kumar RJ. Pyogenic diskitis of the L5-S1 disk space following inadvertent placement of a sacrocolpopexy screw. Int J Gynaecol Obstet. 2010;111:268–9.

10 Hysteropexy

Amr El Haraki and Catherine A. Matthews

Introduction

Hysteropexy is an increasingly popular surgical approach to primary uterovaginal prolapse for appropriately selected women who desire uterine preservation. Patient surveys have demonstrated that between 36% and 60% of women undergoing prolapse surgery in the United States would prefer uterine preservation if given the choice [1]. These preferences may be due to concerns about hormonal changes, preservation of feminine identity, cultural reasons, as well as increased risk of complications related to hysterectomy [2].

Hysteropexy is generally an effective surgical choice. Multiple studies have demonstrated equivalence in terms of surgical success compared with hysterectomy with uterosacral ligament suspension [3–5] and recently, 5-year outcomes of anterior mesh sacrospinous hysteropexy showed superiority to hysterectomy with apical suspension [6]. In the United States, the journey toward hysteropexy was popularized by the widespread use of vaginal mesh kits, as leaving the uterus in situ was associated with a significantly lower risk of vaginal mesh exposure [7]. Through products such as the anterior-apical mesh support system (Uphold™, Boston Scientific, Boston MA) and self-retrieving suture-capture devices that made minimal sacrospinous ligament dissection possible, surgeons became familiar with multiple transvaginal approaches to sacrospinous hysteropexy. After this kit was removed from use in the United States, Overholt et al. demonstrated equivalent results with a similar anterior sacrospinous suture approach without the use of the mesh inlay [8].

Surgical complications favor hysteropexy. Uterine preservation is associated with decreased blood loss and shorter operating time [9]. In a 2020 study assessing 50 women who underwent native tissue SSH through an anterior approach compared with 87 women who underwent vaginal hysterectomy with uterosacral ligament suspension (USLS), we demonstrated comparable short-term success in the study groups, with shorter operative times and fewer serious complications in the hysteropexy group [10].

There are multiple approaches to performing hysteropexy that range from native tissue repair options, such as vaginal sacrospinous or uterosacral hysteropexy to abdominal hysteropexy with or without mesh. Despite avoiding hysterectomy, hysteropexy procedures are not without their own unique complications in addition to common surgical complications that are shared with other procedures. This chapter will focus on surgical decision-making and complications specifically associated with specific methods of hysteropexy.

A. El Haraki (✉) · C. A. Matthews
Urogynecology and Reconstructive Pelvic Surgery, Wake Forest School of Medicine, Winston Salem, NC, USA
e-mail: camatthe@wakehealth.edu

H. B. Goldman, J. Zillioux (eds.), *Complications of Urogynecology and Reconstructive Pelvic Surgery*, https://doi.org/10.1007/978-3-032-00339-3_10

Informed Surgical Choice

The first complication that can arise from hysteropexy is incorrect choice of procedure for a particular patient. Potential areas of pathology that are better served by hysterectomy (with or without oophorectomy) include cervical elongation, recurrent cervical dysplasia, endometrial pathology, such as hyperplasia or endometrial cancer, endometriosis, large uterine leiomyomata, and ovarian disease [11]. On initial presentation, specific questions that should be asked include any history of abnormal cervical cancer screening testing (including HPV testing and pap smear results), abnormal uterine bleeding, and pelvic pain. On examination, besides evaluating for the type and degree of prolapse, attention must be paid to the size of the cervix and uterus.

Potential for Future Malignancy

A unique concern of hysteropexy is leaving behind occult uterine pathology or performing uterine suspension in someone who develops uterine cancer in the future. While the overall risk is low, postmenopausal women with a history of postmenopausal bleeding have the highest risk of occult endometrial pathology. In a retrospective analysis of 1196 women undergoing prolapse repair, 0.3% were found to have malignancy [12]. Similarly, in another study of patients who underwent hysterectomy at the time of prolapse surgery, 0.3% of 681 patients were found to have endometrial cancer. However, 13.3% of women with postmenopausal bleeding despite negative diagnostic evaluation had pathology [13]. Therefore, women with any history of postmenopausal bleeding are not good candidates for uterine preservation. Similarly, for premenopausal women with uterine pathology, such as fibroids or adenomyosis, due to an increased risk for future hysterectomy, we would also recommend against hysteropexy. For obese women with independent risk factors for future endometrial cancer, hysteropexy may also not be the best choice. Cervical cancer is much less common than previously, with HPV vaccination and cervical cancer screening, though consideration should be given to women with inadequate screening or increased risk factors for cervical pathology such as immunosuppression or history of cervical pathology. Finally, women with chronic pelvic pain and concern for endometriosis may be better served by hysterectomy at the time of prolapse repair.

Hemorrhage and Management of Intraoperative Bleeding

Sacrospinous hysteropexy may place patients at higher risk of intraoperative hemorrhage in 0.2–2% of patients [14] due to proximity of the ligament to vascular structures such as the inferior gluteal artery, which passes inferior to the piriformis muscle. Other vascular structures that are in proximity include the inferior gluteal, internal pudendal, vertebral, middle sacral, lateral sacral, and circumflex femoral vessels [15]. Venous injuries from the hypogastric and pudendal venous plexi have been reported in studies as well [16]. One risk factor specific to the sacrospinous dissection involves the typically nonvisual approach commonly used in identifying the point of fixation for the apical suspension. Steps to decrease the risk of this complication involve having intimate knowledge of the space, generous hydrodissection of the surgical spaces, and meticulous hemostasis during dissection to aid in ongoing visualization. Management of hemorrhage during sacrospinous dissection requires a thorough anatomical knowledge of the space and anticipation of this type of complication at the time of procedure. The first steps after recognition of hemorrhage involve communication with the surgical team and staff. Administration of intravenous Tranexamic acid may help decrease any pelvic hemorrhage [17]. We recommend compression for initial management, especially in the case of suspected venous hemorrhage. Depending on the presentation, this compression can be performed directly through the pararectal space or through the vagina [18, 19]. Surgical sponges should be placed in a directed fashion toward the ligament and a retractor can be used to help in adding pressure in that plane. If compression is not effective, direct repair or the use of hemostatic agents may be employed. For direct repair, it is crucial that adequate visualization be first optimized. Once the injured vessel is identified, we recommend the use of laparoscopic clip appliers, as handheld ones would likely be too large to fit into the space. Hemostatic agents such as thrombin, fibrin sealant, or oxidized regenerated cellulose may be used as well. In such cases of hemorrhage, we also recommend leaving in vaginal packing overnight to help with further compression. Postoperatively, if there is suspicion of continued hemorrhage, we recommend computed tomography angiography. Communication with interventional radiology may be warranted in the event of a continued bleed that may be managed with embolization. Adequate fluid resuscitation or transfusion may be needed in the postoperative setting.

Hemorrhage may also occur during uterosacral hysteropexy though this is theoretically less likely in the case of an extraperitoneal dissection. During uterosacral hysteropexy, the major vessels that are in close proximity to the distal uterosacral ligament are the uterine arteries and their branches. It is recommended that the sutures be placed more proximally, as this avoids bleeding from these branches and decreases the risk of ureteral kinking as well. Management of uterosacral hysteropexy hemorrhage involves the typical management of vaginal or abdominal hemorrhage, depending on the approach. Lastly, hemorrhage can be encountered in the case of a sacrohysteropexy or sacrocervicopexy. Depending on the technique employed, this may involve dissection into the broad ligament to tunnel the mesh through or dissection lateral to the cervix for the same reason. During these steps, the uterine arteries and potentially cervical branches are vulnerable to injury. Management of these hemorrhages may be obtained with electrocautery, suturing, or ligation of the uterine artery. In the case that this hemorrhage is uncontrollable, a hysterectomy may ultimately need to be performed, and this is a risk that must be shared with patients at the time of consent.

Ureteral Injury

Avoiding hysterectomy at the time of prolapse repair reduces the risk of ureteral injury in the cardinal ligament but obviously has the same risk of ureteral injury related to the specific apical suspension technique employed. Sacrohysteropexy and sacrospinous ligament hysteropexy have lower risks of ureteral kinking than uterosacral hysteropexy. Ureteral obstruction is one of the most common surgical complications of uterosacral ligament suspension that can happen in 6.2% of cases [19] and is more common with a transvaginal than laparoscopic approach [20]. In one study looking specifically at transvaginal uterosacral ligament hysteropexy, it occurred in 2.5% of patients [21]. This is due to the close proximity of the uterosacral ligament to the ureter, 1.3 to 2.0 cm along the target length in one study [22]. According to the American Urogynecologic Society Consensus Statement [23], cystoscopy is recommended at the end of prolapse repair and helps increase the rate of detection of intraoperative ureteral obstruction, decreasing long-term sequelae associated with injury. Special considerations should be noted depending on patient history, such as history of nephrectomy, double-collecting system, or history of ureteral reimplant. If efflux is absent from one side or both, first one must ensure that the patient is adequately hydrated; that there is sufficient visualization (through IV or oral dye if necessary), and that the patient is in at least a level position. In the case of uterosacral suspension, the suspected suture can be cut while watching for efflux. Since the distal uterosacral ligament is closest to the ureter, we recommend removing or cutting the most distal/lateral/caudad sutures first. If other causes of ureteral obstruction (such as anterior colporrhaphy sutures) have been ruled out, we recommend proceeding with retrograde pyelography or urologic consultation depending on surgeon comfort. After passing a soft, hydrophilic wire, a stent can be used to inject dye and image the ureter to identify the point of injury. If injury is suspected, a stent is passed and left in place for 4–6 weeks [24]. Postoperative ureteral injury may also be recognized. This may be due to a delayed injury due to devascularization, scarring, thermal injury or due to inadequate intraoperative cystoscopy. Patients may present with flank pain, ileus, decreased urinary output, or fevers. Computed tomography urogram is recommended in patients with adequate renal function. If this is recognized in the immediate postoperative period, removal of the offending sutures and stenting may be adequate. If this was more delayed, stenting may not be viable retrograde and patient may need antegrade stenting or nephrostomy with delayed repair of ureteral injury depending on the level and type of injury.

The sacrospinous ligament is further away from the ureter than the uterosacral ligament but kinking may still occur and in one series, it was associated with ureteral obstruction in up to 2.9% of cases [25]. For procedures that involve fixation of the uterus to the sacral promontory, the right ureter can be injured at the pelvic brim due to its close proximity to the promontory; as close as 13 mm in one study [26]. In the case of sacrospinous hysteropexy or abdominal minimally invasive hysteropexy, the management of ureteral obstruction or injury remains similar to the aforementioned approach. Diagnostic cystoscopy is advised at the end of any apical suspension procedure regardless if hysterectomy is performed or not.

Bowel Injury

The risk of bowel injury during open and laparoscopic hysteropexy is not unique to these procedures, so we will focus on the risk of bowel injury in the setting of transvaginal hysteropexy. Rectal injury is known to occur in 0.4–1.7% [27, 28] of sacrospinous ligament fixation, typically associated with the posterior approach to the ligament. This may occur during the initial dissection of the rectovaginal space or during dissection of the pararectal space to expose the sacrospinous ligament. During dissection of the rectovaginal space, injuries may occur to the anterior rectal wall. These can be repaired primarily in at least two layers and patients should be placed on a bowel regimen postoperatively. If the surgeon is comfortable with managing this, the closure is tension-free and the tissues are adequately vascularized, then colorectal surgery consult may not be needed. During suture placement of sacrospinous ligament suspension, the suture may be inadvertently placed in the rectum. This is also true for anchoring devices such that anchors may also be placed in the rectum. We recommend rectal exam following placement of anchor or suture for intraoperative recognition of this inadvertent complication. If removal of the suture is viable then it should be done. In the case of an anchor in the rectum, we would recommend cutting the suture on the vaginal side and removal of the anchor through the rectum so as not to increase the area of damage at the rectal site.

During uterosacral hysteropexy, small bowel obstruction, in which a knuckle of bowel becomes incarcerated into a suspending suture, is a known complication [29]. During a vaginal approach, we recommend packing the bowel away from the site of suture placement and removing the packing prior to tying down the suspension sutures while keeping the patient in steep Trendelenburg. Care should be taken not to otherwise entrap the bowel during colpotomy closure, peritoneal closure, or suspension fixation. During an abdominal approach, direct visualization aids in preventing this. In the case of mesh placement, such as in sacrohysteropexy, we recommend completely retroperitonealizing the mesh to avoid small or large bowel obstruction, which may occur in up to 1.0% of cases [30].

Potential for Pregnancy

In women of childbearing age who elect hysteropexy, there is a risk for future pregnancy. There is a paucity of data examining both pregnancy outcomes as well as recurrence of prolapse following pregnancy in women who have a history of prolapse repair. In one study with 54 women who underwent transvaginal sacrospinous hysteropexy, 8 had pregnancies. All delivered via Cesarean section and through a median follow-up of 45 months, 87.5% of these patients had improvement on their PISQ12 scores and were overall satisfied [31]. In another study that looked at 159 women who underwent laparoscopic hysteropexy using mesh, 8 became pregnant, with 7 out of 8 delivering at term. Of these 7 patients, 6 had stage 0 apical prolapse on exam and 1 had repeat surgery with perineorrhaphy 3 years postoperatively [32]. Given the overall lack of data and the nonurgent nature of prolapse repair, we recommend that hysteropexy be reserved for patients who have completed childbearing.

Mesh-Related Complications

For women undergoing transvaginal hysteropexy with mesh or minimally invasive sacrohysteropexy, mesh complications are relatively uncommon and certainly less than with concomitant hysterectomy [33]. However, vaginal mesh exposure still needs to be monitored, particularly for women with risk factors such as vaginal atrophy and smoking. Small bowel obstruction can occur as an immediate or late complication of sacrohysteropexy. Mesh erosion into the bladder and rectum is uncommon.

Cervical Elongation

Hypertrophic cervical elongation is both a potential contraindication to and complication of hysteropexy procedures other than the Manchester-Fothergill operation. In one study comparing transvaginal uterosacral ligament hysteropexy to hysterectomy plus uterosacral ligament suspension, while anatomic and subjective cure rates were similar, hysteropexy was found to be associated with a higher rate of apical recurrence, particularly due to cervical elongation [34]. A case series by Hyakutake showed cervical elongation in 62.5% of patients who underwent sacrospinous hysteropexy using polypropylene mesh arms. This type of recurrence, if symptomatic, may be treated with a variety of techniques. Depending on the extent and presence of concomitant prolapse in other compartments, this may be treated with a Manchester-Fothergill or simple trachelectomy if uterine preservation is still desired. A loop electrosurgical excision procedure (LEEP) may be an acceptable option depending on the size of the cervix and if there is no need for apical suspension. Finally, a hysterectomy may be a definitive approach to resolving cervical elongation.

Prolapse Recurrence

Cervical elongation, while a consideration following hysteropexy, is not the only presentation of recurrent prolapse following hysteropexy. In one study comparing sacrospinous hysteropexy to apical suspension with hysterectomy, while we showed similar rates of recurrence, patients with anatomic failure all had apical compartment recurrence, with one patient having cervical elongation [10]. In two separate meta-analyses, no major differences in recurrence or reoperation were noted between hysteropexy with apical prolapse repair and hysterectomy with apical prolapse repair [9, 35]. In one of those meta-analyses, hysteropexy was associated with shorter duration, less intraoperative blood loss, and hospitalization. The management of recurrent prolapse following hysteropexy is a shared decision between the patient and surgeon and dependent on the symptom bother as well as the type of prolapse and patient goals. Conservatively, a pessary may be used to manage prolapse or as a first-line treatment. If reoperation were the choice, this may range from a repeat hysteropexy (alternative method such as laparoscopic uterosacral suspension), hysterectomy with apical native tissue suspension or sacrocolpopexy, sacrohysteropexy, or in the case of an isolated compartment recurrence, an isolated repair may be indicated. If the patient is no longer sexually active, colpocleisis might also be a viable option if the anatomy lends itself to this.

Conclusion

Hysteropexy is an important tool in a pelvic surgeon's toolbox for managing uterine prolapse. A clear understanding as to the current and future risks of cervical and uterine pathology can guide surgeons in recommending an individualized patient-centered choice. Through understanding the anatomy of different hysteropexy techniques and understanding the unique complications that may be encountered with these approaches, a urogynecologist can adequately manage these complications and optimize patient outcomes.

References

1. Gutman RE, Woodburn KL. Uterine preservation during pelvic reconstructive surgery. Print; n.d.
2. Jirschele K, Seitz M, Zhou Y, Rosenblatt P, Culligan P, Sand P. A multicenter, prospective trial to evaluate mesh-augmented sacrospinous hysteropexy for uterovaginal prolapse. Int Urogynecol J. 2015;26(5):743–8. https://doi.org/10.1007/s00192-014-2564-x. Epub 2014 Nov 14. PMID: 25394892; PMCID: PMC4544494.
3. Maher C, Feiner B, Baessler K, Schmid C. Surgical management of pelvic organ prolapse in women. Cochrane Database Syst Rev. 2013;2013(4):CD004014.
4. Bradley S, Gutman RE, Richter LA. Hysteropexy: an option for the repair of pelvic organ prolapse. Curr Urol Rep. 2018;19(2):15.
5. Nager CW, Visco AG, Richter HE, et al. Effect of vaginal mesh hysteropexy vs vaginal hysterectomy with uterosacral ligament suspension on treatment failure in women with uterovaginal prolapse: a randomized clinical trial. JAMA. 2019;322(11):1054–65.
6. Gutman RE, Rardin CR, Sokol ER, et al. Vaginal and laparoscopic mesh hysteropexy for uterovaginal prolapse: a parallel cohort study. Am J Obstet Gynecol. 2017;216(1):38.e1–11.
7. Meriwether KV, Antosh DD, Olivera CK, Kim-Fine S, Balk EM, Murphy M, Grimes CL, Sleemi A, Singh R, Dieter AA, Crisp CC, Rahn DD. Uterine preservation vs hysterectomy in pelvic organ prolapse surgery: a systematic review with meta-analysis and clinical practice guidelines. Am J Obstet Gynecol. 2018;219(2):129–146.e2. https://doi.org/10.1016/j.ajog.2018.01.018. Epub 2018 Jan 17. PMID: 29353031
8. Overholt TL, Velet L, Xu M, Dutta R, Matthews CA. Anterior approach sacrospinous hysteropexy: native tissue compared with mesh-augmented repair for primary uterovaginal prolapse management. Int Urogynecol J. 2023;34(10):2603–9. https://doi.org/10.1007/s00192-023-05589-z. Epub 2023 Jul 13. PMID: 37439863
9. He L, Feng D, Zha X, Liao XY, Gong ZL, Gu DQ, Lin YH, Huang L. Hysteropreservation versus hysterectomy in uterine prolapse surgery: a systematic review and meta-analysis. Int Urogynecol J. 2022;33(7):1917–25. https://doi.org/10.1007/s00192-021-04913-9. Epub 2021 Jul 2. PMID: 34213602
10. Plair A, Dutta R, Overholt TL, Matthews C. Short-term outcomes of sacrospinous hysteropexy through an anterior approach. Int Urogynecol J. 2021;32(6):1555–63.
11. Ridgeway BM. Does prolapse equal hysterectomy? The role of uterine conservation in women with uterovaginal prolapse. Am J Obstet Gynecol. 2015;213(6):802–9. https://doi.org/10.1016/j.ajog.2015.07.035. Epub 2015 Jul 28. PMID: 26226554
12. Ackenbom MF, Giugale LE, Wang Y, et al. Incidence of occult uterine pathology in women undergoing hysterectomy with pelvic organ prolapse repair. Female Pelvic Med Reconstr Surg. 2016;22:332–5.
13. Frick AC, Walters MD, Larkin KS, et al. Risk of unanticipated abnormal gynecologic pathology at the time of hysterectomy for uterovaginal prolapse. Am J Obstet Gynecol. 2010;202(507):e1–4.
14. Pahwa AK, Arya LA, Andy UU. Management of arterial and venous hemorrhage during sacrospinous ligament fixation: cases and review of the literature. Int Urogynecol J. 2016;27(3):387–91. https://doi.org/10.1007/s00192-015-2818-2. Epub 2015 Aug 19. PMID: 26282092
15. Barksdale PA, Elkins TE, Sanders CK, Jaramillo FE, Gasser RF. An anatomic approach to pelvic hemorrhage during sacrospinous ligament fixation of the vaginal vault. Obstet Gynecol. 1998;91(5 Pt 1):715–8. https://doi.org/10.1016/s0029-7844(98)00051-9. PMID: 9572217
16. Thompson JR, Gibb JS, Genadry R, Burrows L, Lambrou N, Buller JL. Anatomy of pelvic arteries adjacent to the sacrospinous ligament: importance of the coccygeal branch of the inferior gluteal artery. Obstet Gynecol. 1999;94(6):973–7. https://doi.org/10.1016/s0029-7844(99)00418-4. PMID: 10576185
17. Williams-Johnson JA, McDonald AH, Strachan GG, Williams EW. Effects of tranexamic acid on death, vascular occlusive events, and blood transfusion in trauma patients with significant haemorrhage (CRASH-2) a randomised, placebo-controlled

trial. West Indian Med J. 2010;59(6):612–24. PMID: 21702233
18. Carey MP, Slack MC. Transvaginal sacrospinous colpopexy for vault and marked uterovaginal prolapse. Br J Obstet Gynaecol. 1994;101(6):536–40. https://doi.org/10.1111/j.1471-0528.1994.tb13158.x. PMID: 8018646
19. De Vita D, Giordano S, Piccione E. Management of intraoperative haemorrhage in pelvic organ prolapse repair: a report of two cases. In Vivo. 2011;25(2):275–7. PMID: 21471546
20. Houlihan S, Kim-Fine S, Birch C, Tang S, Brennand EA. Uterosacral vault suspension (USLS) at the time of hysterectomy: laparoscopic versus vaginal approach. Int Urogynecol J. 2019;30(4):611–21. https://doi.org/10.1007/s00192-018-3801-5. Epub 2018 Nov 5. PMID: 30393822
21. Richter LA, Boileau J, Janni M, Tefera E, Iglesia CB. Intraoperative ureteral kinking during uterosacral ligament suspension: effect of training level on occurrence. J Reprod Med. 2016;61(1–2):17–21. PMID: 26995883
22. Siff LN, Jallad K, Hickman LC, Walters MD. Surgical anatomy of the uterosacral ligament Colpopexy. Female Pelvic Med Reconstr Surg. 2018;24(5):380–2. https://doi.org/10.1097/SPV.0000000000000461. PMID: 28727647
23. Cohen SA, Carberry CL, Smilen SW. American Urogynecologic Society Consensus Statement: Cystoscopy at the Time of Prolapse Repair. Female Pelvic Med Reconstructive Surgery. 2018;24(4):258–9. https://doi.org/10.1097/SPV.0000000000000529.
24. Kim JH, Moore C, Jones JS, Rackley R, Daneshgari F, Goldman H, Vasavada S. Management of ureteral injuries associated with vaginal surgery for pelvic organ prolapse. Int Urogynecol J Pelvic Floor Dysfunct. 2006;17(5):531–5. https://doi.org/10.1007/s00192-005-0020-7. Epub 2005 Nov 30. PMID: 16317499
25. Kapoor S, Sivanesan K, Robertson JA, Veerasingham M, Kapoor V. Sacrospinous hysteropexy: review and meta-analysis of outcomes. Int Urogynecol J. 2017;28(9):1285–94. https://doi.org/10.1007/s00192-017-3291-x. Epub 2017 Mar 3. PMID: 28258346
26. Giraudet G, Protat A, Cosson M. The anatomy of the sacral promontory: how to avoid complications of the sacrocolpopexy procedure. Am J Obstet Gynecol. 2018;218(4):457.e1–3. https://doi.org/10.1016/j.ajog.2017.12.236. Epub 2018 Jan 2. PMID: 29305252
27. Demirci F, Demirci O, Dolgun ZN, Karakoç B, Demirci E, Somunkıran A, Iyibozkurt C, Karaalp E. Perioperative complications in abdominal sacrocolpopexy, sacrospinous ligament fixation and prolift procedures. Balkan Med J. 2014;31(2):158–63. https://doi.org/10.5152/balkanmedj.2014.13135. Epub 2014 Jun 1. PMID: 25207189; PMCID: PMC4115928
28. Hoffman MS, Lynch C, Lockhart J, Knapp R. Injury of the rectum during vaginal surgery. Am J Obstet Gynecol. 1999;181(2):274–7. https://doi.org/10.1016/s0002-9378(99)70547-8. PMID: 10454668
29. Unger CA, Walters MD, Ridgeway B, Jelovsek JE, Barber MD, Paraiso MF. Incidence of adverse events after uterosacral colpopexy for uterovaginal and posthysterectomy vault prolapse. Am J Obstet Gynecol. 2015;212(5):603.e1–7. https://doi.org/10.1016/j.ajog.2014.11.034. Epub 2014 Nov 27. PMID: 25434838
30. Wadensweiler P, Whitcomb EL, Jeney SES, Meller D, Moran K, Guaderrama NM, Brueseke T. Bowel obstruction after sacrocolpopexy: a case series. Female Pelvic Med Reconstr Surg. 2021;27(11):e677–80. https://doi.org/10.1097/SPV.0000000000001095. PMID: 34705799
31. Cavkaytar S, Kokanalı MK, Tasdemir U, Doganay M, Aksakal O. Pregnancy outcomes after transvaginal sacrospinous hysteropexy. Eur J Obstet Gynecol Reprod Biol. 2017;216:204–7. https://doi.org/10.1016/j.ejogrb.2017.08.003. Epub 2017 Aug 4. PMID: 28802943
32. Pandeva I, Mistry M, Fayyad A. Efficacy and pregnancy outcomes of laparoscopic single sheet mesh sacrohysteropexy. Neurourol Urodyn. 2017;36(3):787–93. https://doi.org/10.1002/nau.23026. Epub 2016 May 25. PMID: 27224927
33. Chan IS, Chen GY, Shih YC, Jiang LY, Chang YH, Wang TY, Chen YJ. Robot-assisted sacrohysteropexy vs robot-assisted sacrocolpopexy in women with primary advanced apical prolapse: a retrospective cohort study. J Chin Med Assoc. 2023;86(4):418–25. https://doi.org/10.1097/JCMA.0000000000000882. Epub 2023 Mar 2. PMID: 36859778
34. Milani R, Manodoro S, Cola A, Bellante N, Palmieri S, Frigerio M. Transvaginal uterosacral ligament hysteropexy versus hysterectomy plus uterosacral ligament suspension: a matched cohort study. Int Urogynecol J. 2020;31(9):1867–72. https://doi.org/10.1007/s00192-019-04206-2. Epub 2019 Dec 17. PMID: 31848662
35. Porcari I, Zorzato PC, Bosco M, Garzon S, Magni F, Salvatore S, Franchi MP, Uccella S. Clinician perspectives on hysterectomy versus uterine preservation in pelvic organ prolapse surgery: A systematic review and meta-analysis. Int J Gynaecol Obstet. 2024;166(1):173–189. https://doi.org/10.1002/ijgo.15343. Epub 2024 Jan 25. PMID: 38269852. Dietz V, van der Vaart CH, van der Graaf Y, Heintz P, Schrafordt Koops SE. One-year follow-up after sacrospinous hysteropexy and vaginal hysterectomy for uterine descent: a randomized study. Int Urogynecol J. 2010;21(2):209–16. Int Urogynecol J (2023) 34:2603–2609 2609 1 3.

11 Robotic/Laparoscopic Female Pelvic Reconstructive Surgery

Dora Jericevic Schwartz, Lauren Stewart, Dominique Malacarne Pape, and Nirit Rosenblum

Introduction

As the population continues to age, so does the prevalence of medical conditions associated with the advancements of age. Pelvic organ prolapse (POP) is a common condition associated with aging, menopause, prior pregnancy, and vaginal delivery. Across all gynecologic procedures, surgical repair of POP is the most common type of procedure performed in women older than 70 years [1] and is estimated to affect nearly 50% of parous women [2]. It is estimated that 10–15% of all women will undergo surgery for POP or urinary incontinence by age 80, and this is only expected to increase [3].

Minimally invasive sacrocolpopexy (MIS SCP), a mesh-augmented repair, performed with both laparoscopic and robotic-assisted laparoscopic approaches, is regarded as the "gold standard" procedure for correcting symptomatic pelvic organ prolapse. In this chapter, we will discuss the potential complications unique to each step of a MIS SCP and outline strategies to minimize their incidence (Table 11.1). The principles, complications, and management detailed here are applicable to other procedures used to repair POP such as MIS sacrohysteropexy.

In the patient selection section, we will review patient risk factors associated with MIS SCP perioperative complications, focusing on smoking, obesity, and poor glycemic control. In the set-up section, principles of safe positioning and port placement are reviewed to prevent nerve palsy and visceral injury. Pre-sacral hemorrhage is the most significant intraoperative complication of MIS SCP. Techniques for minimizing the risk of pre-sacral hemorrhage and preventing the potential significant morbidity and mortality of major vascular injury should it occur are discussed in the sacral dissection section. Though MIS SCP is performed for post-hysterectomy vaginal vault prolapse, it is often performed when the uterus is present. In the hysterectomy section, we will discuss management of the cervix (supracervical versus total hysterectomy) and implications on mesh exposure, subsequent reoperation, and port site hernia risk. Additionally, the data on bladder and ureteral injury during hysterectomy will be reviewed. Relatedly, in the adnexa section, we discuss surgical management of the fallopian tubes and the decision of whether to perform an oophorectomy, weighing the risk of future malignancy and the potential bone and cardiovascular benefits of keeping the ovaries. In the

D. J. Schwartz · L. Stewart · N. Rosenblum (✉)
Department of Urology, NYU Langone Medical Center, New York, NY, USA
e-mail: dora.jericevic@nyulangone.org; Lauren.stewart@nyulangone.org; Nirit.Rosenblum@nyulangone.org

D. M. Pape
Department of Obstetrics, Gynecology and Urology, New York Medical College, Valhalla, NY, USA
e-mail: dominique.malacarne@nyumc.org

H. B. Goldman, J. Zillioux (eds.), *Complications of Urogynecology and Reconstructive Pelvic Surgery*, https://doi.org/10.1007/978-3-032-00339-3_11

Table 11.1 Step-by-step, minimally invasive (MIS) sacrocolpopexy (SCP) principles, complications, and management

Patient selection	Review patient risk factors associated with MIS SCP perioperative complications, focusing on smoking, obesity, and poor glycemic control
Set-up	Principles of safe positioning and port placement are reviewed to minimize the complications of nerve palsy and visceral injury
Sacral dissection	Review of vascular anatomy and techniques for minimizing the risk of pre-sacral hemorrhage and preventing the potential significant morbidity and mortality of major vascular injury
Hysterectomy	Management of cervix (supracervical versus total hysterectomy) and implications on mesh exposure, reoperation, port site hernia, and genitourinary tract injury
Adnexa	Surgical management of the fallopian tubes and the decision of whether to perform an oophorectomy
Anterior dissection	Cystotomy and vaginotomy prevention and management, particularly in cases of prior hysterectomy or cesarean section
Posterior dissection	Risk factors, prevention, and management of rectal injury
Mesh attachment to the vagina	Suture selection, management of mesh exposure, and transvaginal excision of permanent suture
Mesh attachment to the sacrum	Review of lumbosacral bony anatomy, appropriate suture placement, and workup and management in rare cases of sacral osteomyelitis and pyogenic spondylitis
Peritoneal closure	Prevention of bowel complications from peritoneal closure and the importance of cystoscopy following peritoneal closure
Concomitant midurethral sling	Appropriate preoperative workup and counseling to decrease the risk of worsened postoperative or de novo stress urinary incontinence. Review of the role of urodynamics and the staged sling approach
Postoperative recovery and long-term quality of life	Review of immediate postoperative and delayed bowel complications, prolapse recurrence, persistent pain, and sexual complications

anterior dissection section, we discuss cystotomy and vaginotomy prevention and management, which is particularly important in patients with a prior history of hysterectomy or cesarean section. Though very rare, the posterior dissection section reviews the prevention and management of rectal injury during MIS SCP. The attachment of the mesh section reviews the data on suture selection, and, when a permanent suture is used, management of suture exposure.

Mesh attachment to the sacrum is a critical step of a MIS SCP and though very rare, sacral osteomyelitis and pyogenic spondylitis can occur. We will review the lumbosacral bony anatomy and discuss principles of appropriate suture placement. A peritoneal closure over the mesh is performed by most surgeons and marks the juncture in the case when a cystoscopy is performed. Cystoscopy following completion of MIS SCP is imperative to ensure there has been no injury to the bladder or ureters during the anterior dissection or hysterectomy, as well as no kinking of the ureters from the peritoneal closure. In the concomitant midurethral sling (MUS) section, we discuss occult SUI and the appropriate preoperative workup to decrease the risk of worsened post-operative or de novo stress urinary incontinence. Finally, we review immediate and delayed postoperative bowel complications, prolapse recurrence, persistent pain, and sexual complications.

Patient Selection

Preoperatively, to minimize operative complications of MIS SCP, surgeons should be aware of uterine size, prior abdominopelvic surgeries, colonic disease such as diverticulitis, ureteral anomalies, and sacral and peri-sacral anomalies such as horseshoe kidney.

MIS SCP has the potential to significantly improve quality of life, but it is an elective procedure [4]. Patients should be optimized from a cardiopulmonary and glycemic control (Hemoglobin A1C < 8%) standpoint prior to MIS SCP [5]. Smoking cessation is strongly advised to minimize wound-healing complications [6]. Mesh exposure has been found to be significantly more likely in smokers than in nonsmokers (odds ratio 4.4; $p = 0.01$), [7]. The 4-week postoperative risk for symptomatic venous thromboembolism (VTE) on systematic review and meta-analysis (SRMA) has been found to be 1.5% (0.4–4.6% across VTE risk groups) [8]. All patients should be risk-stratified using the validated Caprini scoring system and have appropriate perioperative VTE prophylaxis to minimize this risk [9].

In POP surgery, obesity is associated with increased blood loss, longer operative times, higher intraoperative complications (specifically conversions to laparotomy), and, in a 2024 SRMA, was associated with a greater likelihood of prolapse recurrence and mesh complications after POP repair [10, 11]. While a strict BMI cutoff for prolapse repair has not been established, for patients who are motivated to lose weight, preoperative referral to weight management can be considered, as modern weight loss strategies can be highly effective, and any degree of weight loss may be expected to improve surgical outcomes. Thus, *patients should be counseled that smoking, obesity, and poor glycemic control have been associated with perioperative complications.*

Set-up

MIS SCP is performed in the low lithotomy and steep Trendelenburg position. As in any MIS, pressure points are padded to prevent peripheral nerve injury and compartment syndrome. The patient should be placed directly on anti-skid material without intervening bedsheets, as the direct contact keeps the patient from slipping during steep Trendelenburg.

Once general anesthesia is induced, the eyes should be taped closed to prevent corneal abrasions, and the patient's face should be padded to prevent trauma from the instruments in the operative field. The patient is placed in the low lithotomy position with care taken to avoid common peroneal and femoral injuries by ensuring the lateral aspect of the knee is padded and avoiding excessive hip flexion, extension, abduction, or external rotation. The arms are tucked securely by the patient's side with the palms facing the body, and the wrists and fingers are protected.

The abdomen is entered in the midline just below the umbilicus. For robotic SCP, the midline entry serves as the camera port. Once insufflation is achieved, the remaining four ports are placed at the level of the umbilicus: two robotic ports on the left hemiabdomen 8–10 cm apart, one lateral to the rectus on the right hemiabdomen, and an 8 mm assistant port at least 3 cm above the anterior superior iliac spine (Fig. 11.1). When SCP is performed using traditional laparoscopy (TL), typically only three lateral ports are required, and all ports can be 5 mm with the exception of a single 8 mm port to allow for suture to enter and exit the abdomen. For many patients, the sacral promontory can be palpated, which may inform superior or inferior adjustments to the described port placement, in addition to prior surgical scars.

A vaginal or uterine manipulator is placed. The patient is placed in steep Trendelenburg, and the small intestine is gently swept out of the pelvis.

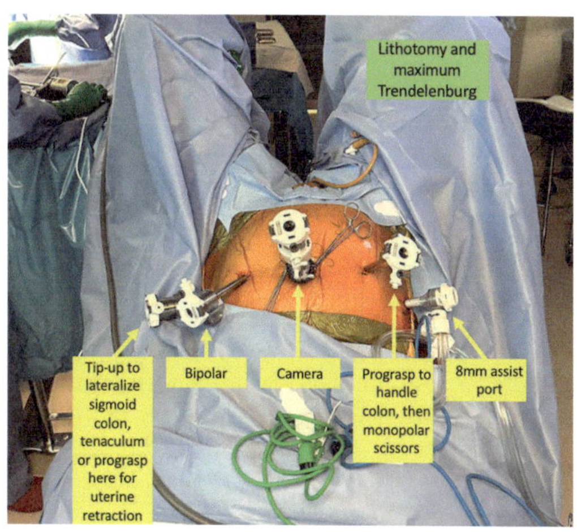

Fig. 11.1 Port placement during robotic sacrocolpopexy

Sacral Dissection

Either the sacral dissection or the hysterectomy is typically performed as the first step of the SCP. Prior to SCP, knowledge of anatomic variations such as a horseshoe kidney, pelvic kidney, or any sacral anomalies, including congenital anomalies, inflammatory diseases of the lumbosacral spine (e.g., sacroiliitis, ankylosing spondylitis), and history of spinal surgery at the lumbosacral levels with anterior hardware is critical as these features can make SCP more difficult or contraindicated.

To maximize exposure of the sacral promontory, the sigmoid colon is lateralized (robotically with the fourth arm or TL with a suture placed through 2–3 sigmoid epiploica and brought through the LLQ abdominal wall lateral and inferior to accessory ports on that side). Pre-sacral hemorrhage is the most significant intraoperative complication of MIS SCP. The normal vascular anatomy associated with the sacral promontory includes the common iliac arteries and veins, the presacral venous plexus, the middle sacral artery (which arises from the abdominal aorta just above its bifurcation into the common iliac arteries), the middle sacral vein (which typically drains into the junction of the common iliac veins), and the lateral sacral arteries that typically arise from the posterior division of the internal iliac artery [12]. Aberrant sacral vasculature is not uncommon [13].

With pneumoperitoneum distorting the appearance of venous vasculature, the most common site of vascular injury is the left common iliac vein, often mistaken for the anterior longitudinal ligament. It may be helpful to perform the sacral dissection under lower intra-abdominal insufflation pressure (i.e., 8–10 mm pressure) to avoid distortion of venous structures overlying the promontory. When intraoperative pre-sacral hemorrhage is encountered, communication with anesthesia and nursing is imperative, as presacral hemorrhage is often difficult to control with bipolar electrocautery, sutures, pressure, and hemostatic agents. In cases of bleeding from smaller sacral vessels, specialized tacks, such as hemostatic clips or bone tacks, can be mechanically driven into the sacrum to occlude bleeding vessels. When larger vessels are injured, the case should be converted to open with vascular surgery assistance. While conversion is undertaken, pressure on the site of sacral bleeding should be maintained. In robotic cases, this is accomplished initially using the robotic arm until the robot is undocked, followed by a laparoscopic instrument until the abdomen is opened.

Hysterectomy

SCP is frequently performed for post-hysterectomy vaginal vault prolapse. In cases where the uterus is present, either a supracervical hysterectomy (SCH) or total hysterectomy (TH) is performed. The differences between the approaches and implications on reoperation for cervical pathology, mesh exposure, and POP outcomes are reviewed and summarized (Table 11.2).

If a SCH is performed, continued surveillance of the cervix is required as per the American College of Obstetricians and Gynecologists (ACOG) Clinical Practice Guidelines [14]. Patients who have a TH at time of SCP, per-

Table 11.2 Differences between total and supracervical hysterectomy in sacrocolpopexy

	Hysterectomy	
	Total	Supracervical
Complication		
Mesh exposure	3–4%	1%
Cervical reoperation for gynecologic pathology	0%	1–5%
Prolapse recurrence	No significant difference	
Dyspareunia	No difference	
Chronic pain	No difference	
Urinary tract injury	0.84%	0.23%
Port site hernia	0.65%	1.30%
Other considerations		
PAP testing	Not needed (typically)	Continue per the American College of Obstetricians and Gynecologists guidelines

formed for indications other than cervical cancer or high-grade cervical dysplasia, do not need continued screening of the vaginal cuff.

With SCH, there is a risk of subsequent trachelectomy for unanticipated gynecologic findings on operative specimen pathology, subsequent cervical dysplasia, prolapse of the cervical stump, cervical fibroids, or abnormal bleeding from the retained cervix. The risk of trachelectomy after SCH ranges between 1% and 5% [15].

If trachelectomy is subsequently recommended for a benign cause, it may be attempted transvaginally, though this can be challenging after SCP when there is excellent apical support. In cases of transabdominal trachelectomy, the entire mesh is typically removed and replaced with new mesh.

In SCP with SCH, the risk of mesh exposure is 1%, while in SCP with TH, the risk of mesh exposure has been found to be higher at 3–4% [15, 16]. However, there are recent studies that suggest there is no difference between groups when using contemporary mesh products [17, 18]. In older studies from the early 2000s, in which heavier weight mesh products were used, rates of mesh exposure are significantly higher among the TH patients, but these figures are not generalizable to present-day urogynecologic practice [19–21] as ultra-lightweight (weight less than 25 g/m^2) and lightweight (25–50 g/m^2) meshes are now standard of care. Intermediate weight (50–80 g/m^2) and heavyweight (greater than 80 g/m^2) meshes have, for the most part, been withdrawn from the market for urogynecologic use. If a mesh exposure is noted after SCP, with lightweight meshes, most cases are managed conservatively with vaginal estrogen and do not require reoperation. The American Urogynecologic Society (AUGS) Committee Opinion on the Management of Mesh and Graft Complications in Gynecologic Surgery states that a trial of vaginal estrogen can be attempted for small (less than 0.5 cm) mesh exposures. Mesh removal surgery should not be performed unless there is a specific therapeutic indication (such as persistent vaginal bleeding and vaginal discharge from mesh exposure refractory to an adequate trial of conservative management). Pelvic pain and dyspareunia may possibly be related to exposed mesh, but symptoms may not respond to mesh removal [22].

Ureteral injury can occur during any hysterectomy, though there is a paucity of the literature to determine the exact ureteral injury rate during minimally invasive prolapse repair specifically. Relatedly, minimally invasive hysterectomy has been associated with a ureteral injury incidence of 0.02–0.54%, which is slightly higher in TH compared to Scheme (0.28% versus 0.12%) [23, 24]. In fact, genitourinary tract injury rates have been found to be 0.84% and 0.23% during TH and SCH, respectively ($p < 0.01$) [23]. Ureteral injury during hysterectomy is most likely to occur during ligation of the ovarian and uterine arteries, as well as during cuff closure in cases of TH. For these reasons, intraoperative cystoscopy is the standard of care to ensure ureteral patency and bladder integrity.

In terms of POP outcomes, reoperation and recurrent POP are similar between groups, though low-level evidence suggests higher rates of anterior compartment prolapse after SCH SCP [25].

In TH SCP, the specimen is extracted vaginally, whereas in SCH SCP, the specimen is extracted through a midline incision. For this reason, the midline port site final incision is typically larger in SCH SCP and is associated with higher rates of port site hernias (1.3% SCH SCP vs 0.65% TH SCP, $p < 0.01$) [17].

Adnexa

Fallopian tubes: Studies have shown that high-grade serous ovarian cancers originate in the fimbrial end of the fallopian tubes [26]. Thus, salpingectomy during hysterectomy is recommended as a preventive measure against ovarian cancer.

Ovaries: Removal of the ovaries is associated with ovarian cancer risk reduction but is also associated with increased cardiovascular and bone health risks in younger women due to the sudden loss of estrogen [27, 28]. Thus, oophorectomy is not routinely performed in average-risk women <65 years as the potential bone and cardiovascular benefits are felt to be outweighed by the risks [29]. If an oophorectomy is performed, the ureter is identified prior to ligation of the infundibulopelvic (IP) ligament as it courses in close proximity to the IP.

Anterior Dissection

The vesicovaginal junction is identified, and the peritoneum overlying the anterior vaginal wall is incised. Using a combination of blunt and sharp dissection, the bladder is dissected off the anterior vaginal wall. This plane is developed toward the bladder neck to create adequate space for mesh fixation such that the entire prolapsed area is suspended. In cases of post-hysterectomy prolapse, and/or prior history of cesarean section, this dissection is often scarred and challenging. Accordingly, a history of prior hysterectomy is associated with a significantly increased odds of lower urinary tract injury on multivariable logistic regression analysis (adjusted odds ratio 162, $p = 0.01$) [30].

The risk of cystotomy during MIS SCP can be minimized by maintaining adequate counter tension during the anterior dissection of the bladder off the vagina. This is achieved with the assistance of a vaginal or uterine manipulator (the former favored in cases of SCH and the latter favored in cases of TH). MIS SCP has been associated with an intraoperative bladder injury rate of 0.4–3.3% and up to 10% in some studies of patients with post-hysterectomy vaginal vault prolapse [31, 32]. However, these studies from a decade ago are felt to overestimate this intraoperative complication given surgeons' advancement on the MIS SCP learning curve. If a cystotomy occurs, following two-layer watertight closure with a negative leak test, interval placement (>6 weeks) of SCP mesh is advised to minimize the risk of mesh bladder erosion and fistulization. Inadvertent vaginotomy/colpotomy can occur during the anterior and posterior dissections. To minimize the risk of vaginal mesh exposure, it is advisable to avoid suturing mesh directly over the colpotomy closure suture line. In addition, a local peritoneal flap can be secured over the repaired colpotomy or cystotomy sites to prevent mesh exposure.

Posterior Dissection

The posterior vaginal wall is identified and the peritoneum in the Pouch of Douglas is incised. The rectum is dissected off the vagina by dissecting through the rectovaginal septum toward the perineal body, although surgeon preference plays a role in the degree of posterior dissection.

Inadvertent rectal injury can occur, though this is a rare complication. Prior history of pelvic surgery, diverticulitis, pelvic inflammatory disease, and endometriosis can make the posterior dissection more scarred and challenging. If rectal injury does occur, it should be repaired together with colorectal surgery assistance, and interval placement (>6 weeks) of SCP mesh is advised to minimize the risk of rectal mesh erosion and fistulization.

Mesh Attachment to the Vagina

With the anterior and posterior dissections complete, the mesh is attached to the anterior and posterior vaginal walls using delayed absorbable (polyglactin, polydioxanone) or permanent suture (polytetrafluoroethylene, polypropylene). Interrupted permanent suture or running absorbable suture are commonly used. At 18-month follow-up, an SRMA found there was no difference in permanent compared with absorbable suture in SCP success rates (proportional anatomic success rate 92% [95% CI 0.88–0.95] vs 96% [95% CI 0.92–0.99]) [30]. Another SRMA also found that absorbable suture yielded similar success rates (anterior, apical, and posterior), but was associated with less suture exposure and less retreatment [31]. A randomized controlled trial, Permanent versus Absorbable Controlled Trial, with 1-year follow-up, found that suture type used for mesh attachment did not influence mesh or permanent suture vaginal exposure rates. The rate of any suture exposure from 3 months to

1 year postoperatively was 2%. While mesh exposure can be managed conservatively with vaginal estrogen, suture exposure is managed with transvaginal excision if symptomatic (bleeding/spotting and copious discharge). This can be done in the clinic by grasping the exposed suture with a tonsil and putting it under tension, such that ideally the entirety of the exposed suture can be cut and removed.

Mesh Attachment to the Sacrum

When placing sacral sutures (typically permanent sutures), the surgeon must avoid the L5-S1 disc space, and the depth of sutures in the anterior longitudinal ligament (ALL) should not exceed 2 mm, the thickness of the ALL itself [33].

The sacral promontory refers to the anterior uppermost part of the sacrum, which is at the superior anterior edge of the first sacral vertebra (top 1/3 of S1). The most forward-projecting point intraoperatively is often referred to as the "sacral promontory," though for most patients this pseudo promontory (most forward-projecting portion of the lumbosacral junction) is the L5-S1 disc space, which is found ~1.5 cm cephalad to the "true" sacral promontory [34].

An MRI study found that the most prominent anterior aspect of the lumbosacral spine is the L5-S1 intervertebral disc space in 73% of women, whereas the remaining 27% of women had their most forward-projecting point at the superior aspect of S1 [35]. The mean height of the L5-S1 disc space was 13.3 mm (4.4–20.6 mm). For those with a non-disk promontory, the anterior height of the S1 vertebrae has been found to be 17–25 mm. As such, we generally place our proximal sacral suspension suture about 10–15 mm below the forward-projecting part of the lumbosacral junction. Additionally, a study of cadavers and computed tomography (CT) scans found a 60-degree average drop between the anterior surfaces of L5 and S1 [34]. This study also confirmed that for most patients, the most visible structure in the "surgical presacral space" is the L5–S1 disc and not the "true" sacral promontory.

Care must be taken to stay in the midline as the first sacral nerve can be expected approximately 3 cm from the upper surface of the sacrum and 1.5 cm from the midline [34].

While rare, postoperative infection of the disc or sacral bone can occur and be severe. Low back pain postoperatively, accompanied by possible fever, possible signs of sepsis, and high clinical suspicion, should prompt immediate lumbosacral imaging: MRI is preferred. The white blood cell count may remain within normal limits, particularly in subacute or chronic cases. C-reactive protein and erythrocyte sedimentation rate should be drawn, the former often used to monitor acute phase/early treatment response and the latter used for the chronic phase/longer term treatment response [36]. This complication requires spine surgery and infectious disease consults, and may require reoperation and removal of all mesh and suture, followed by a prolonged course of broad-spectrum antibiotics.

Peritoneal Closure

It is common practice (performed in >90% of cases) to close the peritoneum over the SCP mesh to prevent mesh-related small bowel obstruction (SBO) [37]. Though the literature is quite limited, it does not support re-peritonealization to reduce bowel complications [38–41]. Re-peritonealization increases operative time by about 20–30 min [39]. When using barbed suture during the peritoneal closure, there must be no exposed barbs as this has been associated with postoperative SBO [42, 43]. Superficial bites of the peritoneum are taken to prevent injury to underlying structures, particularly the right ureter and great vessels. Following re-peritonealization, cystoscopy is imperative to perform to check for ureteral efflux to ensure there is no ureteral kinking from the peritoneal closure, as well as no injury to the urinary tract during the hysterectomy. Several agents may be used to facilitate the visualization of ureteral efflux: (sodium) fluorescein, indocyanine green, indigo carmine, or methylene blue.

Concomitant Midurethral Sling

It is fair to assume that every woman with advanced prolapse is incontinent or has the potential to be incontinent. Thus, screening for stress urinary incontinence (SUI) is pertinent when performing any POP procedure, and if present, a possible concomitant anti-incontinence procedure is discussed. Even without preoperative patient-endorsed SUI, the possibility of de novo SUI after SCP should be discussed, as patients with new leakage after POP repair view it as a complication of surgery if appropriate counseling is not done preoperatively. Ideally, patients should be screened for occult SUI with cough stress test (CST) while the prolapse is reduced to allow for proper counseling and surgical planning. Urodynamic testing is typically not indicated in women with uncomplicated, demonstrable SUI on office evaluation [44].

Management of expectations is critical, and patients should be made aware that MUS placement at the time of POP may be associated with lower SUI cure rates when compared to sling surgery alone [45, 46]. The effect of MUS on urinary outcomes may vary based on the type of POP repair [47]. Moreover, for some patients, SUI may resolve after POP repair [46]. For these reasons, some surgeons counsel patients toward a staged sling placement approach. Most surgeons will place a MUS concurrently at the time of SCP in patients endorsing preop bothersome SUI or with a positive CST. In the final section of postoperative recovery and long-term quality of life, we review the immediate postoperative and delayed bowel complications, prolapse recurrence, persistent pain, and sexual complications.

Postoperative Recovery and Long-Term Quality of Life: Bowel Complications, Prolapse Recurrence, Persistent Pain, Sexual Complications

Bowel Complications

Nausea and emesis should always provoke the question of ileus or SBO. Often this can be managed conservatively with bowel rest and/or a nasogastric tube. In cases of SBO, the decision about return to the operating room is made on a case-by-case basis. While bowel obstruction is rare, overall rates of bowel dysfunction far surpass this at 5–14%, according to a meta-analysis of robotic-assisted sacrocolpopexy [48]. The most common types of dysfunction cited were dyschezia, obstructed defecation, and constipation. It is imperative to place the mesh as flat as possible against the sacral promontory and to avoid attachment to the levator ani musculature in order to decrease anorectal dysfunction postoperatively. Extensive lateral dissection in the rectovaginal septum should be avoided to reduce the risk of rectal denervation injury.

Management of expectations is important in this area. Constipation has been found to be the most frequent reason for patient telephone calls after pelvic organ prolapse surgery [49, 50]. Patients should be counseled that the average time to first bowel movement (BM) is estimated at 3 days after prolapse surgery and that opiate use worsens constipation [51]. Though there is no consensus in the literature for the prevention of postoperative constipation, we typically use a standing regimen of acetaminophen and ketorolac (transitioned to ibuprofen outpatient) with opiates only if needed for breakthrough pain [50]. Additionally, patients are started on a powder laxative (typically polyethylene glycol) 1–2 times daily postoperatively and encouraged to continue this regimen until BMs are regulated.

Prolapse Recurrence

The highest quality data on SCP outcomes is from the open SCP patients enrolled in the CARE trial through the Pelvic Floor Disorders Network. Level 1 evidence has demonstrated that there is similar POP efficacy between robotic and laparoscopic, as well as minimally invasive and open SCP approaches. On a 7-year follow-up in the extended CARE study, one-third of patients have either symptomatic or anatomic failure [52], with approximately 1/4 of patients reporting either or both. Though the definition differs across studies, anatomic failure in the CARE trial was relatively conservative, defined as C > (−2/3 X total vaginal length) (i.e., the vaginal apex descends below the upper third of the vagina) or one of points Ba or Bp greater than 0 cm (i.e., the anterior [Ba] or posterior [Bp] vaginal wall prolapses beyond the hymen). Symptomatic failure was defined as a positive response to 1 or more questions on the Pelvic Organ Prolapse Distress Inventory, or reoperation or pessary for POP. Apical failure is less common after SCP, with recurrent cystocele and distal rectocele occurring more commonly.

Persistent Pain

Although pain and dyspareunia are found to be less common with SCP when compared to vaginal prolapse repairs, these issues still do occur. If persistent de novo pain occurs in the absence of visible mesh exposure, and conservative measures such as analgesics, local hormone therapies, or local anti-inflammatory injections fail, reoperation to remove the mesh may be recommended in select cases. When evaluating these patients, differential diagnosis should include bowel or bladder mesh erosion, suture exposure, lumbosacral discitis, and osteomyelitis. Possible diagnostic tests include cystoscopy, colonoscopy, CT scan, and MRI.

Sexual Complications

MIS SCP is associated with improved postoperative sexual function, increased rates of postoperative sexual activity, and low rates of dyspareunia. Dyspareunia does not necessarily indicate a mesh-related complication. Patients with baseline dyspareunia or pain are more likely to experience persistent dyspareunia after surgery and should be counseled accordingly preoperatively [53].

Conclusions

SCP, whether done via a laparoscopic or robotic route, is an extremely safe, effective, and durable form of surgical repair for POP. Surgeon's understanding of the perioperative and longer term complications associated with MIS SCP helps to decrease the incidence of these complications and increase overall patient satisfaction associated with minimally invasive pelvic floor reconstruction.

References

1. Oliphant SS, Jones KA, Wang L, Bunker CH, Lowder JL. Trends over time with commonly performed obstetric and gynecologic inpatient procedures. Obstet Gynecol. 2010;116(4):926–31.
2. Maher CF, Baessler KK, Barber MD, Cheong C, Consten ECJ, Cooper KG, et al. Surgical management of pelvic organ prolapse. Climacteric. 2019;22(3):229–35.
3. Olsen AL, Smith VJ, Bergstrom JO, Colling JC, Clark AL. Epidemiology of surgically managed pelvic organ prolapse and urinary incontinence. Obstet Gynecol. 1997;89(4):501–6.
4. Lukacz ES, Warren LK, Richter HE, Brubaker L, Barber MD, Norton P, et al. Quality of life and sexual function 2 years after vaginal surgery for prolapse. Obstet Gynecol. 2016;127(6):1071–9.
5. Ringel NE, de Winter KL, Siddique M, Marczak T, Kisby C, Rutledge E, et al. Surgical outcomes in Urogynecology-assessment of perioperative and postoperative complications relative to preoperative hemoglobin A1c-a fellows pelvic research network study. Female Pelvic Med Reconstr Surg. 2022;28(1):7–13.
6. Ban KA, Minei JP, Laronga C, Harbrecht BG, Jensen EH, Fry DE, et al. American College of Surgeons and surgical infection society: surgical site infection guidelines, 2016 update. J Am Coll Surg. 2017;224(1):59–74.
7. Lowman JK, Woodman PJ, Nosti PA, Bump RC, Terry CL, Hale DS. Tobacco use is a risk factor for mesh erosion after abdominal sacral colpoperineopexy. Am J Obstet Gynecol. 2008;198(5):561.e1–4.
8. Lavikainen LI, Guyatt GH, Kalliala IEJ, Cartwright R, Luomaranta AL, Vernooij RWM, et al. Risk of thrombosis and bleeding in gynecologic noncancer surgery: systematic review and meta-analysis. Am J Obstet Gynecol. 2024;230(4):390–402.
9. Gould MK, Garcia DA, Wren SM, Karanicolas PJ, Arcelus JI, Heit JA, et al. Prevention of VTE in nonorthopedic surgical patients: antithrombotic therapy and prevention of thrombosis, 9th ed: American College of Chest Physicians Evidence-Based Clinical Practice Guidelines. Chest. 2012;141(2 Suppl):e227S–e77S.
10. Wen Q, Zhao Z, Wen J, Yang Y, Wang L, Wu J, et al. Impact of obesity on operative complications and outcome after sacrocolpopexy: a systematic review and meta-analysis. Eur J Obstet Gynecol Reprod Biol. 2021;258:309–16.

11. Ringel NE, Lenger SM, High R, Alas A, Houlihan S, Chang OH, et al. Effects of obesity on urogynecologic prolapse surgery outcomes: a systematic review and meta-analysis. Obstet Gynecol. 2024;143(4):539–49.
12. Good MM, Abele TA, Balgobin S, Montoya TI, McIntire D, Corton MM. Vascular and ureteral anatomy relative to the midsacral promontory. Am J Obstet Gynecol. 2013;208(6):486.e1–7.
13. Flynn MK, Romero AA, Amundsen CL, Weidner AC. Vascular anatomy of the presacral space: a fresh tissue cadaver dissection. Am J Obstet Gynecol. 2005;192(5):1501–5.
14. Lawrence JM, Lukacz ES, Nager CW, Hsu JW, Luber KM. Prevalence and co-occurrence of pelvic floor disorders in community-dwelling women. Obstet Gynecol. 2008;111(3):678–85.
15. Kikuchi JY, Yanek LR, Handa VL, Chen CCG, Jacobs S, Blomquist J, et al. Prolapse and mesh reoperations following sacrocolpopexy: comparing supracervical hysterectomy, total hysterectomy, and no hysterectomy. Int Urogynecol J. 2023;34(1):135–45.
16. Nassif J, Yadav GS, Orejuela FJ, Turrentine MA. Rate of mesh erosion after sacrocolpopexy with concurrent supracervical compared with Total hysterectomy: a systematic review and meta-analysis. Obstet Gynecol. 2022;140(3):412–20.
17. Glass Clark S, Bretschneider CE, Bradley MS, Rhodes S, Shoag J, Sheyn D. Risk of postoperative mesh exposure following sacrocolpopexy with supracervical versus total concomitant laparoscopic hysterectomy. Int Urogynecol J. 2024;35(1):207–13.
18. Das D, Carroll A, Mueller M, Kenton K, Lewicky-Gaupp C, Collins S, et al. Mesh complications after total vs supracervical laparoscopic hysterectomy at time of minimally invasive sacrocolpopexy. Int Urogynecol J. 2022;33(9):2507–14.
19. Culligan PJ, Murphy M, Blackwell L, Hammons G, Graham C, Heit MH. Long-term success of abdominal sacral colpopexy using synthetic mesh. Am J Obstet Gynecol. 2002;187(6):1473–80. discussion 81-2.
20. Bensinger G, Lind L, Lesser M, Guess M, Winkler HA. Abdominal sacral suspensions: analysis of complications using permanent mesh. Am J Obstet Gynecol. 2005;193(6):2094–8.
21. Cundiff GW, Varner E, Visco AG, Zyczynski HM, Nager CW, Norton PA, et al. Risk factors for mesh/suture erosion following sacral colpopexy. Am J Obstet Gynecol. 2008;199(6):688.e1–5.
22. Management of Mesh and Graft Complications in. gynecologic surgery. Female Pelvic Med Reconstr Surg. 2017;23(3):171–6.
23. Adelman MR, Bardsley TR, Sharp HT. Urinary tract injuries in laparoscopic hysterectomy: a systematic review. J Minim Invasive Gynecol. 2014;21(4):558–66.
24. Wong JMK, Bortoletto P, Tolentino J, Jung MJ, Milad MP. Urinary tract injury in gynecologic laparoscopy for benign indication: a systematic review. Obstet Gynecol. 2018;131(1):100–8.
25. Myers EM, Siff L, Osmundsen B, Geller E, Matthews CA. Differences in recurrent prolapse at 1 year after total vs supracervical hysterectomy and robotic sacrocolpopexy. Int Urogynecol J. 2015;26(4):585–9.
26. Carlson JW, Miron A, Jarboe EA, Parast MM, Hirsch MS, Lee Y, et al. Serous tubal intraepithelial carcinoma: its potential role in primary peritoneal serous carcinoma and serous cancer prevention. J Clin Oncol. 2008;26(25):4160–5.
27. Jacoby VL, Grady D, Wactawski-Wende J, Manson JE, Allison MA, Kuppermann M, et al. Oophorectomy vs ovarian conservation with hysterectomy: cardiovascular disease, hip fracture, and cancer in the Women's Health Initiative observational study. Arch Intern Med. 2011;171(8):760–8.
28. Parker WH, Broder MS, Chang E, Feskanich D, Farquhar C, Liu Z, et al. Ovarian conservation at the time of hysterectomy and long-term health outcomes in the nurses' health study. Obstet Gynecol. 2009;113(5):1027–37.
29. Parker WH, Broder MS, Liu Z, Shoupe D, Farquhar C, Berek JS. Ovarian conservation at the time of hysterectomy for benign disease. Obstet Gynecol. 2005;106(2):219–26.
30. Welch EK, Dengler KL, Guirguis M, Strauchon C, Olsen C, Von Pechmann W. Risk factors of lower urinary tract injury with laparoscopic sacrocolpopexy. AJOG Glob Rep. 2022;2(1):100035.
31. Anand M, Woelk JL, Weaver AL, Trabuco EC, Klingele CJ, Gebhart JB. Perioperative complications of robotic sacrocolpopexy for post-hysterectomy vaginal vault prolapse. Int Urogynecol J. 2014;25(9):1193–200.
32. Unger CA, Paraiso MF, Jelovsek JE, Barber MD, Ridgeway B. Perioperative adverse events after minimally invasive abdominal sacrocolpopexy. Am J Obstet Gynecol. 2014;211(5):547.e1–8.
33. Florian-Rodriguez ME, Hamner JJ, Corton MM. First sacral nerve and anterior longitudinal ligament anatomy: clinical applications during sacrocolpopexy. Am J Obstet Gynecol. 2017;217(5):607.e1–4.
34. Good MM, Abele TA, Balgobin S, Schaffer JI, Slocum P, McIntire D, et al. Preventing L5-S1 discitis associated with sacrocolpopexy. Obstet Gynecol. 2013;121(2 Pt 1):285–90.
35. Abernethy M, Vasquez E, Kenton K, Brubaker L, Mueller E. Where do we place the sacrocolpopexy stitch? A magnetic resonance imaging investigation. Female Pelvic Med Reconstr Surg. 2013;19(1):31–3.
36. Ghassibi M, Yen TC, Harris S, Si Z, Leary E, Choma TJ. Responsiveness of routine diagnostic tests for vertebral osteomyelitis may be influenced by the infecting organism. Spine J. 2021;21(9):1479–88.
37. Wadensweiler P, Whitcomb EL, Jeney SES, Meller D, Moran K, Guaderrama NM, et al. Bowel obstruction after sacrocolpopexy: a case series. Female Pelvic Med Reconstr Surg. 2021;27(11):e677–e80.
38. Elneil S, Cutner AS, Remy M, Leather AT, Toozs-Hobson P, Wise B. Abdominal sacrocolpopexy for

vault prolapse without burial of mesh: a case series. BJOG. 2005;112(4):486–9.
39. Kulhan M, Kulhan NG, Ata N, Nayki UA, Nayki C, Ulug P, et al. Should the visceral peritoneum be closed over mesh in abdominal sacrocolpopexy? Eur J Obstet Gynecol Reprod Biol. 2018;222:142–5.
40. Mueller MG, Jacobs KM, Mueller ER, Abernethy MG, Kenton KS. Outcomes in 450 women after minimally invasive abdominal sacrocolpopexy for pelvic organ prolapse. Female Pelvic Med Reconstr Surg. 2016;22(4):267–71.
41. Nazik H, Narin MA, Narin R, Dağlıoğlu K, Ünal İ, Tap O, et al. Investigating the clinical significance of mesh peritonization in abdominal vault suspension surgery using a comparative rabbit model. Eur J Obstet Gynecol Reprod Biol. 2014;175:199–204.
42. Limbachiya D, Tiwari R, Kumari R, Aggarwal M. Barbed suture causing acute small bowel obstruction post laparoscopic sacrocolpopexy. Crsls. 2022;9(4)
43. Vahanian SA, Finamore PS, Lazarou G. Delayed small bowel obstruction after robotic-assisted sacrocolpopexy. Female Pelvic Med Reconstr Surg. 2015;21(1):e11–3.
44. Nager CW, Brubaker L, Litman HJ, Zyczynski HM, Varner RE, Amundsen C, et al. A randomized trial of urodynamic testing before stress-incontinence surgery. N Engl J Med. 2012;366(21):1987–97.
45. Osmundsen B, Gregory WT, Denman MA, Adams K, Edwards R, Clark A. Tension-free vaginal tape failure after robotic sacrocolpopexy and tension-free vaginal tape for concomitant prolapse and stress incontinence. Female Pelvic Med Reconstr Surg. 2015;21(5):244–8.
46. Giugale LE, Carter-Brooks CM, Ross JH, Shepherd JP, Zyczynski HM. Outcomes of a staged midurethral sling strategy for stress incontinence and pelvic organ prolapse. Obstet Gynecol. 2019;134(4):736–44.
47. Giugale L, Sridhar A, Ferrante KL, Komesu YM, Meyer I, Smith AL, et al. Long-term urinary outcomes after transvaginal uterovaginal prolapse repair with and without concomitant midurethral slings. Female Pelvic Med Reconstr Surg. 2022;28(3):142–8.
48. Serati M, Bogani G, Sorice P, Braga A, Torella M, Salvatore S, et al. Robot-assisted sacrocolpopexy for pelvic organ prolapse: a systematic review and meta-analysis of comparative studies. Eur Urol. 2014;66(2):303–18.
49. Ramaseshan AS, LaSala C, O'Sullivan DM, Steinberg AC. Patient-initiated telephone calls in the post-operative period after female pelvic reconstructive surgery. Female Pelvic Med Reconstr Surg. 2020;26(10):626–9.
50. Woodbury CF, Coughlin AC, Dubois B, Romanova A. Prevention of postoperative constipation in Urogynecology patients: a systematic review. Urogynecology (Phila). 2023;29(2):175–82.
51. McNanley A, Perevich M, Glantz C, Duecy EE, Flynn MK, Buchsbaum G. Bowel function after minimally invasive urogynecologic surgery: a prospective randomized controlled trial. Female Pelvic Med Reconstr Surg. 2012;18(2):82–5.
52. Nygaard I, Brubaker L, Zyczynski HM, Cundiff G, Richter H, Gantz M, et al. Long-term outcomes following abdominal sacrocolpopexy for pelvic organ prolapse. JAMA. 2013;309(19):2016–24.
53. Ashmore S, Geller EJ, Bretschneider CE. Minimally invasive Sacrocolpopexy: impact on sexual function. Int Urogynecol J. 2024;35:2335.

Colpocleisis

12

Rachel Cline and Alex Gomelsky

Introduction

The world's population is rapidly aging. Between 2010 and 2020, the population ≥ 65 years in the United States saw the largest and fastest growth in any decade since 1880–1890, reaching 55.8 million or 16.8% of the total population in 2020 [1]. Furthermore, the percentage of individuals over the age of 65 in Europe and North America is expected to increase from 18.7% in 2022 to 26.9% in 2050 [2]. During that timeframe, life expectancy is also estimated to increase from 80.4 to 86.1. Worldwide, ~40% of women will experience pelvic organ prolapse (POP), and this proportion is expected to increase as the population ages [3]. As the lifetime risk of undergoing POP surgery in the United States is 12.6%, the demand for pelvic floor services is, not surprisingly, expected to increase by 45% over the next 30 years [4, 5]. Currently, more than 200,000 surgeries are performed annually to address POP, and repairs of apical defects comprise a significant percentage of these surgeries [6, 7]. All these statistics underscore the importance of effective, durable, and safe methods of surgically treating POP in elderly women.

There are two main categories of surgical approaches. The focus of *reconstructive* surgery is to augment and restore vaginal support with the goal of vaginal preservation, while *obliterative* surgery eliminates the potential space of the vagina without compartment-specific reinforcement of the supportive connective tissue layers. With the latter approach, the vaginal cavity is significantly reduced in depth, essentially eliminating the possibility of vaginal coitus. Thus, the chosen surgical approach depends on desired anatomic and functional outcomes, as well as the possibility for future sexual activity.

Colpocleisis is a minimally invasive, obliterative procedure that may be performed with or without uterine preservation. Despite typically high anatomic success rates, adverse sequelae are possible as with any surgical intervention. This chapter will focus on optimizing perioperative outcomes and minimizing postoperative complications in women undergoing colpocleisis.

R. Cline
LSU Health Shreveport School of Medicine, Shreveport, LA, USA

A. Gomelsky (✉)
Department of Urology, University of Florida School of Medicine, Gainesville, FL, USA
e-mail: agomelsky@ufl.edu

H. B. Goldman, J. Zillioux (eds.), *Complications of Urogynecology and Reconstructive Pelvic Surgery*, https://doi.org/10.1007/978-3-032-00339-3_12

History

Denuding and closing a significant portion of the prolapsed vagina was initially described by Gerardin in 1823 and performed by Neugebauer in 1867 [8, 9]. This procedure, also referred to as colpectomy or total colpocleisis, is performed on a woman with significant POP following hysterectomy [Figs. 12.1, 12.2, 12.3 and 12.4]. In 1877, LeFort described uterine-sparing, partial colpocleisis that entailed denuding the middle portion of the anterior and posterior vaginal wall epithelium and then suturing them together, allowing for lateral draining channels [10]. Both techniques have been traditionally reserved for older women who do not desire future vaginal coitus. Likewise, the minimally invasive approach and shorter operative times may be appealing for treating those women who may be poor surgical candidates for reconstructive procedures owing to medical comorbidities.

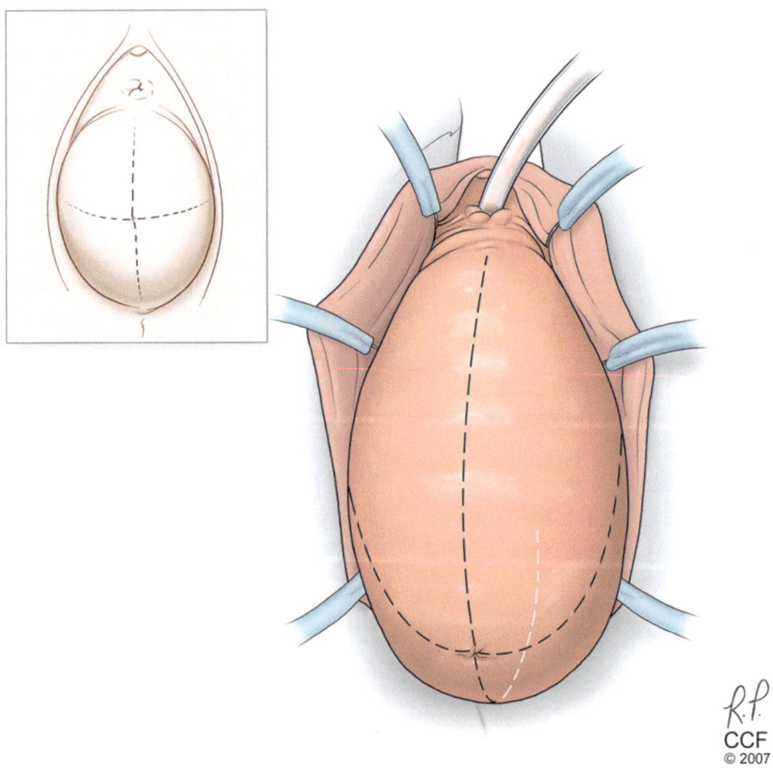

Fig. 12.1 Incisions in the vaginal epithelium are mapped out in a woman with post-hysterectomy vaginal prolapse. Note that the vertical incision stops at least 1.5 cm proximal to the bladder neck

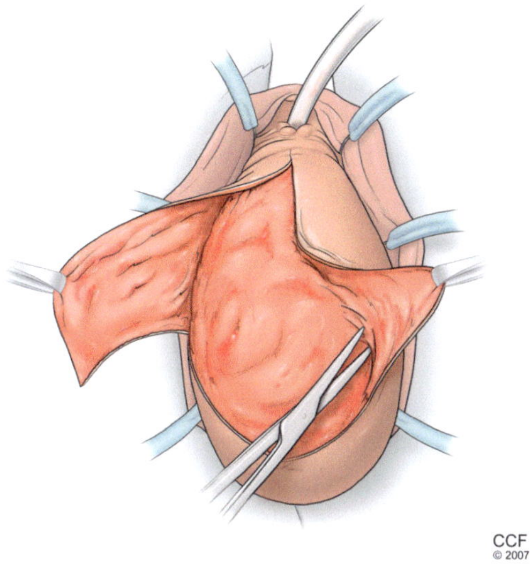

Fig. 12.2 The vaginal epithelium is dissected off the underlying pubocervical fascia, rectovaginal fascia, and any enterocele sac. Care is taken to keep a "thin" plane of dissection to minimize the possibility of injury to the bladder, rectum, or ureters

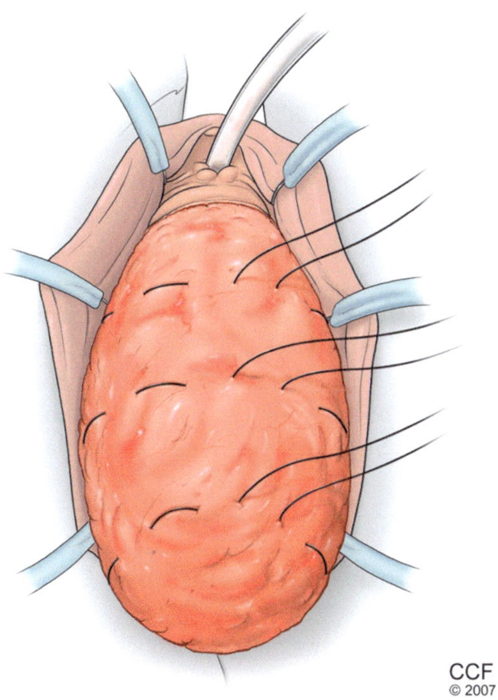

Fig. 12.3 Sequential purse-string delayed absorbable sutures are placed beginning at the apex. The prolapsing segment is reduced as the sutures are tied down

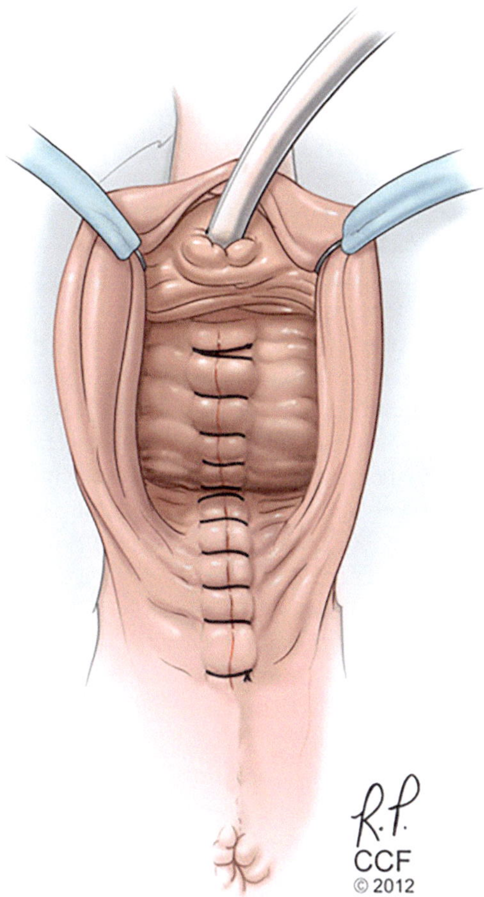

Fig. 12.4 After the pubocervical and rectovaginal fasciae are sutured together, excess vaginal epithelium is removed, and the incision is closed with delayed absorbable sutures

Preoperative Considerations

As the focus of this chapter is the discussion of perioperative complications, it is beyond our scope to describe in detail the nuances of each surgical technique. A thorough assessment of the patient's urogynecologic history and assessment of symptom severity should precede preoperative counseling, as colpocleisis is not indicated in patients with minimal symptoms regardless of the degree of prolapse [11]. It is important to note that preoperative counseling and attentive perioperative management unequivocally decrease the rates of postoperative adverse sequelae. Prior to undergoing a partial colpocleisis, it is recommended that women have their upper genital tract evaluated with either transvaginal ultrasound or endometrial biopsy and a Papanicolaou smear performed to assess for abnormal pathology. Women with preinvasive conditions of the cervix or endometrium and others who require upper genital tract surveillance should be considered for other forms of repair.

If overt stress urinary incontinence (SUI) is present, consideration should be given to a concomitant anti-incontinence procedure. However, women with significant POP may be subjectively continent because the bladder base descent may mechanically kink the urethra [12]. In these cases, SUI is uncovered only after POP reduction is called *occult SUI,* and its incidence in the literature fluctuates significantly (6–80%) [13–18]. The wide range reflects the lack of universal criteria for the diagnosis of occult SUI and the multitude of techniques described for POP reduction [14]. A meta-analysis of 25 studies concluded that the diagnostic accuracy of occult SUI for predicting postoperative SUI differed greatly, likely because of the heterogeneity in the studies [19]. The medians (and ranges) for sensitivity, specificity, positive predictive value, and negative predictive value were 39% (5–100), 86% (57–97), 40% (0–79), and 91% (51–100), respectively. One multi-institutional study from the Netherlands found that women with occult SUI had a higher risk of reporting SUI after POP surgery compared with women without occult SUI [20]. Adding a midurethral sling (MUS) to POP surgery reduced the risk of postoperative SUI and the need for staged treatment in women with occult SUI. Of women with occult SUI undergoing only POP surgery, 13% underwent staged MUS. As such, preoperative urodynamic evaluation with POP reduction should merit consideration in this population. Current data does not recommend placement of a prophylactic sling during colpocleisis to prevent postoperative SUI [21].

Upper urinary tract evaluation is another preoperative consideration. A recent systematic review found that the prevalence of hydronephrosis ranged from 3.5% to 30.6%, and that complete resolution of hydronephrosis was described in 56–83% of patients undergoing surgical treatment for advanced POP [22]. Hence, preoperative renal ultrasonography and postoperative surveillance should also be considered in this cohort.

As most of the postoperative morbidity in the elderly is closely related to surgical stress, a medical and cardiac clearance may be necessary. This will often dictate the method of intraoperative anesthesia, and these surgeries have been successfully performed under both regional and local anesthesia [23, 24]. The ultimate choice of anesthesia is at the discretion of the surgeon, anesthesiologist, and patient. As the incidence of rectal and small bowel injury is very low, a preoperative bowel preparation may be omitted, but should be considered in women with a history of significant constipation or multiple previous vaginal surgeries [25, 26].

Finally, preoperative counseling and a thorough discussion of risks and benefits, as well as options for colpocleisis, should be undertaken. Although long-term anatomic cure rates of colpocleisis are typically >90%, intraoperative and postoperative complications may occur [27]. Additionally, if an anti-incontinence procedure is performed in the same setting, the risks of this surgery should be included in the informed consent process. Furthermore, 10–15% of women experience regret after undergoing colpocleisis and should be counseled appropriately regarding the loss of vaginal depth [28, 29]. Regret rates appear to be lower in sexually inactive patients, with a recent study citing regret rates as low as 0% [30].

Preoperative Considerations

Prophylactic intravenous antibiotics should be given within an hour of surgical "cut" time (first- or second-generation cephalosporin or gentamycin and clindamycin), while 2 h should be allowed for a fluoroquinolone [31]. As rates of deep vein thrombosis (DVT) approach 15% for benign pelvic surgery, a prophylactic strategy should be employed in each operation [32]. Intermittent pneumatic compression (IPC) devices are applied prior to the induction of anesthesia. Also, as age > 60 years by itself places women undergoing colpocleisis into the high-risk category for DVT, consideration should be given to combination therapy with IPC plus low-dose unfractionated heparin (LDUH) or low molecular weight heparin (LMWH), unless the bleeding risk is considered unacceptably high. The presence of additional risk factors, such as smoking, obesity, immobility, estrogen-containing oral contraception or hormone replacement therapy, or heart or respiratory failure, places the woman into the highest risk category, and LDUH or LMWH is strongly recommended [32]. If required, pubic hair should be clipped in the operating room to minimize skin trauma. We prefer to keep an indwelling urethral catheter for continuous drainage during the surgery. A Scott/Lone Star retractor may be of assistance in obtaining exposure. Finally, general tenets, such as cautious intraoperative hydration, minimization of blood loss, meticulous hemostasis, and consideration for transfusion to minimize anemia and cardiac compromise, are imperative adjuncts to any surgical procedure in the elderly population [27].

Intraoperative Considerations

While each surgeon regularly performing these procedures has their own routine to optimize anatomic outcomes and minimize adverse sequelae, we believe that there are several general steps that should be a part of any colpocleisis protocol. First, while the "deep" plane of dissection into the true vesicovaginal space has been historically preferred for the placement of interposition grafts, we keep our plane of dissection superficial to the pubocervical and rectovaginal fasciae. This lessens the possibility of injury to pelvic viscera, urethra, or ureters, as the latter may be rotated forward into the operative field due to significant anterior compartment prolapse. Second, intraoperative stenting with temporary ureteral catheters may potentially lessen the chance of ureteral injury and assist in recognizing such an injury, should one occur. Also, we perform intraoperative cystoscopy with each colpocleisis surgery, regardless of any concomitant anti-incontinence procedure [33]. This step is cost-effective, assists in identifying any bladder injury, and has a sensitivity and specificity for identifying ureteral obstruction of 94.4% and 99.5%, respectively [34, 35]. Prophylactic ureteral stenting was associated with a lower incidence of ureteral injuries during gynecological surgery (pooled OR 0.61, 95% CI: 0.39–0.96), and the number needed to perform ureteral stenting to prevent one ureteral injury was 224 [36]. Rare false negative cases may occur with partial ureteral obstruction. Third, as recommended by Fitzgerald et al., we typically preserve at least 1.5 cm of the anterior vaginal epithelium proximal to the urethrovesical junction [27]. The purpose is to avoid downward traction on the urethra when it is approximated to the posterior vaginal muscularis. Fourth, a concomitant mid-urethral sling (MUS) may be placed through a separate 1 cm suburethral incision to minimize its migration toward the bladder neck. If the patient opts for an autologous pubovaginal sling, a single incision can be used for the sling and colpocleisis. The sling is anchored to the underlying pubocervical fascia to keep it from dislodging. Regardless of sling choice, sling tensioning is performed after the entire POP surgery has been performed. Finally, a levator myorrhaphy or perineorrhaphy (our choice) is performed to decrease the size of the genital hiatus and minimize POP recurrence [27, 37].

Anatomic and Subjective Outcomes

In a PubMed review of the available literature (1996–2004), FitzGerald et al. cited "success" rates of 91–100%, despite the early literature being fraught with poor characterization of preoperative symptoms and inconsistent postoperative follow-up [27]. Outcomes of more recent studies support the low anatomic recurrence rates [38–42]. Anatomical success, defined as POP-Q stage ≤ 1 and no prolapse beyond the hymen, was achieved in 62.5–100% and 87.5–100% of all patients, respectively [43]. In fact, of all surgical procedures for POP, colpocleisis offers the lowest likelihood of reoperation for prolapse and has the lowest risk of long-term reoperation for complications [44]. The overall reoperation risk through 7 years was 7.3% for colpocleisis, 10.4% for uterosacral ligament suspension (USLS), 12.5% for sacrocolpopexy, and 15% for sacrospinous ligament fixation (SSLF) ($p < 0.01$). Reoperation for recurrent POP through 7 years was 2.9% for colpocleisis, 7.3% for sacrocolpopexy, 7.7% for USLS, and 9.9% for SSLF ($p < 0.01$).

Colpocleisis is also associated with high subjective success rates. A recent prospective study assessed quality of life (QoL) in women >65 years of age undergoing obliterative and reconstructive procedures and found significant postoperative QoL improvement without an increase in depression or body image [45]. Vij et al. performed a longitudinal study involving 34 women who underwent colpocleisis with a median follow-up of 3 years and demonstrated that 91% would recommend colpocleisis to a relative or friend [46]. Likewise, in the series by von Pechmann et al., telephone follow-up revealed that 90.3% of patients achieved subjective cure and were either satisfied or very satisfied with how surgery resolved their POP [47]. Finally, Grzybowska et al. cited subjective success in 88–100% of their cohort [43].

Intraoperative Complications

Intraoperative complications encompass hemorrhage and injuries to surrounding structures. Hemorrhagic complications during or after pelvic floor reconstructive surgery are rare [48]. Zebede et al. cited intraoperative complications in 1.6% of their cohort, including bowel injury and hematoma during concomitant suprapubic catheter placement (two patients), small bladder punctures during trocar passage for MUS (2), and uterine injury during hysteroscopic resection of a mass (1) [38]. Higher rates of postoperative adverse indices appear to be strongly associated with concomitant surgery, specifically hysterectomy [27]. Outcomes of two studies, in particular, both revealed low rates of intraoperative complications; however, mean operative times, estimated blood loss, postoperative transfusion rates, and length of stay were significantly higher in the groups undergoing concomitant hysterectomy [26, 47]. Two other studies cited no difference in perioperative sequelae between women undergoing partial and total colpocleisis [49, 50].

Ureteral injury and obstruction have been estimated to occur in 0.3–11% of all types of pelvic reconstructive procedures [51, 52], while the rate of ureteral obstruction during colpocleisis, specifically, is ~4% [34]. Ureteral obstruction is hypothesized to occur from kinking at the trigonal level secondary to anterior vaginal wall distortion, and intraoperative identification of obstruction and injury is imperative to prevent long-term complications requiring staged complex ureteral reconstruction. As vaginal surgery does not allow easy identification of the ureters, cystoscopy after administration of intravenous dye can confirm ureteral and bladder integrity [34]. In one model, oral phenazopyridine and dextrose instillation were the least expensive and most effective agents to aid in the visualization of ureteral patency during intraoperative cystoscopy; however, dextrose use was associated with higher costs owing to a higher rate of adverse reactions (primarily urinary tract infections [UTIs]) [53]. If an obstruction is suspected, removal of the offending suture intraoperatively will relieve the ureteral obstruction in ~90% of cases, whereas other patients may require a ureteral stent for several weeks to allow resolution of the intramural ureteral edema with no residual kinking seen on postoperative imaging [34, 47].

Conversion to laparotomy is a rare event and has been typically associated with concomitant hysterectomy [47]. Whereas vascular injury secondary to a bleeding ovarian vessel at the time of concomitant adnexectomy was reported in one patient, the second laparotomy was due to rupture of a diverticular abscess upon entry into the pouch of Douglas. Furthermore, a proctotomy was identified on a third patient and was repaired without incident [47].

Perioperative and Early Postoperative Complications

While the elderly are at higher risk for complications during vaginal surgery, those women undergoing colpocleisis may experience fewer overall complications. Neither race nor ethnicity appears to be a significant predictor of reoperation or mortality [54]. A recent retrospective analysis of 264,340 women from the Nationwide Inpatient Sample found that the overall in-hospital mortality risk was 0.04% after POP surgery [55]. When compared with women <60 years of age, the odds ratio of mortality in women >80 years of age was 13.6. The overall complication rate was 14.4%, with 20% of women >80 years of age having one or more complications. Those octogenarians who underwent obliterative procedures were less likely to suffer a complication as compared to those receiving reconstructive procedures (17% vs. 24.7%). Nursing home residents demonstrated worse short- and long-term outcomes after POP surgery compared to community dwelling older adults, with the former having statistically significant increased risks for length of hospital stay of ≥3 days (38.9% vs. 18.6%, aRR 2.1, 95% CI: 1.8–2.4), 30-day complications (15.1% vs. 3.8%, aRR 3.9, 95% CI: 2.9–5.3), and 1-year mortality (11.1% vs 3.2%, aRR 3.5, 95% CI: 2.5–4.8) compared to the latter group [56].

A retrospective, multi-institutional study involving 145 medical centers reviewed over 4700 colpocleisis procedures dating from 2002 to 2012 and cited an overall complication rate of 6.82% [57]. Despite 53% of the procedures being performed in octogenarians, the intensive care unit (ICU) admission rate was only 2.8% and there were seven deaths for a mortality rate of 0.15%. Readmissions were uncommon, with an overall 30-day readmission rate of 4.2%. Higher volume centers had lower ICU admission rates and shorter lengths of stay.

In another retrospective review of colpocleisis procedures from the American College of Surgeons NSQIP database, Catanzarite et al. cited an 8.1% overall complication rate within 30 days [58]. The most common complication was UTI in 6.4%, and only 2.1% required a return to the operating room within 30 days. Concomitant sling placement did not increase the 30-day complication rates. In another study of 245 women, postoperative UTI occurred in 34.7% [26].

In the review by Fitzgerald et al., cardiac, thromboembolic, pulmonary, and cerebrovascular postoperative complications occurred in 5% of patients [27]. However, in the studies performed since 1980, the complication rate due to performing surgery on the elderly has decreased to 2%. Complications related to colpocleisis, including transfusion and pyelonephritis, occurred at a rate of 4% and were associated with concomitant hysterectomy as previously mentioned.

Transient postoperative urinary retention (UR) in one study of 172 patients was seen in 55%, with rates of 36.7% with LeFort colpocleisis, 51.5% with posthysterectomy colpocleisis, and 64.9% with colpocleisis with concomitant hysterectomy [59]. Logistic regression revealed an increased risk of postoperative UR if hysterectomy was performed at the time of colpocleisis (OR 2.9, 95% CI: 1.23–6.84; $p = 0.015$). Patient age, prolapse severity, preoperative postvoid residual volume, and concomitant anti-incontinence procedure were not associated with transient UR. In another study, the aOR for postoperative UR in patients with concomitant MUS was 1.68 (95% CI: 0.64–4.41) vs. patients who underwent colpocleisis alone, and this did not reach statistical significance ($p = 0.292$) [60]. Fortunately, after colpocleisis, women had high rates of resolution of UR, regardless of MUS (80.3% vs. 90.6% for colpocleisis alone vs. with MUS; $p = 0.20$). Few women required reoperation for retention (3.1%).

Late Postoperative Complications

During a partial colpocleisis, pyometra, pyocolpos, or pelvic abscess can occasionally occur despite the creation of adequate vaginal channels [61–63]. Meticulous hemostasis cannot be overemphasized. Use of a Bakri balloon has been proposed for dilation of the tunnels in cases of persistent hematocolpos [64]. Gynecologic malignancies are rare after colpocleisis, with fewer than 15 reported in the literature [65].

The impact of colpocleisis on urinary storage and emptying symptoms varies. Long-term UR is rare, with one patient in a large series requiring the use of an indwelling catheter at three months after surgery [25]. No surgery was performed for postoperative voiding difficulty, and no patient underwent sling incision or urethrolysis. In a more recent study, Koski et al. likewise reported that no patients had UR after surgery that required chronic catheterization or reoperation [39]. In a report of their 10-year experience with colpocleisis, Wolff et al. cited similar postoperative UR rates between those undergoing colpocleisis alone and those with MUS (10.1% vs 11.8%, $p = 0.69$) [60].

As mentioned previously, women with overt SUI should be strongly considered for a concomitant anti-incontinence procedure, while an evaluation with POP reduction should be considered for those women who are subjectively stress-continent. De novo postoperative SUI has been postulated to occur due to either the unmasking of occult SUI after POP correction or excessive downward traction on the urethra during approximation to the posterior vaginal muscularis [27]. Whereas earlier authors attempted to modify the LeFort technique by altering the anterior edge of the colpectomy away from the urethral meatus [66, 67], more recent series combined colpocleisis with anti-incontinence procedures [27]. The types of procedures have included suburethral plications, transvaginal bladder neck suspensions, and slings placed at the bladder neck or midurethra [27]. There are no prospective studies comparing one concomitant anti-incontinence procedure with another, and operative choice remains on the experience and discretion of the surgeon.

Interestingly, postoperative SUI may yet occur in women who undergo a concomitant anti-incontinence surgery. In one series of 140 patients, 13% of women who had undergone a concomitant anti-incontinence procedure and 14% of those who only underwent colpocleisis had bothersome SUI one year after colpocleisis [25]. De novo bothersome SUI was uncommon, occurring only in 4% of patients who had an anti-incontinence procedure and in 3% who did not. Of the women that did not seek correction of SUI in the series by Koski et al., four had persistent SUI and one developed de novo SUI [39]. In another retrospective study, 8 of 30 women without preoperative SUI developed de novo SUI after surgery [68]. These findings suggest that the relationship between SUI and POP is dynamic and that, despite treatment of occult SUI, overt SUI may still occur after POP repair. Hence, the ability to properly characterize SUI in the presence of significant POP continues to be inconsistent.

Significant POP may also be related to other urinary storage symptoms and urgency urinary incontinence. In the study by Fitzgerald et al., lower urinary tract symptoms improved at the 3-month follow-up, and improvement was maintained at one year [25]. Fifteen percent of patients at one year described a bothersome urge vs. 41% at baseline. The most common complaint on postoperative UDI-6 was frequency and urgency, and these complaints were present preoperatively [39]. In this study, there was no evidence of postoperative de novo urgency. These findings are corroborated by further significant postoperative improvement in mean IIQ-7 and UDI-6 scores [28]. While colpocleisis is not guaranteed to eliminate all preoperative storage symptoms, it, like other procedures correcting anterior compartment POP, appears to have a beneficial effect [69].

The impact of colpocleisis on bowel function has been infrequently reported; however, the available literature suggests a postoperative improvement in these symptoms [27]. Fitzgerald et al. reported significant improvement on the Colorectal Anal Distress Inventory (CRADI) and Colorectal Anal Impact Questionnaire at 3 and 12 months after surgery [25]. Additionally, Vij et al. reported low postoperative CRADI scores after colpocleisis [46]. Two to five years following colpocleisis, there were no new adverse bowel symptoms reported, with improvement of fecal incontinence in two of nine women and no change in fecal urgency.

Despite appropriate informed consent discussion, the loss of vaginal sexual function following colpocleisis may be associated with regret. One year after surgery, 94% of patients in the study by Fitzgerald et al. were either satisfied or very satisfied with their decision to have vaginal closure [25]. Two percent felt their body looked worse, whereas 10% of women reported improved sexual function following surgery, 3% reported worsening function, and 87% stated it had remained the same. Overall, the regret rate, when reported, ranged from 0% (Reisnauer et al. 2013) to 13% (Winkelman et al. 2020) [29, 47, 70]. In the study by von Pechmann et al., however, four of the eight women expressing some degree of regret after colpocleisis stated they would undergo surgery again, while only one definitely would not [47]. As stated previously, regret in sexually inactive women approaches 0% [30].

Conclusions

Colpocleisis is an effective and minimally invasive method to manage significant POP in the elderly woman who no longer desires vaginal coitus. Intraoperative complications are infrequent and may be minimized by careful dissection and meticulous hemostasis. Morbidity is lower in women undergoing partial colpocleisis. Bothersome urinary, colorectal, and pelvic symptoms are typically alleviated after surgery, and the anatomic recurrence rates are low. Although subjective satisfaction is high, some women may still experience a sense of regret over a vaginal obliterative procedure. Informed consent remains of utmost importance when discussing this procedure as it may have significant implications on a woman's sexual QoL. Proper patient selection and thorough preoperative work-up cannot be overemphasized.

Conflicts of Interest None.

References

1. https://www2.census.gov/library/publications/decennial/2020/census-briefs/c2020br-07.pdf. Accessed 30 Mar 2024
2. United Nations Department of Economic and Social Affairs, Population Division (2022). World Population Prospects 2022: Summary of Results. UN DESA/POP/2022/TR/NO. 3. Accessed 30 Mar 2024
3. Wang B, Chen Y, Zhu X, et al. Global burden and trends of pelvic organ prolapse associated with aging women: an observational trend study from 1990 to 2019. Front Public Health. 2022;10:975829.
4. Wu JM, Matthews CA, Conover MM, et al. Lifetime risk of stress urinary incontinence or pelvic organ prolapse surgery. Obstet Gynecol. 2014;123(6):1201–6.
5. Luber KM, Boero S, Choe JY. The demographics of pelvic floor disorders: current observations and future projections. Am J Obstet Gynecol. 2001;184:1496–501.
6. Nygaard I, Thom DH, Calhoun EA. Chapter 3 urinary incontinence in women. In: Litwin MS, Saigal CS, editors. Urologic diseases in America. US Department of Health and Human Services, public health service, National Institutes of Health, National Institute of Diabetes and Digestive and Kidney Diseases. Washington, DC: US Government Printing Office; 2007. p. 71–103. NIH Publication No. 07–5512.
7. Rooney K, Kenton K, Mueller ER, Fitz Gerald MP, Brubaker L. Advanced anterior vaginal wall prolapse is highly correlated with apical prolapse. Am J Obstet Gynecol. 2006;195(6):1837–40.
8. Gerardin R. Memoire presente a la societe medicale de Metz en 1823. Arch gGen Med. 1825;8:1825.
9. Neugebauer JA. Einige worte uber die mediane vaginalnaht als mittel zur beseitgung des gebarmuttervorfalls. Zentralbl Gynaekol. 1881;5:3–8.
10. LeFort L. Nouveau procede pour la guerison du prolapses uterin. Bull Gene Ther. 1877;92:337–46.
11. Pelvic Organ Prolapse. ACOG practice bulletin, number 214. Obstet Gynecol. 2019;134(5):e126–42.
12. Bump RC, Fantl JA, Hurt WG. The mechanism of urinary continence in women with severe uterovaginal prolapse: results of barrier studies. Obstet Gynecol. 1988;72:291–5.
13. Haylen BT, de Ridder D, Freeman RM, et al. An international Urogynecological association (IUGA)/international continence society (ICS) joint report on the terminology for female pelvic floor dysfunction. Int Urogynecol J. 2010;21:5–26.
14. Haessler AL, Lin LL, Ho MH, et al. Reevaluating occult incontinence. Curr Opin Obstet Gynecol. 2005;17:535–40.
15. Rosenzweig BA, Pushkin S, Blumenfeld D, et al. Prevalence of abnormal urodynamic test results in continent women with severe genitourinary prolapse. Obstet Gynecol. 1992;79:539–42.
16. Gordon D, Groutz A, Wolman I, et al. Development of postoperative urinary stress incontinence in clinically continent patients undergoing prophylactic Kelly plication during genitourinary prolapse repair. Neurourol Urodyn. 1999;18:193–7.
17. Chaikin DC, Groutz A, Blaivas JG. Predicting the need for anti-incontinence surgery in continent

women undergoing repair of severe urogenital prolapse. J Urol. 2000;163:531–4.
18. Reena C, Kekre AN, Kekre N. Occult stress incontinence in women with pelvic organ prolapse. Int J Gynaecol Obstet. 2007;97:31–4.
19. Barbier H, Carberry CL, Karjalainen PK, et al. International Urogynecology consultation chapter 2 committee 3: the clinical evaluation of pelvic organ prolapse including investigations into associated morbidity/pelvic floor dysfunction. Int Urogynecol J. 2023;34(11):2657–88.
20. van der Ploeg JM, Oude Rengerink K, van der Steen A, et al. Dutch Urogynaecology consortium. Vaginal prolapse repair with or without a midurethral sling in women with genital prolapse and occult stress urinary incontinence: a randomized trial. Int Urogynecol J. 2016;27(7):1029–38.
21. Buchsbaum GM, Lee TG. Vaginal obliterative procedures for pelvic organ prolapse: a systematic review. Obstet Gynecol Survey. 2017;72(3):175–83.
22. Siddique M, Ingraham C, Kudish B, et al. Hydronephrosis associated with pelvic organ prolapse: a systematic review. Female Pelvic Med Reconstr Surg. 2020;26(3):212–8.
23. Ardekany MS, Rafee R. A new modification of colpocleisis for treatment of total procidentia in old age. Int J Gynaecol Obstet. 1978;15:358–60.
24. Moore RD, Miklos JR. Colpocleisis and tension-free vaginal tape sling for severe uterine and vaginal prolapse and stress urinary incontinence under local anesthesia. J Am Assoc Gynecol Laparosc. 2003;10:276–80.
25. Diakosavvas M, Thomakos N, Psarris A, et al. Preoperative bowel preparation in minimally invasive and vaginal gynecologic surgery. Sci World J. 2020;2020:8546037.
26. Hill AJ, Walters MD, Unger CA. Perioperative adverse events associated with colpocleisis for uterovaginal and posthysterectomy vaginal vault prolapse. Am J Obstet Gynecol. 2016;214(4):501.e1–6.
27. Fitz Gerald M, Richter H, Siddique S, et al. Colpocleisis: a review. Int Urogynecol J. 2006;17:261–71.
28. Wheeler TL II, Richter HE, Burgio KL, et al. Regret, satisfaction, and symptom improvement: analysis of the impact of partial colpocleisis for the management of severe pelvic organ prolapse. Am J Obstet Gynecol. 2005;193:2067–70.
29. Winkelman WD, Haviland MJ, Elkadry EA. Long-term pelvic floor symptoms, recurrence, satisfaction, and regret following Colpocleisis. Female Pelvic Med Reconstr Surg. 2020;26(9):558–62.
30. Lu M, Zeng W, Ju R, Li S, Yang X. Long-term clinical outcomes, recurrence, satisfaction, and regret after total colpocleisis with concomitant vaginal hysterectomy: a retrospective single-center study. Female Pelvic Med Reconstr Surg. 2021;27(4):e510–5.
31. Lightner DJ, Wymer K, Sanchez J, Kavoussi L. Best practice statement on urologic procedures and antimicrobial prophylaxis. J Urol. 2020;203(2):351–6.
32. Forrest JB, Clemens JQ, Finamore P, et al. AUA best practice statement for the prevention of deep vein thrombosis in patients undergoing urologic surgery. AUA Education and Research, Inc; 2008.
33. Stewart LE, Hall E, Carberry CL. Cystoscopy at the time of incontinence and prolapse surgery. Curr Opin Obstet Gynecol. 2018;30(6):441–5.
34. Gustilo-Ashby AM, Jelovsek JE, Barber MD, et al. The incidence of ureteral obstruction and the value of intraoperative cystoscopy during vaginal surgery for pelvic organ prolapse. Am J Obstet Gynecol. 2006;194(5):1478–85.
35. Luchristt D, Geynisman-Tan J, Mueller MG, Kenton K. Cost-effectiveness analysis of universal cystoscopy at the time of benign laparoscopic hysterectomy. J Minim Invasive Gynecol. 2021;28(8):1470–83.
36. Yanagisawa T, Mori K, Quhal F, et al. Iatrogenic ureteric injury during abdominal or pelvic surgery: a meta-analysis. BJU Int. 2023;131(5):540–52.
37. Welch EK, Dengler KL, Wheat JE, et al. Colpocleisis techniques: an open-and-shut case for advanced pelvic organ prolapse. Urology. 2023;176:252.
38. Zebede S, Smith AL, Plowright LN, et al. Obliterative LeFort colpocleisis in a large group of elderly women. Obstet Gynecol. 2013;121(2 Pt 1):279–84.
39. Koski ME, Chow D, Bedestani A, et al. Colpocleisis for advanced pelvic organ prolapse. Urology. 2012;80(3):542–6.
40. Wang X, Hu C, Chen Y, Hua K. LeFort colpocleisis for recurrent pelvic organ prolapse. Int Urogynecol J. 2020;31(2):381–4.
41. Park JY, Han SJ, Kim JH, et al. Le fort partial colpocleisis as an effective treatment option for advanced apical prolapse in elderly women. Taiwan J Obstet Gynecol. 2019;58(2):206–11.
42. Deffieux X, Thubert T, Donon L, et al. Chirurgie d'occlusion vaginale (colpocléisis) pour prolapsus génital: recommandations pour la pratique clinique [Colpocleisis: guidelines for clinical practice]. Prog Urol. 2016;26(Suppl 1):S61–72.
43. Grzybowska ME, Futyma K, Kusiak A, Wydra DG. Colpocleisis as an obliterative surgery for pelvic organ prolapse: is it still a viable option in the twenty-first century? Narrative review. Int Urogynecol J. 2022;33(1):31–46.
44. Berger AA, Bretschneider CE, Gregory WT, Sung V. Longitudinal reoperation risk after apical prolapse procedures in women aged 65 years and older. Obstet Gynecol. 2024;143(3):411–8.
45. Barber MD, Amundsen CL, Paraiso MF, et al. Quality of life after surgery for genital prolapse in elderly women: obliterative and reconstructive surgery. Int Urogynecol J Pelvic Floor Dysfunct. 2007;18(7):799–806.
46. Vij M, Bombieri L, Dua A, Freeman R. Long-term follow-up after colpocleisis: regret, bowel, and bladder function. Int Urogynecol J. 2014;25(6):811–5.
47. von Pechmann WS, Mutone M, Fyffe J, Hale DS. Total colpocleisis with high levator plication for

the treatment of advanced pelvic organ prolapse. Am J Obstet Gynecol. 2003;189(1):121–6.
48. Cheng W, Bu C, Hong F, et al. Perioperative hemorrhagic complications in pelvic floor reconstructive surgery. Int Urogynecol J. 2019;30(7):1141–6.
49. Ozceltik G, Itil IM, Yeniel AO. Comparison of perioperative outcomes between colpocleisis with hysterectomy and colpocleisis without hysterectomy. J Gynecol Obstet Hum Reprod. 2022;51(9):102456.
50. Ju R, Yang X, Sun XL, et al. Comparison of perioperative conditions between total and partial colpocleisis for elderly patients suffered from severe pelvic organ prolapse. Zhonghua Fu Chan Ke Za Zhi. 2019;54(1):33–7.
51. Stanhope CR, Wilson TO, Utz WJ, et al. Suture entrapment and secondary ureteral obstruction. Am J Obstet Gynecol. 1991;164(6 Pt 1):1513–9.
52. Barber MD, Visco AG, Weidner AC, et al. Bilateral uterosacral ligament vaginal vault suspension with site-specific endopelvic fascia defect repair for treatment of pelvic organ prolapse. Am J Obstet Gynecol. 2000;183(6):1402–11.
53. Askew AL, Myers ER, Dieter AA. Cost-effectiveness of agents used for evaluation of ureteral patency during intraoperative cystoscopy in gynecologic and urogynecologic surgery. Am J Obstet Gynecol. 2022;226(1):100.e1–6.
54. Rodríguez D, Goueli R, Lemack G, et al. Racial and ethnic disparities in pelvic organ prolapse surgery in the United States: an analysis of the ACS-NSQIP clinical registry. Urology. 2023;174:70–8.
55. Sung VW, Weitzen S, Sokol ER, et al. Effect of patient age on increasing morbidity and mortality following urogynecologic surgery. Am J Obstet Gynecol. 2006;194:1411–7.
56. Suskind AM, Zhao S, Boscardin WJ, et al. Comparative outcomes for pelvic organ prolapse surgery among nursing home residents and matched community dwelling older adults. J Urol. 2021 Jan;205(1):199–205.
57. Mueller MG, Ellimootil C, Abernethy MG, et al. Colpocleisis: a safe, minimally invasive option for pelvic organ prolapse. Female Pelvic Med Reconstr Surg. 2015;21(1):30–3.
58. Catanzarite T, Rambachan A, Mueller MG, et al. Risk factors for 30-day perioperative complications after Le fort colpocleisis. J Urol. 2014;192:788–92.
59. DiCarlo-Meacham A, Dengler K, Welch E, et al. Risk factors for urinary retention after Colpocleisis. Female Pelvic Med Reconstr Surg. 2021;27(8):488–92.
60. Wolff BJ, Hart S, Joyce CJ, et al. Urinary retention is rare after colpocleisis and concomitant midurethral sling: a 10-year experience. Int Urogynecol J. 2021;32(3):729–36.
61. Roth TM. Pyometra and recurrent prolapse after Le fort colpocleisis. Int Urogynecol J Pelvic Floor Dysfunct. 2007;18:687–8.
62. McCluskey TC, Stany MP, Hamilton CA. Pyocolpos presenting as a large pelvic mass after total colpocleisis. Am J Obstet Gynecol. 2015;212(1):113.e1–2.
63. Shobeiri SA. Management of pelvic abscess after Le fort colpocleisis. Int Urogynecol J Pelvic Floor Dysfunct. 2006;17:668–9.
64. Yuksel B, Harmanli O, Jones KA. Use of Bakri balloon for treatment of persistent hematocolpos after a LeFort colpocleisis: a case report. Female Pelvic Med Reconstr Surg. 2014;20(5):299–300.
65. Elkattah R, Brooks A, Huffaker RK. Gynecologic malignancies post-LeFort colpocleisis. Case Rep Obstet Gynecol. 2014;2014:846745.
66. Mazer C, Isral SL. The LeFort Colpocleisis; an analysis of 43 operations. Am J Obstet Gynecol. 1948;56(5):944–9.
67. Falk HC, Kaufman SA. Partial colpocleisis: the Le fort procedure; analysis of 100 cases. Obstet Gynecol. 1955;5(5):617–27.
68. Fitz Gerald MP, Brubaker L. Colpocleisis and urinary incontinence. Am J Obstet Gynecol. 2003;189(5):1241–4.
69. Khayyami Y, Elmelund M, Klarskov N. Urinary incontinence before and after pelvic organ prolapse surgery-a national database study. Int Urogynecol J. 2021;32(8):2119–23.
70. Reisnauer C, Oberlechner E, Schoenfisch B, et al. Modified LeFort colpocleisis: clinical outcome and patient satisfaction. Arch Gynecol Obstet. 2013;288(6):1349–53.

Mesh Products in Urogynecology: Past and Present

13

Katherine L. Woodburn

Mesh and other graft materials have been used in female pelvic surgery for decades, with one of the first uses of mesh documented in the early 1970s when Teflon mesh previously used for hernias was used for sacrocolpopexy. Providers continued to use various types of mesh, mostly previously used in hernia repairs, for prolapse and stress incontinence in increasing numbers until the first commercially available mesh transvaginal sling kit was released in 1996. By 2005, approximately 70% of mesh prolapse repairs were using a preconfigured kit and by 2010, over one-third of the 300,000 surgeries performed annually for prolapse used some sort of mesh graft.

However, the use of these various kits and mesh products was not without complication as patients and providers noticed an increase in mesh complications such as pain, dyspareunia, and mesh exposure. In 2008, the Food and Drug Administration (FDA) released a public health notice about the rare but serious complications that could occur with the placement of transvaginal mesh for prolapse and stress incontinence [1]. The second public health notice was released in 2011 with more strongly worded language, including statements like "serious complications associated with surgical mesh for transvaginal repair or pelvic organ prolapse are not rare" and "it is not clear that transvaginal pelvic organ prolapse repair with mesh is more effective than traditional non-mesh repair" [2].

As more patients reported complications and the issues surrounding mesh became part of the public discourse, the FDA mandated aftermarket 522 studies to review the safety of all products in 2012. This resulted in most prolapse mesh kits being removed from the market voluntarily by manufacturers rather than undertake these expensive and time-consuming studies. In 2016, the FDA reclassified transvaginal mesh products for prolapse from class 2 (moderate-risk) to class 3 (high-risk) devices and ultimately, in April 2019, the FDA ordered all transvaginal mesh products for prolapse to stop sales. At this point, only three transvaginal mesh products for prolapse remained on the market—*Uphold Lite, Xenform Soft Tissue Repair System,* and *Restorelle DirectFix Anterior.*

While these changes were made with the safety of patients in mind, one unintended consequence has been that many providers are unfamiliar with historical mesh products, given that majority were removed from the market in the mid-2010s. Unfortunately, providers continue to see complications related to these mesh products, and this lack of familiarity can be detrimental to patient care. Without understanding what mesh product was used, its properties, and anchor points, unfamiliar providers may not fully grasp the implications and risks of surgical excision

K. L. Woodburn (✉)
Department of Urology, Wake Forest School of Medicine, Winston Salem, NC, USA

H. B. Goldman, J. Zillioux (eds.), *Complications of Urogynecology and Reconstructive Pelvic Surgery*, https://doi.org/10.1007/978-3-032-00339-3_13

when indicated for complications. Additionally, many patients do not know what type of mesh product was used or what procedure they underwent. Given that many of the companies who previously manufactured these historical mesh products are either no longer in business or have merged with other companies, finding information on these products can be time-consuming and lead to unverified corners of the Internet.

Knowing these challenges firsthand, a smartphone application was created to address this knowledge gap, serving as an easily accessible database of mesh products used in the treatment of pelvic floor disorders available in the United States [3]. The database was compiled using internet searches, textbooks, original products provided by surgeons, and historical manufacturer materials. Every attempt was made to confirm information, videos, and images with a secondary source and that the list was as comprehensive as possible. While originally created in 2021, the app is a living database, so can be added to and edited as needed. The database may be searched by product name, mesh color, and even years available on the market. This can help narrow down possible mesh products used and procedure type when the patient and provider are uncertain.

The application can be opened on a web browser or smartphone by going to https://vaginal-mesh-catalog-25.glide.page/dl/d0a5f4.

References

1. FDA Public Health Notification: Serious complications associated with transvaginal placement of surgical mesh in repair of pelvic organ prolapse and stress urinary incontinence. Available at: http://www.amiform.com/web/documents-risques-op-coelio-vagi/fda-notification-about-vaginal-mesh.pdf. Published 20 Oct 2008.
2. Urogynecologic Surgical Mesh: Update on the safety and effectiveness of transvaginal placement for pelvic organ prolapse. Available at: https://www.fda.gov/media/81123/download. Published July 2011.
3. Woodburn KL, Cardenas-Trowers OO, Fitzgerald JJ. Mix and mesh: an electronic database of FPMRS mesh products through 2020. Female Pelvic Med Reconstr Surg. 2022;28(6):e154–6. https://doi.org/10.1097/SPV.0000000000001158. Epub 2022 Feb 17. PMID: 35234182.

14 Mesh Prolapse Repair

Farzeen Firoozi, Danni Feng, and Howard B. Goldman

Introduction

The lifetime risk of requiring pelvic surgery for vaginal prolapse or incontinence for a woman in the United States is 20% [1], with a risk for reoperation of 30% [2]. Traditional vaginal repairs for prolapse using only the patient's native tissues have had reported rates of recurrence ranging from 10% to 50% depending on the compartment repaired [3]. In the last 20 years, there have been advancements in pelvic floor reconstructive surgery to create repairs that are reproducible with improved subjective and objective outcomes.

Initial attempts were made to augment transvaginal repairs using biologic grafts or absorbable synthetic mesh during anterior wall augmented repairs. Multiple studies demonstrating the use of porcine dermis graft and absorbable Vicryl mesh showed minimal or no difference in the subjective report of prolapse symptoms. As a result, the use of biologic grafts or absorbable synthetic mesh had been largely abandoned as an alternative for augmenting traditional vaginal repairs of anterior and posterior compartment prolapse.

The use of transvaginal mesh was adapted initially on a large scale after the introduction of synthetic slings for the treatment of urinary incontinence [4]. The use of synthetic mesh slings for urinary incontinence has shown significant efficacy, durability, and safety, and led the way for innovation toward transvaginal mesh prolapse repairs. This was an intuitive step on the progression of improved transvaginal repairs, especially since biologic and absorbable synthetic mesh trials in the past had failed to demonstrate superiority to traditional repairs. The synthetic mesh kit procedures were first approved by the Food and Drug Administration (FDA) in 2003. There were multiple head-to-head trials of synthetic mesh and non-mesh repairs that demonstrated improved objective results and lower recurrence rates in the synthetic mesh group. Therefore, it was widely adopted by surgeons throughout the country.

Controversy arose when the discussion of complications related to mesh use outweighed the benefit of augmenting repairs with synthetic mesh. The main issues are the risks of pain, dyspareunia, poor immunologic response, and mesh extrusion or perforation requiring corrective surgery. Adding significant legitimacy to this side of the debate was the initial white paper published by the FDA in 2008 regarding the use of

F. Firoozi (✉) · D. Feng
The Arthur Smith Institute for Urology, Lenox Hill Hospital, Hofstra Northwell School of Medicine, Northwell Health System, New York, NY, USA
e-mail: ffiroozi@northwell.edu; dfeng1@northwell.edu

H. B. Goldman
Glickman Urological & Kidney Institute, Cleveland Clinic, Cleveland, OH, USA
e-mail: goldmah@ccf.org

H. B. Goldman, J. Zillioux (eds.), *Complications of Urogynecology and Reconstructive Pelvic Surgery*, https://doi.org/10.1007/978-3-032-00339-3_14

transvaginal mesh for both incontinence and prolapse surgery. The overall tone of the report was in keeping with the main concerns, namely, the risk for intra- and postoperative complications. The recommendations included the proper counseling of patients as to the potential risks of mesh use in incontinence and prolapse surgery. An update in July 2011 further expressed the concern for use of synthetic mesh for prolapse surgery, but very clearly separated the use of mesh for urinary incontinence—somewhat of an acknowledgment to the arguments made by many experts that the safety of synthetic mesh slings had been well established over almost two decades of study. Following the FDA warning, the use of transvaginal mesh decreased significantly from 35% in 2008 to 11% in 2017 [5]. The concerns culminated in April 2019 when the FDA banned the manufacturers from selling and distributing surgical mesh kits for transvaginal repair of pelvic organ prolapse. The FDA believed the manufacturers did not demonstrate reasonable assurance of the safety of surgical mesh devices and that there was no conclusive evidence that mesh repairs conferred any greater clinical outcomes. There are a sparse number of surgeons to this day throughout the country who use their own preformed mesh—of which they cut out themselves—for prolapse repairs.

There are two general theories that explain the occurrence of mesh complications. The first is that synthetic mesh implanted in the vagina is simply prone to causing pain, extrusion, or perforation. The other theory is that it is generally a problem with appropriate surgical technique that accounts for mesh complications [6]. We will discuss this portion of the debate in our next section. Regardless, the use of synthetic mesh has shown some utility in augmenting traditional transvaginal repairs of prolapse. A very real aspect of these repairs is the potential intra- and postoperative complications related to the use of mesh. In this chapter, we will review techniques for avoiding complications, recognizing technical issues intraoperatively, and managing complications postoperatively.

Avoiding Complications of Transvaginal Mesh Repairs

Preoperative Considerations

Preoperative preparation of patients for transvaginal mesh repairs begins with optimization of vaginal tissue. We recommend the initiation of vaginal estrogen supplementation 4–6 weeks preoperatively to improve perioperative tissue quality. There are currently many options on the market, including Premarin® cream (Pfizer, New York, NY), Estrace® cream (Allergan, Parsippany, NJ), Vagifem® (Novo Nordisk, Plainsboro, NJ), and E-string® (Pfizer, New York, NY). The continued use of local hormone replacement postoperatively is recommended to maintain tissue quality and to facilitate tissue healing.

Certain patient populations with impaired wound healing or damaged vaginal skin may be at greater risk for mesh extrusion. Patients who have had pelvic radiotherapy, those on steroids, history of diabetes, and smokers are examples of these types of patients. Usah and colleagues evaluated clinical predictors and risk factors for vaginal mesh extrusion. Clinical correlations for vaginal mesh extrusion were vaginal bleeding (60 [16.9] vs. 14 [3.2%], $p < 0.001$), hispareunia (48 [13.5] vs. 15 [3.4%], OR = 4.163, $p < 0.001$), and vaginal discharge (45 [12.6] vs. 18 [4.1%], $p = 0.001$). The risk factors were multiple mesh implantations (218 [67.06] vs. 175 [39.68%], $p < 0.001$) and menopause (314 [88] vs. 364 [82.7%], $p = 0.145$) [7]. Very careful consideration of risk profiles and an acknowledgement of increased rates of extrusion should be undertaken before surgery is performed in this population.

Intraoperative Considerations

A cornerstone of transvaginal mesh repair is developing the proper plane of dissection. Probably, the best way to accomplish this is with copious hydrodissection of the vaginal wall to aid in the actual sharp and blunt dissection that follows. The vaginal wall incision is made through the viscerofascial layer to the potential space (filled with a gelatinous fluid after hydrodissection) between the fascial layer (either pubocervical or prerectal) and the underlying viscera. This plane is much deeper than the typical superficial plane external to the viscerofascial layer used for a traditional repair. If the superficial plane is inadvertently utilized for mesh placement, vaginal wall necrosis and ulceration or extrusion may ensue. In addition to vaginal wall extrusion, the risk for vaginal/pelvic pain and dyspareunia is increased by dissection and mesh placement in too superficial a plane.

Once dissection is complete, hemostasis is of utmost importance. Initial postoperative pain following transvaginal mesh repairs can be secondary to perioperative bleeding. This is typically in the form of a hematoma, which can exert pressure on the vaginal tissues, eliciting pain. In addition to pain, hematomas can also delay healing and promote wound separation. Wound separation in the setting of mesh use may result in extrusion of the synthetic material. For these reasons, it is paramount that adequate hemostasis is achieved at the completion of the case, and a tight vaginal pack is typically placed overnight as well.

Dissection should be adequate to allow the mesh to lie flat over the defect, both side to side and proximal to distal. When a trocar-based system is used, one must take care to make the lateral dissection wide enough to allow the arms to be spread as they pass through that area to avoid bunching of the mesh. Bunching and buckling of the mesh can predispose to pain and extrusion.

Similar to the placement of synthetic mesh slings, the mesh placed during transvaginal repair is meant to be placed without tension. The main reason for this surgical tenet is the avoidance of postoperative vaginal/pelvic pain. Whether a trocar or trocarless kit is used, there should be no tension after completion of mesh placement. This can be done by loosening the arms if they are present and making a releasing incision in the body of the mesh if necessary. Again, the goal is the placement of a tension-free system.

Prior to closure, the practice of vaginal wall trimming (common to traditional repairs) needs to be avoided in transvaginal mesh repairs. Only excoriated areas should be removed, and only in a very judicious fashion. The reasoning behind the minimization of vaginal wall trimming relates to the competency of the wound. A wound under tension has an increased risk of developing a possible separation or compromised coverage of the underlying mesh, predisposing to extrusion of the synthetic graft.

Postoperative Considerations

A Foley catheter and vaginal packing are typically left indwelling at the completion of the case. The vaginal packing serves to tamponade the vagina and reduces the risk of postoperative bleeding and can be removed within 24 h after surgery

Intraoperative Complications

With correct dissection, bleeding involving the vaginal wall or the tissue remaining deep to this dissection plane should be minimal during transvaginal mesh repairs. If bleeding does occur on either the vaginal wall or plane of mesh placement, hemostasis can typically be achieved with electrocautery. If bleeding persists, an absorbable suture placed in figure-of-eight interrupted fashion can be used as a further means of hemostasis. Bleeding can also occur with the passage of external trocars or internal trocars with both anterior and posterior approaches. The first maneuver should be direct compression at the site of bleeding. If bleeding persists, optimal exposure of the site of bleeding is paramount. Typically, the source of bleeding is an aberrant vessel that cannot be managed with compression alone. Once further dissection is performed and exposure of the bleeding vessel is achieved, judicious placement of small clips may be performed to halt further bleeding. Some surgeons use hemostatic agents such as Floseal if there is venous oozing in a deep area where it is difficult to see. If significant bleeding cannot be controlled, packing followed by embolization must be considered.

Another potential intraoperative complication of transvaginal mesh repair is injury to other pelvic organs, including the bladder or rectum. If bladder injury occurs, multilayer closure of the cystotomy should be performed with absorbable suture. A Foley catheter should be left indwelling for approximately 10 days prior to the cystogram for confirmation of bladder healing. If a rectal injury is encountered, consultation with general or colorectal surgery is recommended. The ultimate decision of primary repair of rectal injury versus repair with diversion is at the discretion of the consultant surgeon. With either bladder or rectal injury, placement of mesh at the same setting is discouraged. The main concern for mesh placement would be a risk for mesh perforation of the organ, given compromised tissue healing and infection after an injury.

Evaluation of Mesh Complications

History

There is a litany of complaints that patients can present with after transvaginal mesh repair. In this chapter, we will concentrate on patients who present with mesh extrusions and perforations. In 2010, the International Continence Society (ICS) and International Urogynecological Association (IUGA) created a classification system to help promote a universal language that could be used by all pelvic floor surgeons in order to aid with the reporting of mesh complications. The new classification system uses three components to describe complications related to the use of prostheses/grafts, which include the category (C), time (T), and site (S). The C includes the anatomical site that the graft/prosthesis complication involves and identifies the degree of exposure. More severe complications would involve increasing migration/protrusion into surrounding anatomical structures, opening into surrounding organs, and systemic compromise. The T for the complication is when it is clinically diagnosed. There are three time periods used: intraoperative to 48 h, 48 h to 6 months, and over 6 months. The S selection of this division incorporates the current sites, where the graft/prosthesis complications have been noted.

The first step in taking a history from a patient involves documenting the presenting complaint, which can include dyspareunia, prolonged vaginal discharge, severe incontinence, voiding symptoms, rectal discharge, recurrent prolapse, urinary tract infection (UTI), defecatory dysfunction, and thigh drainage or infection. Vaginal pain and pelvic pain are also presenting complaints, which are covered in another chapter. The temporal relationship between the mesh surgery and the onset of symptoms should be carefully analyzed.

A complete review of symptoms should be performed, specifically those symptoms that have occurred since the time of surgery. If the original case was performed by another surgeon, the preoperative records, operative reports, and any other hospital reports should be reviewed. Any concomitant procedures and intraoperative issues—such as bleeding or injury to pelvic organs or problems that occurred postoperatively, such as prolonged bladder catheterization, blood transfusion, or need for reoperation—should be closely reviewed. These issues tend to signify a complicated postoperative course, which may relate to the complication at hand. Finally, a detailed history of events that followed surgery is useful in any future medical or surgical management of mesh complications. Good documentation of one's findings is critical, as these cases may end up under medicolegal review.

Physical Exam

The focused physical exam involves a complete genitourinary exam. This includes a thorough abdominal and pelvic exam with a pelvic speculum with an internal or external light source. Before the speculum exam, careful initial palpation can be performed to elicit any areas of pain. It is important to perform the digital exam prior to a speculum exam because the discomfort of a speculum can make subsequent localization more difficult. These areas can be associated with folded-over mesh, contracted mesh, or taut arms of the mesh if present. Care should be taken to evaluate each vaginal compartment in mapping out all areas of pain. Often, it is easier to palpate extruded mesh than to see it, and thus a very careful palpation of the entire vaginal surface should be performed.

In terms of the speculum pelvic exam, systematic evaluation of the entire vagina should be carried out. Any areas of mesh extrusion should be documented. If a patient complains of pain over the mesh—the specific sites of pain should be mapped out. Other important findings, such as fistulae, should be evaluated closely. Other urologic testing such as cystoscopy to rule out mesh perforation, cystogram or a colored dye test to confirm the presence of fistula, and urodynamics for bladder dysfunction may also be performed based on presenting symptoms. Those patients who present with rectal bleeding or discharge should be evaluated with proctoscopy.

Management of Mesh Complications

Mesh Extrusion

Complications from transvaginal mesh repairs may present days to years after initial surgery. Vaginal mesh extrusion rate is 5% [8]. This typically occurs as a result of wound separation, infection, or vaginal atrophy. Typically, mesh extrusion noted in the immediate postoperative period, usually within 6 weeks, is a result of wound separation. If the wound does not appear infected, additional attempts at wound closure may be offered under local anesthesia with or without sedation. If the wound appears infected, a short course of antibiotics may rectify the issue, with close observation to ensure closure of the wound. Vaginal estrogens should be applied during this time. If the infection persists, then excision of the exposed area is recommended.

Vaginal mesh extrusion noted more than 6 weeks after surgery may be due to technical error, local infection, vaginal atrophy, or wound separation secondary to hematoma. Initial conservative therapy with local estrogen may be offered in order to avoid reoperation. If conservative therapy fails, partial or complete mesh excision should be pursued. Typically, only the areas of mesh that are involved in an extrusion need to be excised—much of the uninvolved mesh can usually be safely left behind. Some very small extrusions can be excised under local anesthesia in the office by just cutting the exposed portion and allowing the vaginal skin to heal over the area. Many patients with point tenderness can be treated in a similar fashion with just those areas causing tenderness excised—though this is typically done under a deeper anesthetic in the operating room. In such cases, one must carefully map out the areas of pain preoperatively, as there will be no extruded mesh to guide you at the time of operation.

Surgical Technique for Excision of Mesh Extrusion

Under either intravenous sedation or general anesthesia, the patient is placed in the dorsal lithotomy position, and the vagina and lower abdomen are prepped and draped in standard fashion. One percent lidocaine with 1:200,000 epinephrine is used to infiltrate under the vaginal skin around the site of the extrusion. A margin of 2–3 mm of healthy tissue around the site of extrusion should be visualized. Bilateral thick vaginal flaps are created extending at least 2 cm lateral to the visible mesh. One centimeter of skin immediately around the mesh is usually discarded. The mesh is then incised in the midline and dissected off of the bladder or rectum in either direction at least 1–2 cm lateral to where the skin will be closed. It is critical to gently separate the mesh from the underlying bladder or rectum. Typically, sharp or blunt dissection using Kittners, working the underlying tissue off of the mesh, prevents inadvertent injury to the underlying organ. The bottom line is that all the tissue should be left behind and only the mesh removed. Once the lateral extent of the mesh is dissected, the mesh is excised. Excised mesh should be sent off to pathology for additional documentation and confirmation of successful excision to avoid accidentlly only excising scar tissue. It is important to heavily irrigate the wound and obtain meticulous hemostasis prior to closure to prevent recurrence. The vaginal wall is then closed in a single layer, watertight closure with absorbable suture. A running lock suture often works well on vaginal mucosa.

Mesh Perforation

Once mesh perforation of the bladder or rectum has been diagnosed, mapping of the areas of perforation must be documented. Mesh perforation of the bladder is typically seen at the bladder base or lateral bladder walls, where mesh arms can sometimes be found (Fig. 14.1a–h). If the mesh has been in the bladder for an extended period of time, calcification of the synthetic material may occur. We have described the purely transvaginal excision of bladder and rectal mesh perforation as safe and efficacious [9] and feel that often the easiest way to remove the mesh is via the same route it was placed.

Surgical Technique for Excision of Mesh Perforation of the Bladder

Under general anesthesia, the patient is placed in the dorsal lithotomy position, and the vagina and abdomen are prepped and draped in standard fashion. Retrograde pyelograms may be performed to rule out ureteral involvement. If no ureteral involvement is noted, temporary bilateral open-ended ureteral stents are inserted. One percent lidocaine with 1:200,000 epinephrine mixture is infiltrated under the vaginal skin, and an inverted U-shaped incision is made. The vaginal wall is dissected to create an inverted U-flap, which serves as the final layer of closure for the repair (in cases where there is a vesico-vaginal fistula [VVF] closer to the vaginal apex a true [noninverted] U-flap is created with the bottom of the U at the VVF site) (Fig. 14.1a). Dissection of the vaginal skin is performed laterally from the U-flap toward the pelvic sidewall (Fig. 14.1b). When only a small area of mesh has eroded into the bladder, the remainder may be found relatively superficially under the vaginal wall. If a substantial volume of mesh has eroded into the bladder, the mesh may not be as easy to find, and the detrusor muscle may need to be incised vertically in the area of the mesh (which can be determined with cystoscopic guidance) until one comes across it. A right-angle clamp can be used to mobilize the mesh off the bladder in the midline (Fig. 14.1c). An incision is made in the midline of the mesh after which the lumen of the bladder is visible (Fig. 14.1d). Any remaining overlying tissues (superficial to the mesh) are bluntly and sharply dissected. By grasping the midline (incised edge) of the mesh and pulling laterally, the bladder wall underneath the mesh is carefully peeled off using both sharp and blunt dissection. If there is a fistula present, it can be seen in its entirety at this point (Fig. 14.1e). The mesh is incised as far laterally as feasible and removed (Fig. 14.1f). The ureteral catheters can be both palpated and visualized. The mucosal layer is re-approximated using a 3–0 absorbable suture, taking care to stay medial to the ureteral catheters. The detrusor layer is then closed in two nonoverlapping layers using 2–0 Vicryl suture (Fig. 14.1g). The nonoverlapping layers are important to decrease the risk of future refistulization. The anterior vaginal wall is closed with 2–0 Vicryl suture (Fig. 14.1h). Although not mandatory, the open-ended ureteral stents can be replaced with JJ ureteral stents to prevent any potential ureteral obstruction from inflammation and edema involving the bladder. An 18 French Foley catheter is left per urethra.

Another option for the removal of mesh perforation of the bladder would be a transabdominal approach. A Pfannenstiel incision is made in the lower abdomen. The incision is carried down to the level of the rectus fascia using electrocautery. The rectus fascia is incised transversely, and the space of Retzius is entered. The bladder is filled via the indwelling Foley catheter to aid in identification. The bladder is then bivalved with a vertical incision using electrocautery. The mesh can now be visualized. The incision is carried down to the mesh. Bladder flaps are now created lateral to the body of the mesh. The mesh is then excised. The vaginal wall is closed using a 2–0 absorbable suture. A portion of the omentum may be mobilized and placed as an interposition graft between the vagina and bladder. The bladder is then closed in two layers with a 2–0 absorbable suture. An 18 French Foley catheter is left per urethra.

Surgical Technique for Excision of Mesh Perforation of the Rectum

Under general endotracheal anesthesia, the patient is placed in the jackknife position, the perineum and buttocks are prepped and the rectum is cleaned with betadine irrigation. A Hill Ferguson retractor is placed to aid in visualization (Fig. 14.2). Mucosal flaps are developed

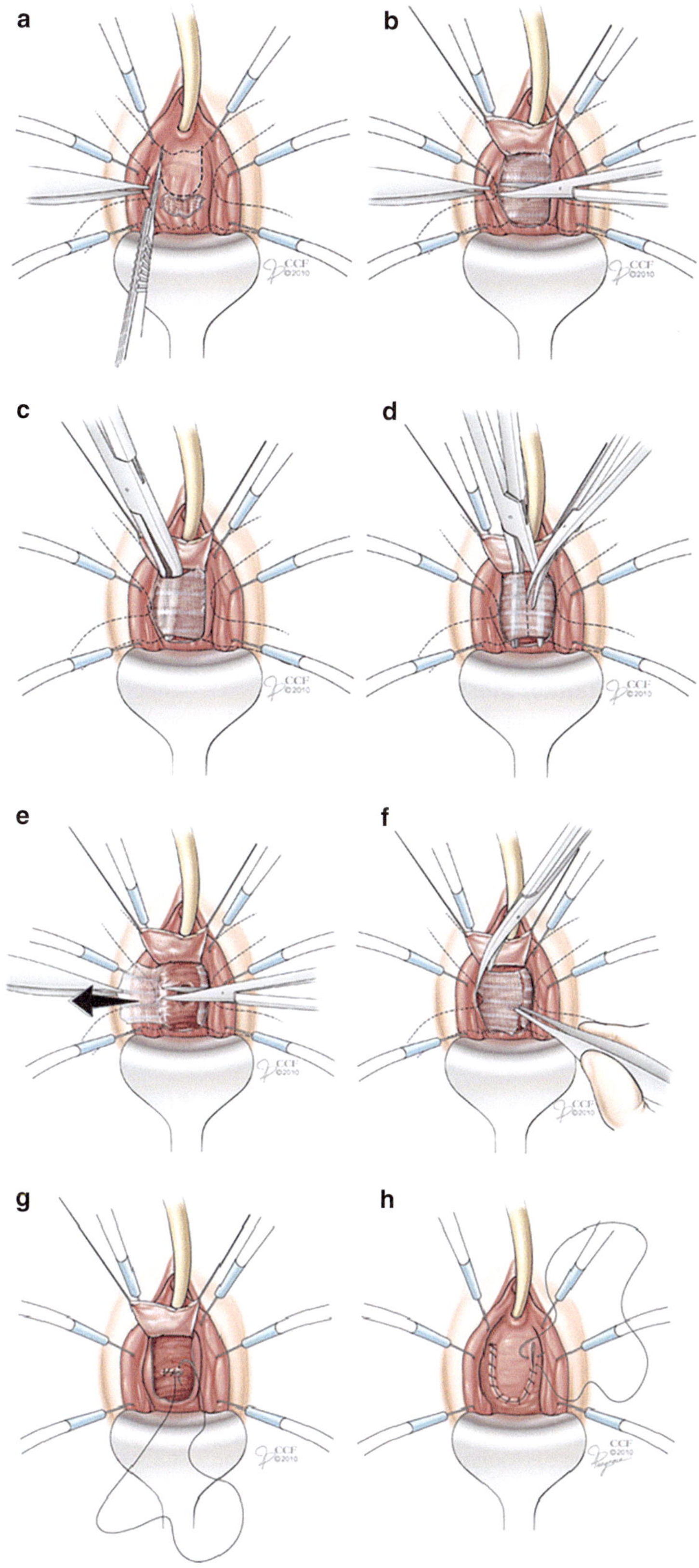

Fig. 14.1 (**a–h**) Excision of transvaginal mesh. (Reprinted with permission, Cleveland Clinic Center for Medical Art & Photography © 2010–2016. All Rights Reserved)

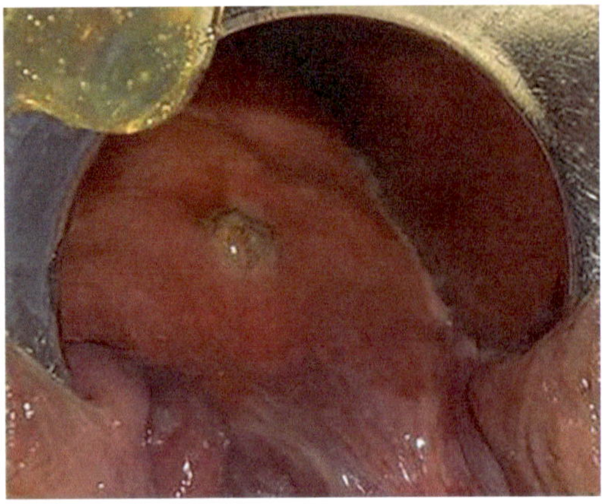

Fig. 14.2 Mesh perforation into the rectum

around the exposed mesh. The mesh is then dissected off the underlying rectal wall and excised. The mucosal flaps are closed with Vicryl suture.

Palpable Tender Mesh Arm in Fornix of Vagina

Occasionally, a patient will note pain near the fornix, and one can palpate a tense arm of mesh at that spot. In such cases, division of the mesh arm may ameliorate the patient's symptoms. Under IV sedation and local or general anesthesia, palpate the arm of interest, inject lidocaine with epinephrine in the vaginal wall overlying it, incise through the vaginal skin at that site, identify and dissect out the mesh arm, and then cut it and close the vaginal skin.

Mesh Complications in Sacrocolpopexy

In terms of apical prolapse, the gold standard has been the abdominal sacrocolpopexy utilizing mesh attached to the vaginal wall. Success rates for managing apical prolapse repairs using mesh via an abdominal route range between 85% and 100% [3]. The safety of this approach has been well established in numerous studies reported over the last several decades [10]. The same complications can arise as discussed above such as vaginal mesh extrusion, visceral mesh perforation, and pain associated with mesh. Additional complications include bowel obstruction, osteomyelitis, and spondylodiscitis. Some intraoperative considerations are hemorrhage, specifically in the presacral area where the middle sacral artery and a rich plexus of veins reside. The plexus of veins can retract when they are injured; therefore, it is imperative to be aware of these potential complications and act in a timely manner. The left iliac vein is at higher risk of injury than the right due to its vertical course closer to the midline [11]. Hemorrhage can be managed with a figure-of-eight sutures, stainless steel thumb tacks, and bone wax.

The same principles of mesh complications as discussed above apply. Of note, mesh complications from sacrocolpopexy more often occur at the apex of the vagina and visceral perforations occur more proximally in the vagina. Therefore, an abdominal approach may be easier and can be performed either open, laparoscopically, or robotically. The rates of bowel perforation and postoperative ileus were 1.6% and 3.6%, respectively, with a median 1.1% of patients requiring reoperation for the obstruction [12]. Sacral osteomyelitis and spondylodiscitis are rare complications, with an incidence of less than 0.001% and can present as low back pain without constitutional symptoms [13]. One-third of patients can experience motor or sensory neurologic deficits, radiculopathy, or loss of anal tone [11]. MRI has a better diagnostic performance and is the gold standard for evaluating early infection [11]. Management ranges from extended antibiotics to excision of the mesh with possible debridement of the infected tissue.

Long-Term Patient Outcomes After Vaginal Mesh Removal

Long-term outcomes and complications of vaginal mesh removal are important, but reports with long-term follow-up are limited. Colby and colleagues conducted a 14-year retrospective case series evaluating patients undergoing vaginal mesh removal. All mesh removals were performed by three board-certified Female Pelvic Medicine and Reconstructive Surgery (FPMRS) surgeons. One hundred and thirteen patients met study criteria with a mean follow-up of 48 months (range of 6–138 months). They found vaginal mesh removal resulted in resolution of pain in

50% of patients and resolution of dyspareunia in 52% of patients [5]. Persistent pain and dyspareunia occurred in 21% and 12%, respectively, but, unfortunately, de novo pain and dyspareunia occurred in 4% and 2% of patients, respectively. After vaginal mesh removal, 84% of patients who had initially complained of recurrent UTI after mesh placement had resolution of their symptoms [5]. Recurrence or persistence of prolapse on one or more compartments beyond the hymen occurred in 25% of patients after vaginal mesh removal, with 20% of patients being symptomatic. Subsequent prolapse repairs occurred in 11% of the patients. A second excision surgery occurred for 29% of patients, while a third and fourth excision surgery were required for 4% and 6% of patients, respectively.

Resolution of symptoms requiring multiple surgical excisions was also found by Warembourg and colleagues, who conducted an 8-year retrospective study with a cohort of 67 patients who had mesh complications. The study found that 15.9% patients required more than one surgical procedure, 11.6% required two procedures, and 4.3% required three interventions [5]. By the 8-year study period, 11.8% of their patients continued to report residual pain. Therefore, long-term pain from vaginal mesh complications is a significant concern that needs to be further studied and addressed.

Conclusion

The use of synthetic mesh for the management of pelvic organ prolapse has been debated for the past few years. At the heart of the controversy lies the concern that complications related to mesh use outweigh the potential benefit of augmenting repairs with mesh. Despite the FDA ban in 2019 on the distribution of surgical mesh kits, urologists continue to deal with transvaginal mesh complications. In our experience, these complications are able to be successfully managed transvaginally with minimal morbidity [14]. We do believe that all who perform transvaginal mesh repairs should be equipped with the surgical skills to manage the potential complications of this surgery.

References

1. Wilkins MF, Wu JM. Lifetime risk of surgery for stress urinary incontinence or pelvic organ prolapse. Minerva Ginecol. 2017;69(2):171–7.
2. Denman MA, Gregory WT, Boyles SH, Smith V, Edwards SR, Clark AL. Reoperation 10 years after surgically managed pelvic organ prolapse and urinary incontinence. Am J Obstet Gynecol. 2008;198(5):555.e1.
3. Maher C, Feiner B, Baessler K, et al. Surgical management of pelvic organ prolapse in women. Cochrane Database Syst Rev. 2010;4:CD004014.
4. Ulmsten U, Petros P. Intravaginal slingplasty (IVS): an ambulatory surgical procedure for treatment of female urinary incontinence. Scand J Urol Nephrol. 1995;29:75–82.
5. Winkelman WD, Modest AM, Richardson ML. U.S. Food and Drug Administration statements about transvaginal mesh and changes in apical prolapse surgery. Obstet Gynecol. 2019;134(4):745.
6. Goldman HB, Fitzgerald MP. Transvaginal mesh for cystocele repair. J Urol. 2010;183:430–2.
7. Khrucharoen U, Ramart P, Choi J, Kang D, Kim JH, Raz S. Clinical predictors and risk factors for vaginal mesh extrusion. World J Urol. 2018;36(2):299–304.
8. Wu PC, Hsiao SM, Chang TC, Chen CH, Lin HH. Clinical outcome and urodynamic changes of tailored transvaginal mesh surgery for pelvic organ prolapse: a mid-term 40 months follow-up. J Formos Med Assoc. 2022;121(12):2424–9.
9. Firoozi F, Goldman HB. Transvaginal excision of mesh erosion involving the bladder after mesh placement using a prolapse kit: a novel technique. Urology. 2010;75:203–6.
10. Maher CF, Feiner B, DeCuyper EM, et al. Laparoscopic sacral colpopexy versus total vaginal mesh for vaginal vault prolapse: a randomized trial. Am J Obstet Gynecol. 2011;204:360.e1–7.
11. Haouari MA, Boulay-Coletta I, Khatri G, et al. Complications of mesh sacrocolpopexy and rectopexy: imaging review. Radiographics. 2023;43(2) https://doi.org/10.1148/rg.220137.
12. Jo YR, Kim JY, Jeon MJ. Significant gastrointestinal morbidity after sacrocolpopexy: the incidence and risk factors. Obstet Gynecol Sci. 2014;57(4):304–9.
13. Stork AM, Giugale LE, Bradley MS, Zyczynski HM. Incidence of sacral osteomyelitis and discitis after minimally invasive sacrocolpopexy. Female Pelvic Med Reconstr Surg. 2021;27(11):672–5.
14. Firoozi F, Ingber MS, Moore CK, et al. Purely transvaginal/perineal management of complications from commercial prolapse kits with the utilization of the new ICS/IUGA prostheses/grafts complication classification system. J Urol. 2012;187(5):1674–9.

15 Retropubic Bladder Neck Suspensions

Menaka Yadav and Elizabeth R. Mueller

Introduction

Open abdominal retropubic procedures for urinary incontinence were widely performed in the United States starting 1950s until the turn of the century, when the use of transvaginal synthetic slings gained popularity [1]. That said, data regarding the success and complications of retropubic suspensions were mostly expert opinion, case series, or underpowered randomized trials until the early 2000s when two large, randomized trials comparing the Burch urethropexy with suburethral slings were published [2, 3]. Since that time, laparoscopic and robotic-assisted laparoscopic retropubic procedures have gained popularity among surgeons due to the mid-urethral sling (MUS) mesh litigation [4]. This chapter will review the retropubic procedures for incontinence and the diagnosis and management of complications that arise from retropubic urethropexy procedures.

M. Yadav
Urogynecology and Reconstructive Pelvic Surgery, Loyola University Chicago Stritch School of Medicine, Maywood, IL, USA

E. R. Mueller (✉)
Professor Emeritus, Urogynecology and Reconstructive Pelvic Surgery, Loyola University Chicago Stritch School of Medicine, Maywood, IL, USA
e-mail: emuelle@luc.edu

Overview of Retropubic Procedures for Incontinence

Retropubic urethropexy procedures generally include the Marshall-Marchetti-Krantz (MMK), the Burch colposuspension, and the paravaginal defect repair. First described by Marshall in 1949, the MMK procedure [5] suspends sutures placed on each side of the bladder neck to the posterior aspect of the pubic bone. This is thought to stabilize the bladder neck and allow abdominal pressures that are being transmitted to the bladder to be equally transmitted to the proximal bladder neck, maintaining continence during stress activities. The MMK procedure was associated with a 20% complication rate and became obsolete when the Burch urethropexy was popularized [6].

The Burch urethropexy was described by John Burch in 1961 as being born out of necessity when the sutures he was trying to place during an MMK kept pulling out of the pubic bone periosteum [7]. After utilizing the arcus tendineus and Cooper's ligament as the point of fixation, he chose the latter based on its consistent presence and inherent strength. Current Burch procedures typically involve bilateral placement of two helical sutures into the vaginal muscularis at the level of the mid-urethra and urethral vesical junction medial to the arcus tendineus fascia pelvis [8]. Each of the four sutures is then placed through the pectineal ligament and tied to elevate the

H. B. Goldman, J. Zillioux (eds.), *Complications of Urogynecology and Reconstructive Pelvic Surgery*, https://doi.org/10.1007/978-3-032-00339-3_15

vaginal wall to the level of the arcus tendineus fascia pelvis.

First described by White in 1909 as a procedure for anterior vaginal prolapse repair, the paravaginal defect repair was popularized for female stress incontinence when the authors reported that reattaching the detached and retracted levator ani fascia to the arcus tendineus resulted in a greater than 90% cure rate [9]. Current clinical evidence does not support the use of the paravaginal defect repair for stress incontinence. It does not have acceptable success rates to justify its use as a stress incontinence procedure.

Key Surgical Techniques in Avoiding Complications

Retropubic procedures require the patient to be prepped and draped in dorsal lithotomy so that the primary surgeon and assistant can have adequate access to the vagina for defining anatomy and providing countertraction. For open procedures, an adequate Pfannenstiel or Cherney incision is made to ensure adequate exposure during dissection of the retropubic space. Alternatively, laparoscopic procedures involve entering the retropubic space either with a transperitoneal or extraperitoneal approach [10]. Once the retropubic space is exposed, the bladder neck can be identified by gentle traction on the Foley catheter. Deflection of the bladder neck and urethra contralaterally prior to elevating the anterior vaginal wall can prevent suture placement in the urethra and bladder [8]. The venous plexus, that can be visualized in the vaginal wall, should be avoided as much as possible since these vessels can be the source of a significant amount of blood loss when sheared during dissection or suture placement.

The goal of both the MMK and the Burch urethropexy is to elevate the vagina to a minimal retropubic position. Care should be taken when tying the sutures as not to cause constriction of the bladder neck and urethra, leading to postoperative urinary obstruction. Numerous authors have described laparoscopic approaches to the Burch [11–13]. While the dissection of the retroperitoneal space is similar, various materials have been used to attach the vaginal wall to Cooper's ligament including sutures, staples, spiral metal tacks, and mesh. Although these materials lend well to the laparoscopic approach, they can be a source of foreign body complications.

Surgical Success

In the seventh edition of the International Consultation on Incontinence, published in 2023, Moore et al. reviewed the literature available on current incontinence procedures and reported that there have been no new randomized trials of open colposuspension since 2017 [14]. The authors state that open colposuspension procedures have comparable short-term subjective and objective outcomes to traditional pubovaginal sling procedures and synthetic MUSs. Pubovaginal slings have better medium- and long-term objective success. They caution, however, that colposuspension procedures are indicated as a primary procedure for stress incontinence and not a salvage procedure for women with recurrent stress incontinence. This recommendation is based on a study of 109 women who were followed for a mean of 14 years with a clinical exam and pad test [15]. The cure rate in primary procedures was 79% versus 61% in women who had a colposuspension for recurrent stress incontinence.

A recent (2019) Cochrane review extracted data from 26 randomized clinical trials enrolling 2271 women with urinary incontinence that included laparoscopic colposuspension in at least one arm of the trials [10]. Thirteen of the trials compared laparoscopic colposuspension to open suspension, nine trials compared laparoscopic colposuspension to MUSs, and the remaining four trials were technique variations (number of sutures and the use of mesh and staples). The authors concluded that subjective cure rates at 18 months were similar for open and laparoscopic colposuspension procedures. They reached the same conclusion for 18-month outcomes comparing the laparoscopic colposuspension using sutures to MUS procedures based on four trials enrolling 256 women. The authors stated there may be a higher subjective cure rate with the use of two sutures bilaterally versus one, but cited that the data was of low quality and based on a single study enrolling 158 women.

Complications

Open Retropubic Urethropexy

Two large, randomized trials comparing the open Burch colposuspension to tension-free vaginal tape and to the fascial sling were published in 2002 and 2007, respectively [3, 16]. The studies randomized 475 women to Burch colposuspension thus providing a solid basis for understanding complications that arise when many different surgeons are performing the procedure.

Ward and Hilton [16] enrolled women from 14 urogynecology and urology centers in the United Kingdom. Women were randomized to the open Burch colposuspension or the tension-free retropubic transvaginal tape (TVT). Exclusion criteria included current need for, or previous history of, surgery for pelvic organ prolapse (POP). One hundred and forty-six women underwent the Burch urethropexy. Women in the study had the following intraoperative and postoperative complications reported at 6 months: urinary tract infection (32%), de-novo detrusor overactivity on urodynamics (11%), wound infection (7%), voiding disorder (7%), bladder injury (2%), deep vein thrombosis (2%), and incisional hernia (2%). Although overall blood loss was higher for the colposuspension, there were no reports of vascular injury or retropubic hematoma in this series. The need for patient catheterization decreased over time, but remained substantial, with 8% of women requiring catheterization after 6 months. Interestingly, there was no statistically significant difference in rates of catheterization and voiding dysfunction compared to TVT.

In 2004, the authors [2] reported the two-year follow-up data. Of the 146 women randomized to Burch urethropexy, 5 (3.4%) underwent surgery for stress incontinence, 7 (4.8%) surgery for POP, and 5 (3.4%) had an incisional hernia repair. At two-years, 4 (2.7%) women continued to catheterize and 3 (2.1%) continued to have symptoms of UTI. On physical exam, the number of women with vault/cervical prolapse increased from 21% preoperatively to 63% at 24 months, and 18% of the women with POP were symptomatic. Over the same 2-year period, vault/cervical prolapse rates increased from 16 to 29% in the TVT arm. In summary, when compared to TVT, Burch colposuspension at 24 months resulted in higher rates of enterocele, voiding dysfunction, and need for catheterization and a 4% lower rate of UTI.

In the Stress Incontinence Surgical Efficacy Trial (SISTEr) [17] involving nine surgical centers in the United States, women were randomized to an open Burch colposuspension or autologous rectus fascial sling. A total of 329 women received a Burch colposuspension; however, 48% of the women had concomitant procedures for pelvic organ prolapse. The following adverse events were reported in women who underwent the Burch colposuspension: cystitis (50%), new onset urge incontinence (3%), incidental cystotomy (3%), surgical wound complications requiring surgery (2.4%), voiding dysfunction >6 weeks (2%), recurrent cystitis leading to diagnostic cystoscopy (1.5%), bleeding (1%), ureteral injury (1%), incidental vaginotomy (0.5%), ureteral vaginal fistula (0.5%), erosion of suture into the bladder (0.5%), and pyelonephritis (0.5%). In summary, compared to a rectus fascial sling, a Burch colposuspension resulted in lower rates of success for stress incontinence and lower rates of cystitis, urge incontinence, and voiding dysfunction.

Marshall-Marchetti-Kranz Procedure

Complications related to the MMK procedure are similar to those mentioned for the Burch colposuspension. In a 1988 review of the literature, Mainprize and Drutz [18] summarized the occurrence of postoperative complications in 2712 patients as follows: wound complications (5.5%), urinary tract infection (3.9%), osteitis pubis (2.5%), direct injury to the urinary tract (1.6%), and ureteral injury (0.1%). Of course, this data is limited, and direct comparisons to the Burch data obtained in a randomized trial would not be advised.

Laparoscopic Colposuspension

Based on the Cochrane review, laparoscopic colposuspension resulted in less pain, shorter inpatient stay, faster return to work, less blood loss, and less time with a catheter when compared to open colposuspension (9 studies, 1117 women) [10]. Operative times were increased by 25 min in procedures that used sutures and 17 min when staples and mesh were used. Bladder perforations were higher in the laparoscopic arm. Similar rates of de novo detrusor overactivity and voiding dysfunction were seen, independent of the surgical approach used.

When compared to MUSs, laparoscopic colposuspension resulted in higher use of analgesics, longer inpatient stays, longer return to work, and longer operative times (four studies, 256 women) [10]. Similar rates of devo detrusor overactivity and voiding dysfunction were reported. Blood loss was not reported in any of the studies and there were no bladder perforations.

Approach to Specific Complications

Intraoperative Complications

Intraoperative Hemorrhage

One of the most anticipated intraoperative complications during a retropubic urethropexy is intraoperative hemorrhage. Risk of hemorrhage can be minimized by assuring adequate exposure of the retroperitoneal space, which includes proper lighting, retraction, and an appropriate length of skin incision. There are numerous vessels that run alongside the bladder and within the vaginal wall. Vaginal wall vessels that are visible can usually be avoided when placing the sutures, and if punctured will often stop bleeding once the sutures are tied into place. When brisk bleeding occurs, direct pressure held for 5 min is often sufficient. Attempts to use metal clips often result in additional shearing of vaginal wall vessels. When packing is insufficient, hemostatic agents may be necessary.

Urinary Tract Injury

The placement of lateral sutures at the level of the bladder neck and mid-urethra can result in ureteral entrapment and proximal urethral injury. A cystourethroscopy should be performed after the Burch suspension is completed to check ureteral patency and look for a foreign body. The detection of brisk ureteral efflux can be aided by giving the patient oral Phenazopyridine just prior to being taken to the operating room.

Postoperative Complications

Urinary Tract Infections

Women who undergo surgical treatment for stress incontinence will most often develop symptoms that are consistent with or mistaken for a UTI. The rates are highest in the first 6 months but do remain between 2% and 9% 24 months after surgery [3, 16]. As a result, it is sensible to require that women with a history of UTI be free of infection prior to undergoing surgery. Women with symptoms of UTI (urgency, frequency, and burning with urination) would benefit by having urine cultures obtained prior to antibiotic treatment to allow for more specific antibiotic treatment but also to document when the symptoms occur with negative cultures. Nonbacterial etiologies include lower urinary tract inflammation, urethral irritation, and irritative voiding symptoms associated with urethral obstruction.

Possible etiologies of recurrent or persistent UTI included incomplete emptying, bacterial colonization from instrumentation and a foreign body in the urinary tract (Fig. 15.1). Women who require catheterization (intermittent or indwelling) should be placed on "treatment" doses of antibiotics once they have stopped using catheters since bacterial colonization occurs often within days of catheter use. Data from the SISTEr trial demonstrate that cystitis rates are highest in the first 6 weeks after surgery [17]. When compared to self-voiders with a cystitis rate of 6%, women who have intermittent or indwelling cath-

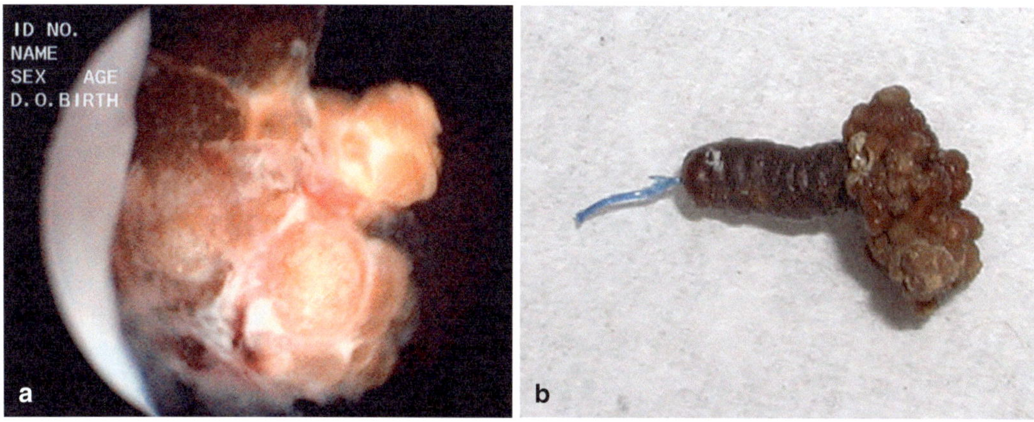

Fig. 15.1 (**a**) Cystoscopic view of a stone at the bladder neck in a patient with pelvic pain and UTIs following a Burch procedure; (**b**) Prolene suture and stone following surgical removal. *(Photographs courtesy of Howard Goldman MD, Cleveland Clinic, OH)*

eters have higher (23% and 13%, respectively) rates of cystitis. In addition, women who undergo voiding trials with post-void residual measurements are often catheterized 2–3 times prior to being discharged thus increasing their risk of colonizing the urinary tract.

When UTIs also present with systemic signs such as fever, chills, and flank pain, upper tract imaging is warranted. The specific imaging depends on the question that needs to be answered. For example, women presenting with febrile UTI and flank pain following an isolated retropubic urethropexy, the imaging question may be "does this patient have ureteral reflux or obstruction?" and a voiding cystourethrogram and renal ultrasound can be ordered. For patients with concomitant prolapse repair, upper tract imaging to assess ureteral patency and cystoscopy to rule out bladder foreign body or cystotomy would be indicated.

Urge Incontinence

In the Ward-Hilton study, 91% of women reported symptoms of bothersome urge incontinence prior to Burch urethropexy that decreased post-procedure to 34% at 6 months and 2 years. On urodynamic testing, the number of women who developed unstable detrusor contractions increased from 1% pre-op to 10% 6-months following a Burch colposuspension. Similarly, persistent urge incontinence was found in 18% of women enrolled in the Burch arm of the SISTEr trial and new onset urge incontinence remained low at 3%.

Possible etiologies of de-novo urge incontinence include UTI, obstructive voiding, and the presence of a foreign body in the lower urinary tract. In women whose symptoms persist after 6 weeks and post-void residuals are normal, conservative treatment for urge incontinence can be considered, including anti-cholinergic and behavioral modifications. A woman who is not responsive or whose symptoms appear severe might benefit from a cystoscopic examination to rule out the presence of a foreign body in the lower urinary tract. Women, who have undergone a laparoscopic Burch procedure and have evidence of a foreign body in the bladder, may have undergone the procedure using metal helical "tackers" to suspend the bladder neck (Fig. 15.2). These are often placed or migrate into the bladder, causing symptoms. If operative notes are not available, then an anterior/posterior and lateral plain x-ray will allow visualization of the offending material.

Uterine or Vaginal Vault Prolapse

In his initial description of the surgical procedure, Burch report the surgical complication of uterine or vaginal vault prolapse. As described previously, 18% of women developed symptomatic prolapse and 4.8% underwent surgical cor-

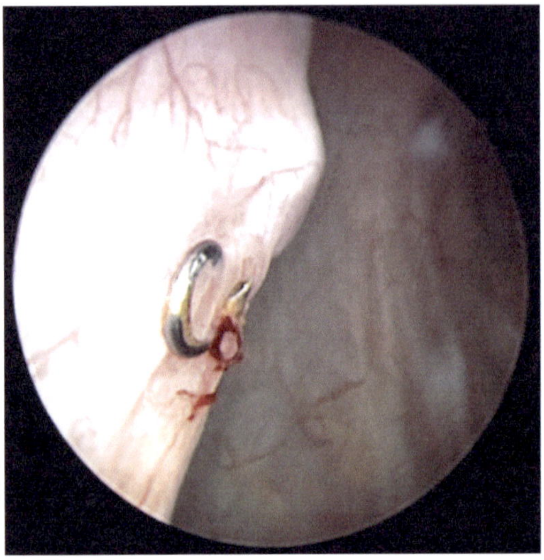

Fig. 15.2 Cystoscopic view of a metal tacker placed during a laparoscopic Burch colposuspension. *(Photograph courtesy of Howard Goldman MD, Cleveland Clinic, OH)*

rection over the 24 months of the Ward–Hilton study [16]. This is believed to be due to the anterior orientation of the vaginal apex. As a result, all women undergoing surgical correction of stress incontinence should have a complete physical exam including the evaluation of vaginal topography ideally in the standing-straining position. Women, who demonstrate apical or uterine descent of greater than 3 cm from optimal position with Valsalva effort, would more likely benefit from a synthetic or autologous suburethral sling since they have not been shown to increase the risk of POP. When a patient is undergoing treatment of POP following an incontinence procedure, care should be taken not to "over-correct" the apical support since this may result in incontinence.

Voiding Dysfunction

Rates of voiding dysfunction following retropubic suspensions vary based on the definitions used, duration of the studies, and whether women with pre-existing voiding dysfunction were excluded from enrollment. The Ward–Hilton study [16] defined a woman as having a voiding dysfunction when two of the three measurements were found on 6-month postoperative urodynamic studies (UDS): peak flow < 15 mL/sec, maximum voiding pressure > 50 cm H2O, and residual volume > 100 mL. Of the women who underwent postoperative UDS, 7% were diagnosed with a voiding dysfunction. Thirty-three percent of women required catheterization (suprapubic, urethral, or intermittent) a week after surgery, and this continued to diminish over time to 13% at 1 month, 8% at 6 months, and 2.7% at 24 months. There were no reports of surgical intervention for voiding dysfunction.

The SISTEr trial also had a gradual return to self-voiding in women undergoing the Burch Procedure. While only 56% of women passed their first voiding trial the authors reported low rates (2%) of voiding dysfunction > 6 weeks after surgery and no surgical revisions for voiding dysfunction in the 329 women who had undergone the Burch procedure. As the series above demonstrates, most voiding dysfunction resolves by 6 weeks and can be treated conservatively with intermittent or indwelling catheterization. In addition, many patients may benefit by undergoing pelvic therapy specifically aimed at pelvic floor relaxation techniques [19].

When obstructive voiding symptoms persist, patients may benefit from filling cystometry and pressure-flow studies to determine if the etiology is obstructive or due to decreased detrusor function. In centers with fluoroscopy, imaging can be helpful. A cystoscopy at the same time would rule out suture placement in the urethra (although this is a rare phenomenon). The etiology is typically obstructive from sutures pulling the bladder neck; sutures placed distally resulting in urethral kinking or scarring of the bladder neck to the back of the pubic bone.

Women who clearly demonstrate obstruction on UDS should be considered for a urethrolysis. In women who have physical exam findings of an indentation of the anterior vaginal wall where sutures have been placed, we consider a transvaginal urethrolysis. For transvaginal urethrolysis, a midline vaginal incision is made ~ mid-urethra and carried to the level of the bladder neck. The dissection continues using sharp and blunt dissection as if making the sling tunnels for a rectus fascial sling. Tissue that is adherent to pubic bone is swept lateral to medial using the surgeon's index finger. Since it is customary in our practice to use a permanent suture, we can palpate the suture as it travels from the proximal urethra and bladder neck to its attachment on the pubic bone (MMK) or Cooper's ligament (Burch). Scissors are then guided to the level of the sutures behind the pubic bone by the surgeon's index finger, and the sutures are transected on each side.

In women who are clearly obstructed and have failed a transvaginal urethrolysis or who do not have a palpable indentation at the level of the bladder neck, a retropubic urethrolysis can be performed. A Pfannenstiel incision is made and carried to the level of the fascia, which is incised two centimeters proximal to the back of the pubic bone. This can also be done laparoscopically. When placing the sutures, the surgeon's nondominant hand is placed into the vagina to assist in locating the sutures that are transected. If the anterior bladder remains fixed to the back of the pubic bone, then this is carefully dissected until the bladder neck and urethra are sufficiently freed to restore a normal degree of mobility.

Anger et al. reported on a retrospective review of 16 women who had symptoms of overactive bladder and/or obstruction following a Burch urethropexy [20]. The study consisted of seven women who had a vaginal approach and nine who underwent the retropubic approach. The groups were not equivalent since 43% in the vaginal group and 55% of the women in the retropubic group performed self-catheterization. Success rates for a return to normal voiding were 66% with the vaginal approach and 100% with retropubic. The authors also reported that overactive symptoms were improved in the retropubic group compared to the transvaginal. They hypothesize that the inability to transect the most proximal sutures through the transvaginal route might result in the lower rates of symptom improvement. That said, most surgeons would agree that the transvaginal approach is less morbid and worth attempting as first-line treatment.

Osteitis Pubis

Osteitis pubis is an inflammatory disease of the pubic symphysis and its surrounding attachments. It occurs in 1–2.5% of MMK procedures but can also occur in any procedure that is in the retropubic space (Fig. 15.3). Symptoms include pubic pain that may be localized to the pubis or radiate to the lower abdomen and thigh. Often, patients adopt a limp and wide-based gait. The diagnosis can be aided using MRI, which can distinguish between osteitis pubis and pelvic osteomyelitis [21]. Medical management includes rest, ice, nonsteroidal anti-inflammatory drugs, physical therapy, and the use of steroids. Patients who are refractory to medical management may benefit from surgical removal of the offending sutures (Fig. 15.3).

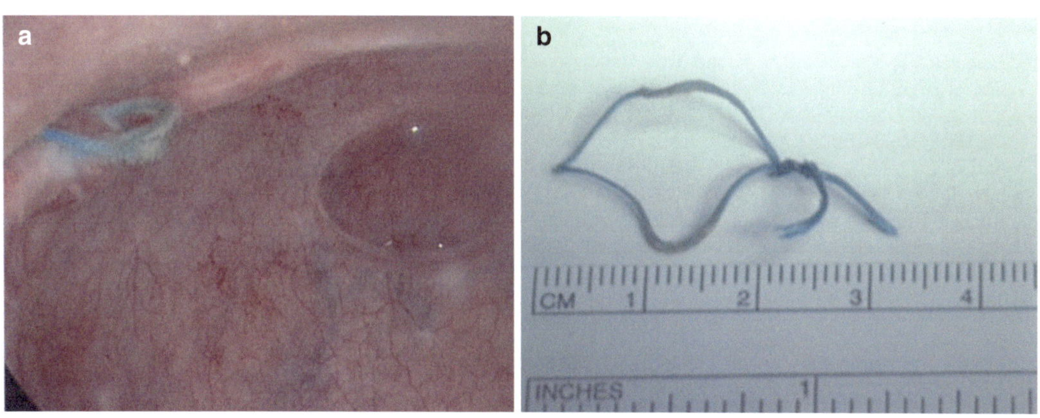

Fig. 15.3 (**a**) Cystoscopic view of suture in the right lateral wall of the bladder placed during open Burch colposuspension 3 years prior. Early postoperative course complicated by osteitis pubis requiring removal of the left-sided suspension sutures. (**b**) Removal of the right bladder wall suture resulted in the resolution of suprapubic pain at rest and ambulation. *(Photographs courtesy of Howard Goldman MD, Cleveland Clinic, OH)*

Summary

With the advent of synthetic MUSs, the retropubic suspensions are often referred to as a procedure of historical interest. However, as we continue to see product liability issue surrounding transvaginally placed surgical mesh, there remains a role for this procedure in the armamentarium of the well-versed pelvic surgeon. It is important to understand potential complications, principles of prevention, and their management strategies.

References

1. Anger JT, Weinberg AE, Albo ME, Smith AL, Kim JH, Rodriguez LV, Saigal CS. Trends in surgical management of stress urinary incontinence among female Medicare beneficiaries. Urology. 2009;74(2):283–7.
2. Ward KL, Hilton P, UK and Ireland TVT Trial Group. A prospective multicenter randomized trial of tension-free vaginal tape and colposuspension for primary urodynamic stress incontinence: two-year follow-up. Am J Obstet Gynecol. 2004;190(2):324–31.
3. Albo ME, Richter H, Brubaker L, Norton P, Kraus SR, Zimmern PE, Chai TC, Zycaynski H, Diokno AC, Tennstedt S, Nager C, Lloyd K, FitzGerald MP, Lemack G, Johnson HW, Leng W, Mallett V, Stoddard AM, Menefee S, Varner RE, Kenton K, Moalli PA, Sirls L, Dandreo K, Kusek JW, Nyberg LM, Steers W. Urinary incontinence treatment network. Burch colposuspension versus fascial sling to reduce urinary stress incontinence. N Engl J Med. 2007;365(21):2143–55.
4. Zacche MM, Mukhopadhyay S, Giarenis I. Changing surgical trends for female stress urinary incontinence in England. Int Urogynecol J. 2019;30(2):203–9.
5. Marshall VF, Marchetti AA, Krantz KE. The correction of stress incontinence by simple vesico-urethral suspension. Surg Gynecol Obstet. 1949;88:281–90.
6. De Vries AM, Heesakkers JPFA. Contemporary diagnostics and treatment options for female stress urinary incontinence. Asian J Urol. 2018;5(3):141–8.
7. Burch J. Urethrovaginal fixation to Cooper's ligament for correction of stress incontinence, cyctocele and prolapse. Am J Obstet Gynecol. 1961;81:281–90.
8. Tappy E, Pan E, Corton M. Robotic Burch colposuspension: anatomical and technical considerations. Int Urogynecol J. 2023;34(7):1653–7.
9. Richardson AC, Edmonds PB, Williams NL. Treatment of stress urinary incontinence due to paravaginal fascial defect. Obstet Gynecol. 1981;57:357–62.
10. Freites J, Stewart F, Omar MI, Mashayekhi A, Agur WI. Laparoscopic colposuspension for urinary incontinence in women. Cochrane Database Syst Rev. 2019;12(12):CD002239.
11. Wallwiener D, Grischke E, Rimbach S, Maleika A, Bastert G. Endoscopic retropubic colposuspension: "Retziusscopy" versus laparoscopy - a reasonable enlargement of the operative spectrum in the management of recurrent stress incontinence? Endosc Surg Allied Technol. 1995;3:115–8.
12. Ross J. Two techniques of laparoscopic Burch repair for stress incontinence: a prospective, randomized study. J Am Assoc Gynecol Laparosc. 1996;3(3):351–7.
13. Zullo F, Palomba S, Piccione F, Morelli M, Arduino B, Mastrantonio P. Laparoscopic Burch colposuspension: a randomized controlled trial comparing two transperitoneal surgical techniques. Obstet Gynecol. 2001;98(5 Pt 1):783–8.
14. Moore K, Athanasiou S, Chen Z, Gomelsky A, Gomes C, Harding C, Peyronnet C, Rovner E, Serati M, Smith A, Tomoe H. Surgery for urinary incontinence in women. In: Cardoza L, Rovner E, Wagg A, Wein A, Abrams P, editors. Incontinence. 7th ed. Bristol: ICI-ICS. International Continence Society; 2023.
15. Alcalay M, Monga A, Stanton S. Burch colposuspension: a 10-20 year follow up. Br J Obstet Gynaecol. 1995;102:740–5.
16. Ward K, Hilton P, United K, Ireland Tension-free Vaginal Tape Trial Group. Prospective multicentre randomised trial of tension-free vaginal tape and colposuspension as primary treatment for stress incontinence. Br Med J. 2002;325(7355):67.
17. Chai T, Albo M, Richter H, Norton P, Dandreo K, Kenton K, Lowder J, Stoddard A. Complications in women undergoing burch colposuspension versus autologous rectus fascial sling for stress urinary incontinence. J Urol. 2009;181:2192–7.
18. Mainprize TC, Drutz HP. The Marshall-Marchetti-Krantz procedure - a critical review. Obstet Gynecol Surv. 1989;43:724–9.
19. Smith PP, Appell RA. Functional obstructed voiding in the neurologically normal patient. Curr Urol Rep. 2006;7(5):346–53.
20. Anger JT, Amundsen CL, Webster GD. Obstruction after Burch colposuspension: a return to retropubic urethrolysis. Int Urogynecol J Pelvic Floor Dysfunct. 2006;17(5):455–9.
21. Knoeller SM, Uhl M, Herget GW. Osteitis or osteomyelitis of the pubis? Acta Orthop Belg. 2006;72(5):541.

16 Pain Related to Transvaginal Mesh Placed for Stress Urinary Incontinence and Pelvic Organ Prolapse

Tyler Trump, Ashley B. King, and Howard B. Goldman

Introduction

In 2008, after receiving numerous claims related to complications associated with transvaginal mesh, the Food and Drug Administration (FDA) released a safety communication related to these materials. A follow-up report in 2011 stated that "serious complications associated with surgical mesh for transvaginal repair of POP are not rare" [1]. The focus of this safety communication was on transvaginal mesh for pelvic organ prolapse repair (TVM/POP), not that used for stress urinary incontinence (SUI).

In response, the American College of Obstetricians and Gynecologists (ACOG) and the American Urogynecologic Society (AUGS) jointly published a position statement on mesh used for prolapse repair. ACOG and AUGS recommended that patients are counseled appropriately regarding risks and alternatives and the surgeons have proper training on the specific devices implanted. They also stress the importance of proper data collection on outcomes [2]. To contrast mesh used for SUI, The Society of Urodynamics, Female Pelvic Medicine and Urogenital Reconstruction (SUFU), and AUGS also released a position statement in 2014 in support of synthetic midurethral slings, which was most recently updated in 2021 [3].

As time has passed and long-term complications related to mesh placement have come to light, societies have responded by publishing guidance regarding these complications. In 2017, ACOG and AUGS published a committee opinion with the objective of guiding the general obstetrician-gynecologist on management of simple mesh complications as well as guidance on when to refer to appropriate specialists for further evaluation and management [4]. Following this, in 2020, AUGS in collaboration with the International Urogynecological Association (IUGA) published guidance for management of mesh related complications for the specialist [5].

Various complications can occur after transvaginal mesh placed for either SUI or pelvic prolapse; however, this chapter will focus on persistent pain after mesh placement for SUI and pelvic prolapse, including vaginal pain, dyspareunia, suprapubic pain, and thigh pain.

T. Trump (✉)
Center for Urogynecology and Reconstructive Pelvic Surgery, Glickman Urological Institute, Cleveland Clinic, Cleveland, OH, USA
e-mail: trumpt@ccf.org

A. B. King
Woodlands Medical Specialist, Department of Urology, Center for Female Pelvic Medicine and Reconstructive Surgery, Pensacola, FL, USA

H. B. Goldman
Glickman Urological & Kidney Institute, Cleveland Clinic, Cleveland, OH, USA

H. B. Goldman, J. Zillioux (eds.), *Complications of Urogynecology and Reconstructive Pelvic Surgery*, https://doi.org/10.1007/978-3-032-00339-3_16

Classification of Complications

In 2011, IUGA and ICS developed a classification system for complications related to grafts used in female pelvic surgery. The classification system is outlined in Fig. 16.1. Category 1 includes cases where there is no exposure of mesh in the vagina, but the mesh is prominent because of folding or wrinkling, or there is mesh contracture or shrinkage. Mesh exposure in the vagina is further characterized and differentiated from perforation of viscera. Complaints of pain are divided into pain provoked by vaginal exam alone, pain during sexual activity, pain during physical activity, and spontaneous pain [6].

- General Description
  - Vaginal: no separation
  - Vaginal: ≤ 1cm exposure
  - Vaginal: larger >1 cm, or any extrusion
  - Urinary Tract: compromise or perforation
  - Rectal or Bowel: compromise or perforation
  - Skin and/or Musculoskeletal: complications including discharge, pain, lump or sinus tract formation
  - Patient: compromise including hematoma or systemic compromise
- Category
  - Asymptomatic
  - Symptomatic
  - Infection
  - Abscess
- Time (clinically diagnosed)
  - T1: Intraoperative to 48 hours
  - T2: 48 hours to 2 months
  - T3: 2 months to 12 months
  - T4: over 12 months
- Site
  - S1: Vaginal: area of suture line
  - S2: Vaginal: away from area of suture line
  - S3: Trocar passage (excluding intra-abdominal)
  - S4: Other skin or musculoskeletal site
  - S5: Intra-abdominal
- Subclassification of Pain
  - Asymptomatic or no pain
  - Provoked pain only (during vaginal examination)
  - Pain during intercourse
  - Pain during physical activities
  - Spontaneous pain

Fig. 16.1 IUGA/ICS joint terminology and classification of the complications related directly to the insertion of prostheses. (Reprinted with permission of John Wiley and Sons from Haylen et al. [6])

Evaluation of Patient

Evaluation of a patient with vaginal, suprapubic, or thigh pain after transvaginal mesh placement starts with a thorough history and physical exam. During history, it is important to determine if the patient had any chronic pain prior to mesh placement, as this is important in counseling about success after mesh removal. Obtaining details regarding the original surgery, as well as any prior mesh excisions, is important. Reviewing the prior operative notes, if they can be obtained, and understanding the details of the implanted material and index operation is critical, even if the procedure was not part of the surgeon's training. Many surgeons may not be aware of the characteristics and attachment points of the transvaginal prolapse and sling meshes that were used. Chapter 13 gives a nice overview of the majority of the meshes that were used and should be reviewed. Descriptive information regarding the location of pain, type of pain, and any alleviating or aggravating factors should be well documented.

On physical exam, a thorough abdominal exam, vaginal exam, and thigh exam are important. Assessing for any pain or tenderness along the expected trajectory of any mesh placed should be done with palpation—in general, pain related to the mesh implant is reproducible on examination [5]. Often, exposures are best detected with finger palpation although visualization can be helpful. The levator muscles should also be palpated to try to differentiate levator spasm from pain related to the mesh although the former could develop in reaction to the latter. Rectal exam should be performed to assess tone and evaluate for pain or mesh perforation. Cystoscopy may be utilized to rule out bladder or urethral perforation. Urodynamics may be indicated depending on the other presenting symptoms; however, if mesh excision is planned for pain, then urodynamics may not be indicated.

Vaginal Pain and Dyspareunia

Synthetic Midurethral Slings

Vaginal exposure, vaginal pain, dyspareunia, and sexual function outcomes after midurethral sling placement are extremely intertwined and difficult to tease out in the literature. The most recent Cochrane review reports an overall exposure rate of 0.4% in transobturator cases and 1.5% in retropubic cases [7]. The 5-year data from the TOMUS trial showed no difference in exposure rate between retropubic and transobturator slings, with an overall exposure rate of 1.7% at 5 years [8].

Dyspareunia rates range from 4.3% in larger reviews [9] to 14.5% in smaller series [10]. One finding after the TOT sling that has been reported is paraurethral banding. Some have thought that this could lead to worsening pain and dyspareunia; however, this has not been supported in the literature [11].

Sexual function generally improves after sling placement, although this can be related to decreased coital incontinence. However, de novo dyspareunia and urgency incontinence negatively impact sexual function [12, 13]. Some studies have shown similar improvement in sexual function after both retropubic and transobturator slings; however, the 5-year data from the TOMUS trial does show greater improvement in sexual function after transobturator sling [8].

Transvaginal Mesh for Pelvic Organ Prolapse Repair

Rates of vaginal exposure after TVM/POP vary; however, in the Cochrane Review from 2024, the overall mesh vaginal exposure rate was 11.8% [14] but has been quoted as high as 20% in some series [15]. Vaginal exposure does not always correlate with dyspareunia or vaginal pain.

Bontje et al. reported their series of 84 patients who underwent a Prolift graft. None of the patients with dyspareunia had a mesh exposure [16]. Other studies have also demonstrated dyspareunia rates to be similar among patients with and without a mesh exposure [17]. De novo dyspareunia rates after TVM/POP vary, ranging as high as 16.7% [18]. According to the Cochrane Review, there is no difference in dyspareunia rates between native tissue suture-based repairs and TVM/POP [14].

The effect of TVM/POP on overall sexual function is controversial. Altman et al. reported on a series of 261 patients who underwent an anterior, posterior, or total Prolift mesh prolapse repair. Of the 105 who were sexually active prior to the procedure, overall sexual function declined; however, dyspareunia rates were not significantly changed. The decline in sexual function was related more to behavioral or emotional domains. The authors also found that anatomic success did not correlate with improved sexual function [19]. Others have found no effect on sexual function [20].

Risk Factors

Vaginal pain and dyspareunia after transvaginal mesh placement can be related to mesh exposure or may present without any mesh exposure. Separating this causality in the literature is difficult. However, risk factors for mesh exposure include increased intraoperative blood loss [21], lower BMI [21], and smoking [22]. Sirls et al. performed a retrospective review of 335 women who underwent mesh augmented prolapse repair to assess for risk factors for mesh exposure. Overall exposure rate was 8.1% with a median time to detection of exposure of 96 days. Lower BMI and increased blood loss were associated with mesh exposure, but no other risk factors were identified, including age, smoking history, menopause, diabetes, steroids, past surgery, or prolapse stage [21].

There has been an assumption that postmenopausal status would lead to worsening pain after mesh placement. The literature on this is limited; however, Long et al. examined the effect of menopausal status on changes in sexual function after mesh augmented prolapse repair [23]. Contrary to the expected outcome, they found that sexual function worsened in the premenopausal group compared to the postmenopausal group and that anatomic success was not correlated with improvements in sexual function. However, it should be noted that there was a significant minority of patients in the postmenopausal group on estrogen replacement. In addition, although most of the total patients were postmenopausal, only 30% of the postmenopausal group were sexually active and completed follow-up compared to 89% of the premenopausal group.

Another concern brought up in the FDA communication was the role that mesh contraction plays. Some have found that mesh length in the patients who reported vaginal pain and de novo OAB was significantly decreased by about 1 cm compared to patients without these complaints [24]. However, it is important to remember that several series, including the most recent Cochrane review, found no difference in dyspareunia rates after mesh or native tissue prolapse repair [14]. Other studies have shown more dyspareunia after mesh augmented prolapse repair compared to native tissue repair. Anger et al. utilized a 5% random sample of Medicare beneficiaries who underwent prolapse repairs with and without mesh from 2007 to 2008. These were compared to patient who underwent prolapse repair without mesh from 1998 to 2000. They found that failures within 1 year requiring reoperation were higher in the non-mesh group; however, the mesh group was more likely to report dyspareunia and pelvic pain [25].

Prevention

Despite the removal of vaginal mesh kits from the market in many parts of the world, prevention is still relevant, as in some countries these types of kits are still in use. While nothing can completely prevent complications from occurring, a number of strategies can help minimize the risk of pain after mesh surgery. Dissection must be carried out in the proper plane (most experts suggest the proper plane is deep to the pubocervical fascia). If the dissection is too superficial, then the patient is at increased risk of exposure and potentially vaginal pain. The mesh should be placed to avoid any tension on the mesh body or arms. Good hemostasis is also important, as hematoma formation and drainage can lead to wound separation and exposure. Knowledge of the anatomic borders and staying within them is vital.

Treatment

Treatment depends somewhat on whether there is vaginal pain and dyspareunia (or partner-related pain) with or without vaginal exposure. However, overall treatment options include medical management, physical therapy, and surgical intervention.

To treat vaginal pain and dyspareunia without vaginal exposure, NSAIDS, pain medications, neuroleptics, and muscle relaxants can be utilized alone or with pelvic floor physical therapy. Botulinum toxin A has been used to improve pain related to levator spasm; however, insurance coverage can be difficult in some cases, as it is not an FDA-approved treatment for pelvic pain. Transvaginal trigger-point injections with local anesthetic and triamcinolone into the levators is an alternative. Pudendal nerve blocks can be performed in patients with pudendal neuralgia.

If a patient fails more conservative treatment options, then mesh excision can be performed. Typically, in the face of pain and vaginal exposure, excision is favored; however, topical estrogen cream and other more conservative treatments can be attempted depending on the size of exposure and degree of pain. Treatment with topical estrogen alone is generally reserved for small (<1 cm) solitary exposures. If there is no resolution after 3 months of therapy with estrogen, then patients should be counseled that resolution is unlikely, and surgical management should be discussed [5].

Office-based trimming is often performed as an initial treatment strategy, but the long-term success of this strategy is thought to be low. Patients may wish to undergo office-based trimming as an initial step due to its relatively low risk profile, but they should be counseled at this time regarding more definitive surgical therapy should their symptoms persist or recur. In one series of patients undergoing surgical removal of their mesh, nearly 3/4th of patients (73%) reported that they underwent previous office-based trimming that ultimately was unsuccessful [26].

Technique for Mesh Excision

Typical mesh excision can be performed transvaginally as previously described [27]; although in the case of ureteral involvement or an anterior bladder perforation, transabdominal repair may be necessary. Typically, if the excision is done for pain, then a wider excision is performed than for vaginal exposure alone; however, the focus of dissection should be on the areas that cause pain with palpation as determined on physical exam. Further details of transvaginal mesh removal are contained in the corresponding chapter.

Outcomes of Surgical Excision

Resolution rates of vaginal pain and dyspareunia vary in the literature. Many series quote a resolution rate around 50%; however, this varies from 13% to 100% resolution [28, 29, 30, 31]. The series, which showed resolution of dyspareunia in only 13% after mesh excision, found on multivariate analysis that complete excision, de novo overactive bladder symptoms after initial placement, and obesity correlated with improvement in symptoms. Patients who developed de novo OAB symptoms after the original surgery showed improvement of these symptoms after excision. As far as the relationship between obesity and improved symptoms, the authors proposed a possible role of elevated estrogen from peripheral conversion in the adipose tissue as leading to improved healing [30]. One series found that patients who had mesh exposure were more likely to have improvements in pain after excision, but the difference was not statistically significant. The authors also found that a history of chronic pain led to a higher risk of worsening or unchanged symptoms [32].

Recurrence of SUI after sling excision for pain ranges from 2% to 56%. One study focusing on pain after MUS placement identified no statistically significant difference in rate of recurrent SUI among patients undergoing complete mesh removal compared to partial mesh removal [33]. Recurrence of prolapse occurs in 5–29% of patients with higher rates of recurrence after complete excision of TVM/POP [34]. Some series report low complications rates after transvaginal excision; however, others report slightly higher complication rates. Tijdink et al. performed a retrospective series of 73 patients who underwent TVM/POP excision. Overall, intraoperative and postoperative complication rates were 5% and 16%, respectively. Intraoperative complications included three bowel injuries and one case of bilateral ureteral injury, which was diagnosed postoperatively with anuria. The patient underwent bilateral ureteral reimplantation after diagnosis [34]. Counseling the patient is very important, including possible lack of improvement in pain, possibly worsening of symptoms, recurrent incontinence or prolapse depending on the type and degree of mesh excised, visceral injury, significant bleeding, ureteral injury requiring abdominal surgery, and fistula formation.

Suprapubic Pain

Risk Factors

Fisher et al. performed anatomic dissection to illustrate possible nerve injuries that are at risk with TVT placement. The ilioinguinal and iliohypogastric nerves can be injured if the trocar is passed too laterally. The ilioinguinal nerve is involved in sensation to the skin over the pubic symphysis, groin, labia, and inner thigh. The iliohypogastric has similar sensory function over the pubic symphysis and groin. The pudendal nerve has branches under the pubic bone and if one passes the trocar scraping the edge of the pubic bone (often done to avoid bladder injury), these branches can be involved. Injury to the pudendal branches can lead to localized pain or perineal pain [35]. In addition, obturator neuralgia has been reported from a lateral passage of TVT trocar [36]. Therefore, it appears that suprapubic pain after retropubic sling placement can be reduced by proper passage of the trocars.

Treatment

Overall, rates of persistent suprapubic pain after sling placement appear low at around 2.3% [37]. However, when pain persists, treatment options include NSAIDS, pain medications, and neuroleptics. Local anesthetic injection can be utilized. If a patient fails more conservative treatment options, then mesh excision can be performed. If there is concurrent vaginal pain, a vaginal excision alone may be considered first. However, if this does not relieve the suprapubic pain or if there is isolated suprapubic pain, then excision of the suprapubic arms can be performed either open or laparoscopically [36, 38].

Technique for Suprapubic Dissection

Suprapubic dissection can be performed open or laparoscopically (with or without robotic assistance). If performed open, the dissection is extraperitoneal; however, if done laparoscopically or robotically, either an extraperitoneal or intraperitoneal approach can be done. The laparoscopic approach gives outstanding visualization, while the use of robotic assistance provides much improved ergonomics and the ability to dissect the mesh arms through the rectus fascia via the intraperitoneal approach.

Open excision can be done through an infraumbilical or Pfannenstiel incision. The rectus muscles are split, and the space of Retzius is developed. The mesh arm is localized by palpation and visualization in the expected location of passage. The arm can then be dissected off the pubic bone down through the endopelvic fascia and then in the opposite direction out to the level of the skin. In some cases, it can be difficult to identify the mesh arms. Bladder injury should be avoided; however, if a bladder injury occurs during dissection, it can be repaired from this approach.

For a laparoscopic or robotic-assisted approach, a midline periumbilical camera port can be placed as well as two working ports, each about 8 cm lateral and 2 cm caudal to the midline port. Additional assistant ports can also be utilized. The approach is similar to the open technique; however, with an intraperitoneal approach, the space of Retzius must be exposed. This is done by incising the peritoneum above the pubic symphysis and then dividing the median umbilical ligaments and the urachus. The bladder can then be dropped down to obtain adequate exposure. To perform the surgery via an extraperitoneal approach, balloon dilation may be performed first to develop the space of Retzius. With the laparoscopic approach, the visualization is such that it is typically quite simple to identify and dissect the mesh arms.

An alternative approach can be done if a vaginal dissection is performed concomitantly. The vaginal arms can be dissected through the endopelvic fascia and then bluntly peeled off the pubic bone up to the rectus fascia. Then, with an instrument on the mesh, the tip of the instrument can be advanced around the pubic bone toward the fascia. Through a small suprapubic incision, the tip of the instrument can be palpated, and the mesh can be dissected free where it passes through the fascia. Cystoscopy is prudent after excision to rule out any bladder injury.

Thigh Pain

Transobturator Sling

The risk of persistent thigh pain is higher after transobturator slings compared to retropubic slings. In the TOMUS trial, at the 12 month follow-up, neurologic symptoms were higher in the transobturator group compared to the retropubic group (9.4% vs 4.0%) [39]. At 5 year follow-up, two women in the transobturator group reported persistent thigh pain [8]. Others have reported rates of persistent thigh pain at 5 years of 32.8% [40].

Risk Factors

Two main factors that may contribute to the development of persistent thigh pain are patient positioning at the time of sling placement and the technique of transobturator sling placement. Two cadaver studies have emphasized the importance of proper patient positioning to increase the distance between mesh placement and the branches of the obturator nerve. Hinoul et al. showed in a cadaveric study that the exit site of the TVT-O is variable and affected by the positioning of the legs during trocar placement. They recommended hyperflexion to maximize trocar distance from the obturator nerve branches [41].

Hubka et al. also analyzed the effect of leg position during the TVT-O procedure on proximity to the branches of the obturator nerve in both properly positioned and malpositioned cadavers. The malpositioned bodies were placed with the legs at 30° to the horizontal plane versus the properly positioned bodies with legs at 90° to the horizontal plane. All the legs were abducted 30° to the sagittal plane. In the malpositioned group of both formalin embalmed bodies and fresh frozen bodies, the mean distance from all the branches of the obturator nerve was less than 1 cm, and there was direct contact with the nerve noted three times in this group of 19 bodies. In the properly positioned fresh frozen bodies, the mean distance from the obturator nerve was over 2 cm, and no direct contact with the nerve was noted [42].

Others have looked at the impact of body mass index on the risk of persistent pain after transobturator mesh placement. Cadish et al. performed a retrospective study of all patients who underwent TVT-O sling placement. A total of 219 TVT-O slings were reviewed. The overall rate of postoperative thigh or hip pain was 15.5% with an average follow-up of 1.6 months. There was equal incidence of right-sided, left-sided, and bilateral groin pain. The rate of postoperative groin pain was higher in normal-sized women versus obese patients (21.0% versus 10.3%). The authors propose several explanations for these findings, including increased adipose tissue serving as a barrier to surrounding nerves or possible increased attention during positioning by the care team in obese patients. However, the study is limited by the retrospective nature, which lacked a direct, standardized routine assessment of postoperative groin pain [43]. In addition, surgeons who have done thigh dissections can attest to the fact that there is no fat between the obturator membrane, pubic bones, and muscles of the medial thigh compartment. This study and the cadaver studies discussed above all focused on the TVT-O, presumably because one has less control over the exit site with "inside-out" slings than "outside-in" slings.

Treatment

Similar to other mesh-related pain, treatment options for thigh pain include NSAIDS, pain medications, physical therapy, and local anesthetic injection. If a patient fails more conservative treatment options, then mesh excision can be performed. Vaginal dissection can be attempted initially to see if that alone relieves thigh pain. However, if pain persists or if there is isolated thigh pain, then thigh dissection can be performed to remove the thigh portion of the mesh.

Technique for Thigh Dissection

The technique of thigh dissection can be performed in a similar fashion as described by Wolter et al. and King et al. [44, 45] If a vaginal mesh excision is planned concomitantly, then vaginal dissection can be performed first. The vaginal portion should be left intact to use as an aid in the thigh dissection. For the thigh dissection, an incision is marked 1–2 cm lateral to the inferior pubic ramus. The incision is approximately 6–8 cm in length (Fig. 16.2). After incision, dissection is carried down to the gracilis muscle, which is then cut as close to the inferior pubic ramus as possible (Fig. 16.3). The remaining muscle layers are cut and then reflected in a similar fashion, including the adductor brevis and obturator externus. Occasionally, the mesh is found more easily and then can be traced to the obturator membrane without dividing all the muscle layers. However, typically localizing the mesh arm can be difficult and is aided by knowledge of the typical route of passage, visualization of any scar from the initial groin incision, close inspection for mesh fibers, and palpation. Often, the mesh can be palpated as an aberrant band before it is seen. This author often digitally explores the muscles and typically can palpate the mesh, after which it can be exposed. The mesh arm can be located in an aberrant location, complicating dissection (Fig. 16.4). Once the sling has been identified, it is dissected to the obturator membrane. The arm should be freed from the inferior pubic ramus if possible—this can be extremely difficult as the mesh is often completely adherent where it passes the bone at the anteromedial portion of the obturator fora-

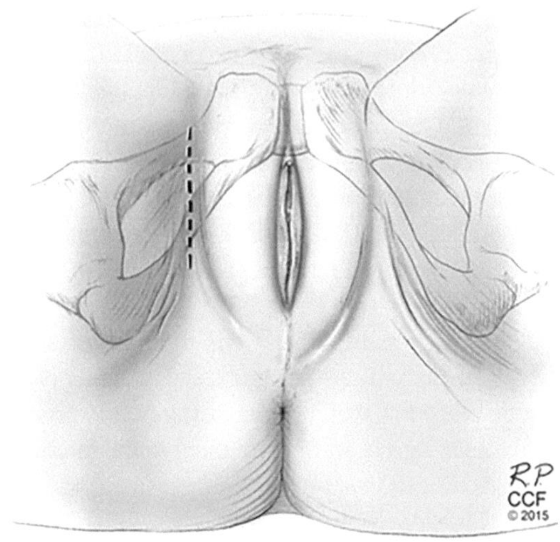

Fig. 16.2 Incision for thigh dissection to remove TOT tape. (Reprinted with permission, Cleveland Clinic Center for Medical Art & Photography © 2015–2016. All Rights Reserved)

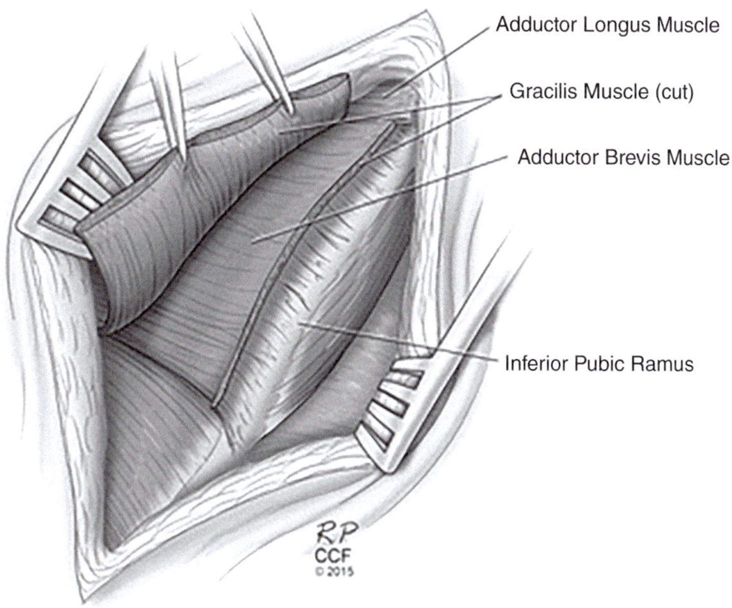

Fig. 16.3 Gracilis muscle has been cut to reveal Adductor Brevis Muscle below. (Reprinted with permission, Cleveland Clinic Center for Medical Art & Photography © 2015–2016. All Rights Reserved)

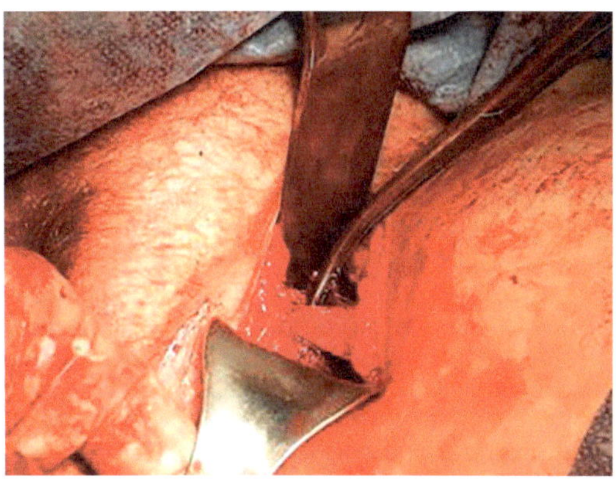

Fig. 16.4 Thigh portion of mesh above the adductor longus tendon. Surgical clamp is grasping portion of mesh

men. The dead space is closed, and the skin incision is closed after placing a bulb suction drain.

Outcomes

The data is limited; however, some series have shown improvement with conservative management, including local anesthetic and nerve blocks [46, 47]. In addition, there are three series of eight patients who underwent thigh dissection, which showed improvement after mesh excision. Rigaud et al. found that at a mean follow-up of 6.4 months pain scores improved from 7 (± 1.7) to 3.5 (± 3.3). There was a trend toward greater improvement in the TOT group who underwent thigh dissection compared to patients who underwent transvaginal excision alone. No complications were noted [48].

Reynolds et al. performed a multicenter, retrospective study of eight patients who had undergone thigh dissection to remove transobturator mesh arms from either transobturator slings or mesh placed for pelvic organ prolapse repair. With an average follow-up of 6 months, five patients reported a cure [49]. Overall, the data is very limited regarding thigh dissection and likely should be limited to centers with experience performing this procedure [45].

After doing many of these procedures, it is the author's practice to tell patients that in 1/3 the pain will completely or almost completely disappear, in 1/3 they will have significant improvement, and in 1/3 they may have no or only limited improvement.

Conclusion

While the majority of patients do not have pain after mesh-based procedures, pelvic floor surgeons must be equipped to deal with this when it arises. In the patients who do suffer from persistent vaginal pain, dyspareunia, suprapubic pain, or thigh pain, there is significant associated morbidity. As pelvic floor surgeons, the goal is to be able to counsel our patients appropriately regarding either mesh placement or mesh excision and to have the technical expertise to try to help relieve pain as best we can.

Dunn et al. interviewed 84 women treated for mesh-related complications. The authors identified three different experiences that characterized these women. One was "cascading health problems" where the women were very hopeless and overwhelmed by multiple health problems. Other women were "settling for a new normal," while others had suffered complications but had undergone surgery or medical intervention which allowed them to return to their previous state of health [50]. As pelvic reconstructive surgeons, it is our responsibility to understand the surgical procedures these patients have undergone, understand the pathophysiology driving their symptoms, and provide them with up-to-date treatment options to best restore their quality of life. We believe this chapter provides a framework for clinicians to best deal with these situations.

References

1. US Food and Drug Administration. (2011, July 13). FDA safety communication: update on serious complications associated with transvaginal placement of surgical mesh in repair of pelvic organ prolapse. Available at http://www.fda.gov/MedicalDevices/Safety/AlertsandNotices/ucm262435.htm. Accessed Feb 22, 2016.
2. Committee on Gynecologic Practice. Vaginal placement of synthetic mesh for pelvic organ prolapse. Female Pelvic Med Reconstr Surg. 2012;18:5–9.
3. Goldman HB. Joint position statement on midurethral slings for stress urinary incontinence. Neurourol Urodyn. 2022;41:31–4. https://doi.org/10.1002/nau.24838.
4. Committee Opinion No. 694. American College of Obstetricians and Gynecologists. Management of mesh and graft complications in gynecologic surgery. Obstet Gynecol. 2017;129:e102–8.
5. Developed by the Joint Writing Group of the American Urogynecologic Society and the International Urogynecological Association, Rardin Charles R, Duckett Jonathan Milani Alfredo L, Pavan Lucilia Ines Rogo-Gupta Lisa Pavan Lucila Ines Twiss Christian O. Joint position statement on the management of mesh-related complications for the FPMRS specialist. Int Urogynecol J. 2020;31(4):679–94.
6. Haylen BT, Freeman RM, Swift SE, Cosson M, Davila GW, Deprest J, Dwyer PL, Fatton B, Kocjancic E, Lee J, Maher C, Petri E, Rizk DE, Sand PK, Schaer GN, Webb R. An International Urogynecological Association (IUGA)/International Continence Society (ICS) joint terminology and classification of the complications related directly to the insertion of prostheses (meshes, implants, tapes) and grafts in female pelvic floor surgery. Neurourol Urodynam. 2011;30:2–12.
7. Ford AA, Rogerson L, Cody JD, Aluko P, Ogah JA. Mid-urethral sling operations for stress urinary incontinence in women. Cochrane Database Syst Rev. 2017;7(7):CD006375. https://doi.org/10.1002/14651858.CD006375.pub4. Accessed 19 March 2024.
8. Kenton K, Stoddard AM, Zyczynski H et al. for the Urinary Incontinence Treatment Network. 5-year longitudinal followup after retropubic and transobturator mid urethral slings. J Urol. 2015;193:203–10.
9. Stanford EJ, Paraiso MF. A comprehensive review of suburethral sling procedure complications. J Minim Invasive Gynecol. 2008;15:132–45.
10. Mazouni C, Karsenty G, Bretelle F, Bladou F, Gamerre M, Serment G. Urinary complications and sexual function after the tension-free vaginal tape procedure. Acta Obstet Gynecol Scand. 2004;83:955–61.
11. Cholhan HJ, Hutchings TB, Rooney KE. Dyspareunia associated with paraurethral banding in the transobturator sling. Am J Obstet Gynecol. 2010;202:481.e1–5.
12. Serati M, Salvatore S, Uccella S, Zanirato M, Cattoni E, Nappi RE, Bolis P. The impact of the mid-urethral slings for the treatment of stress urinary incontinence on female sexuality. J Sex Med. 2009;6:1534–42.
13. Zyczynski HM, Rickey L, Dyer KY, et al. Sexual activity and function in women more than 2 years after midurethral sling placement. Am J Obstet Gynecol. 2012;207:421.e1–6.
14. Yeung E, Baessler K, Christmann-Schmid C, Haya N, Chen Z, Wallace SA, Mowat A, Maher C. Transvaginal mesh or grafts or native tissue repair for vaginal prolapse. Cochrane Database of Systematic Reviews. 2024;3(3):CD012079. https://doi.org/10.1002/14651858.CD012079.pub2. Accessed 15 July 2024.
15. Miller D, Lucente V, Babin E, Beach P, Jones P, Robinson D. Prospective clinical assessment of the transvaginal mesh technique for treatment of pelvic

organ prolapse—5-year results. Female Pelvic Med Reconstr Surg. 2011;17:139–43.
16. Bontje HF, Van de Pol G, Van der Zaag-Loonen HJ, Spaans WA. Follow up of mesh complications using the IUGA/ICS category—time—site coding classification. Int Urogynecol J. 2014;25:817–22.
17. Deffieux X, De Tayrac R, Huel C, Bottero J, Gervaise A, Bonnet K, Frydman R, Fernandez H. Vaginal mesh erosion after transvaginal repair of cystocele using Gynemesh or Gynemesh-soft in 138 women: a comparative study. Int Urogynecol J. 2007;18:73–9.
18. Lowman JK, Jones LA, Woodman PJ, et al. Does the Prolift system cause dyspareunia? Am J Obstet Gynecol. 2008;199:707.e1–6.
19. Altman D, Elmer C, Kiilholma P, Kinne I, Tegerstedt G, Falconer C. Sexual dysfunction after trocar-guided transvaginal mesh repair of pelvic organ prolapse. Obstet Gynecol. 2009;113:127–33.
20. Brandao DR, da Silveira S, Haddad JM, de Jarmy-DI Bella ZIK, Nastri F, Kawabata MGM, da Silva Carramao S, Rodrigues CA, Baracat EC, Auge APF. Multicenter, randomized trial comparing native vaginal tissue repair and synthetic mesh repair for genital prolapse surgical treatment. Int Urogynecol J. 2015;26:335–42.
21. Sirls LT, McLennan GP, Killinger KA, Boura JA, Fischer M, Nagaraju P, Peters K. Exploring predictors of mesh exposure after vaginal prolapse repair. Urogynecology. 2013;19(4):206–9.
22. Araco F, Gravante G, Sorge R, Overton J, De Vita D, Primicerio M, et al. The influence of BMI, smoking, and age on vaginal erosions after synthetic mesh repair of pelvic organ prolapses. A multicenter study. Acta Obstet Gynecol Scand. 2009;88(7):772–80.
23. Long C-Y, Hsu C-S, Wu M-P, Lo T-S, Liu C-M, Tsai E-M. Comparison of the changes in sexual function of premenopausal and postmenopausal women following transvaginal mesh surgery. J Sex Med. 2011;8:2009–16.
24. Rogowski A, BienKowski P, Tosiak A, Jerzak M, Mierzejewski P, Baranowski W. Mesh retraction correlates with vaginal pain and overactive bladder symptoms after anterior vaginal mesh repair. Int Urogynecol J. 2013;24:2087–92.
25. Anger JT, Khan AA, Eilber KS, Chong E, Histed S, Wu N, Pashos CL, Clemens JQ. Short-term outcomes of vaginal mesh placement among female medicare beneficiaries. Urology. 2014;83:768–73.
26. Abbott S, Unger CA, Evans JM, Jallad K, Mishra K, Karram MM, et al. Evaluation and management of complications from synthetic mesh after pelvic reconstructive surgery: a multicenter study. Am J Obstet Gynecol. 2014;210(2):163–e1.
27. Firoozi F, Ingber MS, Moore CK, Vasavada SP, Rackley RR, Goldman HB. Purely transvaginal/perineal management of complications from commercial prolapse kits using a new prostheses/grafts complication classification system. J Urol. 2012;187:1674–9.
28. Skala CE, Renezeder K, Albrich S, Puhl A, Laterza RM, Naumann G, Koelbl H. Mesh complications following prolapse surgery: management and outcome. Eur J Obstet Gynecol Repro Bio. 2011;159:453–6.
29. Crosby EC, Abernethy M, Berger MB, DeLancey JO, Fenner DE, Morgan DM. Symptom resolution after operative management of complications from transvaginal mesh. Obstet Gynecol. 2014;123:134–9.
30. Hokenstad ED, El-Nashar SA, Blandon RE, Occhino JA, Trabuco EC, Gebhart JB, Klingele CJ. Health-related quality of life and outcomes after surgical treatment of complications from vaginally placed mesh. Female Pelvic Med Reconstr Surg. 2015;21:176–80.
31. Ridgeway B, Walters MD, Paraiso MFR, et al. Early experience with mesh excision for adverse outcomes after transvaginal mesh placement using prolapse kits. Am J Obstet Gynecol. 2008;199:703.e1–7.
32. Danford JM, Osborn DJ, Reynolds WS, Biller DH, Dmochowski RR. Postoperative pain outcomes after transvaginal mesh revision. Int Urogynecol J. 2015;26:65–9.
33. Misrai V, Roupret M, Xylinas E, Cour F, Vaessen C, Haertig A, Richard F, Chartier-Kastler E. Surgical resection for suburethral sling complications after treatment for stress urinary incontinence. J Urol. 2009;181:2198–203.
34. Tijdink MM, Vierhout ME, Heesakkers JP, Withagen MIJ. Surgical management of mesh-related complications after prior pelvic floor reconstructive surgery with mesh. Int Urogynecol J. 2011;22:1395–404.
35. Fisher HW, Lotze PM. Nerve injury locations during retropubic sling procedures. Int Urogynecol J. 2011;22:439–41.
36. Ramanathan A, Bryant S. Obturator neuropathy after retropubic tension-free vaginal tape placement. Obstet Gynecol. 2015;125:62–4.
37. Brubaker L, Norton PA, Albo ME et al. for the Urinary Incontinence Treatment Network. Adverse events over two years after retropubic or transobturator midurethral sling surgery: findings from the Trial of Midurethral Slings (TOMUS) study. Am J Obstet Gynecol. 2011;205:498.e1–6.
38. Miklos JR, Moore RD, Chinthakanan O. Obturator neuralgia: a rare complication of tension-free vaginal tape sling—complete resolution after laparoscopic tension-free vaginal tape removal. J Minim Invasive Gynecol. 2015;22:548.
39. Richter HE, Albo ME, Zyczyski HM et al. for the Urinary Incontinence Treatment Network. Retropubic versus transobturator midurethral slings for stress incontinence. N Engl J Med. 2010;362:2066–76.
40. Petri E, Ashok K. Comparison of late complications of retropubic and transobturator slings in stress urinary incontinence. Int Urogynecol J. 2012;23:321–5.

41. Hinoul P, Vanormelingen L, Roovers J, et al. Anatomical variability in the trajectory of the inside-out transobturator vaginal tape technique (TVT-O). Int Urogynecol J. 2007;18:1201–6.
42. Hubka P, Nanka O, Martan A, et al. Anatomical study of position of the TVT-O to the obturator nerve influenced by the position of the legs during the procedure: based upon findings at formalin-embalmed and fresh-frozen bodies. Arch Gynecol Obstet. 2011;284:901–5.
43. Cadish LA, Hacker MR, Dodge LE, Dramitinos P, Hota LS, Elkadry EA. Association of body mass index with hip and thigh pain following transobturator midurethral sling placement. Am J Obstet Gynecol. 2010;203(508):e1–5.
44. Wolter CE, Starkman JS, Scarpero HM, Dmochowski RR. Removal of transobturator midurethral sling for refractory thigh pain. Urology. 2008;72(461):e1–3.
45. King A, Tenggardjaja C, Goldman HB. Prospective evaluation of the effect of thigh dissection for removal of transobturator midurethral slings on refractory thigh pain. J Urol. 2016;195; epub.
46. Parnell BA, Johnson EA, Zolnoun DA. Genitofemoral and perineal neuralgia after transobturator midurethral sling. Obstet Gynecol. 2012;119:428–31.
47. Roth TM. Management of persistent groin pain after transobturator slings. Int Urogynecol J. 2007;18:1371–3.
48. Rigaud J, Pthin P, Labat J, et al. Functional results after tape removal for chronic pelvic pain following tension-free vaginal tape or transobturator tape. J Urol. 2010;184:610–5.
49. Reynolds WS, Kit LC, Kaufman MR, Karram M, Bales G, Dmochowski RR. Obturator foramen dissection for excision of symptomatic transobturator mesh. J Urol. 2012;187:1680–4.
50. Dunn GE, Hansen BL, Egger MJ, Nygaard I, Sanchez-Birkhead AC, Hsu Y, Clark L. Changed women: the Long-term impact of vaginal mesh complications. Female Pelvic Med Reconstr Surg. 2014;20:131–6.

Autologous Fascial Slings

17

Yu Zheng, Paholo Barboglio Romo, and J. Quentin Clemens

Introduction

The autologous fascia pubovaginal sling (PVS) was popularized in 1978 by McGuire and Lytton to address female stress urinary incontinence (SUI) caused by low urethral closing pressure or fixed (immobile) urethra that may be scarred from prior surgical interventions, leading to intrinsic sphincter deficiency (ISD) [1]. This technique involves using the patient's own tissue, typically fascia from the rectus abdominis or fascia lata, to create a supportive sling for the urethra. The popularity of the PVS declined with the advent of mid-urethral synthetic slings (MUSS), which offered the advantages of reduced operative time and fewer comorbidities associated with fascia harvest. However, controversies surrounding transvaginal mesh implants, including FDA warnings about their potential risks, have led to a resurgence of interest in the autologous PVS technique [2, 3]. The procedure remains an excellent anti-incontinence surgery and can still be considered as a first-line anti-incontinence treatment in women who want to avoid synthetic material. In addition, autologous tissue slings are commonly utilized in complex reconstructive cases where the vaginal tissue quality is poor and there is a high risk of synthetic mesh exposure (e.g., urethral diverticulum, urethrovaginal fistula, prior failure to MUSS, history of radiation or intentionally obstructing slings for neurogenic bladders). The purpose of this chapter is to provide a comprehensive overview of the complications associated with autologous PVS and to discuss the most effective strategies for mitigating and managing these complications. Complications, listed in Table 17.1, can be classified based on their temporal relationship to the procedure, distinguishing between intraoperative, perioperative, and chronic postoperative issues.

Y. Zheng (✉)
Department of Urology, Brigham and Women's Hospital, Boston, MA, USA
e-mail: yzheng20@bwh.harvard.edu

P. B. Romo · J. Q. Clemens
Department of Urology, University of Michigan, Ann Arbor, MI, USA

H. B. Goldman, J. Zillioux (eds.), *Complications of Urogynecology and Reconstructive Pelvic Surgery*, https://doi.org/10.1007/978-3-032-00339-3_17

Table 17.1 Adverse events from surgical management of female stress urinary incontinence

Perioperative Genitourinary
Bladder and urethral injury
Gastrointestinal (GI)
Bowel injury
Vascular
Bleeding complications (with and without surgical intervention)
Deep venous thrombosis (DVT)
Neurological
Nerve injury
Chronic pelvic pain
Delayed Genitourinary
Urethral erosion
Voiding dysfunction—de novo urinary urgency
Transient and persistent Urinary retention
Infectious
Urinary tract infection (UTI)
Wound Complications
Seroma
Hematoma
Hernia
Cellulitis
Persistent leg pain

Intraoperative Complications

Bladder Injury

The incidence of bladder perforations occurs in 1.5–3.3% of cases [4]. Bladder injuries can be sustained when developing the space of Retzius and dissecting the bladder off the pubis. This step is generally performed with blunt dissection, but the presence of scarring from previous surgeries or anti-incontinence procedures can increase the risk of bladder injury. Inadvertent bladder injuries can be minimized by dissecting directly on the pubis, just lateral to the insertion of the rectus muscle bodies. In cases where the space of Retzius is significantly scarred, using sharp dissection to separate the bladder from the pubic bone can help prevent tearing of the bladder. Bladder injuries that occur during the retropubic dissection should be identified and repaired, as these injuries tend to be large. Generally, a two-layer bladder closure with absorbable suture and a Foley catheter placement for 5–10 days, depending on the size of the bladder injury, is recommended.

Bladder injuries can also occur when a sling suture carrier is introduced into the retropubic space to deliver the sling sutures from the vaginal incision to the abdominal incision. We typically use a long, curved clamp with a fairly sharp tip (Crawford clamp) for this maneuver, but other instruments such as Stamey needle or Raz needle are also commonly used. At the time of passage to minimize the risk of bladder injuries, the clamp is kept in direct continuity with the back of the pubis at all times, and a finger is positioned within the ipsilateral aspect of the vaginal incision, adjacent to the urethra. This allows for direct tactile control as the instrument tip is passed through the endopelvic fascia and minimizes the degree of "blind" passage. During this time, a Foley catheter should be placed in the bladder to ensure that it is empty. As recommended by the American Urological Association (AUA) Guideline, we perform cystoscopy after passage of the instruments to rule out injury to the urinary tract [5]. Use of a 70-degree lens allows for a thorough evaluation of the entire bladder and urethra. If a clamp is noted to be in the bladder, it is withdrawn and repositioned, and repeat cystoscopy is performed. Injuries from clamp passage do not require formal repair, although it may be prudent to maintain bladder drainage with a Foley catheter for a few days postoperatively.

Bladder injuries can be missed and present at a later date with voiding symptoms (Fig. 17.1). A retrospective review of delayed genitourinary injuries after sling surgeries identified two autologous rectus fascia sling bladder erosions encountered in the bladder dome. Both patients presented with urge incontinence and were diagnosed at 4 and 9 days after surgery. The slings were removed cystoscopically and the patients did well with adequate continence outcomes [6].

Urethral Injury

Urethral injuries during PVS surgeries are rare but can occur during the vaginal dissection or the passage of the sling suture carrier [7–9]. Injuries to the urethra or bladder neck can occur if the

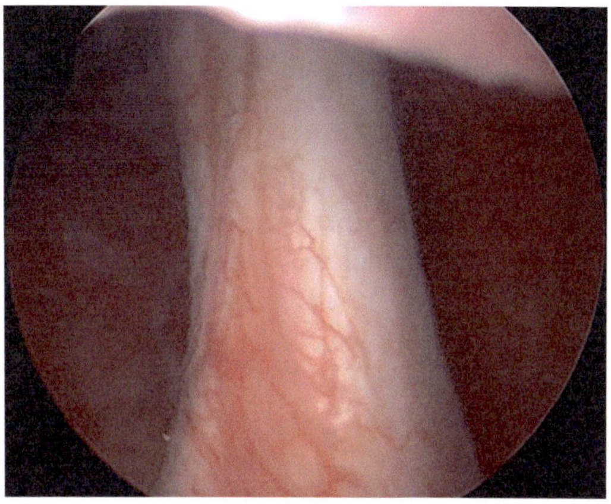

Fig. 17.1 Cystoscopic view of autologous fascia perforation at the 2 o'clock position from the bladder dome that was diagnosed 3 months after surgery on a patient with irritative urinary symptoms (de novo urgency)

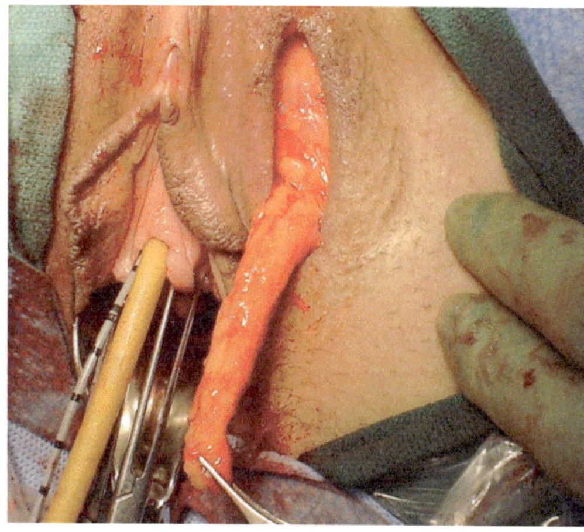

Fig. 17.2 Adipose tissue labial (Martius) flap with an inferior pedicle

vaginal dissection is too deep into the periurethral fascia or if the retropubic space is dissected too medially. In these occasions, primary repair with absorbable suture is recommended. Patients with a history of prior vaginal surgery, radiation, or poorly estrogenized vaginal wall can distort the dissection planes, leading to urethral injuries. Unlike mesh sling surgeries, PVS procedures can proceed after a urethral injury occurs [7]. After the urethral injury is repaired, the autologous PVS sling can still be placed since the presence of the autologous fascia does not increase the risk of urethrovaginal fistula development after urethral perforation [7, 10]. In fact, the autologous sling then provides another layer to the repair. If the urethral injury is large or the tissue quality is poor, a Martius flap can be interposed between the urethra and the sling (Fig. 17.2). Urethral perforations by the sling suture carrier can be managed with a Foley catheter for a few days after repair, but larger perforations that occurred during the vaginal dissection may require a longer Foley catheter duration of 2–3 weeks after repair.

Vaginal Perforations

Similar to synthetic slings, vaginal perforation is a potential complication during autologous PVS placement that can occur when the sling suture carrier inadvertently penetrates the vaginal wall during its passage from the retropubic space into the vagina. Given the excellent biocompatibility of the autologous fascial sling, there is essentially no risk of fascial sling exposure or extrusion if the vaginal wall is inadvertently perforated [11, 12]. Vaginal perforations can be simply managed by removing the sling suture carrier and repassing the instrument to the proper location. Suturing the perforation may be necessary to close the defect, achieve hemostasis, and promote healing. Once the instrument is repositioned in the appropriate location and the vaginal wall perforation site is repaired, the surgeon can complete the procedure in the standard fashion without significant deviation from standard postoperative measures.

Vascular Complications

It is not uncommon to encounter venous bleeding from the vaginal epithelium during the vaginal portion of the procedure. For this reason, we will typically harvest the sling from the rectus fascia or fascia lata prior to proceeding with the vaginal dissection. Vaginal bleeding can be minimized by entering the correct surgical plane superficial to the periurethral fascia. Vasoconstrictor agents such as epinephrine or vasopressin are commonly injected into the vaginal wall to facilitate the dissection before making the incision, but we are aware of no data that demonstrate that this maneuver significantly reduces the amount of bleeding. Most vaginal bleeding stops after the sling is placed and the incision is closed. Therefore, the most effective maneuver to stop vaginal bleeding is to expeditiously proceed with the procedure rather than attempt to identify and cauterize or ligate bleeding sources. In rare cases with brisk venous bleeding, placement of absorbable figure-of-eight sutures through the vaginal mucosa at the vaginal fornices can help to control bleeding. A vaginal gauze pack is typically placed postoperatively and is left in place overnight to maintain pressure and prevent bothersome oozing from the incision. Using these maneuvers, the reported blood transfusion rate is approximately 2%, although these rates include concomitant procedures and likely overestimate the transfusion rate for autologous PVS procedures performed in isolation [4, 8, 10].

Clinically significant retroperitoneal bleeding generally responds to conservative management with pelvic rest, serial bloodwork to monitor hemoglobin trends, and blood transfusions if necessary. In patients with evidence of persistent postoperative bleeding, such as hemodynamic instability or persistent transfusion requirement, a CT scan of the pelvis can help to identify the presence and extent of a pelvic or retroperitoneal hematoma and may help to determine the bleeding source (Fig. 17.3). Selective angiography and embolization can be considered to address active bleeding. Elard and colleagues reported a case where they were able to control bleeding from an inferior vesical artery with selective embolization [13].

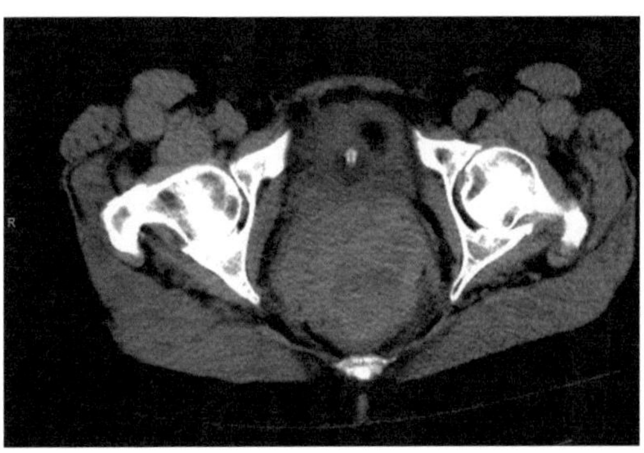

Fig. 17.3 CT scan shows a retroperitoneal hematoma likely associated with retropubic dissection or instrument passage

Surgical intervention is typically avoided in the early phase, as the hematoma itself provides tamponade, and opening the retroperitoneal space during active bleeding can lead to catastrophic hemorrhage. However, large hematomas may cause significant bladder deviation, resulting in bothersome symptoms such as urinary urgency, frequency, and dysuria. If these symptoms become severe and significantly impact quality of life, surgical evacuation of the hematoma can be considered. Hematomas can be aspirated by interventional radiology if CT scans demonstrate significant liquefication of the hematoma. Alternatively, the prior Pfannenstiel incision and rectus fascia are opened, and the hematoma is evacuated. After irrigation, bleeding sites are identified and addressed. A drain can be left in the retroperitoneal space if there is concern of ongoing bleeding.

Bowel Injury

Bowel injury can occur while mobilizing the superior leaf of the rectus fascia during the abdominal dissection. If there is a large amount of scarring in this area due to previous surgery, we favor using scissors rather than electrocautery for this dissection. Placing patients in steep Trendelenburg can help minimize the risk of bowel injury and entry into the peritoneum. If the peritoneum is entered, it is closed after the fascia is adequately mobilized. Bowel injury can also occur during retropubic passage of the clamp, especially if there has been prior pelvic surgery and the peritoneum extends deep into the pelvis. In rare cases, entry into the peritoneum may be necessary to clearly identify the anatomy and ensure that the clamps can be passed safely.

Postoperative Complications

Severe postoperative complications, including myocardial infarction, pulmonary embolism, deep vein thrombosis, and death, are extremely uncommon after PVS procedures [4, 10]. The most prevalent postoperative complications include voiding dysfunction, wound complications, and urinary tract infections (UTIs).

Voiding Dysfunction

Voiding dysfunction after PVS surgery is a significant concern, with reported incidence rates ranging from 3% to 35% [4, 10]. De novo urinary urgency and urgency incontinence are particularly common, affecting 3–18.5% of patients [14, 15]. These patients should be evaluated with a post-void residual to rule out urinary retention as a cause of these symptoms. De novo urinary urgency after PVS is theorized to be due to the increased bladder outlet pressure or disruption of the autonomic nervous system near the bladder neck during the sling placement [16]. These symptoms are initially managed conservatively with behavioral changes (timed voiding, double voiding), pelvic floor physical therapy, or medications such as anticholinergics or beta-3 agonists and tend to resolve within several months post-procedure [11, 17]. However, refractory cases may require more advanced interventions, including sacral neuromodulation or botulinum toxin bladder injections. Some studies suggest that patients with a history of prior pelvic organ prolapse surgery or detrusor underactivity may be at increased risk for developing voiding dysfunction after PVS [10, 14].

In those with persistent symptoms (longer than 3 months), it is crucial to evaluate for bladder outlet obstruction (BOO) caused by the PVS as an underlying factor for urinary urgency and urgency incontinence. The diagnosis of BOO in female patients can be difficult and subtle. In addition to urinary urgency, some patients may complain of urinary hesitancy, decreased stream, straining to void, or needing to shift positions to void. Pelvic examination may show a hyper-suspended urethra at the urethrovesical junction (Swan neck deformity) that suggests obstruction, but the exam can be normal as well. Post-void residual measurement is important to assess bladder emptying, but a low post-void residual does not rule out BOO, as the bladder can compensate by generating a large enough force to overcome the obstruction to fully empty the bladder. Videourodynamics can be extremely helpful in the diagnosis of BOO from a PVS. In females, BOO is suggested by the presence of a sustained detrusor contraction (> 25 mmH2O) with low flow values (<12 ml/s) [18]. In addition, the use of fluoroscopic imaging to demonstrate the location of the obstruction and the upstream dilation of the urethra (Fig. 17.4) has been shown to be highly predictive of BOO in women [19]. Patients with symptomatic BOO from a PVS should be offered urethrolysis and/or sling division.

Urinary Retention

Intermittent self-catheterization (ISC) is generally taught to all patients who undergo a PVS surgery, given the transient urinary retention that many patients experience postoperatively. The average duration of urinary retention after autologous PVS is 10 days [20, 21]. Contemporary PVS outcomes series suggest acute urinary retention rates of 12–33% while chronic urinary retention requiring surgery or catheterization is <5% [21, 22]. ISC should be performed as frequently as necessary in order to maintain bladder volumes of less than 500 ml. Patients are instructed to stop catheterization when residual bladder volumes are less than 150 ml. If ISC is not possible, placement of a suprapubic tube can be considered at the time of autologous PVS to allow for postoperative voiding trials. Studies have suggested that risk factors for urinary retention after PVS surgery include over-tensioning of the sling as well as baseline detrusor underactivity. A lax sling height (measured from the knot of the suture to the rectus fascia) of less than 40 mm and a preoperative detrusor pressure (Pdet) of less than 12 cm H2O on preoperative urodynamics may be

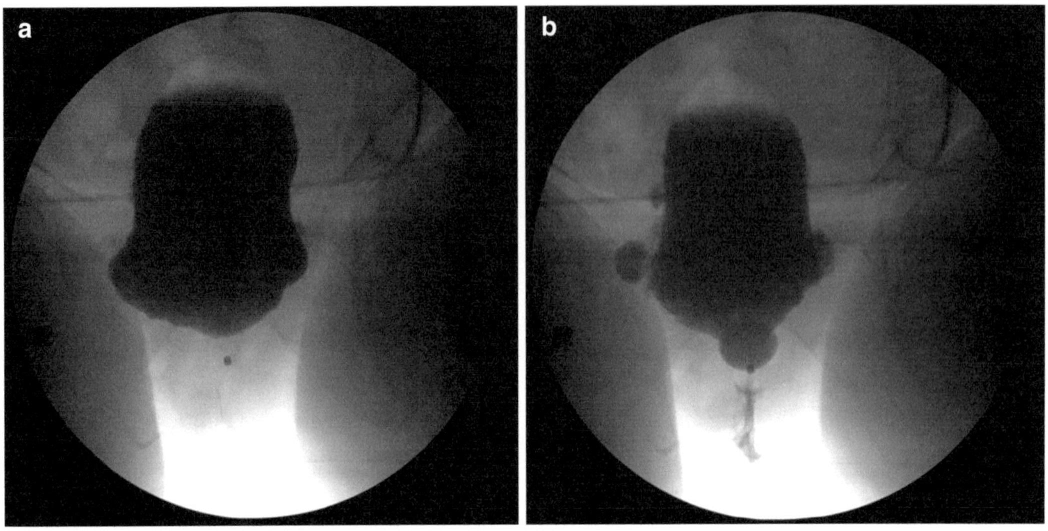

Fig. 17.4 Fluoroscopic images during filling (left) and voiding (right). Note the very prominent dilation of the bladder neck and urethra during voiding, to the level of the obstruction

predictive of urinary retention after PVS that will require ISC or urethrolysis [23, 24].

Sling Revision/Urethrolysis

In patients with persistent urinary retention or those found to have symptomatic BOO, the decision to offer revision of the sling or urethrolysis is individualized, depending on the trajectory of symptoms and patient preferences (Fig. 17.5). Recurrent stress incontinence can occur in 17–54% of women after PVS revision, which may be an unacceptably high risk of recurrent stress incontinence to some women, and they may choose to continue ISC [25]. Early revision of the sling (3–6 week period) can be considered in patients who are in complete urinary retention. To do this, the vaginal incision is reopened and the autologous sling is identified. A right-angled clamp is placed between the sling and the periurethral tissue, and gentle caudal traction is applied to loosen the sling from the endopelvic fascia. The sling is generally not divided in early revisions. If sling revision surgery is performed later on (3–6 months), it is generally recommended to isolate and divide the autologous sling. The prior anterior vaginal wall incision is opened to identify the proximal urethra and bladder neck. The sling should be superficial to the periurethral fascia. A right-angle clamp can be used to gently isolate the sling anterior to the urethra, and then the sling is divided midline. The vaginal wall is then closed and Foley catheter is removed. Success rates of sling division are reportedly 84–92% with less comorbidities compared to a formal urethrolysis [26, 27].

For sling revisions performed after 6 months, the sling may be inconspicuous, and a urethrolysis of the lateral periurethral tissues is often required. Urethrolysis can be performed from a retropubic [28], infrapubic (suprameatal), or vaginal approach [29], and reported success rates vary from 65% to 93%. Urethrolysis can be successful in patients who continue to be obstructed from the PVS even after a prior sling incision has been performed. In our practice, a transvaginal approach is performed through an inverted U incision in the anterior vaginal wall, with dissection proceeding medial to lateral until identifying the sling as described by McGuire [29]. Allis clamps are placed on each lateral border of the sling, and dissection is carried up to the endopelvic fascia. The sling is divided at this level without getting into the retropubic space after the urethra has been cleared with the passage of a

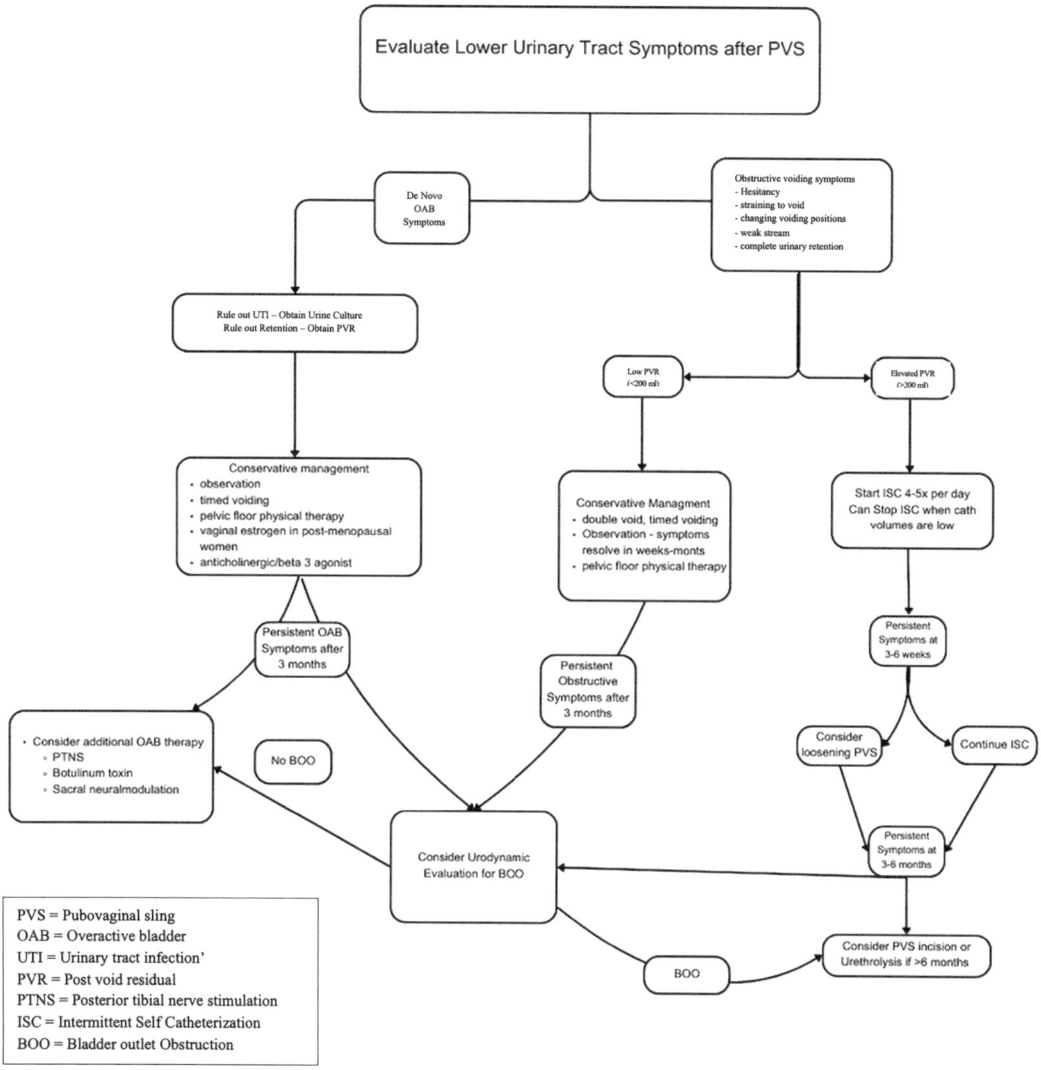

Fig. 17.5 Evaluation and management of voiding dysfunction after PVS

right-angle instrument as aforementioned. If no release is observed at the time of lysis of the sling or the PVS cannot be identified, then a urethrolysis is recommended. This procedure starts with a standard transvaginal urethrolysis in which the lateral sling attachments to the endopelvic fascia are sharply divided with scissors. This dissection should be conducted along the medial aspect of the ischiopubic ramus in order to prevent injury to the urinary tract. Often dissection of the lateral urethral attachments allows for adequate urethral mobility and resolution of the obstruction, but in cases of recurrent BOO after urethrolysis, further dissection is conducted anteriorly, between the urethra and the overlying pubis [30]. Staying just under the pubis maintains the dissection at the level of the midurethra, and prevents injury to the bladder. Once the circumferential dissection is complete, we wrap a Martius flap around the urethra to prevent postoperative scarring. A Crede maneuver, as described by Amunsden, can be helpful when there is a question about the necessity of further urethrolysis [31].

Urethral Erosion

There are isolated reports in the literature of urethral "erosions" following autologous PVS placement, but most of these occurred after a traumatic catheterization or other event, suggesting that catheter trauma rather than erosion was the etiology [32]. Other reports occurred in the early postoperative period, suggesting intraoperative urethral injury may have occurred [33, 34]. The vast majority of these injuries can be managed conservatively with urethral catheterization to permit wound healing.

Wound Complications

Wound complications associated with fascia harvest for PVS procedures can vary depending on the source of the fascia. Either the rectus fascia or fascia lata is harvested for PVS procedures with comparable continence outcomes with either tissue source. It can be challenging to harvest rectus fascia in patients with a scarred abdomen from prior surgeries or after abdominoplasty. Fascia lata may offer decreased wound complications but increased operative time due to the need to reposition the patient after the fascia is harvested or persistent leg pain. Peng et al. compared PVS with rectus fascia vs. fascia lata and found less wound complications, such as seroma and infections, in the fascia lata group (0% vs 14.3%) [35]. Interestingly, their series noted no significant difference in operating time between the two types of fascial harvest. A prospective study of 29 patients evaluating the cosmetic and functional outcome of fascia lata harvest demonstrated that 34% of patients reported discomfort at the harvest site, but this was generally mild [36]. Harvesting rectus fascia carries about a 1% risk of ventral hernias and up to 15% risk of seromas, hematomas, and wound infections [4, 35]. Judicious intraoperative evaluation for hemostasis and irrigation of the wound prior to closure can minimize these wound complications. Although there are risks and benefits to both the rectus fascia and fascia lata, the decision of which type of fascia to use for a PVS is ultimately up to the surgeon preference.

Nerve Injury

Significant pain, dysesthesia, or evidence of motor dysfunction in the immediate postoperative period suggests a nerve injury. These are most commonly associated with prolonged surgical procedures and are therefore more likely if the autologous PVS is performed concomitantly with other surgeries. Table 17.2 describes the most common nerve injuries that are encountered during pelvic surgery [37]. The obturator nerve can be injured when passing the instrument in the retropubic space. Patients with obturator nerve injuries will typically report hip pain and/or weakness during hip adduction. Depending on the type of injury, adduction of her thigh could be absent or simply impaired. These symptoms can usually be managed conservatively with pain control and physical therapy, but severe and intractable pain may require surgical exploration and removal or repositioning of the sling.

Chronic pain in the groin or the pelvic area after autologous PVS is not commonly reported in the literature, and we are aware of no reports where a sling was removed or urethrolysis was performed to address isolated pain symptoms after autologous sling placement. It is common for patients to report unilateral discomfort on one side of the Pfannenstiel incision, which can persist for weeks. We surmise that this may be due to self-limited irritation from the dissection or from the sling sutures.

Urinary Tract Infections

The incidence of UTIs after PVS surgery is 2.5–6.3% [4, 10]. However, diagnosing UTIs in this context can be particularly challenging due to the overlapping symptoms with overactive bladder that can emerge postoperatively. Symptoms such as urinary urgency, frequency, and discomfort can mimic those of a UTI, mak-

Table 17.2 Types of nerve injury during pubovaginal sling

Nerve	Motor	Sensation	Cause	Treatment
Femoral	Knee extension	Front and inner sides of the thigh, shin, and arch of the foot	Retroperitoneal hematoma, positioning injury, and direct pressure at the time of the surgery	Consider exploration/evacuation if a large hematoma and significant symptoms; Physical therapy
Ilioinguinal	None	Mons pubis, labia majora	Direct injury, supra/para-vesical hematoma, pressure from retractors	Consider evacuating the hematoma or exploring early post-op. Nerve could be caught during fascia closure or, less commonly, by the string/sling. Physical therapy; consider trigger point injections
Genitofemoral	None	Upper anterior thigh (femoral branch)	Retroperitoneal hematoma, injury when positioning or passing an instrument	Consider evacuating retroperitoneal hematoma; Physical therapy
Lateral femoral cutaneous	None	Lateral thigh	When harvesting fascia lata, extrinsic compression over the groin area	Physical therapy
Obturator	Thigh adduction	Medial thigh	Direct injury in the retroperitoneal tunnel or retroperitoneal hematoma	Consider releasing the sling in the first 24 h if no major hematoma and significant neuropraxia; Physical therapy

ing it difficult to distinguish between the two conditions. This diagnostic ambiguity can lead to misdiagnosis and inappropriate treatment. Additionally, patients who commence ISC after PVS often become colonized with bacteria. In these cases, routine urine cultures are not recommended, as they can result in the overtreatment of asymptomatic bacteriuria. Treating asymptomatic bacteriuria in patients using ISC can lead to unnecessary antibiotic use, which may contribute to antibiotic resistance and other complications. Thus, careful clinical evaluation and a judicious approach to testing and treatment are essential in managing UTIs after PVS surgery.

Conclusion

The autologous PVS is an effective treatment for women with complex SUI and for those who wish to avoid the use of synthetic materials. Major perioperative complications are rare. Transient urinary retention occurs very frequently following the surgery; patients should be made aware of this before surgery, and a clear plan should be implemented to manage this postoperatively. Lower urinary tract symptoms are also common postoperatively, and these usually resolve with time. Evaluation of persistent postoperative urinary symptoms is focused on determining if urinary obstruction is present.

References

1. Mcguire EJ, Lytton B. Pubovaginal sling procedure for stress incontinence. J Urol. 1978;119(1):82–4. https://doi.org/10.1016/s0022-5347(17)57390-5.
2. Rac G, Younger A, Clemens JQ, et al. Stress urinary incontinence surgery trends in academic female pelvic medicine and reconstructive surgery urology practice in the setting of the food and drug administration public health notifications. Neurourol Urodyn. 2017;36(4):1155–60. https://doi.org/10.1002/nau.23080.
3. Sharma JB, Thariani K, Deoghare M, Kumari R. Autologous fascial slings for surgical management of stress urinary incontinence: a come back. J Obstet Gynaecol India. 2021;71(2):106–14. https://doi.org/10.1007/s13224-020-01408-3.
4. Schimpf MO, Rahn DD, Wheeler TL, et al. Sling surgery for stress urinary incontinence in women: a systematic review and metaanalysis. Am J Obstet Gynecol. 2014;211(1):71.e1–71.e27. https://doi.org/10.1016/j.ajog.2014.01.030.
5. Kobashi KC, Vasavada S, Bloschichak A, et al. Updates to surgical treatment of female stress urinary incontinence (SUI): AUA/SUFU guideline (2023). J

Urol. 2023;209(6):1091–8. https://doi.org/10.1097/JU.0000000000003435.
6. Clemens JQ, Delancey JO, Faerber GJ, Westney OL, McGuire EJ. Urinary tract erosions after synthetic pubovaginal slings: diagnosis and management strategy. Urology. 2000;56(4):589–94.
7. McCoy O, Vaughan T, Nickles SW, et al. Outcomes of autologous fascia pubovaginal sling forpatients with transvaginal mesh related complications requiring mesh removal. J Urol. 2016;196(2):484–9. https://doi.org/10.1016/j.juro.2016.02.2976.
8. Khan ZA, Nambiar A, Morley R, Chapple CR, Emery SJ, Lucas MG. Long-term follow-up of a multicentre randomised controlled trial comparing tension-free vaginal tape, xenograft and autologous fascial slings for the treatment of stress urinary incontinence in women. BJU Int. 2015;115(6):968–77. https://doi.org/10.1111/bju.12851.
9. Albo ME, Richter HE, Brubaker L, Norton P, Kraus SR, Zimmern PE, et al. Burch colposuspension versus fascial sling to reduce urinary stress incontinence. N Engl J Med. 2007;356:2143–55.
10. Grigoryan B, Kasyan G, Pushkar D. Autologous slings in female stress urinary incontinence treatment: systematic review and meta-analysis of randomized controlled trials. Int Urogynecol J. 2024;35(4):759–73. https://doi.org/10.1007/s00192-024-05768-6.
11. Lee D, Murray S, Bacsu CD, Zimmern PE. Long-term outcomes of autologous pubovaginal fascia slings: is there a difference between primary and secondary slings? Neurourol Urodyn. 2015;34(1):18–23. https://doi.org/10.1002/nau.22502.
12. Wadie BS, Edwan A, Nabeeh AM. Autologous fascial sling vs polypropylene tape at short-term followup: a prospective randomized study. J Urol. 2005;174(3):990–3. https://doi.org/10.1097/01.ju.0000169492.96167.fe.
13. Elard S, Cicco A, Salomon L, et al. Embolization for arterial injury incurred during tension-free vaginal tape procedure. J Urol. 2002;168(4 Pt 1):1503. https://doi.org/10.1016/S0022-5347(05)64492-8.
14. Asthanasopoulos A, Gyftopoulos K, McGuire EJ. Efficacy and preoperative prognostic factors of autologous fascia rectus sling for treatment of female stress urinary incontinence. Urology. 2011;78:1034–8.
15. Milose JC, Sharp KM, He C, Stoffel J, Clemens JQ, Cameron AP. Success of autologous pubovaginal sling after failed synthetic mid urethral sling. J Urol. 2015;193(3):916–20. https://doi.org/10.1016/j.juro.2014.09.038.
16. Mitsui T, Tanaka H, Moriya K, Kakizaki H, Nonomura K. Clinical and urodynamic outcomes of pubovaginal sling procedure with autologous rectus fascia for stress urinary incontinence. Int J Urol. 2007;14(12):1076–9. https://doi.org/10.1111/j.1442-2042.2007.01909.x.
17. Chen J, Li B, Peng L, Shen H, Luo D. Autologous pubovaginal sling for recurrent stress urinary incontinence after two or more failed synthetic midurethral sling. Eur J Obstet Gynecol Reprod Biol. 2022;272:213–6. https://doi.org/10.1016/j.ejogrb.2022.03.024.
18. Defreitas GA, et al. Refining diagnosis of anatomic female bladder outlet obstruction: comparison of pressure-flow study parameters in clinically obstructed women with those of normal controls. Urology. 2004;64(4):675–9. discussion 679–81.
19. Nitti VW, Raz S. Obstruction following anti-incontinence procedures: diagnosis and treatment with transvaginal urethrolysis. J Urol. 1994;152(1):93–8. https://doi.org/10.1016/s0022-5347(17)32825-2.
20. Morgan TO Jr, Westney OL, McGuire EJ. Pubovaginal sling: 4-YEAR outcome analysis and quality of life assessment. J Urol. 2000;163(6):1845–8. https://doi.org/10.1016/s0022-5347(05)67557-x.
21. Yang PS, Delpe S, Kowalik CG, Reynolds WS, Kaufman MR, Dmochowski RR. Risk factor of De Novo urgency and urge incontinence after autologous fascia pubovaginal sling. Res Rep Urol. 2021;13:591–6. Published 2021 Aug 14. https://doi.org/10.2147/RRU.S321955Zaragoza.
22. Moorman M, Chew L. Ultra long-term follow-up of the autologous pubovaginal sling for stress incontinence: results at 23 years. Urology. 2024;185:44–8. https://doi.org/10.1016/j.urology.2023.12.001.
23. Preece P, Chan G, O'Connell H, Gani J. Optimising the tension of an autologous fascia pubovaginal sling to minimize retentive complications. Neurourol Urodyn. 2019;38:1409–141.
24. Natale F, Illiano E, Zucchi A, Balzarro M, La Penna C, Costantini E. Transobturator mid-urethral sling in females with stress urinary incontinence and detrusor underactivity: effect on voiding phase. Int Urogynecol J. 2019;30:1519.
25. Thiel DD, Pettit PD, McClellan WT, Petrou SP. Long-term urinary continence rates after simple sling incision for relief of urinary retention following fascia lata pubovaginal slings. J Urol. 2005;174(5):1878–81. https://doi.org/10.1097/01.ju.0000177493.41432.77.
26. Goldman HB. Simple sling incision for the treatment of iatrogenic urethral obstruction. Urology. 2003;62(4):714–8. https://doi.org/10.1016/s0090-4295(03)00569-7.
27. Nitti VW, Carlson KV, Blaivas JG, Dmochowski RR. Early results of pubovaginal sling lysis by midline sling incision. Urology. 2002;59(1):47–52. https://doi.org/10.1016/s0090-4295(01)01559-x.
28. Carr LK, Webster GD. Voiding dysfunction following incontinence surgery: diagnosis and treatment with retropubic or vaginal urethrolysis. J Urol. 1997;157(3):821–3.
29. Foster HE, McGuire EJ. Management of urethral obstruction with transvaginal urethrolysis. J Urol. 1993;150(5 Pt 1):1448–51. https://doi.org/10.1016/s0022-5347(17)35805-6.
30. Scarpero HM, Dmochowski RR, Nitti VW. Repeat urethrolysis after failed urethrolysis for iatrogenic obstruction. J Urol. 2003;169(3):1013–6. https://doi.org/10.1097/01.ju.0000042452.65641.05.

31. Amundsen CL, Guralnick ML, Webster GD. Variations in strategy for the treatment of urethral obstruction after a pubovaginal sling procedure. J Urol. 2000;164(2):434–7.
32. Golomb J, Groutz A, Mor Y, Leibovitch I, Ramon J. Management of urethral erosion caused by a pubovaginal fascial sling. Urology. 2001;57(1):159–60.
33. Handa VL, Stone A. Erosion of a fascial sling into the urethra. Urology. 1999;54(5):923. https://doi.org/10.1016/s0090-4295(99)00276-9.
34. Webster TM, Gerridzen RG. Urethral erosion following autologous rectus fascial pubovaginal sling. Can J Urol. 2003;10(6):2068–9.
35. Peng M, Sussman R, Escobar C, Palmerola R, Pape D, Smilen S, Rosenblum N, Brucker B, Peyronnet B, Nitti V. Rectus fascia versus fascia Lata for autologous fascial pubovaginal sling: a single-center comparison of perioperative and functional outcomes. Female Pelvic Med Reconstr Surg. 2020;26(8):493–7. https://doi.org/10.1097/SPV.0000000000000761.
36. Johnson C, Vollstedt A, Nakatsuka H, Orzel J, Takacs EB. Cosmetic and functional impact of fascia lata harvest for use in surgery for stress urinary incontinence. Neurourol Urodyn. 2024;43(5):1185–91. https://doi.org/10.1002/nau.25462.
37. Wilson M, Ramage L, Yoong W, Swinhoe J. Femoral neuropathy after vaginal surgery: a complication of the lithotomy position. J Obstet Gynaecol. 2011;31(1):90–1. https://doi.org/10.3109/01443615.2010.528082.

18 Synthetic Midurethral Slings: Urinary Tract Sequelae

Karla Rebullar, Natalie Pace, Elizabeth Timbrook Brown, Joshua A. Cohn, Melissa R. Kaufman, William Stuart Reynolds, and Roger R. Dmochowski

Introduction

Female stress urinary incontinence (SUI) is estimated to affect half of all adult women [1]. Despite the pervasiveness of SUI, surgical treatment options were historically limited to invasive therapies such as pubovaginal slings, suspension-type procedures, or retropubic urethropexies until the development of the midurethral sling (MUS) [2]. The MUS is currently considered by many to be the standard of care for the treatment of SUI due to the minimal morbidity, rapid convalescence, short operative time, and long-term efficacy [3]. The 2023 American Urological Association (AUA) Guideline on the surgical management of SUI characterizes MUS as retropubic (RMUS), transobturator (TMUS), single-incision (SIS), or adjustable slings. The AUA Guidelines conclude that well-conducted long-term randomized controlled trials (RCTs) are necessary to compare the different kinds of MUS, and no clear superior one can be established from the current literature [4].

Complications from MUS surgery unique to the use of polypropylene mesh may occur, including chronic pelvic pain, dyspareunia, and mesh exposure, which are the most common, as well as mesh contracture, neuromuscular injury, and/or organ perforation (see Chap. 19). In addition, there can be significant urinary tract sequelae such as urinary tract injury, de novo urgency and/or urgency urinary incontinence (UUI), urinary obstruction, and/or urinary tract infection (UTI). As a result of these complications and the ensuing morbidity, it is imperative that providers have a high index of suspicion for intraoperative and postoperative complications.

K. Rebullar · N. Pace · M. R. Kaufman · W. S. Reynolds · R. R. Dmochowski (✉)
Department of Urologic Surgery, Vanderbilt University Medical Center, Nashville, TN, USA
e-mail: karla.rebullar@vumc.org; natalie.pace@vumc.org; roger.dmochowski@vumc.org

E. T. Brown
MedStar Health Department of Urology, MedStar Georgetown University Hospital, Washington, DC, USA

J. A. Cohn
Division of Urology, Fox Chase Cancer Center, Philadelphia, PA, USA

Preventing Urinary Tract MUS Complications

Complications can be minimized by adhering to fundamental surgical practices during the MUS insertion. These include appropriate knowledge of pelvic and vaginal anatomy; careful vaginal dissection and hemostasis; diligence during the passage of the sling trocars to avoid injury or perforation to the bladder, urethra, vaginal tissue, or groin structures; appropriate tensioning (i.e., "tension-free") during sling deployment; and, prudence for identifying intraoperative

H. B. Goldman, J. Zillioux (eds.), *Complications of Urogynecology and Reconstructive Pelvic Surgery*, https://doi.org/10.1007/978-3-032-00339-3_18

complications. According to the standards in the AUA Guideline, intraoperative cystoscopy should always be performed at the time of sling placement. The AUA Guideline also states that an MUS should not be placed in the presence of a urethrotomy [4].

Diagnosing Mesh-Related Urinary Tract Sequelae

To evaluate a patient with a potential mesh-related urinary tract complication, the clinical evaluation should begin with a detailed clinical history. Providers should maintain a high index of suspicion as mesh-related complications can be subtle and difficult to identify. Patients should be assessed for voiding dysfunction, hematuria, urinary incontinence, and recurrent UTIs, as well as vaginal discharge or bleeding, pelvic/groin pain, dyspareunia, or "hispareunia" (painful intercourse secondary to a mesh exposure that is reported by the male partner) [5]. Standardized questionnaires can also be utilized to assess baseline symptomatology and monitor improvement throughout subsequent therapies. A complete surgical history—including the clinical time course of symptom presentation and information about previous treatments—should also be obtained. Acquiring the previous operative records is paramount to confirm the type of mesh and previous surgical approach.

A physical exam, including a thorough abdominal and pelvic exam, should be performed. Attention should be directed at identifying vaginal discharge or bleeding, scar tissue contraction or banding, reproducible areas of tenderness or discomfort, granulation tissue, or foreign body exposure. At times, an exam under anesthesia may be required to ensure a complete examination, especially if significant pain or difficult body habitus are present. A urinalysis should be obtained to assess for hematuria and/or UTI, with urine culture, if indicated. Measuring post-void residual (PVR) urine volumes can identify incomplete emptying or urinary retention.

Cystourethroscopy should always be performed if there is any suspicion of a mesh-related complication. This can identify a mesh perforation within the urethra or bladder. Urodynamics (UDS) should be performed for patients who present with voiding dysfunction, which may identify iatrogenic BOO or de novo or persistent detrusor overactivity. Videourodynamics (VUDS) may also be helpful to identify urethral narrowing or kinking and associated proximal urethral dilation at the level of the MUS during a sustained detrusor contraction [6, 7].

While imaging has not been routinely employed in this setting, translabial ultrasonography has been utilized to aid in both preoperative and intraoperative identification of the sling. Staack and colleagues compared the clinical versus definitive operative findings of 51 women undergoing surgical MUS excision. The study was able to accurately locate the position of the mesh sling and identify the type (retropubic vs. transobturator) [8].

Managing Urinary Tract MUS Complications

Intraoperative Complications

Urinary Tract Injury

The lower urinary tract (LUT) is at risk for injury during any portion of the MUS procedure, and, if unrecognized, can have significant ramifications. Specifically, passage of the MUS trocars may cause injury to the bladder, urethra, or bladder neck. The urethra can also be injured during the vaginal dissection. Though rare, ureteral injury can occur with passage of the MUS trocar near the trigone or with the vaginal dissection. Patients with an unrecognized LUT injury can develop mesh perforations in the urethra or bladder, urethrovaginal or vesicovaginal fistulae, gross hematuria, bladder stones, pelvic pain, and recurrent UTIs. As such, it is paramount that these injuries be identified intraoperatively. The rate of urinary tract injury with a trocar at the time of surgery ranges from 2.7% to 23.8% [9].

To assess for LUT injury, intraoperative cystoscopy should always be performed with 70° and 30° lenses after trocar passage and with the trocars in place. The bladder should be fully filled to achieve complete expansion. The bladder, as well as the bladder neck and urethra, should be carefully inspected along the trocar course. Urethroscopy can be difficult in women due to short urethral length, but diligence is required as urethral perforation can be subtle and poorly visualized. Ureteral patency should also be documented by identifying efflux of clear urine, and, if there is concern for injury, a retrograde pyelogram should be performed: a JJ stent should be placed if extravasation occurs.

In an attempt to prevent LUT injuries, the MUS trocars should only be passed after the bladder is fully drained. A rigid urethral guide can be used to gently deflect the urethra to the contralateral side while the ipsilateral trocar is passed through the paraurethral space. If a bladder injury does occur during trocar placement, the offending trocar should be removed and repassed (Fig. 18.1). A Foley catheter may be left in place if there is concern for a large bladder defect, but a small trocar puncture site typically closes without difficulty, and prolonged catheterization is unnecessary. As aforementioned, if a urethral injury occurs either during the vaginal dissection or with passage of the MUS trocar, mesh sling placement should be aborted [4]. The urethral defect should be closed primarily, and an indwelling Foley catheter is left in place for healing.

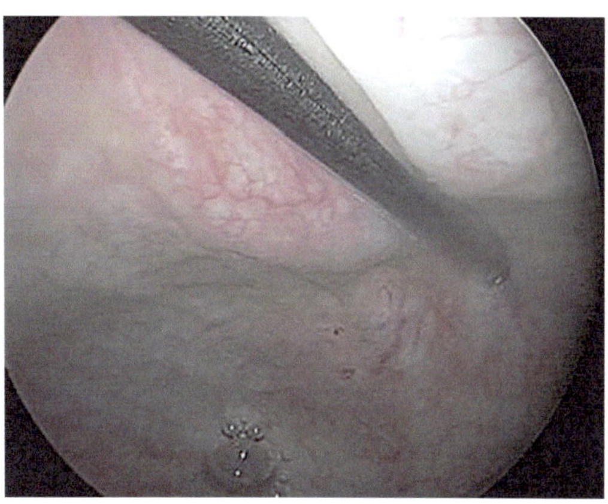

Fig. 18.1 Cystoscopic view of MUS trocar passed through the bladder wall. The offending trocar should be carefully withdrawn and repassed

Postoperative Complications

Urinary Tract Infection

In a 2023 systematic review involving 30 registries and over 700,000 MUS cases, Farag and colleagues reported de novo UTI in 6.19% of cases. [10]. Patients with typical symptoms of a UTI, such as frequency, urgency, and/or hematuria, should be evaluated with a urine culture. Those with severe, recurrent, or persistent symptoms may warrant a more thorough investigation, including blood cultures, cross-sectional imaging, PVR, UDS, or cystoscopy when clinically appropriate. Abscesses, urinary obstruction, foreign bodies, sling perforation, or stones should all be included in the differential [11].

The AUA best practice policy statement on urologic procedures and antimicrobial prophylaxis recommends a single dose of antibiotics for vaginal surgery [12]. However, a recent RCT of 149 patients by Jackson and colleagues evaluated the benefit of adding a 3-day antibiotic course postoperatively for patients undergoing vaginal surgery for SUI. Patients were randomized to a 3-day postoperative placebo ($n = 75$) or nitrofurantoin (100 mg two times a day) ($n = 74$). Overall, 37 (24.8%) women were diagnosed with a UTI within the 6-week postoperative study period. The incidence was significantly lower in the treatment arm (17.6%) compared to placebo (32%) ($p = 0.04$) [13]. In contrast, a retrospective study of 112 subjects by Wu and colleagues found no significant difference in postoperative UTI rates between the group without postoperative prophylactic antibiotics and those who did receive antibiotics (14% versus 16%, $p = 0.82$) [13].

Lower Urinary Tract Dysfunction

Lower urinary tract dysfunction or overactive bladder (OAB) can occur after placement of an

MUS in patients without any previous OAB symptomatology. De novo urge incontinence or UUI is often transient and may resolve spontaneously. In such cases, patients should be counseled and reassured. However, persistent symptoms requiring intervention can occur in a quarter of patients [15]. In the aforementioned systematic review by Farag and colleagues, de novo lower urinary tract symptoms were reported in 4.37% of cases [10]. In a series of 463 patients, Holgren and colleagues reported de novo urgency in 14.5% of patients undergoing an MUS. Older age and parity were identified as significant risk factors for developing de novo urgency [16]. Lee and colleagues also evaluated risk factors for developing de novo urgency or UUI. The study identified 358 women with SUI or mixed urinary incontinence who underwent an MUS. De novo urgency occurred in 27.7% of patients, and de novo UUI occurred in 13.7%. Intrinsic sphincteric deficiency, previous surgery for SUI or pelvic organ prolapse (POP), colposuspension, and/or preexisting detrusor overactivity increased the risk of postoperative urgency or UUI [17].

Reversible causes of de novo urgency/UUI should be evaluated and treated accordingly. A recent review by Abraham and Vasavada cited that de novo urgency occurs in 6% of patients and modifiable causes include postoperative UTI (7.4–14.7%), BOO (1.9–19.7%), and perforation of the urinary tract (0.5–5%), with 0–28% of cases occurring due to idiopathic etiologies [18]. Conversely, it has also been proposed that an MUS can actually improve OAB symptoms. A study by Segal and coworkers retrospectively reviewed 98 MUS patients and found that approximately 57% of patients with OAB demonstrated resolution of their symptoms, while only 4.3% reported de novo OAB [19].

Treatment options for post-MUS urgency or UUI are similar to those for uncomplicated OAB and include behavioral modification such as bladder training and fluid management; pelvic floor muscle training; pharmacotherapy with antimuscarinics or beta-3 agonists; and noninvasive options such as Botulinum toxin injections, sacral neuromodulation, and implantable/percutaneous tibial nerve stimulation. The updated AUA Guideline for OAB has eliminated the concept of stepwise progression from least invasive to most invasive management and instead proposes shared decision-making in treatment selection. [20]. Of note, a recent study by Serati and coworkers found that in the setting of de novo OAB after an MUS, solifenacin had significantly lower efficacy compared to controls without prior procedure for SUI [21]. OnabotulinumtoxinA, however, showed similar efficacy in a prospective study of 102 women comparing those with idiopathic OAB (n = 53) to women with de novo OAB post-MUS (n = 49) in a study by Miotla and colleagues [22].

Bladder Outlet Obstruction

BOO can present in a variety of ways and, as a result, the true incidence is difficult to accurately assess. The rate of urinary retention (catheter dependency for at least 28 days) is estimated to occur after 1–10% of MUS [4, 23]. Additionally, patients may also complain of de novo frequency and urgency, UUI, hesitancy, straining to void, weak stream, incomplete emptying, dysuria, or recurrent UTIs. Pressure-flow UDS and a PVR may be used to assess BOO. Currently, however, there is no consistent index value for BOO in women, and the absence of “high pressure, low flow” on UDS does not rule out iatrogenic obstruction [24, 25].

Treatment options for BOO vary widely according to individual patient factors, sling type, and patient or surgeon preference. Surgical intervention is often necessary, including sling loosening, sling incision, sling excision, or urethrolysis (infrapubic, retropubic, or transvaginal) [26]. Nonsurgical therapies may be offered for transient obstruction, such as self-intermittent catheterization (SIC) or indwelling catheterization [23]. Often times, residual edema after the procedure can lead to urinary retention. Spontaneous voiding should occur within 1 week, and 66–100% of temporary voiding dysfunction resolves by 6 weeks [14, 27].

If the patient cannot void at that time, loosening the sling has been reported in the literature.

Advocates of this technique recommend making a small vaginal incision along the previous suture line. A right-angle clamp is then placed behind the sling and steady downward traction is applied to gently loosen the MUS [28]. Care must be taken to avoid urethral injury when passing the clamp between the overtensioned MUS and the periurethral fascia. This has been described in an office setting under a local anesthetic, but maximizing vaginal exposure in the operating room can be advantageous. There are several reports that show some benefit of urethral dilation [14, 29]; however, there are concerns about the trauma induced by the dilation and the potential for urethral scarring and mesh perforation.

If the obstructing sling is well incorporated into the vaginal tissue, a sling incision can also be performed [30]. Once a vaginal incision is made over the previous suture line, the rough tissue overlying the MUS can typically be palpated. A cystoscope or urethral sound may be inserted into the urethra with upward traction to assist with identification of the MUS. The overlying granular tissue can be visualized, or a tight, band-like structure can be identified. A right-angle clamp is then carefully inserted behind the sling and spread gently open (Fig. 18.2). Once the right-angle clamp is completely behind the sling, a scalpel is used to incise the MUS complex. This should be done with extreme caution to prevent urethral injury. The cut edges of the sling will then retract due to the tension release, and the suburethral portion of the sling may then also be excised to prevent erosion [10]. Typically, this technique is done within the first 3 months of surgery. After 3 months, the MUS is fixed along its entire course, and a midline sling incision might not achieve the desired release or sling relaxation [31].

When the clinical presentation is especially delayed, a formal sling excision should be performed. This technique is best employed with an inverted, U-shaped anterior vaginal wall flap, with the base located at the bladder neck and the apex at the urethra. This incision maximizes exposure for the lateral dissection along the pubocervical fascia. If the MUS complex is identifiable at this juncture, the sling may be transected. The dissection is then carried as lateral as possible along the sling to safely remove the maximum amount of mesh (Fig. 18.3). This should be done judiciously as there can be significant bleeding and/or organ injury within the transobturator or retropubic spaces.

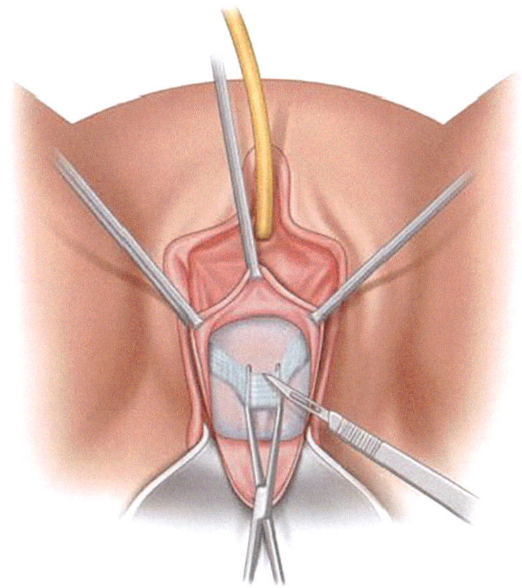

Fig. 18.2 Isolation of the MUS complex with a right-angle clamp

If the sling is not easily identifiable, the endopelvic fascia may be perforated with Metzenbaum scissors to enter the retropubic space. Using a combination of blunt and sharp dissection, the sling can often be identified laterally and then transected and excised. In such cases, a partial or total urethrolysis may also be required. With careful, blunt dissection, the urethra is freed from its attachments anteriorly to the pubic bone and proximally to the bladder neck (Fig. 18.4).

If adequate vesicourethral mobility cannot be achieved, a sling excision and urethrolysis can be performed from a retropubic approach [11]. This can allow for complete removal of the retropubic mesh arms. A low midline or Pfannenstiel incision is made, and the space of Retzius is adequately developed. Any retropubic and prevesical adhesions are sharply incised, and all visible sling material is transected and removed (Fig. 18.5). Observation of free-flowing urine by Crede maneuver can confirm a complete ure-

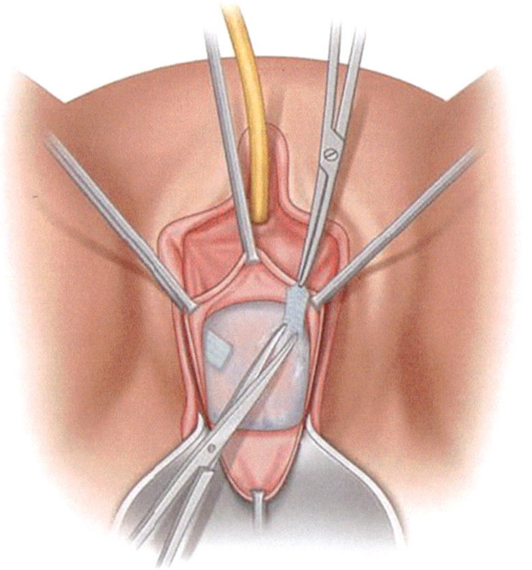

Fig. 18.3 After the MUS is transected, the mesh arms are isolated, and the dissection is carried laterally to remove the maximum amount of mesh that is safely possible

throlysis. In the original description, an omental pedicle flap is interposed between the urethra and the pubic bone to prevent readherence [11].

In the setting of an MUS, cure rates for urethrolysis are variable, as much of the initial data are extrapolated from pubovaginal slings (Table 18.1). The earlier literature for suspension procedures and bladder neck slings suggests that the rate of recurrent SUI is low. In a 2001 review by Klutke et.al, 17 out of 600 women required reoperation due to retention and BOO after MUS. They reported performing a sling release at a mean of 64 days post-MUS surgery. Hundred percentage had resolution of symptoms and voided to completion, and 16 out of 17 (94%) remained continent [49]. In another retrospective review of 9040 women who had MUS, 50% of the 48 women who underwent sling lysis remained continent [50]. However, a recent study

Fig. 18.4 Transvaginal approach for urethrolysis

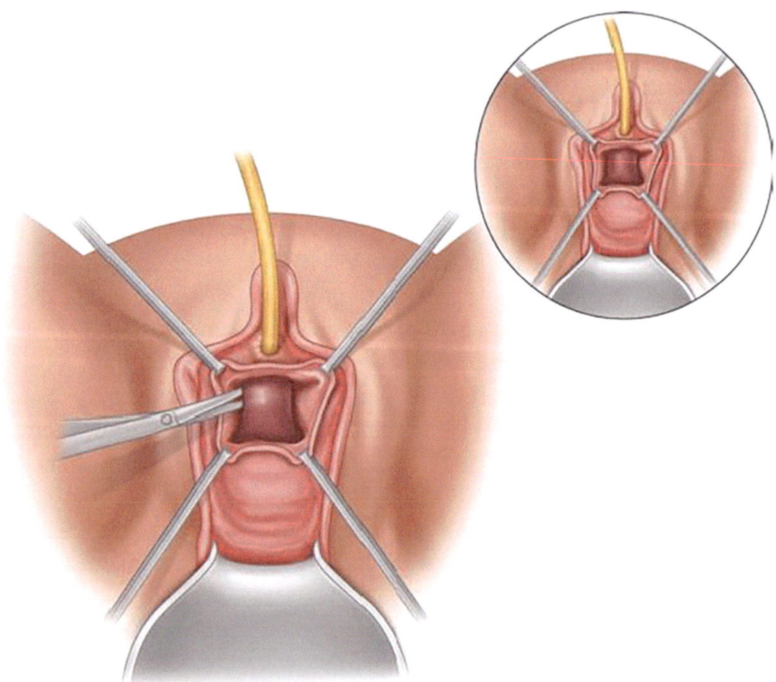

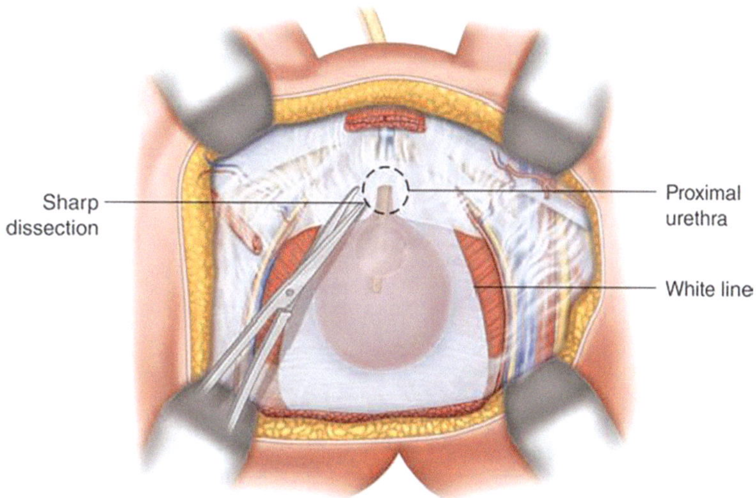

Fig. 18.5 Retropubic approach for urethrolysis

Table 18.1 Results of delayed surgical intervention for BOO after anti-incontinence procedures

Investigators	Patients (*n*)	Initial anti-incontinence procedure	Surgical approach	Mean time to intervention (months)	Overall success (%)	Recurrent SUI (%)
Webster and Kreder [32]	15	SP	RP lysis	8	93	13
Scarpero et al. [26]	24	PVS, SP	RP lysis	9	92	18
Petrou and Young [33]	12	MUS, PVS	RP lysis	19	83	18
Petrou et al. [34]	32	PVS, SP	SM lysis	–	67	3
Carr and Webster [35]	54	PVS, SP	RP lysis 65%	15	78	14
			TV lysis 28%			
			SM lysis 7%			
Starkman et al. [36]	40	PVS	TV lysis 90%	22	82	15
			RP lysis 10%			
Anger et al. [37]	16	SP	TV lysis 44%	11	78	11
			RP lysis 56%	14	43	14
Austin et al. [38]	18	PVS, SP	TV lysis	>6	69	6
Amundsen et al. [39]	32	MUS, PVS	TV lysis 75%	10	94	13
			TV SI 25%			
Carey et al. [40]	23	MUS, PVS, SP	TV lysis	14	87	13
Foster and McGuire [41]	48	PVS, SP	TV lysis	26	65	0

(continued)

Table 18.1 (continued)

Investigators	Patients (*n*)	Initial anti-incontinence procedure	Surgical approach	Mean time to intervention (months)	Overall success (%)	Recurrent SUI (%)
Nitti and Raz [42]	42	PVS, SP	TV lysis	54	71	0
Cross et al. [43]	39	PVS, SP	TV lysis	11	72	3
Goldman et al. [44]	32	PVS, SP	TV lysis	14	84	19
McCrery et al. [45]	55	MUS, PVS, SP	TV lysis	34	87	16
Nitti et al. [46]	19	MUS, PVS	TV SI	11	84	17
Abraham et al. [47]	107	Mus		22	24	49
		TOT 43%	TV SI 21%			
		RP 57%	TV SE 79%			
Yoost et al. [48]	39	MUS	TV SI	29	63	28

Lysis urethrolysis, *MUS* synthetic midurethral sling, *PVS* pubovaginal (bladder neck) sling, *RP* retropubic, *SE* sling excision, *SI* midline sling incision, *SM* suprameatal, *SP* suspension-type procedures, *TOT* transobturator, *TV* transvaginal

of 107 MUS patients evaluated the rate of recurrent SUI after surgical intervention for BOO. In the 107 patients, recurrent SUI occurred in 49%: significant bother was reported in 83%, leading 14% of the women to undergo a subsequent anti-incontinence procedure [47].

It has been postulated that delayed surgical intervention of BOO may not necessarily improve micturition, and long-standing obstruction of the urethra can have an irreversible impact. In fact, persistent voiding dysfunction after urethrolysis has been reported in the literature. In a series by Starkman and coworkers, approximately 50% of patients reported persistent OAB symptoms following urethrolysis. The study evaluated 40 patients with obstructive urinary symptoms, 36 of whom reported OAB symptomatology at presentation. After urethrolysis, 56% reported refractory OAB and were continued on antimuscarinics postoperatively, with eight ultimately undergoing sacral neuromodulation [36, 51]. As such, prompt diagnosis of BOO and early intervention are imperative.

Mesh-Related Pain and Sexual Dysfunction

Pelvic pain is another recognized postoperative complication of synthetic MUS. Chronic pelvic pain, defined as pain persisting more than 6 months [52], that is attributable to transvaginal mesh surgery, is highly variable and reported between 0% and 30% [53]. In a recent review article, Shah and Baldani reported overall pelvic/groin pain rates of 0%–16.6% [54].

Mesh-induced pain can present as pelvic, vaginal, or buttock pain. Pain is commonly related to the obturator and/or pudendal nerve distribution, as these nerves are especially susceptible to injury from the trocar passage, leading to neuralgia. Other mechanisms that can cause pain include sling tensioning and involvement of pelvic muscles.

The degree of sexual dysfunction reported in the literature for women undergoing MUS surgery varies widely. In a 2004 study of 71 women followed prospectively, 14.5% developed dyspareunia and 5.4% reported decreased libido postoperatively [55]. In a more recent 2010 study, however, a lower rate of 3% was reported for de novo dyspareunia [56].

Interestingly, the resolution of incontinence after MUS surgery has been shown to improve sexual function in women. A randomized trial showed the rate of dyspareunia decreased from 34% to 13% 5 years after MUS surgery [57]. Similarly, in a retrospective study of 136 women after MUS surgery, Bekker et al. found that 21.3% reported improved sexual intercourse postoperatively [58].

Initial management of mesh-induced pelvic pain involves conservative measures such as transvaginal estrogen and referral to a pain specialist and/or pelvic floor physiotherapy. However, the failure rate of conservative management is high, and many patients eventually receive surgical intervention [52]. There is sparse evidence to support pelvic floor physiotherapy for mesh-related pain, and alternative interventions should not be delayed if patients experience no improvement. Review of the literature shows that MUS removal can lead to pain relief in approximately 60–80% of women [59]. There is conflicting evidence in the literature on the amount of mesh that is required to be removed for pain resolution—with some case series showing no difference in partial versus complete resection [60]. In a recent retrospective cohort of 55 women who had mesh-induced pain, Fuentes et al. reported pain resolution in 67% after undergoing sub-urethral sling removal only [59]. The American Urogynecologic Society (AUGS) Joint Position Statement recommends partial vaginal mesh excision for those with focal vaginal pain at the sling, and complete vaginal excision only if the pain persists. For those with groin pain, a similar approach is recommended; however, for those with retropubic pain, extravaginal mesh excision, i.e., removal of the retropubic portions of the mesh +/− vaginal mesh excision, is recommended [60].

Notably, more serious mesh-related complications such as infection, perforation/erosion, and fistula can present as pelvic pain and dyspareunia. Thus, it is imperative to rule these out prior to establishing a sole diagnosis of mesh-induced pelvic pain.

Mesh Perforation and Urinary Fistula

Pelvic surgeons should always maintain a high index of suspicion for LUT mesh perforation (Fig. 18.6), as it can present with variable symptomatology. In a retrospective review by Osborn and coworkers, 27 patients were identified to have a postoperative MUS perforation (bladder perforation n = 12, urethral perforation n = 15). Of these, 11/27 (41%) presented with irritative voiding symptoms, 7/11 (26%) with incontinence, 4/11 (15%) with vaginal pain, and 2/11 (7%) with either recurrent UTIs or dyspareunia [61]. Cystourethroscopy is diagnostic in confirming the mesh perforation into the urethral lumen or bladder.

The true incidence of mesh perforations is unknown, but it is estimated to be 0.7–5% for retropubic slings and 0–0.5% for transobturator slings [17, 61]. It is also unclear whether a mesh perforation results from a missed LUT injury at the time of the procedure or from progressive erosion of the mesh over time [10]. Various etiologies leading to mesh perforation include

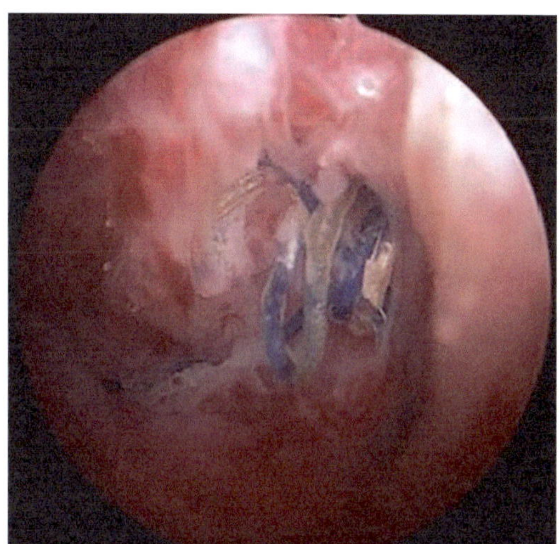

Fig. 18.6 Cystoscopic view of MUS perforation within the urethra

extensive vaginal dissection resulting in devascularization of the urethra, sling tension, missed trocar injury at the time of MUS placement, traumatic catheterization or dilation, or compromised urethral vascularity, such as from estrogen deficiency or radiation therapy [10].

Mesh perforation typically mandates surgical excision; however, this may be performed in a variety of approaches. For a small, isolated mesh segment within the urinary tract, endoscopic management has been described with scissors, holmium laser, or transurethral resection [62, 63]. However, most mesh perforations require a transvaginal and/or abdominal exploration and excision, closure of the urinary tract, and postoperative urinary drainage.

For a urethral or bladder neck mesh perforation, a transvaginal mesh excision is performed. Prior to incision, complete cystourethroscopy verifies the location of the urinary tract mesh. Then, similar to a vaginal mesh excision, an inverted, U-shaped anterior vaginal wall flap is created to maximize exposure. The pubocervical fascia is dissected laterally, and the endopelvic fascia is perforated with Metzenbaum scissors. A cystoscope or urethral sound may be inserted into the urethra to assist with the identification of the MUS. Once the sling is identified, the mesh is carefully transected and removed from within the urethra or bladder neck. The bladder and/or urethral mucosa is then repaired with a fine, absorbable suture in a running fashion. The vaginal incision should be closed in several layers, if possible, with an absorbable suture. Depending on the location of the defect within the urinary tract, an interposition graft—such as a Martius, vaginal, or omental flap—can be employed. An indwelling catheter is left in place for prolonged urinary drainage.

An abdominal mesh excision maximizes exposure for a mesh perforation within the bladder dome, wall(s), or trigone. A low midline or Pfannenstiel incision is made, and the space of Retzius is adequately developed. A cystotomy may be required to visualize and adequately remove the mesh arm(s) from the bladder mucosa. Care should be taken to observe ureteral efflux as a ureteral neocystotomy may also be required. Once the mesh is completely excised, the cystotomy is repaired with an absorbable suture and closed in multiple layers. Again, prolonged urinary drainage with an indwelling catheter is necessary for healing. A concomitant transvaginal excision may also be required to remove the suburethral component of the sling. Shah and coworkers described a series of 21 patients with mesh perforation after MUS who underwent a transvaginal or transvaginal/transabdominal mesh excision, urinary tract reconstruction, and concomitant pubovaginal sling with autologous rectus fascia. Of these, 100% had complete resolution of their presenting symptoms. All of the patients with mesh perforations of the bladder were continent, and 10/14 (71.5%) with urethral perforations were continent postoperatively [64].

Unrecognized or untreated mesh perforations can lead to fistula formation; fistulae can also develop after attempts to treat prior mesh complications. Blaivas and Mekel reported a series of 10 women who presented with urinary fistulae after MUS placement. Patients presented with SUI (70%), unaware incontinence (50%), OAB (40%), pelvic pain (30%), and voiding symptoms (20%). Of these, 7/10 underwent a successful fistula repair. A urinary diversion was performed in one patient, while the other 9/10 underwent primary repair with an interposition graft (Martius flap, omental flap, bladder wall flap, or autologous sling) [65]. In this series, the majority of patients had a successful repair, but results can be quite variable.

For more details on mesh exposure and perforation, and their sequelae, please see Chap. 19.

Long-Term Sequelae

Unfortunately, despite multiple attempts at surgical revision, complications from MUS can be quite morbid. Blaivas and colleagues reported a retrospective review of 47 women with a surgical history of at least one operation to correct MUS complications [66]. With a mean follow-up of 3 years, 72% of patients had a successful outcome after the first procedure. Of the 13 patients with treatment failure, 9 patients underwent a total of 14 salvage operations. Another study by Hansen and colleagues evaluated 111 patients with vaginal mesh complications. Of these, 37% were MUS patients (mean 2.4 years prior) presenting to the tertiary care facility for further intervention. Results from the administered, validated questionnaire showed patients commonly reported problems with their "emotional health" or "feeling frustrated," suggesting that these sequelae can significantly impact a patient's quality of life [67]. As such, prior to any procedure for the management of an MUS complication, preoperative counseling should include a thorough discussion of realistic outcomes.

Recurrent or Persistent SUI After MUS Surgery

Factors such as poor patient selection, errors in surgical technique, or incorrect choice of procedure can lead to persistent SUI despite MUS. Recurrence of SUI after a period of resolution can occur due to patient-associated factors such as age and obesity. The rate of reoperation for these women is estimated to be 6% [68].

Similar options exist for treatment of recurrent or persistent SUI: conservative management, repeat anti-incontinence procedure (urethral bulking, colposuspension, MUS, autologous pubovaginal sling [PVS]). In a retrospective analysis of 6914 MUS, 165 women underwent a repeat procedure for recurrent SUI—98 MUS and 67 urethral bulking procedures; 11 out of 98 (11.2%) and 26 out of 67 (38.8%) failed [69]. The same study reported an expected success rate of 62–89% for repeat MUS. More recent studies have shown favorable results for urethral bulking agents for recurrent SUI post-MUS. A 2022 systematic review of 11 studies reported a pooled value of cure and improvement rate of 84% and 80% for Macroplastique and Bulkamid, respectively [70]. Similarly, a Norwegian registry study reported a 72.9% negative stress test and 73.7% satisfaction rate for patients who received polyacrylamide hydrogel periurethral bulking after a failed MUS surgery [71]. Risk factors for failure of a repeat MUS procedure include lack of urethral mobility and preoperative intrinsic sphincter deficiency (ISD) [31].

Autologous PVS remains an alternative option for persistent or recurrent SUI. The PVS is placed in a location that is different from that of the MUS, making it advantageous. However, there remains the disadvantage of harvest site morbidity and postoperative voiding dysfunction.

What Every Woman Should Be Told

The Current State of the MUS

The plethora of MUS complications, in addition to those reported from transvaginal mesh (TVM) use in the treatment of POP, led the Food and Drug Administration (FDA) to issue a Public Health Notification in 2008 to inform patients of adverse events related to the use of mesh placed in the urogynecology setting. In 2011, the FDA released a Safety Communication, which reported complications with TVM for POP, but did not include TVM for SUI. Subsequently, in 2013, the FDA updated its recommendations regarding the use of TVM for SUI, asserting that the currently marketed, multi-incision, polypropylene MUS are safe and effective with a positive risk-to-benefit profile. The FDA reaffirmed these findings in 2019 [72].

Similarly, The Society of Urodynamics, Female Pelvic Medicine and Urogenital Reconstruction (SUFU), and the AUGS issued a joint position statement in 2014, updated in 2021, strongly supporting the use of polypropylene mesh for the treatment of SUI, maintaining that the MUS procedure is safe, effective, and remains the standard of care for the treatment of SUI. The 2021 update emphasizes the more recent FDA update in 2019 reaffirming MUS as safe and effective, and added the support from the European Commission inquiry for continued use of synthetic slings for SUI [73]. Additionally, the AUA position statement on the use of vaginal mesh for the surgical treatment of SUI states that the restriction of the use of synthetic multi-incision MUS would be a disservice to women who choose surgical correction of SUI [74]. It is noteworthy that patients who present without complaints of mesh-related symptomatology and report no mesh-related complications should not undergo surgical revision unless bothersome symptoms develop [72].

Nevertheless, there has been a plethora of litigation surrounding the placement of mesh for POP and SUI. Legal action has been taken against hospitals, surgeons, and mesh manufacturers [75]. Consequently, it is imperative that physicians provide and document clear, unambiguous informed consent that includes specific mesh-related risks when discussing any procedure involving mesh. The AUA, SUFU, and International Urogynecological Association (IUGA) all have issued detailed guidelines for consenting patients [73, 74, 76]. Additionally, the FDA published their own guidelines for obtaining informed consent for mesh-related procedures stating: providers should inform patients that (1) implantation of surgical mesh is permanent, and that some complications associated with mesh may require additional surgery that may or may not correct the complication; and (2) there is potential for serious mesh-related complications that can have an effect on quality of life, including dyspareunia, scarring, and vaginal wall narrowing [72]. The FDA strongly advises that providers explicitly state to patients that mesh will be used in surgery and recommends that written information about the specific mesh product be given to the patient. The AUA also specifies that surgeons wishing to perform synthetic sling procedures should: (1) undergo rigorous training in the principles of pelvic surgery and anatomy, (2) be properly trained in specific sling techniques, and (3) be able to recognize and manage complications associated with synthetic mesh sling placement [77].

Conclusions

Urinary tract complications after MUS are not rare. The MUS should be inserted according to the standard guidelines by an experienced surgeon to reduce the incidence of complications. However, if a patient reports persistent or worsening lower urinary tract symptoms, providers should have a high index of suspicion for mesh-related urinary tract sequelae. Unfortunately, these complications, such as de novo OAB, BOO, sexual dysfunction, mesh-related pain, mesh perforation, and fistula formation, are not always reversible and can be quite debilitating for patients. Despite the MUS complication profile, the FDA, AUA, SUFU, AUGS, and IUGA all continue to support the MUS for the surgical treatment of SUI.

References

1. Reynolds WS, Dmochowski RR, Penson DF. Epidemiology of stress urinary incontinence in women. Curr Urol Rep. 2011;12(5):370–6.
2. Anger JT, Weisenberg AE, Albo ME, et al. Trends in surgical management of stress urinary incontinence among female Medicare beneficiaries. J Urol. 2009;74(2):283–7.
3. Wood L, Anger J. Urinary incontinence in women. BMJ. 2014;349:g4531.
4. Kobashi KC, Vasavada S, Bloschichak A, Hermanson L, Kaczmarek J, Kim SK, et al. Updates to surgical treatment of female stress urinary incontinence (SUI): AUA/SUFU guideline (2023). J Urol. 2023;209:1091–8.
5. Mohr S, Kuhn P, Mueller MD, et al. Painful love-"hispareunia" after sling erosion of the female partner. J Sex Med. 2011;8(6):1740–6.
6. Murray S, Haverkorn RM, Koch YK, et al. Urethral distortion after placement of synthetic mid urethral sling. J Urol. 2011;185(4):1321–6.
7. Nitti V, Tu LM, Gitlin J. Diagnosing bladder outlet obstruction in women. J Urol. 1999;161:1535–40.
8. Staack A, Vitale J, Ragavendra N, et al. Translabial ultrasonography for evaluation of synthetic mesh in the vagina. Urology. 2014;83:68–74.
9. Richter HE, Albo ME, Zyczynski HM, et al. Retropubic versus transobturator midurethral slings for stress incontinence. NEJM. 2010;362(22):2066–76.
10. Farag F, Osman NI, Pang KH, Castro-Diaz D, Chapple CR, Cruz F, et al. Complications of synthetic midurethral slings: is there a relevant discrepancy between observational data and clinical trials? Eur Urol Focus. 2023 [cited 2024 Apr 1]. Available from: https://www.eu-focus.europeanurology.com/article/S2405-4569(23)00244-4/fulltext.
11. Chang-Kit L, Kaufman M, Dmochowski R. Complications of biologic and synthetic slings and their management. In: Goldman H, editor. Complications of female incontinence and pelvic reconstructive surgery. London: Springer; 2013.

12. Lightner DJ, Wymer K, Sanchez J, et al. Best practice statement on urologic procedures and antimicrobial prophylaxis. J Urol. 2020;203:351.
13. Jackson D, Higgins E, Bracken J, et al. Antibiotic prophylaxis for urinary tract infection after midurethral sling: a randomized controlled trial. Female Pelvic Med Reconstr Surg. 2013;12(3):137–41.
14. Wu E, Kuehl TJ, Danford JM, Bird ET, Yandell PM. Postoperative prophylactic antibiotics for retropubic mid-urethral slings. Int Urogynecol J. 2022;33:897–902.
15. Mishra VC, Mishra N, Karim OMA, et al. Voiding dysfunction after tension-free vaginal tape: a conservative approach is often successful. Int Urogynecol J. 2005;16:210–5.
16. Holgren C, Nilsson S, Lanner L. Frequency of de novo urgency in 463 women who had undergone tension-free vaginal tape (TVT) procedure for genuine stress urinary incontinence-a long term follow-up. Obstet Gynecol. 2007;132:121–5.
17. Lee J, Dwyer P, Rosamilla A. Which women develop urgency or urgency urinary incontinence following midurethral slings? Int Urogynecol J. 2013;24:47–54.
18. Abraham N, Vasavada S. Urgency after sling: review of the management. Curr Urol Rep. 2014;15:400.
19. Segal J, Vassallo B, Kleeman S, et al. Prevalence of persistent and de novo overactive bladder symptoms after the tension-free vaginal tape. Obstet Gynecol. 2004;104(6):1263–9.
20. Cameron AP, Chung DE, Dielubanza EJ, et al. The AUA/SUFU guideline on the diagnosis and treatment of idiopathic overactive bladder. J Urol Published online April 23, 2024. https://doi.org/10.1097/JU.0000000000003985. https://www.auajournals.org/doi/10.1097/JU.0000000000003985.
21. Serati M, Braga A, Sorice P, et al. Solifenacin in women with de novo overactive bladder after tension free obturator vaginal tape-is it effective? J Urol. 2014;191:1322–6.
22. Miotla P, Futyma K, Cartwright R, et al. Effectiveness of botulinum toxin injection in the treatment of de novo OAB symptoms following midurethral sling surgery. Int Urogynecol J. 2016;3(27):393–8.
23. Patel B, Kobashi K, Staskin D. Iatrogenic obstruction after sling surgery. Nat Rev Urol. 2012;9:429–34.
24. Shah S, Nitti V. Diagnosis and treatment of obstruction following anti-incontinence surgery-urethrolysis and other techniques. In: Cardozo L, Staskin D, editors. Textbook of female urology and urogynecology, vol. II. 3rd ed. London: Informa Healthcare; 2010. p. 749–62.
25. Aponte MM, Shah SR, Hickling D, et al. Urodynamics for clinically suspected obstruction after anti-incontinence surgery in women. J Urol. 2013;190(2):598–602.
26. Lee D, Bacsu C, Zimmern P. Meshology: a fast-growing field involving mesh and/or tape removal procedures and their outcomes. Expert Rev Med Devices. 2015;12(2):201–6.
27. Scarpero HM, Dmochowski RR, Nitti VW. Repeat urethrolysis after failed urethrolysis for iatrogenic obstruction. J Urol. 2003;169:1013–6.
28. Nguyen JN. Tape mobilization for urinary retention after tension-free vaginal tape procedures. Urology. 2005;66:523–6.
29. Hong B, Park S, Kim HS, Choo M. Factors predictive of urinary retention after a tension-free vaginal tape procedure for female stress urinary incontinence. J Urol. 2003;170:852–6.
30. Goldman HB. Simple sling incision for the treatment of iatrogenic urethral obstruction. Urology. 2003;62:714–8.
31. Gomelsky A, Dmochowski RR. Slings: autologous, biologic, synthetic, and mid-urethral. In: Campbell-Walsh Urology. 12th ed. WB Saunders Co. pp. 2830–76.
32. Webster GD, Kreder KJ. Voiding dysfunction following cystourethopexy: its evaluation and management. J Urol. 1990;144:670–3.
33. Petrou SP, Young PR. Rate of recurrent stress urinary incontinence after retropubic urethrolysis. J Urol. 2002;167:613–5.
34. Petrou SP, Brown JA, Blaivas JG. Suprameatal transvaginal urethrolysis. J Urol. 1999;161:1268–71.
35. Carr LK, Webster GD. Voiding dysfunction following incontinence surgery: diagnosis and treatment with retropubic or vaginal urethrolysis. J Urol. 1999;161:1535–40.
36. Starkman J, Duffy J, Wolter C, et al. The evolution of obstruction induced overactive bladder symptoms following urethrolysis for female bladder outlet obstruction. J Urol. 2008;179:2028–3.
37. Anger JT, Amundsen CL, Webster GD. Obstruction after Burch colposuspension: a return to retropubic urethrolysis. Int Urogynecol J Pelvic Floor Dysfunct. 2006;17(5):455–9.
38. Austin P, Spryropoulos E, Lotenfoe R, et al. Urethral obstruction after anti-incontinence surgery in women: evaluation, methodology, and surgical results. Urology. 1996;47:890–4.
39. Amundsen CL, Buralnick ML, Webster GD. Variations in strategy for the treatment of urethral obstruction after a pubovaginal sling procedure. J Urol. 2000;164:434–7.
40. Carey JM, Chon JK, Leach GE. Urethrolysis with Martius labial fat pad for iatrogenic bladder outlet obstruction. Urology. 2003;61:21–5.
41. Foster HE, McGuire EJ. Management of urethral obstruction with transvaginal urethrolysis. J Urol. 2005;150:1448–51.
42. Nitti V, Raz S. Obstruction following anti-incontinence procedures: diagnosis and treatment with retropubic or vaginal urethrolysis. J Urol. 1997;157:821–3.
43. Cross CA, Cespedes RD, English SF, et al. Transvaginal urethrolysis for urethral obstruction after anti-incontinence surgery. J Urol. 1998;159:1199–201.

44. Goldman HB, Rackley PR, Appell RA. The efficacy of urethrolysis without resuspension for iatrogenic urethral obstruction. J Urol. 1999;161(1):196–8.
45. McCrery R, Appell R. Transvaginal urethrolysis for obstruction after antiincontinence surgery. Int Urogynecol J Pelvic Floor Dysfunct. 2007;18(6):627–33.
46. Nitti VW, Carlson KV, Blaivas JG, et al. Early results of pubovaginal sling lysis by midline sling incision. Urology. 2002;59:47–51.
47. Abraham N, Makovey I, King A, et al. The effect of time to release of an obstruction synthetic mid-urethral sling on repeat surgery for stress urinary incontinence. Neurourol Urodyn. 2015. epub ahead of print.
48. Yoost T, Rames R, Lebed B, et al. Predicting for post-operative incontinence following sling release. Int Urogynecol J. 2011;22:665.
49. Klutke C, Siegel S, Carlin B, Paszkiewicz E, Kirkemo A, Klutke J. Urinary retention after tension-free vaginal tape procedure: incidence and treatment. Urology. 2001;58:697–701.
50. Laurikainen E, Kiilholma P. A nationwide analysis of transvaginal tape release for urinary retention after tension-free vaginal tape procedure. Int Urogynecol J Pelvic Floor Dysfunct. 2006;17:111–9.
51. Starkman JS, Duffy J, Wolter C, et al. Refractory overactive bladder after urethrolysis for bladder outlet obstruction: management with sacral neuromodulation. Int Urogynecol J. 2008;19:277–82.
52. Campbell F, Collett BJ. Chronic pelvic pain. Br J Anaesth. 1994;73:571–3.
53. Lee D, Chang J, Zimmern PE. Iatrogenic pelvic pain: surgical and mesh complications. Phys Med Rehabil Clin N Am. 2017;28(3):603–19.
54. Shah HN, Badlani GH. Mesh complications in female pelvic floor reconstructive surgery and their management: a systematic review. Indian J Urol. 2012;28:129–53.
55. Mazouni C, Karsenty G, Bretelle F, Bladou F, Gamerre M, Serment G. Urinary complications and sexual function after the tension-free vaginal tape procedure. Acta Obstet Gynecol Scand. 2004;83:955–61.
56. Stav K, Dwyer PL, Rosamilia A, Schierlitz L, Lim YN, Chao F, et al. Repeat synthetic mid urethral sling procedure for women with recurrent stress urinary incontinence. J Urol. 2010;183:241–6.
57. Ward KL, Hilton P, UK and Ireland TVT Trial Group. Tension-free vaginal tape versus colposuspension for primary urodynamic stress incontinence: 5-year follow up. BJOG. 2008;115:226–33.
58. Bekker M, Beck J, Putter H, Venema P, Lycklama à Nijeholt A, Pelger R, et al. Sexual function improvement following surgery for stress incontinence: the relevance of coital incontinence. J Sex Med. 2009;6:3208–13.
59. Fuentes JL, Finsterbusch C, Christie AL, Zimmern PE. Mesh sling arm removal for persistent pain after an initial vaginal suburethral mesh sling removal procedure. Female Pelvic Med Reconstr Surg. 2021;27(5):e522–7.
60. Developed by the Joint Writing Group of the American Urogynecologic Society and the International Urogynecological Association. The AAGL endorses this document. The Society of Gynecologic Surgeons supports this document. Individual contributors are noted in the acknowledgment section. Joint Position Statement on the Management of Mesh-Related Complications for the FPMRS Specialist. Female Pelvic Med Reconstr Surg. 2020;26(4):219–32.
61. Osborn D, Dmochowski R, Harris C, et al. Analysis of patient and technical factors associated with midurethral sling mesh exposure and perforation. Int J Urol. 2014;21:1167–70.
62. Oh TH, Ryu DS. Transurethral resection of intravesical mesh after midurethral sling procedures. J Endourol. 2009;181(5):2198–202.
63. Dounouchtsis SK, Lee F, Bramwell D, et al. Evaluation of holmium laser for managing mesh/suture complications of continence surgery. BJUI. 2011;108:1472–8.
64. Shah K, Nikolavsky D, Gilsdorf D, et al. Surgical management of lower urinary mesh perforation after mid-urethral polypropylene mesh sling: mesh excision, urinary tract reconstruction and concomitant pubovaginal sling with autologous rectus fascia. Int Urogynecol J. 2013;24:2111–7.
65. Blaivas J, Mekel G. Management of urinary fistulas due to midurethral sling surgery. J Urol. 2014;192:1137–42.
66. Blaivas J, Purohit R, Weinberger J, et al. Salvage surgery after failed treatment of synthetic mesh sling complications. J Urol. 2013;190(4):1281–6.
67. Hansen B, Dunn G, Norton P, et al. Long-term followup of treatment for synthetic mesh complications. Female Pelvic Med Reconstr Surg. 2014;20(3):126–30.
68. Zimmern PE, Gormley EA, Stoddard AM, Lukacz ES, Sirls L, Brubaker L, et al. Management of recurrent stress urinary incontinence after burch and sling procedures. Neurourol Urodyn. 2016;35:344–8.
69. Gaddi A, Guaderrama N, Bassiouni N, Bebchuk J, Whitcomb EL. Repeat midurethral sling compared with urethral bulking for recurrent stress urinary incontinence. Obstet Gynecol. 2014;123:1207–12.
70. Braga A, Caccia G, Papadia A, et al. Urethral bulking agents for the treatment of recurrent stress urinary incontinence: a systematic review and meta-analysis. Maturitas. 2022;163:28–37. https://doi.org/10.1016/j.maturitas.2022.05.007.
71. Myhr SS, Rakovan M, Schiøtz HA. Periurethral injection with polyacrylamide after previous TVT surgery. Int Urogynecol J. 2022;33(4):1017–22. https://doi.org/10.1007/s00192-021-04891-y.
72. U.S. Food & Drug Administration. Considerations about surgical mesh for SUI. Available at: https://www.fda.gov/medical-devices/urogynecologicsurgical-mesh-implants/considerations-about-surgical-mesh-sui.

73. AUGS-SUFU position statement on mesh midurethral slings for SUI. https://www.augs.org/assets/1/6/AUGS-SUFU_Joint_Publication.pdf.
74. American Urologic Association (AUA) position statement on the use of vaginal mesh for the surgical treatment of stress urinary incontinence. 2012. www.auanet.org/education/vaginal-mesh-for-sui.cfm.
75. Kuhlmann-Capek M, Kilic G, Shah A, et al. Enmeshed in controversy: use of vaginal mesh in the current medicolegal environment. Female Pelv Med Reconstr Surg. 2015;21(5):241–3.
76. Miller D, Milani AL, Sutherland SE, et al. Informed surgical consent for a mesh/graft-augmented vaginal repair of pelvic organ prolapse. Consensus of the 2nd IUGA grafts roundtable: optimizing safety and appropriateness of graft use in transvaginal pelvic reconstructive surgery. Int Urogynecol J. 2012;23(Suppl 1):33.
77. Kobashi KC, Vasavada S, Bloschichak A, et al. Updates to surgical treatment of female stress urinary incontinence (SUI): AUA/SUFU guideline (2023). J Urol. 2023;209(6):1091–8.

19 Synthetic Midurethral Slings: Exposure and Perforation

Priyanka Gupta, Brandee Spitnale, Natalie Gaines, and Larry T. Sirls

Abbreviations

BMI	Body mass index
FSFI	Female Sexual Function Index
IUGA/ICS	International Urogynecological Association/International Continence Society
MUS	Midurethral sling
PFPT	Pelvic floor physical therapy
RCT	Randomized clinical trial
RP	Retropubic
SIS	Single-incision sling
SUI	Stress urinary incontinence
TO	Transobturator
TOMUS	Trial of Midurethral Slings
TUR	Transurethral resection
TVT	Transvaginal tape

P. Gupta (✉) · B. Spitnale
Department of Urology, University of Michigan, Ann Arbor, MI, USA
e-mail: guptapr@med.umich.edu; brandebr@med.umich.edu

N. Gaines
Amarillo Urology Associates, Amarillo, TX, USA

L. T. Sirls
Corewell Health William Beaumont University Hospital, Bloomfield Hills, MI, USA

Introduction

Urinary incontinence is a quality of life condition, and the potential complications of surgical treatment are important to consider due to their impact on surgical decision-making. Since its description by Ulmsten and Petros in 1995, the mesh midurethral sling (MUS) has revolutionized the treatment of stress urinary incontinence (SUI) [1]. Outcomes are excellent, with reported long-term success rates of 43–92% for transobturator and 51–88% for retropubic slings [2]. In the United States there has been a near doubling of SUI surgical procedures between 1979 and 1997, and this same trend continued into 2009 [3]. The excellent results, prompt return to normal activities, and low complication rates (Table 19.1) quickly pushed MUS to the forefront of surgical procedures chosen for SUI treatment. However, sling procedures can result in immediate surgical injury to the vaginal wall, urethra, bladder, or surrounding organs, and the use of mesh introduces the concept of delayed mesh-related complications, like vaginal wall exposure and adjacent organ perforation.

Urogynecological Association/International Continence Society (IUGA/ICS) published a consensus on mesh complications terminology in 2011 [4]. The generic term "erosion" should be avoided, as it implies a wearing away by friction or pressure, and it does not represent the clinical presentations encountered. IUGA/ICS

H. B. Goldman, J. Zillioux (eds.), *Complications of Urogynecology and Reconstructive Pelvic Surgery*, https://doi.org/10.1007/978-3-032-00339-3_19

Table 19.1 Reported vaginal wall exposure rates and mesh perforation rates of mesh midurethral sling surgery

	Retropubic	Transobturator	Single-incision
Vaginal wall mesh exposure	2.04%[a]	2.07%[a]	Similar to slings; RR 0.61, 95% CI 0.47–0.97[a]
Bladder injury	0.7–15.7%[a]	0–1.4%[a]	0.8%[c]
Urethral injury	0–0.3%[a]	0–1.7%[a]	<4%[b]
Bowel injury	0–0.35%[a]	0%[a]	0.8%[c]

[a]Ford 2017 [2]
[b]Nambiar 2023 [5]
[c]Barber 2012 [6]

instead suggested the use of the term *exposure* to represent vaginal mesh that is visible or palpable through the separated mucosa at the original vaginal incision site, whereas the term *extrusion* was suggested to represent the delayed process whereby mesh gradually passes through the vaginal wall. However, these definitions were suggested after many reports were already published in the literature, and the events of mesh exposure vs. extrusion can be difficult to distinguish. Therefore, *in this chapter, we will use the term mesh exposure to describe mesh that is visible or palpable through the vaginal wall mucosa, whether at the incision site or elsewhere, at any time point. Mesh perforation will describe a delayed event where mesh has entered an adjacent hollow organ, either the urinary tract (urethra or bladder) or the bowel. Trocar injury will refer to the recognized passage of the sling trocar through the vaginal wall, or into the urethra, bladder, or bowel at the time of sling placement.*

The astute reader must be careful to distinguish between the two different types of publications reporting on MUS complications. One group of studies and meta-analyses reports complications from index surgeries, and a second group of publications reports symptoms identified in patients referred to a regional center for management of complications. The former are felt to represent "real world" complication rates, whereas the latter are affected by selection bias, because patients referred to these institutions have more complicated sling problems requiring expert management.

Midurethral Sling Surgery Uses Less Vaginal Dissection

All MUS procedures, including retropubic (RP), transobturator (TO), or single-incision slings (SIS), are "tension-free." They provide support under the hypermobile urethra only during times of increased abdominal pressure, leading to "dynamic kinking" of the urethra, which prevents leakage of urine. The transvaginal tape (TVT) was the first MUS [1], and it requires a less extensive dissection than the traditional fascial pubovaginal sling. The traditional pubovaginal sling dissection requires a wide vaginal incision and subsequent periurethral mobilization to permit passage of the surgeon's finger (not just a narrow trocar) into the retropubic space. This allows for controlled guidance of the sling passage needle from the suprapubic incision onto the surgeon's finger as it is passed behind the pubic bone and delivered through the vaginal incision. Precise control of the needle minimizes the chance of inadvertent bladder injury. In contrast, the TVT is a trocar-based device that places a piece of mesh tape retropubically through a limited vaginal incision and exits through a small suprapubic skin incision. The vaginal-to-suprapubic trocar passage is also called the "bottom-up" approach. The TVT procedure introduced "blind" passage of the trocar through the retropubic space, as it is not passed directly on the surgeon's finger. This blind passage resulted in increased bladder and bowel injury, and by 2001, these complications helped to promote the development of the TO sling. The TO sling follows a lateral vector, the natural curve of the vaginal wall, to pass the sling through the obturator fossa, which allows it to avoid the blind retropubic pass [7]. With subsequent development of the "top-down" retropubic sling in 2001 and then the "inside-out" transobturator sling in 2003, four different methods of placing a MUS were available (RP: "bottom-up" and "top-down"; TO: "inside-out" and "outside-in"), each with its own benefits and complication profiles, secondary to their different vectors of passage. The SIS sling was FDA approved in 2006. It was designed to have the benefits of lateral vector passage, like a TO sling, but to avoid passage through the adductor muscle complex of the thigh, which is associated with rare pain complications.

This chapter will review MUS complications and their management, with a specific emphasis on two main concepts:

1. Mesh exposure, defined as exposed mesh visible or palpable through the full-thickness vaginal wall at either the incision site or a separate site. These may be early or delayed.
2. Mesh perforation, very early presentation may represent a technical error of sling trocar placement through the urethra, bladder, or bowel, and when delayed, it may represent more patient-specific tissue healing factors. While these complications are uncommon overall, a clear understanding of the sling-specific and patient-specific risk factors and the utility of prompt diagnosis and appropriate treatment is critical for the pelvic reconstructive surgeon.

Mesh Exposure

Mesh exposure, defined as exposed mesh visible or palpable through the full-thickness vaginal wall, is rare after MUS, occurring in 0–4.4% of patients [8–15]. Mesh exposure occurs secondary to a combination of patient and technical factors. Patient factors include body habitus, poor tissue ingrowth, and poor wound healing. Technical factors include folding or wrinkling of the sling, sling tension, sling material properties, and iatrogenic vaginal wall injury [13, 16]. While increasing age is not a risk factor for mesh exposure [17], younger age is a risk factor for the need for surgical intervention for vaginal mesh exposure, with women 18–39-years old at the highest risk [18]. Younger women may be more sexually active, experience vaginal spotting, dyspareunia, or partner dyspareunia, which prompts evaluation and secondary surgery [18].

Synthetic slings behave differently from autologous, allograft, and xenograft slings. The polypropylene mesh sling is a permanent foreign body that may expose the patient to long-term complications. Biomechanical properties of the sling material play a crucial role in vaginal mesh exposure. Although various materials have been used for sling surgery, the literature strongly supports the use of the Amid Classification Type I mesh, a macroporous, weaved monofilament polypropylene mesh [19]. Type I mesh has a large pore size that allows for tissue ingrowth and incorporation into the surrounding tissue, which minimizes sling encapsulation and infection [20, 21]. Historical use of non-Type I mesh products, with their smaller pore size, resulted in poor tissue incorporation into the mesh, more encapsulation, and subsequently higher rates of vaginal mesh infection and exposure. Examples include ObTape® and Uratape®, with reported mesh exposure rates of 19% and 12%, respectively [16, 22].

Mesh Exposure Reflects the RP and TO Vectors of Placement

Vector differences when passing the RP and TO sling trocars are directly related to the different rates and locations of vaginal wall mesh exposure. The increased incidence of mesh exposure with TO slings reflects the "smile" sling vector traveling from the midurethra, coursing laterally along the anterior vaginal wall, and passing toward the obturator foramen. At the lateral vaginal sulcus, there is a potential for thinning of the vaginal wall, either due to individual patient anatomy or the surgeon's dissection, and this may lead to mesh exposure. The RP sling has a "U" vector, which travels underneath the urethra, then directly behind the pubic bone. It does not travel laterally along the anterior vaginal wall. RP slings have a lower rate of mesh exposure than TO slings because passage of the RP sling avoids the lateral vaginal sulci [23, 24]. Mesh exposure after an RP sling most commonly occurs in the midline at the incision site.

Both RP and TO slings have two different entry points and trajectories: either from the vaginal incision to the outside skin ("bottom-up" RP sling and "inside-out" TO sling) or from the outside skin to the vaginal incision ("top-down" RP sling and "outside-in" TO sling). Because each courses laterally, both TO approaches still carry the risk of vaginal perforation at the lateral vaginal sulcus. In 341 women who underwent TO sling, Abdel-Fattah et al. reported an increased risk of vaginal wall mesh exposure with the "outside-in" technique. Only 3 of 20 lateral sulcus injuries occurred after "inside-out" TO slings versus 17 of 20 after "outside-in" TO slings ($p = 0.001$) [25]. Similar results were noted by But in 2008 [26]. The reason for the increased exposure rate with the "outside-in" approach may be due to the additional dissection required to allow a finger to receive the TO trocar at the pubic bone. It may also be secondary to the relative lack of three-dimensional orientation when receiving the sling trocar entering from the groin crease. This is in contrast with the "inside-out" technique, in which the surgeon places the trocar in a precise and controlled position under direct vision relative to the vaginal wall and urethra.

The SIS, or "mini-sling," follows the same vector as the TO sling; however, due to its shorter length, it only reaches the obturator internus membrane. Because it has a similar lateral vector of passage along the anterior vaginal wall as the TO sling, SIS has a rate of mesh exposure of 1.3% (95% CI 0.8–1.9), comparable to the TO sling [27].

In a 2014 meta-analysis, the rate of vaginal wall perforation by TO sling was 2.8% (95% CI 2.2–3.5%), whereas the rate of vaginal wall perforation by the RP sling was 0.73% (95% CI 0.40–1.2%) [27]. The Trial of Midurethral Slings (TOMUS), a high-quality multicenter RCT of 597 women, reported that the recognized vaginal wall trocar or perforation rate at the time of surgery was 4.4% with TO sling and 2% with RP sling, and the mesh exposure rates on follow-up were 1.3% with TO sling and 0.7% with RP sling [15].

Surgical Tips to Minimize the Risk of Vaginal Wall Mesh Exposure

Optimal vaginal wall thickness during dissection is essential to avoid urethral or vaginal wall thinning and to minimize vaginal wall trocar perforation. Hydrodissection is performed prior to incision with 10 cc of saline at the midurethra, and hydrodissection may be performed laterally to the vaginal sulcus for the TO sling. This hydrodissection creates a submucosal space that can facilitate the creation of the optimal plane. We place the vaginal wall over the midurethra under tension using a toothed forceps to help the 18-gauge injection needle find a surgical plane at an appropriate depth. Early vaginal wall blanching means the injection is too superficial, and a lack of an obvious injection bleb means the hydrodissection is too deep. Direct visualization and palpation of the sling trocar trajectory during all phases of passage are critical to inform the surgeon of vaginal wall thickness.

If inadvertent perforation of the lateral vaginal mucosa is noted, a new deeper access for the sling trocar is created using Metzenbaum scissors, and the sling trocar is repassed into the new path with thicker vaginal wall coverage. The vaginal wall perforation should be closed with an absorbable suture. In TOMUS, perforation of the vaginal epithelium managed by operative repair and replacement of the sling led to no short- or long-term complications at two years [15].

Another potential risk factor for mesh exposure is postoperative formation of a vaginal wall hematoma. The hematoma may either cause incisional pressure, resulting in reopening of the incision, or it may cause mucosal separation with mesh exposure as the hematoma liquefies and drains. Good mucosal closure may minimize delayed mucosal separation, and if the vaginal dissection has caused more bleeding than normal, some surgeons will try to minimize the vaginal wall hematoma by placing a vaginal pack that is removed in the recovery room after 1–2 hours.

Key Points: Prevention and Management of Vaginal Wall Perforation

- Prevention
  - Adequate hydrodissection
    - Transobturator sling, hydrodissection laterally to sulcus
  - Confirm vaginal wall thickness by palpation
- Management
  - Identification is key
  - Remove trocar, create deeper plane, beware of urethra, replace trocar
  - Close vaginal wall injury with 3-0 Vicryl

Clinical Presentation of Vaginal Wall Mesh Exposure

Vaginal wall mesh exposure may be early or delayed and has a variety of presentations. A patient may be asymptomatic, with the sling visible or palpable only on physical examination. The symptomatic patient may have vaginal spotting or discharge, vaginal pain, dyspareunia, and/or partner dyspareunia. Additionally, persistent SUI may be found in those with mesh exposure [64]. Because symptoms can be nonspecific, one must have a high index of suspicion with any postoperative sling patient.

Symptoms may begin within a few weeks to a few months after the procedure. Osborn et al. found that patients who had mesh exposure presented at a median of 6 months from the time of their initial surgery [28]. The most common symptom was vaginal bleeding (20/50 women), reported as intermittent spotting increasing after intercourse. Vaginal discharge was reported in 3/50, 18/50 had dyspareunia, and 20/50 women had vaginal pain. Kokanali reported that the most common presenting symptom of vaginal wall mesh exposure was the patient feeling the mesh on self-examination [29]. In the authors' experience, when patients report vaginal pain or dyspareunia, we are also concerned that the sling may be too tight and are careful to evaluate for evidence of pelvic floor muscle dysfunction/spasm.

According to a 2013 review of 188,454 index patients who underwent MUS placement, the risk of surgical removal or revision due to mesh exposure increases throughout the first four years after surgery, from 1.3% at 1 year to 2.1% at four years postoperatively. After that time, the rate of surgical intervention for mesh exposure remains around 2.5% [18]. These findings are consistent with the 5-year results from the TOMUS, which reported a 1.7% rate of mesh exposure [30].

The RP MUS has been extensively studied, with average follow-up greater than 10 years in several publications. These studies inform the clinician that there is a continued, but small, risk for vaginal mesh exposure. In the Nordic study, only one of 46 women who did not have mesh exposure at 7 years and returned for the 17-year physical examination had mesh exposure [31]. Similarly, Svenningsen reported a 0.6% mesh exposure rate at a mean follow-up of almost 11 years [32]. The longest published TO sling follow-up study reported 2/61 women had vaginal mesh exposure at 5 years, and, importantly, both were recognized on the 1-year exam [33].

Clinical Evaluation of Mesh Exposure

A thorough pelvic examination is typically adequate to diagnose vaginal mesh exposure. Careful visual inspection of the entire anterior vaginal wall and the lateral sulcus should be methodically performed, making special note of the location of the vaginal wall incision. The urethra should then be methodically palpated, beginning in the midline and extending laterally to each sulcus, feeling for a lateral exposure. Careful examination of the lateral vaginal fornices is particularly important after a TO or SIS. Mesh may not readily be visualized but may only be palpated as a grainy, superficial structure, sometimes with a sharp edge.

Inspection and palpation of the suprapubic and bilateral lower quadrants and each groin crease should also be performed, looking for any evidence of early or delayed wound issues, such as tenderness, inflammatory changes, drainage, or a potential fistula tract. In the patient who is difficult to examine, vaginoscopy with a cystoscope, with manual compression of the labia to permit filling of the vagina, may allow visualization of mesh exposure, though this technique is more commonly used to look for proximal vaginal wall mesh exposure after prolapse surgery.

The use of imaging may be considered in cases where there is a degree of suspicion for additional complications or as an addition to cystoscopy. One study found that translabial ultrasound and transvaginal ultrasound have high sensitivity and specificity for detecting bladder exposure (98–100%, respectively) [65]. Translabial ultrasound, however, can be technically challenging, and results may vary. Further studies are needed to elucidate the utility of these modalities.

Management of Vaginal Wall Mesh Exposure

Once exposed vaginal mesh is recognized, there are multiple appropriate treatment strategies based on the patient's quality of life and expectations. If the patient is asymptomatic, particularly if she is not sexually active, observation may be appropriate. While the addition of vaginal estrogen is commonplace, a paucity of literature exists demonstrating the efficacy of estrogen replacement therapy for complete regrowth of the vaginal epithelium over the exposed mesh. In 2009, Higgins et al. evaluated the effect of vaginal estrogen in an ovariectomized rabbit vagina model with mesh implantation. Estrogen supplementation did show some beneficial effects, including reversal of vaginal atrophy and increased deposition of collagen into the mesh [34]. In the authors' experience, vaginal estrogen can make the mucosa more vascular and healthy, as well as reduce the size of the exposure, but *very rarely* will it result in complete coverage of the mesh exposure.

Type I mesh allows for excellent tissue ingrowth and typically remains uninfected even when exposed. Thus, exposed mesh that is well-incorporated can be left intact and re-covered with vaginal epithelium with minimal risk of infection. However, if the mesh has folds, wrinkles, or any ridges, excision and revision may be necessary to reduce the risk of repeat exposure. Some older non-type I mesh slings may be found free-floating without any tissue incorporation (Fig. 19.1), and sometimes with obvious infection. These slings need to be excised until healthy tissue is seen investing and surrounding the sling. In the authors' practice, complete sling removal is not commonly needed unless the sling is clearly not incorporated into the tissue, suggesting possible infection, which is an unusual finding with type I mesh. More extensive mesh removal along the course of the vaginal wall may be considered if the initial attempt at mesh trimming and vaginal mucosal flap coverage has failed. However, extensive retropubic, obturator, or groin dissection to remove all portions of the sling is typically unnecessary. In the case reports of these extensive procedures, very specific indications were present.

If a patient is symptomatic from her mesh exposure, operative intervention is reasonable. Location of the procedure, whether in the office or in the operating room, is dependent on surgeon's experience, the patient's tolerance, and the size and location of the exposure. Myers et al. successfully managed small exposures less than 5 mm via an office-based excision, while exposures 6 mm to 1 cm were managed in the operat-

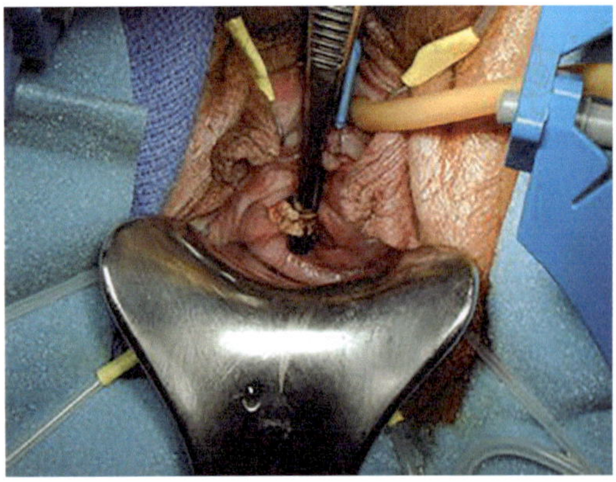

Fig. 19.1 Midurethral sling mesh exposure through vaginal wall. Note this non-type I mesh is not well incorporated and is free-floating with calcifications. The mesh will need to be resected back to where it is well incorporated into the tissue

ing room [35]. Small midline exposures may be managed in the office by experienced surgeons. Local anesthetic is infiltrated around the exposure, and an incision is made from the mesh exposure into the surrounding healthy tissue. If significant inflammatory or granulation tissue is present, an elliptical excision of the granulated vaginal mucosal edge may be needed to expose healthy tissue that can then be mobilized. Once the extent of the exposure is clarified, and a healthy vaginal wall exposed, dissection superficial to the mesh but under the vaginal mucosa helps to create mobile vaginal wall flaps to provide tension-free coverage of the exposed mesh. The Finnish nationwide review reported that 10/1455 MUS procedures had mesh exposure [9]. Three of these patients were managed without surgical intervention, four patients had the mesh re-covered with mobilized vaginal mucosa, and two patients required partial mesh excision.

Recurrent SUI may occur after mesh removal. The incidence of this may vary depending on the amount of sling removed. In a study by Karmakar et al, 1 in 3 women developed SUI following partial or complete removal of the sling and required further surgery. In this study, 33/2823 patients at a tertiary urogynecology center in Australia with MUS had mesh exposure. Twenty of these patients were managed with partial excision of the suburethral portion of the MUS. In these patients, the vagina around the erosion was excised and mobilized, with 2–3 cm of sling removed. Eleven patients with sling conservation had mobilization of the sling and surrounding tissues, with vagina closure following. Of the 20 women with sling excision, 5 had a concomitant continence procedure with no recurrent SUI, and 5 of the remaining 15 required further surgery for SUI. Of the 11 women with sling conservation, 7 required a second procedure for recurrent exposure [66]. Some surgeons may perform a concomitant SUI procedure at the time of mesh removal; however, if considering this, the authors recommend ensuring the periurethral tissue is healthy and no urethral injury has occurred during removal.

Mesh excision can improve sexual function. In Kuhn et al., the sexual function in women with MUS mesh exposure was evaluated pre- and postoperatively with the Female Sexual Function Index (FSFI) [36]. Of 21 exposures, 18 had mesh re-coverage with vaginal mucosa. Two patients had recurrent exposure, one had repeat vaginal closure, and the other had partial sling excision and vaginal closure. Importantly, FSFI domains of desire, arousal, lubrication, satisfaction, and pain improved significantly.

The authors recommend leaving well-incorporated exposed mesh in situ and covering it with vaginal epithelium. An absorbable suture, such as a 3-0 VICRYL®, is used to close the mobilized vaginal wall in a tension-free manner. The patient should abstain from intercourse or tampon use for several weeks to permit healing. If the patient has a large exposure (> 1 cm), exposure at the lateral vaginal sulcus, or if the surgeon's comfort dictates, we prefer surgical management in the operating room with better retraction and exposure. Removal of a portion of the sling can be performed if indicated. The patient should be counseled on the risks and benefits of removing or covering only the exposed mesh versus excision of a larger section of the sling. It is important to recognize that removal of a large section of the sling does risk injury to the urethra and recurrence of stress incontinence. If a large section of an RP sling is to be removed, the sling can be incised and dissected laterally to the urethra behind the pubic bone. Chasing the RP sling into the retropubic space is done only with bladder or other adjacent organ injury that demands a more aggressive approach. Because it requires extensive dissection behind the pubic bone, which is difficult to perform vaginally, complete removal of an RP sling from the retropubic space usually requires a concurrent open or laparoscopic/robotic approach.

Similarly, the TO sling can be traced laterally behind the pubic bone to its path through the obturator internus muscle. Removing the TO sling from the obturator fossa or groin crease/adductor muscles should only be done in the rare patient who has significant symptoms, such as pelvic floor muscle or adductor muscle pain. Dissection past the obturator internus from the vaginal approach can be difficult and may be associated with bleeding that is difficult to control. Therefore, if complete removal is indicated, a groin crease or medial thigh counter incision may be needed. SIS sling removal is similar to the vaginal approach of TO sling removal.

Key Points: Management of Vaginal Mesh Exposure

- Asymptomatic and not sexually active: consider observation
- Symptomatic
  - Exam
    - Confirm location
    - Identify all exposed mesh
  - Surgical intervention
    - Resection
      - Remove inflamed mucosa surrounding exposed mesh
      - Remove wrinkled, folded, or prominent mesh
      - Remove "free-floating" poorly incorporated mesh
    - Closure
      - Mobilize vaginal wall to allow tension-free closure
      - Close with 3-0 SAS

Mesh Perforation: Adjacent Organs

Bladder

Bladder Injury Is Higher with the RP Sling

Bladder perforation is more common with RP slings due to the blind pass and trajectory of the retropubic trocar behind the pubic bone. Most current literature describes bladder trocar injury at the time of the index surgery. A 2015 meta-analysis reported a 3.2% rate of bladder perforation with RP sling, significantly higher than the TO sling rate of 0.2% (OR 5.72, CI 2.94–11.12, $p < 0.0001$) [37]. The TOMUS trial, which consisted of high-volume fellowship-trained surgeons practicing at teaching institutions, reported a 5% rate of bladder perforation and 1% urethral perforation rate with the RP sling compared to 0% bladder and 0% urethral perforation with the TO sling [15]. The rate of bladder or urethral trocar injury with TO surgery in other randomized studies is reported between 0 and 1.3% [15, 38]. Interestingly, Tamussino reported that 9/10 bladder injuries occurred with the "outside-in" TO trocar technique [39].

Several risk factors are associated with bladder perforation. First, as with any procedure, there is a learning curve, so proper training and surgeon experience are important. Stav et al. reported that 32/34 (94%) bladder perforations were by surgeons who had performed fewer than 50 slings ($p < 0.0001$). All but one of these perforations was by an RP sling, and the route of trocar insertion ("top-down" or "bottom-up") did not affect risk [40]. History of prior abdominal or pelvic surgery that may scar the retropubic space can increase the risk of bladder perforation, including colposuspension, cesarean section, or prior anti-incontinence surgery. Diabetes mellitus is a medical comorbidity that may increase the risk of bladder perforation. Chen noted an increased risk of mesh perforation into the bladder in diabetic patients, possibly related to their poor wound healing abilities [41]. Interestingly, several series have reported decreased rates of bladder perforations with RP slings in patients with BMI > 30 kg/m^2 [40, 42, 43]. The protective mechanism may be that the retropubic fat pushes the bladder away from the pubic bone, shielding the bladder from the trocar.

Prevention of Bladder Injury

To minimize the risk of bladder perforation, the bladder must have an indwelling Foley catheter and be empty prior to sling placement. Ulmsten's original paper on the RP sling describes hydrodissection behind the pubic bone by injecting 60–70 cc of local anesthesia through a spinal needle suprapubically on the left and right sides [1]. When placing an RP sling, we will inject 20 cc of saline through a spinal needle behind the pubic bone on both the right and left side to hydrodissect the retropubic space and help push the bladder away from the pubic bone. Careful technique is then required to pass the curved trocar directly behind the bone, keeping the tip of the trocar directly against the bone as a guide, regardless of whether the approach chosen is "top-down" or "bottom-up."

Finding a Bladder Injury

The AUA states that cystoscopy should be considered a standard component of any surgical implantation of a sling [44]. Intraoperative bladder perforation is most reliably recognized with cystoscopy. If bladder injury is recognized at the time of cystoscopy, management consists of trocar replacement and repeat cystoscopy to confirm the proper location. When using a rigid cystoscope, it is important to use a 70-degree lens and have a reasonably full bladder to reduce the risk of a bladder fold that may hide a bladder injury. Of note, Cetinel et al. reported normal cystoscopy in two patients with bladder perforation. In those cases, the trocars were removed, and cystoscopy fluid began to leak from the suprapubic incisions [45]. In the series by Zyczynski et al., patients who sustained trocar bladder injury that was recognized cystoscopically at the time of retropubic MUS underwent sling removal and replacement at the time of the index surgery. They found that trocar injury was not associated with overall success, voiding dysfunction, recurrent urinary tract infection (UTI), or urge urinary incontinence [46]. No study has shown a link between recognized bladder trocar injury and postoperative bleeding, hematoma, or subsequent mesh perforation into the bladder or urethra. Thus, in patients with inadvertent bladder perforation, which is recognized and corrected at the index surgery, both the surgeon and the patient can be reassured that there are no long-term sequelae.

Management of Mesh Perforation of the Bladder

Patients who present at a later date with a bladder perforation most commonly sustained an unrecognized trocar perforation at the time of index surgery. They may present at any time after the index surgery with a variable symptomatology, including irritative voiding symptoms, recurrent UTI, bladder stones, or hematuria. Unlike asymptomatic vaginal wall mesh exposure, mesh perforation of the bladder should not be observed. As with any other foreign body in the bladder, the mesh can encrust, leading to stone formation (Fig. 19.2).

Small areas of bladder mesh may be managed with endoscopic techniques, including endoscopic scissors, transurethral resection (TUR), and holmium laser ablation. However, a separate abdominal, laparoscopic, or robotic approach to the retropubic space is often necessary to completely remove all mesh. Oh et al. reported successful deep TUR of transvesical mesh, with excision into the perivesical fat, in 13/14 patients with an 18-month follow-up [47]. Holmium laser excision of transvesical mesh has been reported by several authors [48, 49]. We would consider endoscopic removal of mesh only in cases with a small amount of mesh in the bladder and prefer open surgical removal with bladder or urethral reconstruction for a definitive single operation.

The open approach for removing mesh perforating the bladder can be vaginal or abdominal

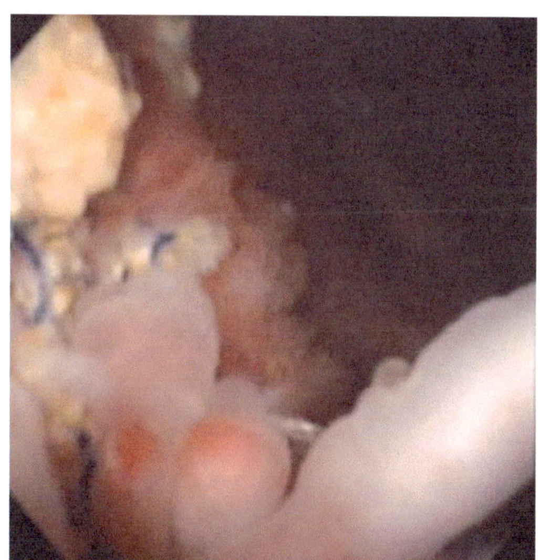

Fig. 19.2 Cystoscopic view of midurethral sling mesh perforation just inside the bladder, below the trigone (though ureteral orifices not seen in photo), with stones that have encrusted the mesh

(either open, laparoscopic, or robotic). Mesh perforating the bladder below the trigone is often accessible via a transvaginal approach. Supratrigonal perforations may require an abdominal approach. Cystoscopy is important to assess the proximity of the ureteral orifices to the perforation and to help guide the surgical approach. If the mesh perforation incorporates the ureteral orifice, or is within 5–10 mm, the patient may need an abdominal approach as well as a ureteral reimplant. During abdominal approach for mesh perforation, it may be necessary to open the bladder for exposure and to assure complete mesh removal (Fig. 19.3). This approach also permits placement of additional tissue for coverage, such as omentum, as per the surgeon's discretion.

There is a paucity of the literature that describes approaches other than open incisions. Fong et al. describe that regardless of the robotic approach, they all begin with an open vaginal incision in which mesh is identified and dissected as far cephalad as possible under vision. Then, with a transvaginal robotic-assisted approach, free-floating ports were used to dissect out the remaining mesh. Authors noted that the free-floating ports were preferred over a GelPoint mini due to difficulty maintaining an air seal in the vaginal cavity, and insufflation with gas was not required with adequate retraction. Alternatively, a transabdominal robotic-assisted removal of a mispositioned retropubic sling is also described, in which the transvaginal portion of the sling is passed into the pelvic cavity by the bedside surgeon through the endopelvic fascia. Ultimately, complete mesh removal was achieved in 60% of patients, another 33% with near complete or partial mesh removal achieved, and a few complications [67].

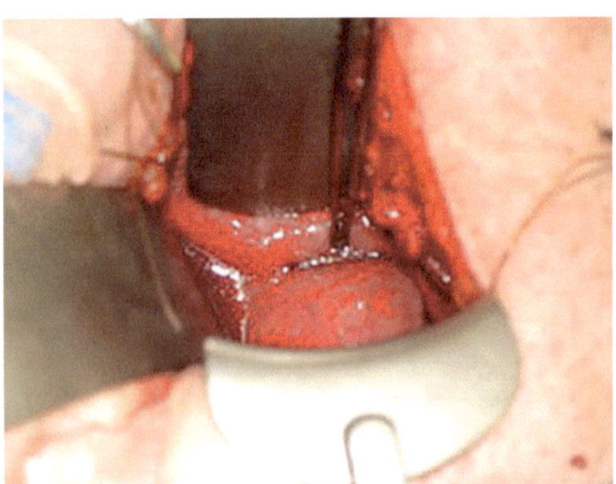

Fig. 19.3 Abdominal approach to supratrigonal mesh perforation of the bladder. The bladder has been opened for exposure. Careful evaluation of the ureteral orifices is required

When using a vaginal approach, an inverted U-shaped incision exposes the urethra, bladder neck and floor to permit removal all of the mesh within or near the bladder, which is the primary surgical goal. The mesh is identified and traced to the site of the bladder perforation. Complete sling removal will require a cystotomy, but usually the entire sling does not need to be removed. After careful closure of the cystotomy, the surgeon may use a Martius or other flap for additional coverage. Another advantage of the

Key Points: Management of Bladder Trocar Injury

- Prevention
  - Confirm empty bladder
  - Hydrodissection of retropubic space
  - Careful technique to hug pubic bone with RP trocar
- Identification
  - Careful cystourethroscopy
    - Look for hematuria/clot
    - Fill bladder completely—folds can hide mesh
- Management
  - Immediate recognition
    - Remove, replace trocar
    - Repeat cystoscopy to confirm placement
    - Foley per surgeon discretion
  - Delayed recognition
    - Location/access guides approach
      - Above trigone/through trigone
        - Evaluate proximity to ureteral orifices
        - May require combined vaginal/abdominal approach
          - Ureteral reimplantation?

- Below the trigone
  - Vaginal approach with inverted U-shaped incision
  - Follow mesh into bladder/cystotomy
  - Widely resect mesh
  - Close cystotomy

inverted U-shaped incision is that closure avoids overlapping suture lines, helping to minimize the risk of vesicovaginal fistula.

Urethra

Urethral Injury Is Less Common but Can Be More Complex

Urethral injuries are uncommon, occurring in 0.2–0.3% of MUS surgeries [40, 50]. The urethra can be injured during dissection or trocar placement, or delayed mesh perforation can occur secondary to technical factors or tissue characteristics. Patient factors that increase the risk of urethral perforation include previous surgery with scarring, any condition causing poor vascularity, including a history of radiation, estrogen deficiency, or urethral atrophy. Technical factors predisposing to delayed urethral perforation include over-tensioning of the sling, dissecting too deeply into the urethral wall, and placement of the sling trocar partially through the urethral wall at the time of surgery. Importantly, urethral dilation postoperatively to loosen an obstructive sling is not only ineffective at relieving obstruction but has also been reported to cause urethral perforation [7].

Prevention of Urethral Injury

The same surgical technique described to minimize vaginal wall mesh exposure also protects against urethral injury. The bladder is emptied with an indwelling Foley catheter. Midurethral hydrodissection is performed with 10 cc of saline. For the TO sling, hydrodissection can also be performed laterally to the vaginal sulcus. A toothed forceps is used to tension the vaginal wall over the midurethra, permitting easy entry of the 18-gauge injection needle into the proper surgical plane at an appropriate depth. Early vaginal wall blanching means the injection is too superficial; lack of an injection bleb indicates the hydrodissection is too deep. Hydrodissection creates a submucosal plane that helps to find proper vaginal wall thickness and avoids urethral thinning or injury. Direct visualization and palpation of the sling trocar trajectory with frequent palpation of the urethra (via palpation of the indwelling urethral catheter) informs the surgeon of proper urethral wall thickness during all phases of trocar passage.

Finding a Urethral Injury

Urethral mesh perforation is diagnosed with cystourethroscopy (Fig. 19.4). Flexible cystoscopy or the short-beaked 17-French "female" rigid cystoscope sheath is used (Fig. 19.5). The shorter length of this rigid cystoscope sheath permits fluid flow and urethral distention very close to the lens, which allows the surgeon to more carefully inspect the shorter female ure-

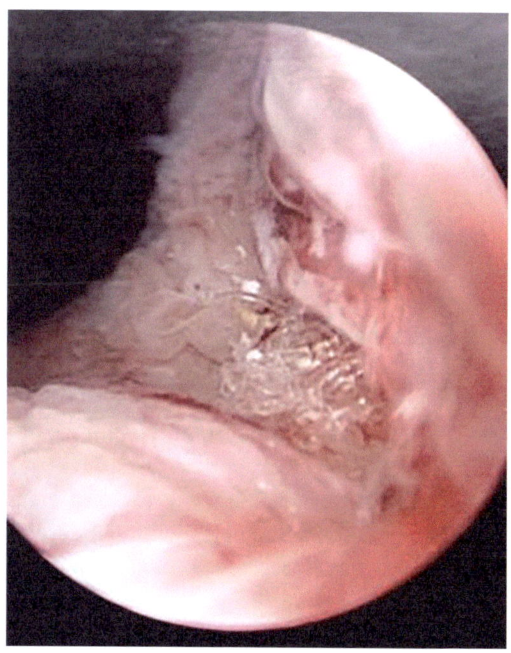

Fig. 19.4 Cystoscopic view of midurethral sling mesh at the proximal urethra. This location is amenable to open transvaginal excision with primary urethral repair

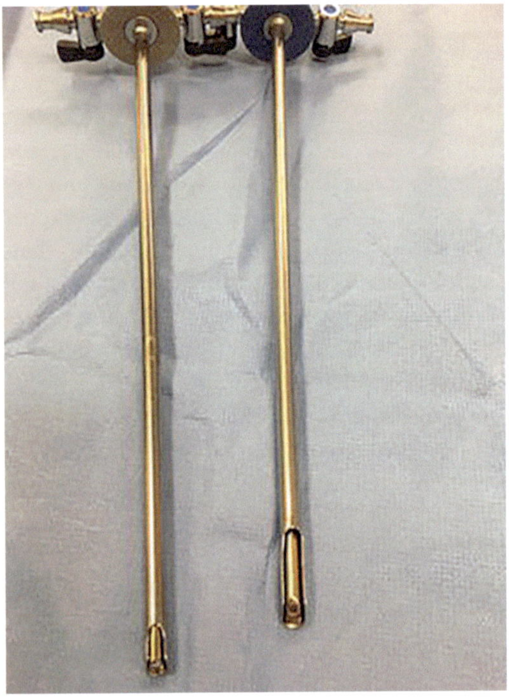

Fig. 19.5 Short-beaked 17-French "female" cystoscope sheath, seen on the left, compared to standard rigid cystoscope sheath on the right. The short "beak" allows fluid flow closer to the lens, allowing excellent distension and careful inspection of the shorter female urethra

thra. Unlike bladder or vaginal injury at the time of the initial surgery, if urethral injury is recognized at the time of index surgery, proper management includes sling removal and urethral repair. The primary surgeon must also decide at that time whether to proceed with concomitant sling placement. The authors prefer aborting the sling procedure if there is a urethral injury and allowing complete healing before attempting a second procedure.

Delayed urethral mesh perforation may present with a variety of nonspecific voiding symptoms. Sergouniotis reported that 77% of patients presented with de novo urgency [51], whereas Velemir reported that the most common presenting symptom was obstructed voiding [52]. Other less specific symptoms that may indicate urethral injury include recurrent urinary tract infection, urinary retention, recurrent incontinence, or hematuria. Less commonly, the patient presents with continuous incontinence, indicating a urethrovaginal fistula. The timing of presentation is variable. Amundsen reported that the diagnosis is typically made within 1 year of surgery, with a mean time from surgery to symptoms of 9 months [53], whereas in Hammad et al., 30% of the urethral injuries were diagnosed more than 1 year after index surgery [54].

Management of Urethral Mesh Perforation

Management options for delayed urethral perforation include a variety of endoscopic techniques or open transvaginal excision. The authors prefer transvaginal surgical excision as a first-line treatment. However, the literature also supports endoscopic management as the initial step for a small urethral mesh perforation. Successful endoscopic removal of urethral mesh is not definitive and does not ensure that all mesh is removed. There may be a risk of recurrent urethral mesh perforation that will require additional procedures for removal.

Reported endoscopic techniques include using hysteroscopic scissors through a cystoscope [55], electrosurgical resection, and use of the holmium laser. Jo et al. compared transurethral electrosurgical resection to holmium laser in patients with urethral and bladder mesh perforations and saw higher success rates after TUR, but TUR was also associated with subsequent vesicovaginal fistula development [56]. If endoscopic treatment fails, the next step in the management of urethral mesh perforation is a transvaginal approach and mesh excision with urethral repair.

A systematic review by Karim et al. showed that in patients with bladder or urethral mesh erosion following incontinence procedures, the success rate with laser excision of mesh was 67–92% and with endoscopic excision (with electric loop or laparoscopic scissors) was 80–98%, with many patients in both groups requiring repeat procedures. The most common complication rate was SUI, with 21% of patients experiencing SUI in both groups [68].

An inverted U-shaped incision via an open transvaginal approach provides excellent exposure to the urethra and bladder neck. The goal is to completely remove the mesh from the area of

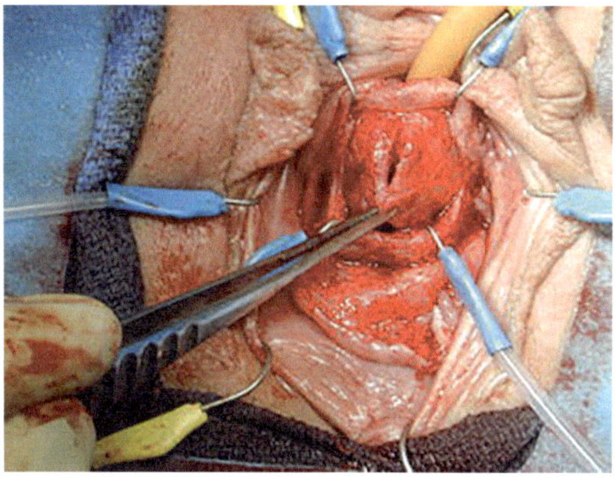

Fig. 19.6 Urethrotomy after urethral perforation and mesh removal. Forceps are approximating the longitudinal urethral wall opening that will be closed vertically, the periurethral fascia (retracted by blue stays) will be closed transversely, followed by closure of the vaginal wall U-shaped incision, seen lying at the 6-o'clock position. This multilayered closure with non-overlapping suture lines will minimize the risk of urethrovaginal fistula

the urethral injury and subsequent repair. Layered closure should avoid overlapping suture lines, minimizing the risk of urethrovaginal fistula (Fig. 19.6). The RP sling is grasped and dissected back behind the pubic bone until it enters the retropubic space. A TO sling should be followed laterally where it courses under the pubic rami. The mesh arms traveling behind the pubic bone or through the obturator foramen are not removed unless there are other special circumstances, such as poorly incorporated mesh suggesting infection. Prior to closure of the vaginal incision, a Martius flap may be used for additional coverage, based on the surgeon's discretion, followed by an indwelling urethral catheter drainage for 7–14 days. Some surgeons will place a fascial sling in the same setting to manage potential recurrent SUI.

There is limited data to support concomitant autologous fascia pubovaginal sling (AF-PVS) placement versus staged placement after initial mesh repair, though one study by McCoy et al. showed there was no statistical difference in objective success between the two groups. In this study, 30 patients underwent concomitant mesh excision and AF-PVS placement compared to 16 who underwent staged AF-PVS after their last mesh excision (with a mean of 7 months since the last mesh excision). Additionally, the authors highlight the potential selection bias in that those undergoing staged AF-PVS were more likely to have severe issues and tended to have mesh erosion into the GU tract (63% vs 17%, $p = 0.003$) [69]. The authors do not favor the placement of any type of sling at the same time as urethral mesh removal to allow for optimal healing of the initial repair.

Key Points: Management of Delayed Urethral Perforation

- Diagnosis
  - Cystoscopy with short-beaked cystoscope sheath
- Treatment
  - Inverted U-shaped incision
  - Remove mesh from urethra, resect mesh from urethra/bladder location
  - Close urethra with 3-0 or 4-0 SAS
  - Consider use of Martius flap
  - Foley catheter × 7–14 days +/− VCUG

Women with delayed urethral perforation should be counseled extensively on the increased risk of persistent SUI after urethral repair. In Colhoun et al., 4/5 patients reported persistent SUI at a mean of 54 months postoperatively; 2/5 underwent pelvic floor physical therapy (PFPT); 1/5 underwent pubovaginal sling placement; 1/5 underwent both PFPT and pubovaginal sling placement; and 1 remained incontinent and declined any additional intervention [57].

Bowel

Sling Perforation of the Bowel

Bowel injury during MUS placement is exceedingly rare, reported in 0–0.04% of cases [30, 58, 59]. All reported bowel injuries have occurred after the RP sling, which is intuitive, considering that the TO sling avoids the abdominal cavity. Typically, bowel injuries occur in patients with a history of prior abdominal or pelvic surgery and adhesions of the bowel to the pelvis. Most commonly, the patient presents within hours to several days after surgery with abdominal pain, nausea, vomiting, decreased urine output, other signs of peritonitis, and possibly passage of bowel contents through the suprapubic trocar sites. However, patients can have significantly delayed and atypical presentations. Some patients may not have signs or symptoms of peritonitis at presentation [60], and Elliott reported an asymptomatic patient whose bowel injury was found incidentally [61]. Chelvaratnam and Phillips both describe patients who presented years after their RP sling. One report describes a patient with symptoms of diarrhea and right-sided abdominal pain who was found to have the RP sling perforated into the ascending colon [62]. Another patient presented with a de novo small bowel obstruction whose laparotomy showed that the sling had penetrated the peritoneum and caused inflammation near the terminal ileum, leading to local adhesions and bowel obstruction [63]. Bowel injury in the patient with peritoneal signs may be confirmed with free infra-diaphragmatic air on plain abdominal x-ray. In a patient with a less clear or more insidious clinical course, a CT scan of the abdomen and pelvis and/or colonoscopy is appropriate. In one case report, a sigmoid colon perforation was found following retropubic TVT mesh placement on colonoscopy after the patient presented within a 4-month period after surgery; this was managed with laparotomy and partial tape removal [70].

Treatment consists of abdominal exploration to remove the mesh and perform bowel repair. While Meschia and Elliott both report laparoscopic management, others prefer laparotomy to evaluate and repair the bowel, irrigate the abdomen, and evacuate spilled bowel contents. The mesh is localized and excised back to the retroperitoneal space, with closure of the peritoneal defect. The injured bowel may require resection and primary repair as per the surgeon's judgment. The patient is managed hemodynamically and placed on broad-spectrum antibiotics. Others may elect for observation if the patient is asymptomatic, the perforation is small, and is found incidentally years after initial sling placement, such as during routine colonoscopy [71].

To prevent potential bowel injury, de Almeida recommends preoperative CT in high-risk patients to permit localization of the bowel and to evaluate for any pelvic adhesions, or one can choose to place a TO instead to avoid the pelvis and any bowel injury [60]. Overall, the risk of bowel injury remains low but is an important consideration when choosing which sling procedure to perform in a given patient.

Key Points: Prevention of Bowel Injury

- Risk factors: prior abdominal or pelvic surgery
- Consider CT abdomen/pelvis
- Surgical technique
  - Choose another approach—TO or SIS instead of RP
  - Hydrodissection of retropubic space
  - Careful technique to hug pubic bone with RP trocar

Conclusion

Midurethral mesh slings are the gold standard treatment for surgical management of female SUI. The complications are acceptably low, but the surgeon must be properly trained and maintain a surgical volume to remain competent. MUS surgeons must practice surgical techniques that minimize these complications, and importantly, be able to recognize and manage or refer complications of vaginal wall mesh exposure and adjacent organ injury when encountered.

References

1. Ulmsten U, Petros P. Intravaginal slingplasty (IVS): an ambulatory surgical procedure for treatment of female urinary incontinence. Scand J Urol Nephrol. 1995;29(1):75–82.
2. Ford AA, Rogerson L, Cody JD, Aluko P, Ogah JA. Mid-urethral sling operations for stress uri-

nary incontinence in women. Cochrane Database Syst Rev. 2017;7:CD006375. https://doi.org/10.1002/14651858.CD006375.pub4.
3. Jonsson Funk M, Levin PJ, Wu JM. Trends in the surgical management of stress urinary incontinence. Obstet Gynecol. 2012;119(4):845–51.
4. Haylen BT, Freeman RM, Swift SE, et al. An International Urogynecological Association (IUGA)/International Continence Society (ICS) joint terminology and classification of the complications related directly to the insertion of prostheses (meshes, implants, tapes) and grafts in female pelvic floor surgery. Neurourol Urodyn. 2011;30(1):2–12.
5. Carter E, Johnson EE, Still M, Al-Assaf AS, Bryant A, Aluko P, Jeffery ST, Nambiar A. Single-incision sling operations for urinary incontinence in women. Cochrane Datab Syst Rev 2023;10:CD008709. https://doi.org/10.1002/14651858.CD008709.pub4. Accessed 07 Sept 2024.
6. Barber MD, Weidner AC, Sokol AI, et al. Single-incision mini-sling compared with tension-free vaginal tape for the treatment of stress urinary incontinence: a randomized controlled trial. Obstet Gynecol. 2012;119(2 Pt 1):328–37.
7. Delorme E. Transobturator urethral suspension. Mini-invasive procedure in the treatment of stress urinary incontinence in women. Prog Urol. 2001;11(6):1306–12. French.
8. Karram MM, Segal JL, et al. Complications and untoward effects of the tension-free vaginal tape procedure. Obstet Gynecol. 2003;101(5):929–32.
9. Kuuva N, Nilsson CG. A nationwide analysis of complications associated with the tension-free vaginal tape (TVT) procedure. Acta Obstet Gynecol Scand. 2002;81(1):72–7.
10. Rodríguez LV, Raz S. Prospective analysis of patients treated with a distal urethral polypropylene sling for symptoms of stress urinary incontinence: surgical outcome and satisfaction determined by patient driven questionnaires. J Urol. 2003;170(3):857–63.
11. Levin I, Groutz A, Gold R, et al. Surgical complications and medium-term outcome results of tension-free vaginal tape: a prospective study of 313 consecutive patients. Neurourol Urodyn. 2004;23(1):7–9.
12. Tsivian A, Kessler O, Mogutin B, et al. Tape related complications of the tension-free vaginal tape procedure. J Urol. 2004;171(2 Pt 1):762–4.
13. Kobashi KC, Govier FE. Management of vaginal erosion of polypropylene mesh slings. J Urol. 2003;169(6):2242–3.
14. Jonsson Funk M, Siddiqui NY, Kawasaki A, et al. Long-term outcomes after stress urinary incontinence surgery. Obstet Gynecol. 2012;120(1):83–90.
15. Richter HE, Albo ME, Zyczynski HM, et al. Retropubic versus transobturator midurethral slings for stress incontinence. N Engl J Med. 2010;362(22):2066–76.
16. Domingo S, Alamá P, Ruiz N, et al. Diagnosis, management and prognosis of vaginal erosion after transobturator suburethral tape procedure using a non-woven thermally bonded polypropylene mesh. J Urol. 2005;173(5):1627–30.
17. Kim J, Lucioni A, Govier F, et al. Worse long-term surgical outcomes in elderly patients undergoing SPARC retropubic midurethral sling placement. BJU Int. 2011;108(5):708–12.
18. Jonsson Funk M, Siddiqui NY, Pate V, et al. Sling revision/removal for mesh erosion and urinary retention: long-term risk and predictors. Am J Obstet Gynecol. 2013;208(1):73.e1–7.
19. Amid PK. Classification of biomaterials and their related complications in abdominal wall hernia surgery. Hernia. 1997;1:15–21.
20. Dietz HP, Vancaillie P, Svehla M, et al. Mechanical properties of urogynecologic implant materials. Int Urogynecol J Pelvic Floor Dysfunct. 2003;14(4):239–43.
21. Slack M, Sandhu JS, Staskin DR, et al. In vivo comparison of suburethral sling materials. Int Urogynecol J Pelvic Floor Dysfunct. 2006;17(2):106–10.
22. Karsenty G, Boman J, Elzayat E, et al. Severe soft tissue infection of the thigh after vaginal erosion of transobturator tape for stress urinary incontinence. Int Urogynecol J Pelvic Floor Dysfunct. 2007;18(2):207–12.
23. Deffieux X, Daher N, Mansoor A, et al. Transobturator TVT-O versus retropubic TVT: results of a multicenter randomized controlled trial at 24 months follow-up. Int Urogynecol J. 2010;21(11):1337–45.
24. Novara G, Galfano A, Boscolo-Berto R, et al. Complication rates of tension-free midurethral slings in the treatment of female stress urinary incontinence: a systematic review and meta-analysis of randomized controlled trials comparing tension-free midurethral tapes to other surgical procedures and different devices. Eur Urol. 2008;53(2):288–308.
25. Abdel-Fattah M, Ramsay I, Pringle S, et al. Evaluation of transobturator tapes (E-TOT) study: randomised prospective single-blinded study comparing inside-out vs. outside-in transobturator tapes in management of urodynamic stress incontinence: short term outcomes. Eur J Obstet Gynecol Reprod Biol. 2010;149(1):106–11.
26. But I, Faganelj M. Complications and short-term results of two different transobturator techniques for surgical treatment of women with urinary incontinence: a randomized study. Int Urogynecol J Pelvic Floor Dysfunct. 2008;19(6):857–61.
27. Schimpf MO, Rahn DD, Wheeler TL, et al. Sling surgery for stress urinary incontinence in women: a systematic review and metaanalysis. Am J Obstet Gynecol. 2014;211(1):71.e1–27.
28. Osborn DJ, Dmochowski RR, Harris CJ, et al. Analysis of patient and technical factors associated with midurethral sling mesh exposure and perforation. Int J Urol. 2014;21(11):1167–70.
29. Kokanali MK, Doğanay M, Aksakal O, et al. Risk factors for mesh erosion after vaginal sling procedures for urinary incontinence. Eur J Obstet Gynecol Reprod Biol. 2014;177:146–50.

30. Kenton K, Stoddard AM, Zyczynski H, et al. 5-year longitudinal followup after retropubic and transobturator mid urethral slings. J Urol. 2015;193(1):203–10.
31. Nilsson CG, Palva K, Aarnio R, et al. Seventeen years' follow-up of the tension-free vaginal tape procedure for female stress urinary incontinence. Int Urogynecol J. 2013;24(8):1265–9.
32. Svenningsen R, Staff AC, Schiøtz HA, et al. Risk factors for long-term failure of the retropubic tension-free vaginal tape procedure. Neurourol Urodyn. 2014;33(7):1140–6.
33. Groutz A, Rosen G, Gold R, et al. Long-term outcome of transobturator tension-free vaginal tape: efficacy and risk factors for surgical failure. J Womens Health (Larchmt). 2011;20(10):1525–8.
34. Higgins EW, Rao A, Baumann SS, et al. Effect of estrogen replacement on the histologic response to polypropylene mesh implanted in the rabbit vagina model. Am J Obstet Gynecol. 2009;201(5):505.e1–9.
35. Myers DL, LaSala CA. Conservative surgical management of Mersilene mesh suburethral sling erosion. Am J Obstet Gynecol. 1998;179(6 Pt 1):1424–8.
36. Kuhn A, Burkhard F, Eggemann C, et al. Sexual function after suburethral sling removal for dyspareunia. Surg Endosc. 2009;23(4):765–8.
37. Seklehner S, Laudano MA, Xie D, et al. A meta-analysis of the performance of retropubic mid urethral slings versus transobturator mid urethral slings. J Urol. 2015;193(3):909–15.
38. Porena M, Costantini E, Frea B, et al. Tension-free vaginal tape versus transobturator tape as surgery for stress urinary incontinence: results of a multicentre randomised trial. Eur Urol. 2007;52(5):1481–90.
39. Tamussino K, Hanzal E, Kölle D, et al. Transobturator tapes for stress urinary incontinence: results of the Austrian registry. Am J Obstet Gynecol. 2007;197(6):634.e1–5.
40. Stav K, Dwyer PL, Rosamilia A, et al. Risk factors for trocar injury to the bladder during mid urethral sling procedures. J Urol. 2009;182(1):174–9.
41. Chen HY, Ho M, Hung YC, et al. Analysis of risk factors associated with vaginal erosion after synthetic sling procedures for stress urinary incontinence. Int Urogynecol J Pelvic Floor Dysfunct. 2008;19(1):117–21.
42. Bohlin KS, Ankardal M, Pedroletti C, et al. The influence of the modifiable life-style factors body mass index and smoking on the outcome of mid-urethral sling procedures for female urinary incontinence. Int Urogynecol J. 2015;26(3):343–51.
43. Lovatsis D, Gupta C, Dean E, et al. Tension-free vaginal tape procedure is an ideal treatment for obese patients. Am J Obstet Gynecol. 2003;189(6):1601–4.
44. Dmochowski RR, Blaivas JM, Gormley EA, et al. Update of AUA guideline on the surgical management of female stress urinary incontinence. J Urol. 2010;183(5):1906–14.
45. Cetinel B, Demirkesen O, Onal B, et al. Are there any factors predicting the cure and complication rates of tension-free vaginal tape? Int Urogynecol J Pelvic Floor Dysfunct. 2004;15(3):188–93.
46. Zyczynski HM, Sirls LT, Greer WJ, et al. Findings of universal cystoscopy at incontinence surgery and their sequelae. Am J Obstet Gynecol. 2014;210(5):480.e1–8.
47. Oh TH, Ryu DS. Transurethral resection of intravesical mesh after midurethral sling procedures. J Endourol. 2009;23(8):1333–7.
48. Ogle CA, Linder BJ, Elliott DS. Holmium laser excision for urinary mesh erosion: a minimally invasive treatment with favorable long-term results. Int Urogynecol J. 2015;26:1645–8.
49. Giri SK, Drumm J, Flood HD. Endoscopic holmium laser excision of intravesical tension-free vaginal tape and polypropylene suture after anti-incontinence procedures. J Urol. 2005;174(4 Pt 1):1306–7.
50. Clemons JL, Weinstein M, Guess MK, et al. Impact of the 2011 FDA transvaginal mesh safety update on AUGS members' use of synthetic mesh and biologic grafts in pelvic reconstructive surgery. Female Pelvic Med Reconstr Surg. 2013;19(4):191–8.
51. Sergouniotis F, Jarlshammar B, Larsson PG. Urethral complications after tension-free vaginal tape procedures: a surgical management case series. World J Nephrol. 2015;4(3):396–405.
52. Velemir L, Amblard J, Jacquetin B, et al. Urethral erosion after suburethral synthetic slings: risk factors, diagnosis, and functional outcome after surgical management. Int Urogynecol J Pelvic Floor Dysfunct. 2008;19(7):999–1006.
53. Amundsen CL, Flynn BJ, Webster GD. Urethral erosion after synthetic and nonsynthetic pubovaginal slings: differences in management and continence outcome. J Urol. 2003;170(1):134–7.
54. Hammad FT, Kennedy-Smith A, Robinson RG. Erosions and urinary retention following polypropylene synthetic sling: Australasian survey. Eur Urol. 2005;47(5):641–7.
55. McLennan MT. Transurethral resection of transvaginal tape. Int Urogynecol J Pelvic Floor Dysfunct. 2004;15(5):360–2.
56. Jo DJ, Lee YS, Oh TH, et al. Outcomes of transurethral removal of intravesical or intraurethral mesh following midurethral sling surgery. Korean J Urol. 2011;52(12):829–34.
57. Colhoun A, Rapp DE. Long-term outcomes after repair of transurethral perforation of midurethral sling. Female Pelvic Med Reconstr Surg. 2016 Apr 6. [Epub ahead of print].
58. Meschia M, Busacca M, Pifarotti P, et al. Bowel perforation during insertion of tension-free vaginal tape (TVT). Int Urogynecol J Pelvic Floor Dysfunct. 2002;13(4):263–5.
59. Tamussino KF, Hanzal E, Kölle D, et al. Tension-free vaginal tape operation: results of the Austrian registry. Obstet Gynecol. 2001;98(5 Pt 1):732–6.
60. de Almeida SH, Brandina R, Dall'Aqua V. Small-bowel obstruction and bladder injury due to retro-

pubic sling malposition in the peritoneal cavity. Int Urogynecol J. 2013;24(8):1411–2.
61. Elliott JE, Maslow KD. Remote discovery of an asymptomatic bowel perforation by a mid-urethral sling. Int Urogynecol J. 2012;23(2):243–5.
62. Chelvaratnam U, Terlevich A. An unusual case of abdominal pain and diarrhea. Tension-free vaginal tape eroding into the ascending colon. Gastroenterology. 2015;149(2):296–7.
63. Phillips L, Flood CG, Schulz JA. Case report of tension-free vaginal tape-associated bowel obstruction and relationship to body habitus. Int Urogynecol J Pelvic Floor Dysfunct. 2009;20(3):367–8.
64. Siblini T, Baracy M, Kulkarni S, et al. Midurethral sling mesh exposure confers a high risk of persistent stress urinary incontinence. Int Urogynecol J. 2024;35:1177–82.
65. Frigerio M, Barba M, Marino G, Volonte S, Cola A. Pelvic floor ultrasound evaluation in the diagnosis of exposure of synthetic implanted materials in the lower urinary tract. Int J Gynaecol Obstet. 2023;163(3):834–9. https://doi.org/10.1002/ijgo.14933. Epub 2023 Jun 18.
66. Karmakar D, Dwyer PL, Nikpoor P. Mid-urethral sling revision for mesh exposure-long-term outcomes of two surgical techniques from a comparative clinical retrospective cohort study. BJOG. 2020;127(8):1027–33. https://doi.org/10.1111/1471-0528.16149. Epub 2020 Feb 27
67. Fong E, Yao HH, Zargar H, Connell HE. Early experience of transabdominal and novel transvaginal robot-assisted laparoscopic removal of transvaginal mesh. J Endourol. 2022;36(4):477–92. https://doi.org/10.1089/end.2021.0520.
68. Karim SS, Pietropaolo A, Skolarikos A, Aboumarzouk O, Kallidonis P, Tailly T, de Coninck V, Keller EX, Somani BK. Role of endoscopic management in synthetic sling/mesh erosion following previous incontinence surgery: a systematic review from European Association of Urologists Young Academic Urologists (YAU) and Uro-technology (ESUT) groups. Int Urogynecol J. 2020;31(1):45–53. https://doi.org/10.1007/s00192-019-04087-5. Epub 2019 Aug 29. PMID: 31468095; PMCID: PMC6949195.
69. McCoy O, Vaughan T, Nickles SW, Ashley M, MacLachlan LS, Ginsberg D, Rovner E. Outcomes of autologous fascia Pubovaginal sling for patients with transvaginal mesh related complications requiring mesh removal. J Urol. 2016;196(2):484–9. https://doi.org/10.1016/j.juro.2016.02.2976. Epub 2016 Mar 17.
70. Huang X, Jiang H, Xie L. Case report of sigmoid colon perforation and colocutaneous fistula due to retropubic midurethral sling placement for stress urinary incontinence. BMC Urol. 2020;20(1):33. https://doi.org/10.1186/s12894-020-00600-x. PMID: 32197605; PMCID: PMC7082911.
71. Cohen SA, Goldman HB. Mesh perforation into a viscus in the setting of pelvic floor surgery—presentation and management. Curr Urol Rep. 2016;17:64. https://doi-org.proxy.lib.umich.edu/10.1007/s11934-016-0621-3.

20 Mini-Slings: Unique Issues

Kristina A. Burger, Dina A. Bastawros, and Michael J. Kennelly

Abbreviations

AJOG	American Journal of Obstetrics and Gynecology
AUGS	American Urogynecologic Society
ICS	International Continence Society
IUGA	International Urogynecological Association
MUS	Midurethral sling
PGI-I	Patient Global Impression of Improvement questionnaire
RCT	Randomized controlled trial
SIMS	Single-incision mini-sling
SUFU	Society of Urodynamics, Female Pelvic Medicine & Urogenital Reconstruction
SUI	Stress urinary incontinence
TOT	Transobturator tape
TVT	Tension free vaginal tape
UI	Urge incontinence

K. A. Burger (✉) · M. J. Kennelly
Urogynecology and Reconstructive Pelvic Surgery, Atrium Health Wake Forest Baptist, Charlotte, NC, USA
e-mail: michael.kennelly@atriumhealth.org

D. A. Bastawros
Urogynecology and Reconstructive Pelvic Surgery, Novant Health Pelvic Health Center, Winston-salem, NC, USA

Introduction

The synthetic midurethral sling (MUS) is the most extensively studied surgical procedure for the treatment of stress urinary incontinence (SUI) [1]. Regardless of the route of placement, the MUS has been shown to be highly effective and safe [1] and has been endorsed by the American Urogynecologic Society (AUGS) and the Society of Urodynamics, Female Pelvic Medicine & Urogenital Reconstruction (SUFU) as the standard of care for the treatment of SUI [2]. However, the MUS procedure is not without risk. As with all surgical procedures, bleeding, infection, and damage to nearby structures such as the bowel, bladder, and urethra are possible. Additionally, de novo vaginal or extravaginal pain as well as mesh exposure are unique complications of the MUS procedure. In an attempt to minimize these risks, the single-incision mini-sling (SIMS) was developed as an alternative minimally invasive treatment for SUI that could potentially be performed in an ambulatory office setting.

The design of these SIMS is aimed at providing fewer complications. SIMS are shorter in length and thus have less mesh than the traditional MUS. Additionally, these slings only require a single vaginal incision. SIMS are anchored to various structures within the obturator space, thus avoiding "blind" passage through the retropubic and obturator spaces. Table 20.1 summarizes the various characteris-

H. B. Goldman, J. Zillioux (eds.), *Complications of Urogynecology and Reconstructive Pelvic Surgery*, https://doi.org/10.1007/978-3-032-00339-3_20

Table 20.1 Characteristics of currently available single incision incision mini-slings

	Needleless®	Solyx™	Altis®	Ophira™	Desara® One
Manufacturer	Neomedic International (Terrassa, Spain)	Boston Scientific (Somerville, NJ)	Coloplast (Humbleback, Denmark)	Promedon (Córdoba, Argentina)	Caldera Medical (Westlake Village, CA)
Year introduced	2007	2009	2012	2012	2020
Trajectory	Transobturator	Transobturator	Transobturator	Transobturator	Transobturator
Fixation point	Obturator internus muscle	Obturator internus muscle	Obturator membrane	Obturator internus muscle	Obturator internus muscle
Fixation tips	Pocket positioning, no anchor tips	Permanent polypropylene anchors	Permanent polypropylene anchors	Multipoint fishbone-like polypropylene tips	Permanent polypropylene anchors
Tensioning method	Bidirectional	By advancement, prior to device release	Bidirectional even after device release	By advancement, prior to device release	Bidirectional, prior to device release
Mesh size (cm)	11.4 × 1.2	9 × 1.1	7.75 × 1.1	10.2 × 0.9	9.05 × 1.1
Mesh weight	60 g/m^2	100 g/m^2	70 g/m^2	69 g/m^2	105 g/m^2
Mesh thickness	0.4 mm	0.66 mm	0.3 mm	–	0.69 mm
Pore size (approximate)	55% porosity	1182 μm	550 × 170 μm	500–1000 μm	1000 μm
Color	Clear	Clear and blue	White	Clear with blue midline circle	Blue
Needle	None	One needle and driver	Two needle introducers	One needle and driver	One needle and driver
Needle diameter (mm)	N/A	3.81	–	2.2	2.4
Needle disengagement	N/A	One step	One step	One step	One step
Midline mark	Yes	Yes (on introducer)	No	Yes	Yes (on introducer)
FDA approved	Yes	Yes	Yes	No	Yes
522 completed	Yes	Yes	Yes	No	No

tics of SIMS currently available. While many SIMS are no longer available due to product discontinuation, Table 20.2 summarizes historically available SIMS, as many patients may have these devices implanted and reconstructive surgeons may need to manage complications related to these products [3]. This chapter will focus on the unique aspects associated with SIMS. While portions of the following chapter describe SIMS as a group, each SIMS is unique and should be evaluated on its own merits due to differences in design as further described in Table 20.1.

Table 20.2 Characteristics of historically available single incision mini-slings

	TVT-Secur™	MiniArc™	Ajust™	MiniArc Precise™
Manufacturer	Ethicon (Somerville, NJ)	Astora Women's Health (Eden Prairie, MN)	Bard (Covington, GA)	Astora Women's Health (Eden Prairie, MN)
Year introduced	2006	2007	2009	2010
Year discontinued	2012	2016	2016	2016
Trajectory	Transobturator or retropubic	Transobturator	Transobturator	Transobturator
Fixation point	Obturator internus muscle ("hammock") or urogenital diaphragm ("U")	Obturator internus muscle	Obturator membrane	Obturator internus muscle
Fixation tips	Absorbable 2 cm fixating tips coated with PDS™ and Vicryl™	Permanent self-fixating tips	Permanent self-fixating polypropylene anchors	Permanent self-fixating tips that are tapered and reinforced
Tensioning method	Only by advancement, prior to device release	Optional redocking feature	Bidirectional independent adjustment	Only by advancement, prior to device release
Intraoperative tightening	No	Yes (optional redocking feature)	Yes (and loosening)	Yes (optional redocking feature)
Mesh size (cm)	1.1 × 8	1.1 × 8.5	1.2 × 5	1.1 × 8.5
Needle	Two needles and driver	One needle and driver	One needle driver and flexible stylet	One needle and driver
Needle diameter (mm)	8	2.3	5	2.3
Needle disengagement	Two step	One step	One step	One step
Midline mark	No	Yes	Yes	Yes
Pull-out force (lb)	1.9	5.5	6.56	5.75

Preoperative Considerations

While many SIMS have at one time been available, there are four currently available (Tables 20.1 and 20.2). Each currently available option differs in various ways; however, they are all lightweight type 1 polypropylene mesh devices, and all are placed via a horizontal transobturator trajectory. To date, there is no published research evaluating the safety or efficacy of the Desara ® One SIMS.

In general, other than the proposed benefits of a single vaginal incision and a smaller amount of mesh compared to a full-length sling, there are certain patient considerations that may make a SIMS preferable. For patients with extensive abdominal surgeries and possible intra-abdominal adhesions, SIMS may be preferred to the retropubic sling as the trocars do not penetrate the retropubic space. Additionally, for patients with high body mass index, SIMS may be preferred as the length of the full-length MUS may not be long enough to reach the skin adequately. Finally, for patients with significant medical comorbidities prohibiting general anesthesia, SIMS can be placed under local anesthesia.

Initially, there was concern regarding the efficacy of the SIMS due to data showing significantly lower cure rates compared to the first SIMS, TVT-Secur ™ (Ethicon, Somerville, New Jersey, USA) [4]. The TVT-Secur device utilized a poor fixation method, an absorbable fleece material, and is no longer on the market due to voluntary cessation of production by Ethicon in

2012. However, more recent data on newer SIMS devices, excluding the TVT-Secur device, have been published, illustrating similar efficacy of the SIMS to the traditional full-length MUS [5]. The largest systematic review and meta-analysis to date on SIMS is the 2023 Cochrane Review, which included 62 studies with 8051 women. In this review, excluding those studies including the TVT-Secur device, SIMS were likely as effective as traditional full-length slings at 12 months. Long-term efficacy still needs to be determined [5].

Perioperative Considerations

The general surgical procedure is similar among all SIMS, with some particular differences. Typically, after local anesthetic is utilized for hydrodissection, a full-thickness vertical midline incision underneath the midurethra is completed to accommodate the width of the sling. Periurethral dissection is then performed bilaterally in the direction of eventual trocar placement. The sling is then placed underneath the midurethra utilizing trocars, and cystourethroscopy is performed to confirm the absence of lower urinary tract injury. The sling is then positioned to support the urethra, and the vaginal incision is closed [6]. Each currently available SIMS has various differences, particularly with anchor loading and deployment. After anchor deployment into the obturator membrane, the Altis ® device (Fig. 20.1) is adjustable via the dynamic anchor technology; this is the only currently available SIMS that is adjustable after anchor deployment. The Desara ® One (Fig. 20.2) implant is loaded onto the introducer until a click is felt, indicating complete engagement. The anchor is deployed into the obturator internus muscle by pressing down on the introducer release buttons. The Needless ® (Fig. 20.3) device does not utilize traditional anchors, but instead utilizes a pocket positioning and anchoring system which is guided into and expanded within the obturator internus muscle with a hemostat. The Ophira ® (Fig. 20.4) device has multiple fixation points along its self-fixating arms and has blue loosening sutures at each base to allow for correction of excessive tensioning. Finally, the Solyx ® (Fig. 20.5) device is tensioned by delivery device advancement and retraction.

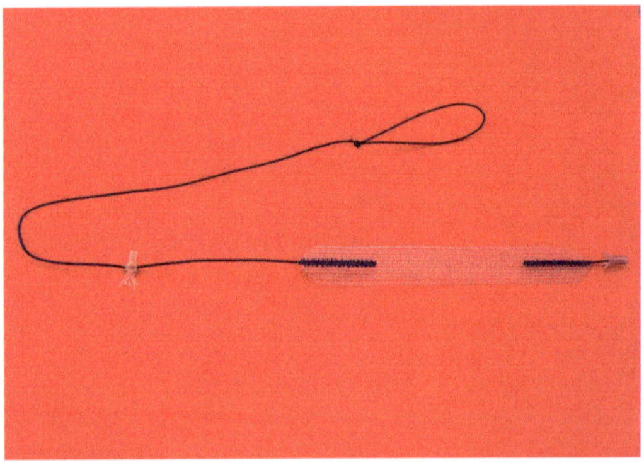

Fig. 20.1 Altis ®. The Altis's 1.1 × 7.75 cm polypropylene mesh is placed through the obturator membrane with self-fixating anchors. Post-insertion adjustments can be made related to the fixed anchor [manufactured by Coloplast, Minneapolis, Minnesota, USA]

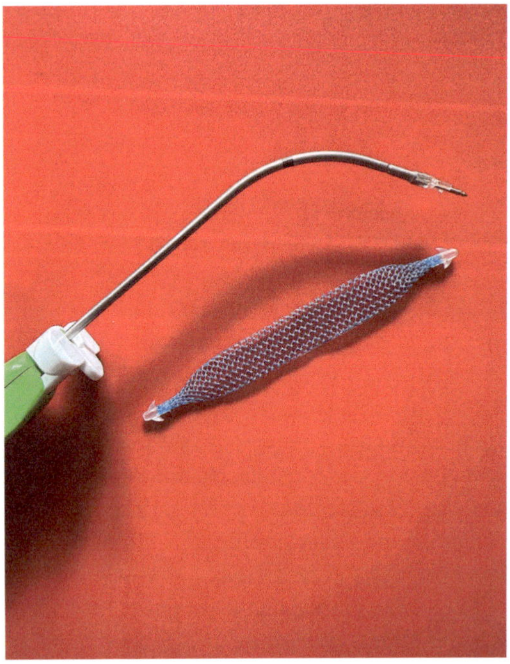

Fig. 20.2 Desara ® One. The Desara One 9.05 × 1.1 mesh is secured into the obturator internus muscle via permanent polypropylene anchors [manufactured by Caldera Medical, Westlake Village, CA]

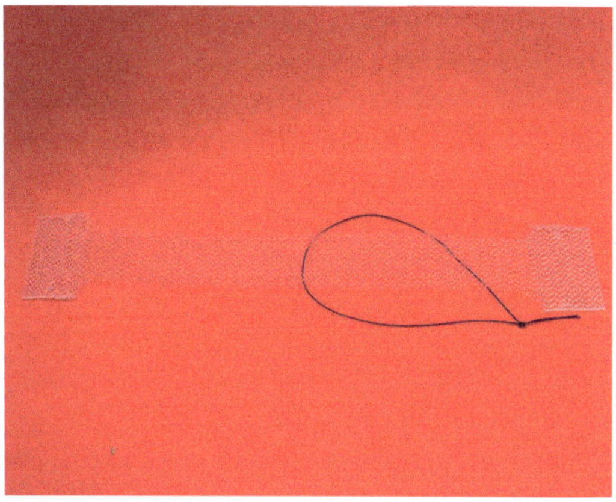

Fig. 20.3 Needless ® System. The Needleless 1.4 × 12 cm polypropylene mesh is placed in the obturator internus fascia without any anchor tips [manufactured by Neomedic International, Terrassa, Spain]

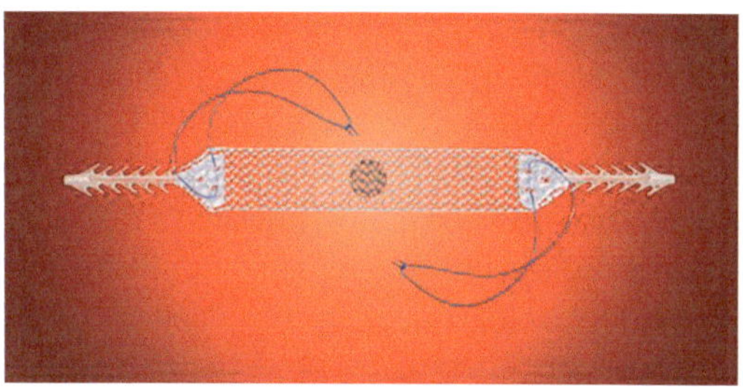

Fig. 20.4 Ophira ™ Mini Sling. The Ophira Mini Sling System's 0.9 × 10.2 cm polypropylene mesh uses several self-fixating tips placed in the obturator internus membrane with a 2.2 cm needle [manufactured by and image provided courtesy of Promedon, Cordona, Argentina]

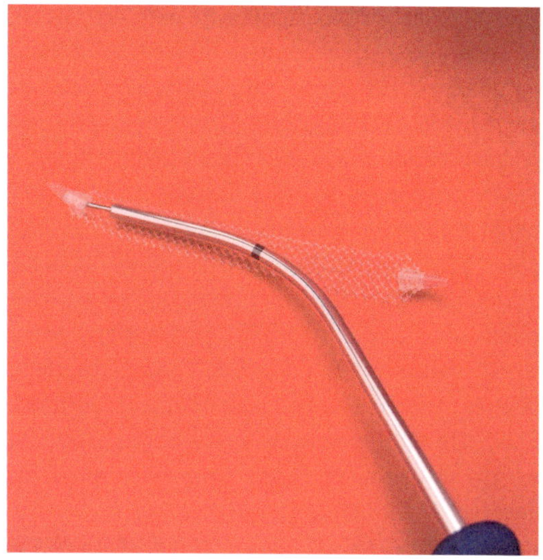

Fig. 20.5 Solyx ™ Single Incision System. The Solyx's 9 × 1.1 cm polypropylene mesh with fused carrier barbs is placed in the obturator internus muscle with a snap-fit delivery device [manufactured by Boston Scientific Corporation, Natick, Massachusetts, USA]

Postoperative Considerations

SIMS were designed to decrease the complications inherent in 3-incision full-length MUS sling procedures. By only requiring a single vaginal incision and by not passing through various muscles within the groin (obturator externus, adductor brevis, and gracilis muscles), SIMS placement should decrease the frequency and severity of groin pain experienced after full-length midurethral slings (MUS). Additionally, the lack of mesh distal to their anchor sites would decrease residual mesh in the superficial groin should a SIMS mesh need to be removed. Additionally, while not currently available, the design of retropubic SIMS avoided blind passage through the retropubic space, therefore decreasing the possibility of bladder or bowel perforation. More recent data support the overall safety of these devices [5]. However, despite these benefits, SIMS are still associated with various issues of which the reconstructive surgeon should be aware. The following is a description of various issues that may be experienced after SIMS placement. Given all of these issues also pertain to the standard full-length MUS, we will attempt to compare rates of various issues experienced with SIMS to those of MUS.

Failure to Correct SUI

The ability of a SIMS to subjectively or objectively cure SUI compared to a full-length MUS is likely dependent on the type of SIMS, type of comparative MUS, surgeon factors, and patient factors. Many early studies comparing SIMS initially focused largely on the TVT-Secur ™ device, which showed lower rates of cure compared to the MUS [4]. Given these results, the TVT-Secur ™ device is no longer on the market. Similarly, studies evaluating the efficacy of other historically available SIMS no longer on the market showed conflicting results. For example, Basu and Duckett implemented one of the first prospective randomized trials comparing the MiniArc ™ SIMS (American Medical Systems, Minnetonka, Minnesota, USA) to Advantage TVT ™ (Boston Scientific, Natick, Massachusetts, USA) which showed higher subjective and objective failure rates at 6 and 12 months in the SIMS group [7].

However, more recent studies on SIMS show more promising results. At this time, single-incision slings have been extensively studied and are likely as effective as full-length MUS to cure incontinence at 1 year, as shown by the most recent Cochrane Systematic Review on SIMS operations specifically when comparing against full-length transobturator slings [5]. This systematic review reports that "there is little to no difference in subjective cure or improvement of incontinence at 12 months post-surgery between single-incision slings and transobturator slings (RR 1.00, 95% CI 0.97 to 1.03; 17 studies, 2359 participants; high-certainty evidence)." There are less trials evaluating subjective cure or improvement for longer durations of time and in comparison to other types of anti-incontinence procedures [5].

Each SIMS has different characteristics including fixation points within the pelvis, tensioning method, and mesh size (Table 20.1), which may slightly alter their effectiveness. Altis ® has been shown to be effective within 3 [8] and 8 years [9] for the treatment of SUI. In a retrospective single-arm trial by Morciano et al., Altis ® showed an objective cure rate of 88.7% at 36 months, as defined by cough stress test (CST) and urodynamic evaluation [8]. Altis ® additionally showed a subjective success rate of 86.9% at 36 months as measured by the Patient Global Impression of Improvement (PGI-I) questionnaire [8]. The efficacy remains high over time with an overall success rate of 73.3% at a median follow-up of 8 years as defined by no self-reported SUI symptoms or reintervention [9]. Most recently, Altis ® has also been compared to retropubic MUS in a randomized controlled trial (RCT) published in the American Journal of Obstetrics and Gynecology (AJOG) by Matthews et al. In this trial, Altis ® was found to be noninferior to the retropubic sling group with comparable rates of persistent bothersome SUI and retreatment rates [10]. Similarly, Solyx ™ (Boston Scientific, Somerville, NJ) has been shown to be effective in various studies. In a prospective, nonrandomized, parallel cohort study by White et al., treatment success was similar between Solyx ™ and Obtryx II ™ (MUS, Boston Scientific, Somerville, NJ) at 36 months, at 90.4% and 88.9%, respectively. Treatment success was defined as composite negative CST and subjective improvement by PGI-I [11]. Another SIMS, Ophira ™ (Promedon, Córdoba,

Argentina) has also been shown to be noninferior to MUS. In a randomized noninferiority controlled trial, Ophira ™ was found to have similar objective (86.4% vs 84.4%) and subjective (83.3% vs 81.3%) cure rates when compared to TOT MUS after 4-year follow-up [12]. Overall, the current data is promising for the efficacy of SIMS, though long-term data is necessary. Additionally, stratification of efficacy based on preoperative SUI severity may also guide reconstructive surgeons in deciphering whether a SIMS or MUS is best for their patient.

Rate of Reoperation

A different way to evaluate efficacy after surgical management of SUI is the rate of reoperation. While some studies combine all reasons for reoperation together, this measure can still be useful to understand instances of significant complications that cannot be managed conservatively. At this time, it is unclear whether SIMS has a higher rate of reoperation for persistent or recurrent SUI or for mesh revision. This is true when comparing SIMS to transobturator MUS as well as retropubic MUS [5]. Pooled analysis of randomized clinical trials is inconclusive, and evaluation of individual studies is contradictory. In one randomized clinical trial comparing SIMS to MUS, while not powered to detect statistical difference, more patients underwent repeat surgical treatment in the SIMS group (8.7% vs 4.6%) including surgery for urinary incontinence (4.3% vs 2.3%), pain (2.5% vs 0.8%), and mesh exposure (2.5% vs 1.1%) [13]. While not statistically different, a randomized clinical trial comparing Ophira ™ to the outside-in TOT Unitape T Plus (Promedon, Córdoba, Argentina) showed higher rates of reoperation for SUI in the SIMS group at 36 months (10.1% vs 3.3%, $p = 0.172$) [14]. Alternatively, a randomized clinical trial comparing Needleless ® to the inside-out KIM transobturator MUS (Neomedic International, Terrassa, Spain) showed similar rates of reoperation for mesh revision and urinary incontinence, though numbers of these complications were small [15]. Overall, it appears that the rate of reoperation for any reason after SIMS or MUS procedure is generally low, but it is challenging to comment on whether they are equivalent or not at this time.

De Novo Urge Incontinence

Many patients often present with a picture of mixed urinary incontinence. In general, it is reasonable to treat urge incontinence (UI) prior to stress incontinence in order to prevent worsening UI symptoms as well as isolate urge incontinence postoperatively caused by sling placement. Currently, it is unclear if there are similar rates of de novo urge incontinence following SIMS compared to MUS [5]. When looking at individual studies, it may denote similar rates of de novo urge incontinence between the groups [14]. The largest body of RCT literature reporting on de novo urge incontinence as a secondary outcome is on Needleless ® and Ophira ™. RCTs comparing Needleless ® with transobturator MUS show no difference in de novo urge incontinence rates [15–18]. Similarly, randomized clinical trials comparing Ophira ™ to transobturator MUS show no difference in de novo urge incontinence rates [12, 19, 20]. While nonrandomized, data also suggest that de novo urge urinary incontinence does not differ between Solyx ™ and Obtryx ™ [11].

De novo urge incontinence may be triggered by various characteristics of sling surgery. Close proximity of the SIMS to the urethra [21] or close proximity of the mesh to the detrusor muscle in the case of a retropubic MUS could cause irritation, leading to urge incontinence. Additionally, while type 1 lightweight polypropylene mesh is superior to other materials, it is still a permanent device, potentially leading to a natural foreign body reaction, irritation of surrounding tissue, and de novo urge incontinence.

Urinary Retention

Urinary retention due to bladder outlet obstruction is a significant risk that surgeons must be cognizant of when placing and positioning MUS and SIMS. When tensioning these slings, they should be placed in order to allow for support underneath the urethra with stress maneuvers while minimizing the probability of obstruction. However, despite the goal of placing slings optimally, urinary retention may still result. The rates of urinary retention following retropubic midurethral sling placement have been quoted between 4% and 8% with reported rates of about half of this after transobturator placement [1]. Single-incision slings likely result in similar or even decreased rates of urinary retention compared to traditional MUS [5]. In general, there appear to be low and comparable rates of urinary retention with various SIMS procedures including Altis ® [8, 9], Needleless® [15–18, 22], Ophira ™ [12, 20], and Solyx ™ [11] devices. The rates of urinary retention quoted in these studies are most commonly in the 1–3% range.

Management of postoperative urinary retention depends on the severity and duration of retention. A majority of instances of urinary retention following sling surgery are temporary and can be managed conservatively. Often, temporary urinary retention following sling surgery can be secondary to a variety of etiologies, including pain, anesthesia, opiates, and localized swelling. Typically, these instances of temporary urinary retention can be managed with indwelling Foley catheter placement for 1–3 days. For urinary retention that is persistent or profound, sling loosening or lysis may be required. The decision of when to perform one of these procedures is controversial. There is some evidence to suggest that patient satisfaction, recurrent SUI, and voiding dysfunction may be improved if early sling loosening is performed instead of delayed sling lysis [23–25].

Mesh Exposure

Utilization of a permanent mesh material for treatment of prolapse has come under a significant amount of scrutiny within the last decade, predominantly due to increased risks of pain and mesh exposure with questionable improvements in outcome. This scrutiny led to the 2019 FDA order for the cessation of manufacturing and marketing of mesh for the transvaginal repair of pelvic organ prolapse [26]. Despite this, mesh for the treatment of SUI has been shown to be efficacious with low complication rates, including mesh exposure. However, it is still necessary for the reconstructive surgeon to understand and disclose the possibility of mesh exposure following MUS and SIMS placement. The term "mesh exposure" with a description of where the mesh exposure is located is the preferred terminology, as other terms such as "erosion," "extrusion," and "perforation" have been used inconsistently and are nonspecific [27]. Further guidance regarding the classification of mesh complications is available via the International Continence Society–International Urogynecological Association (ICS-IUGA) Classification System for Mesh Complications, which is also available as an online calculator at https://www.ics.org/complication. In general, the rate of mesh exposure in the first year following a MUS is about 1%, with a cumulative 9-year risk of up to about 5% [28, 29]. It is likely that single-incision slings have similar rates of mesh exposure to traditional MUS [5].

There are various device, patient, and surgeon factors that increase the risk of mesh exposure. All currently available single-incision slings are lightweight type 1 polypropylene products that have been shown to be better tolerated with lower rates of mesh exposure [30]. There are various differences in mesh weight, porosity, and other factors that can further be seen in Table 20.1, which may affect the risk of mesh exposure. Various patient factors may increase mesh exposure rates, such as smoking, immunosuppressive medication use, and uncontrolled diabetes [31, 32], though there is little data supporting these risk factors. Finally, there are various technical factors at the time of sling placement that may increase the risk of exposure. Higher surgeon volume may mitigate exposure rates [33]. Full-thickness dissection, placement of mesh so that there is no curling, bunching, or undue tension, excellent hemostasis, and full-thickness vaginal mucosal re-approximation are all techniques employed at the time of MUS and SIMS placement to decrease the risk of mesh exposure.

Women with vaginal mesh exposure may present with multiple symptoms or may be completely asymptomatic. Common complaints of mesh exposure include vaginal spotting or discharge, pain, dyspareunia, and partner dyspareunia [34]. A thorough pelvic exam is indicated to identify mesh exposure with a low threshold to incorporate in-office vaginoscopy and cystoscopy for a complete evaluation. Sometimes, a pelvic exam under anesthesia may be necessary in order to fully identify mesh exposure sites in the event there is high clinical suspicion without any evidence on office examination [34].

Management of mesh exposure varies depending on symptoms, size, and location. For asymptomatic small, less than 1 cm, vaginal exposures, observation is reasonable with or without vaginal estrogen. If symptoms are associated with these small vaginal exposures, office trimming is appropriate to offer, though persistent or recurrent mesh exposure is common, and resection and reclosure of the vaginal epithelium in the operating room is typically employed. If a mesh exposure is located within the urethra, bladder, or other surrounding structures, surgical resection and repair of the affected organ is appropriate [27].

Dyspareunia and Pain

Pain and dyspareunia are recognized postoperative complications that can occur with standard full-length retropubic and transobturator MUS. Pain may be experienced in the suprapubic area, groin, vagina, pelvis, lower abdomen, and urethra. In particular, the transobturator MUS may lead to higher rates of groin pain [35], though typically this pain will resolve within 6 months [1]. One benefit of SIMS is a decrease in postoperative groin pain compared to the full-length transobturator MUS. This advantage has been supported by the literature, with women experiencing less pain with SIMS between 30 days and 12 months compared to transobturator MUS [5]. A difference in the rates of dyspareunia between SIMS and MUS is less clear [5].

The rate of reoperation for pain after full-length MUS procedures is low [36], ranging between 1% and 3% at 9 years [28, 29]. However, reconstructive surgeons should be aware of this complication in order to properly counsel their patients. In particular, it is prudent to evaluate for and identify preexisting pelvic pain in women seeking treatment for SUI, as pelvic pain and pelvic pain conditions are relatively common. If pelvic pain is identified preoperatively, care must be taken to ameliorate pain with the assistance of pelvic floor physical therapy prior to proceeding with surgery. Patients should be counseled that any pelvic surgery, including MUS and SIMS placement, can not only cause pain and dyspareunia, but can also exacerbate existing pain if present. If a patient presents postoperatively with pain, conservative therapy with pelvic floor physical therapy and analgesic and/or steroid injections may be trialed initially, but these patients may require surgical excision with good reported success rates [27].

Conclusions

Single-incision slings were developed to mitigate risks inherent in traditional MUS, such as visceral injury and groin pain. As all currently available SIMS have a horizontal trajectory, injury to the bowel is avoided. Additionally, given the single-incision nature, pain, particularly groin pain seen in the traditional transobturator MUS, is mitigated. Original reports evaluating SIMS showed a lack of efficacy compared to MUS, particularly driven by the TVT-Secur ™. The limited efficacy of the TVT-Secur ™ may be due to its poorly designed absorbable fixation tips [4]. Newer SIMS with stable fixation systems have been shown to have improved efficacy, as shown by likely comparable rates of subjective and objective improvement to their MUS counterparts [5]. Ultimately, each patient must be evaluated individually and their unique patient factors considered when determining the optimal surgical management for the treatment of SUI. The differences inherent between MUS and SIMS, as well as among different SIMS, can guide the reconstructive surgeon to choose the best surgical procedure for each patient, balancing the unique issues surrounding SIMS.

References

1. Ford AA, Rogerson L, Cody JD, Aluko P, Ogah JA. Mid-urethral sling operations for stress urinary incontinence in women. Cochrane Database Syst Rev. 2017;2017:7. https://doi.org/10.1002/14651858.CD006375.pub4.
2. AUGS-SUFU Joint Publication. Joint position statement on midurethral slings for stress urinary incontinence. Female Pelvic Med Reconstr Surg. 2021;27(12):707–10.
3. Woodburn KL, Cardenas-Trowers OO, Fitzgerald JJ. Mix and mesh: an electronic database of FPMRS mesh products through 2020. Female Pelvic Med Reconstr Surg. 2022;28:e154–6.
4. Nambiar A, Cody JD, Jeffrey ST, Aluko P. Single-incision sling operations for urinary incontinence in women. Cochrane Database Syst Rev. 2017;2017:7. https://doi.org/10.1002/14651858.CD008709.pub3.
5. Carter E, Johnson EE, Still M, Al-Assaf AS, Bryant A, Aluko P, et al. Single-incision sling operations for urinary incontinence in women. Cochrane Database Syst Rev. 2023;2023:10. https://doi.org/10.1002/14651858.CD008709.pub4.
6. AUGS-IUGA Joint Publication. Joint report on terminology for surgical procedures to treat stress urinary incontinence in women. Female Pelvic Med Reconstr Surg. 2020;26:162–72.
7. Basu M, Duckett J. A randomized trial of retropubic tension-free vaginal tape versus a mini-sling for stress incontinence. BJOG. 2010;117:730–5.
8. Morciano A, Marzo G, Caliandro D, Fachechi G, Alessia G, Campagna G, et al. Altis ® adjustable single incision sling system for treatment of intrinsic sphincteric deficiency: a 3-year follow-up observational study. Urogynecology. 2022;28:500–5.
9. Gromicho A, Dias J, Araújo D, Rodrigues R, Bou Kheir G, Ferraz L. Long-term outcomes of Altis ® single-incision sling procedure for stress urinary incontinence. Int Urogynecol J. 2022;33:717–22.
10. Matthews C, Rardin CR, Sokol A, et al. A randomized trial of retropubic vs single-incision sling among patients undergoing vaginal prolapse repair. Am J Obstet Gynecol. 2024;231(2):261.e1–261.e10.
11. White AB, Kahn BS, Gonzalez RR, et al. Prospective study of a single-incision sling versus a transobturator sling in women with stress urinary incontinence: 3-year results. Am J Obstet Gynecol. 2020;223:545.e1–11.
12. Huser M, Hudecek R, Belkov I, Horvath I, Jarkovsky J, Tvarozek S. Safety and efficacy of single incision sling versus midurethral sling in the treatment of stress urinary incontinence: a randomized controlled trial. Urogynecology. 2023;29:113–20.
13. Abdel-Fattah M, Cooper D, Davidson T, Kilonzo M, Hossain M, Boyers D, et al. Single-Incision Mini-Slings for Stress Urinary Incontinence in Women. N Engl J Med. 2022;386:1230–43.
14. Pascom AL, Djehdian LM, Bortolini MA, Jarmy-Di Bella ZI, Delroy CA, Tamanini JT, et al. Randomized controlled trial comparing single-incision mini-sling and transobturator midurethral sling for the treatment of stress urinary incontinence: 3-year follow-up results. Neurourol Urodyn. 2018;37(7):2184–90.
15. Dogan O, Kaya AE, Pulatoglu C, Basbug A, Yassa M. A randomized comparison of a single-incision needleless (Contasure-needleless) mini-sling versus an inside-out transobturator (Contasure-KIM) midurethral sling in women with stress urinary incontinence: 24 month follow up results. Int Urogynecol J Pelvic Floor Dysfunct. 2018;29(9):1387–95.
16. Amat I, Tardiu L, Martínez Franco E, Laïlla Vicens JM. Contasure-Needleless compared with transobturator-TVT for the treatment of stress urinary incontinence. Int Urogynecol J. 2011;22(7):827–33.
17. Fernandez-Gonzalez S, Martinez Franco E, Lin Miao X, Amat TL. Contasure needleless compared with Monarc for the treatment of stress urinary incontinence. Int Urogynecol J. 2017;28(7):1077–84.
18. Gaber ME, Borg T, Samour H, Nawara M, Reda A. Two new mini-slings compared with transobturator tension-free vaginal tape for treatment of stress urinary incontinence. A 1 year follow up randomized controlled trial. J Obstet Gynaecol Res. 2016;42(12):1773–81.
19. Jurakova M, Huser M, Belkov I, Janku P, Hudecek R, Stourac P, et al. Prospective randomized comparison of the transobturator mid-urethral sling and the single-incision sling among women with stress urinary incontinence: 1-year follow-up study. Int Urogynecol J. 2016;27(5):791–6.
20. Maturana AP, Palos CC, Ghersel FR, Fernandes CE, Oliveira E. Randomized controlled trial comparing minisling with transobturator sling for the treatment of stress urinary incontinence. Int Urogynecol J. 2019;31(9):1925–31.
21. Taner CE, Okay G, Göklü Y, Başoğul Ö, Başoğul N. Perioperative and postoperative complications after Ophira mini sling operations. Arch Gynecol Obstet. 2015;291:341–6.
22. Chen YG, Zhang YG, Zhang W, Li X, Wang X. Clinical value of needleless sling in treatment of female stress urinary incontinence. World J Clin Cases. 2020;8(18):4043–50.
23. Brennard EA, Tang S, Birch C, Robert M, Kim-Fine S. Early voiding dysfunction after midurethral sling surgery: comparison of two management approaches. Int Urogynecol J. 2017;28:1515–26.

24. Pinsard M, Fauconnier A, D'Halluin F, et al. Comparison of early loosening vs delayed section of mid-urethral slings for postoperative voiding dysfunction. Int Urogynecol J. 2023;34:675–81.
25. Maldonado DV, Wymer KM, Gebhart JB, et al. Cost-effectiveness analysis of early sling loosening versus delayed sling lysis in the management of voiding dysfunction after midurethral sling placement. Female Pelvic Med Reconstr Surg. 2022;28:e103–7.
26. FDA.gov [Internet]. FDA takes action to protect women's health, orders manufacturers of surgical mesh intended for transvaginal repair of pelvic organ prolapse to stop selling all devices. [cited 2019 April 16]. Available from: https://www.fda.gov/news-events/press-announcements/fda-takes-action-protect-womens-health-orders-manufacturers-surgical-mesh-intended-transvaginal.
27. Joint position statement on the management of mesh-related complications for the FPMRS specialist. Female Pelvic Med Reconstr Surg. 2020;26:219–32.
28. Berger AA, Tan-Kim J, Menefee SA. Long-term risk of reoperation after synthetic mesh midurethral sling surgery for stress urinary incontinence. Obstet Gynecol. 2019;134:1047.
29. Gurol-Urganci I, Geary RS, Mamza JB, et al. Long-term rate of mesh sling removal following midurethral mesh sling insertion among women with stress urinary incontinence. JAMA. 2018;320:1659.
30. Cundiff GW, Varner E, Visco AG, et al. Risk factors for mesh/suture erosion following sacral colpopexy. Am J Obstet Gynecol. 2008;199:688.e1–5.
31. Ortega MV, Bangura M, Ayati E, et al. Association between hemoglobin A_1c and midurethral sling complications in diabetic women: a cohort study. Female Pelvic Med Reconstr Surg. 2021;27:159–62.
32. Ringel NE, de Winter KL, Siddique M, et al. Surgical outcomes in urogynecology—assessment of perioperative and postoperative complications relative to preoperative hemoglobin A_1c—A Fellows Pelvic Research Network Study. Female Pelvic Med Reconstr Surg. 2022;28:7–13.
33. Brennand EA, Quan H. Evaluation of the effect of surgeon's operative volume and specialty on likelihood of revision after mesh midurethral sling placement. Obstet Gynecol. 2019;1333:1099–108.
34. Nazemi TM, Kobashi KC. Complications of grafts used in female pelvic floor reconstruction: mesh erosion and extrusion. Indian J Urol. 2017;23(2):153–60.
35. Latthe PM, Foon R, Toozs-Hobson P. Transobturator and retropubic tape procedures in stress urinary incontinence: a systematic review and meta-analysis of effectiveness and complications. BJOG. 2007;114:522–31.
36. Armengaud C, Fauconnier A, Drioueche H, et al. Serious complications and recurrences after retropubic vs transobturator midurethral sling procedures for 2682 patients in the VIGI-MESH register. Am J Obstet Gynecol Forthcoming. 2024;230(4):428.e1–428.e13.

21 Female Urethral Reconstructive Surgery

Rajveer S. Purohit, Camille Torres, and Jerry G. Blaivas

Introduction

Female urethral reconstruction is an uncommon surgery for urethral strictures, urethral diverticula, or urethral tissue loss (e.g., fistulas). Consequently, there is significantly less data regarding outcomes and prevention of complications compared to male urethral reconstruction. However, conclusions can be drawn from available sources and anecdotal experience. Complications can be minimized with careful preoperative assessment and focus on principles of surgical technique and approach. Intraoperative complications include hemorrhage and bladder or ureteral injury. Early postoperative complications include infection, flap or graft necrosis, and late complications include stricture or fistula recurrence, sphincteric incontinence, urethral obstruction, and overactive bladder (OAB). In addition, complications of ancillary procedures such as a Martius flap or buccal graft may occur.

R. S. Purohit (✉) · J. G. Blaivas
Icahn School of Medicine at Mount Sinai Hospital, Department of Urology, New York, NY, USA

C. Torres
Crane Center for Transgender Surgery, Austin, USA

Preoperative Assessment

Many complications from urethral reconstructive surgery are preventable because the elective nature of most of these surgeries permits careful preoperative surgical planning. Minimizing the risk of complications begins with a focused, but detailed history, physical examination of the urethral defect and vagina, assessment of urethral sphincter and detrusor function, and exclusion of concomitant urethral obstruction, vesicovaginal or ureterovaginal fistula, and ureteral obstruction. Many patients who require urethral reconstruction have had prior surgery, so it is important to either obtain the operative reports or discuss the surgery with the previous surgeon. It is particularly important to determine if a foreign body such as mesh is in or near the wound. One of our patients failed a urethral reconstruction because of retained mesh at the site of a urethrovaginal fistula. Neither the patient nor the surgeon knew that a mesh sling had been done previously. This unfortunate case emphasizes the need for obtaining an accurate surgical history.

Preoperative physical examination should be performed with a comfortably full bladder. Particular attention should be paid to the health of the vaginal tissue. In patients with vaginal atrophy and post-radiation changes, preoperative estrogen cream may improve the quality of vaginal tissue. A careful speculum examination of the entire vaginal wall should assess the presence of

H. B. Goldman, J. Zillioux (eds.), *Complications of Urogynecology and Reconstructive Pelvic Surgery*, https://doi.org/10.1007/978-3-032-00339-3_21

sling erosion. Granulation tissue, drainage from a sinus tract, and fistula are tell-tale signs of erosion.

In cases of urethral damage from previous vaginal or urethral surgery, the vaginal tissue is often scarred, fibrotic, and ischemic. The extent of urethral tissue loss, the integrity of the vaginal tissue, adequacy of the vasculature, and the need for advancement, lateral, or pedicle skin flaps should be assessed preoperatively (Figs. 21.1 and 21.2). Bimanual pelvic exam should focus on the presence of urethral masses or pelvic organ prolapse. When incontinence is observed from the urethral meatus, and a fistula is suspected, the examination should be repeated with a finger occluding the meatus to observe leakage from the fistula itself.

Videourodynamics may show urethral obstruction, sphincteric incontinence, low bladder compliance, impaired detrusor contractility, or detrusor overactivity secondary to urethral damage. The voiding cystourethrogram (VCUG) is a critical component in preoperative evaluation of the diseased urethra. In patients with urethral obstruction, the VCUG demonstrates the site, and for those with strictures, its length and location in relation to the bladder neck. If the urethral stricture is located in the distal third of the urethra or at the meatus, imaging typically reveals ballooning of the bladder neck on voiding (Fig. 21.3). In addition, residual diverticular contrast after voiding may help confirm and clarify the anatomy of the diverticula to aid in surgical planning.

Other imaging techniques like MRI and delayed CT with contrast may be useful to distinguish abscess, cyst, tumor, and urethral diverticulum in patients with periurethral masses, to assess foreign bodies, and to rule out additional injury to the urinary tract following pelvic trauma.

Cystourethroscopy with a flexible cystoscope will confirm a urethral stricture, the presence of a foreign body, including suture or sling material, and evaluate the extent of the fistula. It can also evaluate the remainder of the urethra, particularly the length and viability of the proximal urethra. In patients with tight meatal stenosis or urethral stricture where a complete cystourethroscopy cannot be performed, a voiding cystourethrogram (VCUG) is critical to evaluate the extent of the urethral stricture. At the time of surgery, if needed, we perform a cystoscopy with a semi-rigid ureteroscope, which can often atraumatically

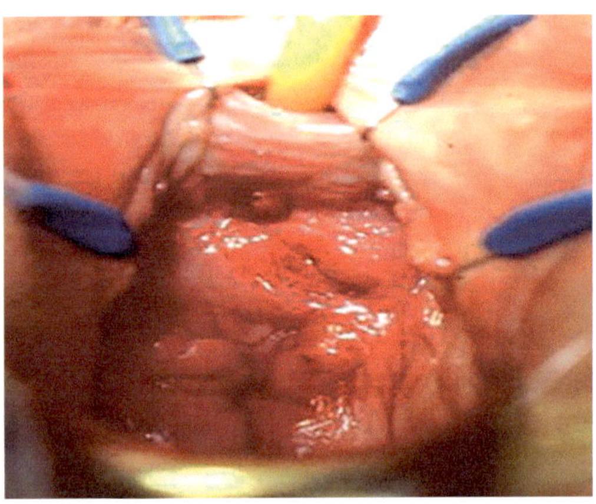

Fig. 21.1 Inspection of the anterior vaginal wall in a woman with a seemingly straightforward urethrovaginal fistula. She underwent a simple repair with vaginal wall flaps and a Martius flap, but the fistula recurred within 3 weeks. At secondary repair, a mesh sling was encountered and excised. Neither the patient nor the surgeon knew that mesh had been used in a prior anti-incontinence operation. (Courtesy of J.G. Blaivas)

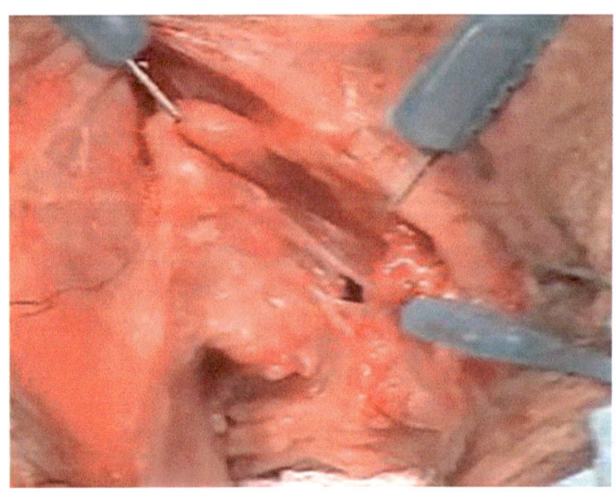

Fig. 21.2 Inspection of the anterior vaginal wall in a woman who had previously undergone an extensive urethral reconstruction after excision of a sterile periurethral abscess that formed after injection of calcium hydroxylapatite (Coaptite) for sphincteric incontinence refractory to two mesh slings. Despite the obvious stricture, she had severe sphincteric incontinence as well. At the time of surgery, after incising the stricture, the proximal urethra was only about 2 cm in length, just barely large enough to accept an autologous fascial sling. (Courtesy of J.G. Blaivas)

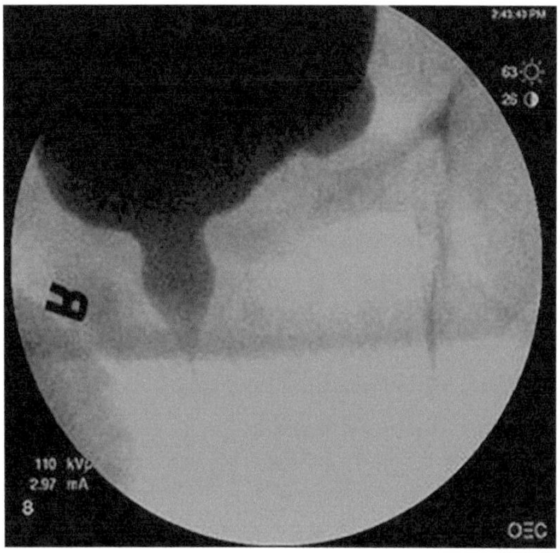

Fig. 21.3 Voiding cystourethrogram in this patient confirms a distal urethral stricture. There is almost no possibility of sphincteric injury during reconstructive surgery that is limited to the distal urethra, so either a ventral or dorsal approach may be considered. (Courtesy of J.G. Blaivas)

navigate past a stricture and confirm details of the proximal urethra.

Prior to the urethroplasty for stricture, ideally, the patient should have avoided dilation or endoscopic management for at least 3 months [1]. The concept of urethral rest stems from having a stable stricture, which permits the surgeon to visualize the full extent of the disease. In our experience, recurrence is often at the margins of the repair site, suggesting that the extent of the stricture was underappreciated at the time of urethroplasty, likely from recent instrumentation.

Principles of the Surgical Technique

The choice of surgical technique is dictated by a number of factors including (1) the experience and expertise of the surgeon, (2) the desires of the patient, (3) the patient's age and comorbidities, (4) lower urinary tract and renal function, (5) the presence of concomitant conditions such as pelvic organ prolapse or abdominal or pelvic disease requiring surgical correction, (6) prior abdominal and pelvic surgical procedures, and (7) sexual function.

1. *The surgeon*: Urethral reconstruction ranges from simple ventral incision and meatotomy for distal urethral strictures to full-length dorsal buccal grafts for longer strictures to neourethral reconstruction with local vaginal wall flaps reinforced with Martius flaps and occasionally, gracilis, thigh, or rectus flaps. Few of these procedures are learned in residency or fellowship; most of the expertise is garnered over decades of experience in tertiary referral centers. In our judgment, the most demanding part of the expertise is decision-making both before and during the surgery. With the exception of proximal dorsal buccal mucosal grafts for strictures, ventral bladder neck reconstruction, and complex urethral diverticula, the technical aspects of the surgery are usually straightforward. With these caveats in mind, it is up to the individual surgeon to decide whether he or she possesses the requisite surgical expertise for each individual patient. In some instances, referral to a reconstructive expert is prudent.
2. *The patient*: For practical purposes, the damaged urethra presents one or more of three potential problems—incontinence, urethral obstruction, and pelvic pain. Surgical treatment of incontinence and pain is entirely elective; whereas, untreated urethral obstruction may portend urinary retention or upper tract damage and even renal failure. Further, the success rate for treating urethral obstruction and sphincteric incontinence is very high—over 90%, while the success rate for pelvic pain and overactive bladder is far less. Keeping these facts in mind, it is important that the patient be apprised of the pros and cons of surgical intervention and that the decision about how to proceed is based on realistic expectations for success, failure, and complications.
3. *Patient age and comorbidities*: Age and comorbidities are factors insofar as the patient's life expectancy and ability to withstand the morbidity of surgery that could last as long as 4–6 h should be taken into account, although excessive blood loss during surgery is rare. The decision to undergo elective

surgery is based on a complex calculus involving factors such as the bother to the patient, risk of complications if no surgery is pursued versus the likelihood of success and duration of recovery based on the patient's preoperative age and comorbidities. For example, in an elderly patient with minimal bother from a urethrovaginal fistula and difficulty with ambulation, the improvement in quality of life may not be worth the risks of surgery and the morbidity of recovery to the patient. In addition, the surgeon should consider the extent to which advanced age, lichen sclerosus, concomitant medical conditions, or prior radiation treatment may impair vascularity and viability of adjacent vaginal or labial tissue when considering a local flap for urethroplasty.

4. *Urinary tract function*: It is axiomatic that lower urinary tract function is an essential component of decision-making in planning surgery. As a general rule, we believe it is most prudent to treat sphincteric incontinence as part of the reconstructive procedure, although some surgeons prefer a staged operation. Low bladder compliance and detrusor overactivity often improve after successful surgery, so they are not addressed at the same time, except in rare circumstances when due to multiple surgeries or radiation. In these instances, urinary diversion rather than urethral reconstruction might be considered (Fig. 21.4).
5. *Concomitant conditions*: When concomitant conditions such as vesicovaginal fistula, urethral diverticulum, and localized urethral cancer are present, the decision about how to proceed should be made on a case-by-case basis, taking particular care to assess the potential impact on flap or graft survival if more than one procedure is done at a time.
6. *Prior surgery*: It is important to know what prior pelvic surgeries the patient has undergone, particularly if mesh has been used for prior repairs. As a general rule, as much mesh as can be safely removed should be taken; when that is not feasible, it is important that all mesh be at least removed from the urethra and bladder when there has been erosion. In patients complaining of pain, it is best to remove all mesh from the affected side whenever possible, but this can be extremely challenging in patients who have undergone Transobturator Tape or prolapse repairs.
7. *Sexual function*: It is essential that the patient's desires about postoperative sexuality be discussed and incorporated into surgical planning and informed consent. The literature about sexual complications of urethral reconstructions is rudimentary at best, but dyspareunia can occur after any of these operations. When maintaining sexual function is a factor, special attention must be paid to ensuring adequate vaginal size of at least two loose finger breaths to a depth of at least 8 cm.

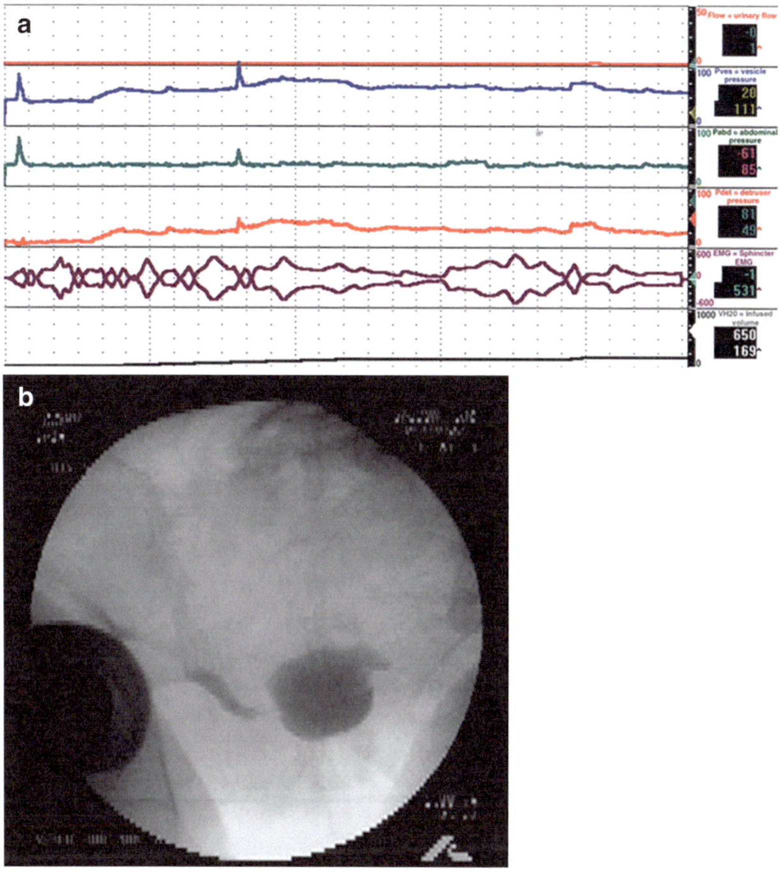

Fig. 21.4 Videourodynamic study in a 72-year-old woman who underwent anterior prolapse repair and TVT sling complicated by colovesical and urethrovaginal fistula. She subsequently underwent unsuccessful attempts at surgical repair of these defects and presented with refractory urge incontinence as well as sphincteric incontinence and colovesical fistula. She had arthritis that precluded self-catheterization through the urethra. Because of the findings described below, she underwent continent urinary diversion instead of another attempt at lower urinary tract reconstruction. (**a**) Urodynamic tracing demonstrates severe low bladder compliance (2 mL/cm H_2O) at a bladder volume of only 50 mL. Note that each time infusion is stopped, detrusor pressure falls. (Courtesy of J.G. Blaivas). (**b**) Cystogram reveals a tiny bladder with right vesicoureteral reflux. The colovesical fistula and sphincteric incontinence were not visualized. (Courtesy of J.G. Blaivas)

Surgical Techniques

Before proceeding with the vaginal incision, it is critical to choose the site and shape of the initial incision for the urethral reconstruction. We have previously described several methods of urethral reconstruction for stricture, and in the majority of the cases, the repair can be accomplished with a single transvaginal operation [2].

All surgical approaches follow the same rules: fine, sharp dissection is preferable, and homeostasis is maintained. Sharp dissection permits the development of correct planes and excision of the dense fibrotic tissue and may prevent inadvertent injury to the bladder or sphincter. The urethra should be opened proximally enough to clearly see the extent of the urethral stricture when present. If the edges of the stricture are uncertain, we place progressively larger bougie-a-boule sounds into the urethra past the area of suspected stricture. As the sound is pulled back, it will catch on the stricture. If a stricture is present, the urethrotomy is extended until the bougies can be withdrawn without resistance and healthy viable tissue is encountered proximal to the stricture site. In addition to aiding visualization, attention to homeostasis may prevent hematoma and breakdown of the suture lines. When excessive bleeding is encountered, pressure should be applied until the bleeding stops or bleeding vessels individually clamped and sutured or coagulated, preferably with bipolar energy. Frantic efforts to control hemorrhage without clearly identifying the bleeding vessels may lead to unnecessary injury to adjacent organs.

In preparing for vaginal surgery, the patient is placed in a dorsal lithotomy position with the least degree of Trendelenburg that is necessary for adequate exposure. Draping should permit access to the vagina as well as the abdominal area (when concomitant surgery is planned). At the onset of surgery, if possible, the bladder is drained via a transurethral catheter, and palpation of the balloon allows identification of the bladder neck. If suprapubic cystotomy, pubovaginal sling, or rectus fascia graft is planned, these should be done prior to the vaginal reconstructive surgery to avoid subsequent damage to the reconstruction during dissection for these procedures. For pubovaginal slings, though, the sutures should not be tied until the reconstruction has been completed so that tension can be judged.

In cases of minimal urethral disruption, such as small urethrovaginal fistula or diverticulum, the defect can be circumscribed and closed over a catheter with tension-free, interrupted 4′0 or 5′0 absorbable monofilament sutures. An inverted U anterior vaginal wall flap is usually adequate for closure, but sometimes a lateral vaginal flap may be more appropriate.

If urethral injury is extensive and sufficient vaginal wall tissue exists, vaginal wall flaps may be considered. Flap-based urethroplasty techniques have been demonstrated to be effective and improve the outcome in urethrovaginal fistulas, and also are an option for female urethral strictures that are distal to the sphincter mechanism [3–5]. In one such technique, the anterior vaginal wall can be mobilized, and a rectangular incision around the urethral defect is made. A lateral vaginal wall flap is advanced, rolled over the catheter, and sutured to the contralateral side, without tension, to form the entire posterior urethral wall. However, if the extent of urethral injury and lack of vaginal tissue preclude simple repair, use of an advancement flap may be required. Another choice is to create a labia minora flap. An oval-shaped incision is made in an adjacent hair-free portion of the labia minora and carried through the underlying tissue, and a pedicle is raised on a posterior- or anterior-based blood supply. This island flap is tunneled beneath the vaginal wall, rotated, and sutured over the catheter, so the vaginal epithelial surface creates the inner wall of the urethra. Rarely, it is not possible to close the defect in the vaginal wall primarily, and, in such instances, it is possible to create a labia majora flap to cover the wound. We have rarely needed a gracilis flap and have never used any other major kind of flap (rectus, Singapore, etc.), but of course, those are available if needed [2].

Urethral damage associated with erosion of synthetic material poses unique considerations, and the repairs can be even more challenging [6]. Most authors agree that eroded synthetic slings require complete removal of the sling from the urethra and bladder. The literature on the surgical management of erosions suggests midline anterior vaginal wall incision at the erosion site, bilateral dissection into the retropubic space, and removal of the entire synthetic sling including sutures, and, when possible, bone anchors if they were used [7]. In our experience, especially with transobturator techniques, attempting to remove all of the sling leads to difficult and morbid surgery and should probably be reserved for those who failed at the first attempt. Once the sling has been excised, the urethra can usually be repaired primarily. If this is not feasible, any of the techniques described above may be considered.

For patients with recurrent urethral strictures, ventral urethroplasty using vaginal and labial skin flaps is an option, but our preferred technique is dorsal onlay buccal mucosal graft. This approach can be utilized in almost all patients with urethral strictures and an intact bladder neck and urinary sphincter mechanism with low risk of urinary incontinence. Our dissection is carried just deep to the urethral mucosa and superficial to the vascular plexus that surrounds the urethra. Methylene blue placed in the urethra prior to beginning surgery aids in the identification of the urethral mucosa. This dorsal dissection minimizes both bleeding and injury to the sphincter. Using this dorsal plane for dissection, we have been able to repair strictures that extend to the bladder neck [8, 9]. Ventral urethrotomy approaches risk urethral sphincter damage and de novo urinary incontinence when the stricture involves the proximal urethra or when sphincteric incontinence was present preoperatively. In cases of documented preoperative sphincteric incontinence, the dorsal approach also offers easier access to the bladder neck and permits an easier concomitant anti-incontinence procedure.

Unlike the dorsal approach, ventral urethroplasty may redirect the urethra and the urinary stream anteriorly or posteriorly. When the urethra is too short, a vaginally directed urinary stream that causes post-void dribbling may occur. In some patients, there has been spontaneous resolution; in others, reconstructive surgery to lengthen the urethra may be required [10]. If the urethra is too long, there may be an excessive anteriorly directed stream, and the patient may actually void over the toilet bowl. This is easily corrected with a ventral meatotomy.

Vaginal tissue from the labia minora has been reported as a free inlay graft with minimal short-term complications [11]. We commonly utilize this approach with a labia minora free graft in urethral lengthening in transgender men with placement of a dorsal labial minora free graft and a contralateral ventral labia minora rotational flap during urethroplasty for metoidioplasty. Similarly, in cisgender women, several groups have proposed a dorsal onlay urethroplasty using labia minora skin graft [12] or vestibular flap [13]. The dorsal technique has several advantages, but requires different surgical expertise, utilizing many of the surgical principles derived from urethral reconstruction in men. A surgical plane is developed between the urethra and the overlying clitoral cavernous tissue. Care should be taken during the dissection of the dorsal urethra to avoid injury to the clitoral bulb, body, or crura, and the clitoral neurovascular bundle and to minimize excessive bleeding. The clitoro-urethrovaginal complex is supplied by pudendal neurovascular bundles, which arise from pelvic side walls and bifurcate into clitoral and perineal divisions. The clitoral neurovascular bundle ascends along the ischiopubic ramus and adjacent clitoral crura on both sides, runs under the surface of the symphysis pubis in the midline, and then travels along the cephaled surface of the clitoral body toward the glans (Fig. 21.5). The nerves of the clitoral neurovascular bundle are not large enough to be seen on the MRI. However, the histological dissections show that they accompany the vessels [14].

From a practical standpoint, it is fairly straightforward to avoid these structures during the dissection by confining the dissection to the dorsal urethra. We are neither aware of any reports of injury to the clitoral structures, nor have there been any reports of orgasmic changes. Our experience corroborates these findings.

During the dissection, troublesome bleeding can be encountered if the dissection is too deep, but we caution against blind coagulation or suture ligature. All that is usually necessary is to place a gauze pack between the dorsal urethra and pubis, extending into the retropubic space for compression. Alternatively, use a lone-star retractor and placement of the yellow stays underneath the vascular complex typically compresses and stops bleeding. Positioning the graft on the dorsal surface preserves the intact ventral midurethra and provides a better vascular bed for a graft. In addition, there is less risk of fistula formation and graft sacculation. In our judgment, doing so minimizes the likelihood of requiring an incontinence procedure. However, unlike the ventral approach, dorsal dissection is infrequently performed in pelvic reconstructive surgery, and for some surgeons, the anatomy is not well known. Further, some pelvic surgeons may be unfamiliar with the techniques of graft reconstruction that are done much more commonly in men.

Although vaginal surgery is the most commonly utilized approach and excellent for mid to

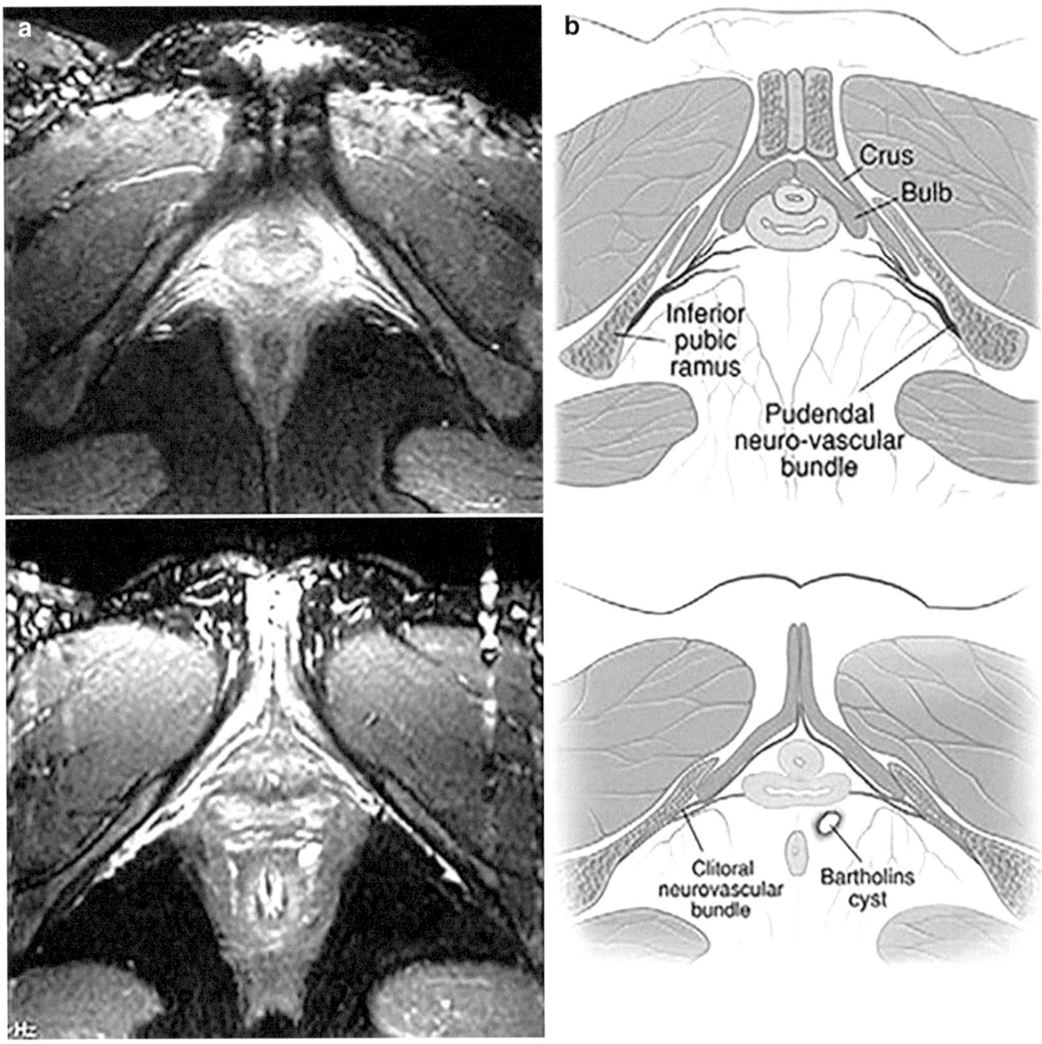

Fig. 21.5 (**a**) MRI of the clitoris in the axial section, as seen on the left, shows divisions of the pudendal neurovascular bundle, which arises from the pelvic side wall and bifurcates into the perineal and clitoral neurovascular bundles. The vascular component of the bundle and cavernous tissue is bright white due to the fat saturation technique. Muscles and bones appear as dark structures. (**b**) On the right is an artist's rendition of the images. (Reprinted with permission from the Journal of Urology [9])

distal urethral pathologies, there is an alternative approach when patients have a proximal dorsal urethral diverticulum or cases with complex horseshoe circumferential diverticulum, which may extend into the retropubic space. Mozafarpour et al. [15] and Sivarajan et al. [16] present their case reports describing the feasibility of urethral diverticulectomy in cases where a vaginal approach would be difficult due to the proximity of the diverticulum. This approach allows for better visualization of the urethral neck with minimal dissection of the urethra and therefore decreased risk of damaging the sphincter.

Use of a Graft and Potential Complications

One of the challenges of urethral reconstruction is achieving a long and stricture-free lumen that allows nonobstructive voiding and maintains continence. Due to the variable etiology of the urethral pathology, local tissue may not be available for the urethral repair. In cases of extensive posttraumatic or postsurgical urethral fibrosis, lichen sclerosus, congenital malformations, and recurrent urethral strictures, reconstructing the urethra with a free graft provides an alternative to a vaginal flap or bladder flap.

Various graft urethroplasty techniques have been proposed in small series. These techniques can be complicated and require knowledge and experience with processing and tissue transfer.

Buccal mucosa grafts are commonly used in male urethral reconstructive surgery and have been shown to be successful in the construction of the neourethra in female pediatric patients [17]. The buccal mucosa graft has been applied to female urethral strictures using both dorsal and ventral approaches [8–10, 18].

In our experience, buccal mucosa graft is an option in patients with previously failed reconstructive surgery and urethral stricture recurrence. It is also our treatment of choice for proximal urethral strictures in women who do not have a current or past history of sphincteric incontinence because we believe that there is no need for anti-incontinence surgery when the dorsal approach is used. Buccal mucosa has several advantages: is easy to harvest, is resilient to infection, and is already accustomed to a moist environment. Properties like elasticity and thick epithelium make it easy to handle [19]. It has the ability to supplement the native urethral plate to form a conduit that closely resembles a normally functioning urethra with low risk of sacculation and diverticulum formation. In addition, buccal grafts have a panlaminar vascular plexus, which eases graft take to the recipient bed. In animal studies, extensive neovascularization in the subepithelial layer was evident 3 weeks after surgery, followed by inflammation and minimal fibrosis at 6 weeks [20]. Supple urethral coaptation can be accomplished by buccal mucosa graft and may play a role in achieving continence after urethral reconstruction [17]. The graft is harvested from the buccal mucosa inferior to Stensen's duct, which is identified adjacent to the second upper molar. The graft typically measures between 2 and 2.5 cm wide and 2–5 cm in length, depending on the amount of tissue needed. The graft is defatted and anastomosed to the urothelium after urethrotomy. To maximize outcomes after free grafts, ensuring adequate vascularity of the donor bed is necessary. Typically, the vascular plexus around the urethra is adequate for graft survival. The graft must be anastomosed to the recipient bed using monofilament absorbable sutures. In order to allow possible postoperative contraction of the graft, it should be trimmed to a slightly larger size than the urethral defect or stricture.

Serious complications associated with harvesting buccal mucosa graft are rare; the literature describes generally minor complications such as post-op oral pain and/or numbness and wound contraction, which manifests as a sensation of tightness when the mouth is open [21, 22]. In male reconstructive surgery, complications reported include donor site wound pain, swelling, damage to Stensen's duct, postoperative perioral numbness, and infection. According to data from male case series, 59% of patients developed short-term numbness after surgery, which persisted in 16% beyond 1 year [21]. Major complications of buccal grafts are uncommon; however, the possibility of a mental nerve neuropathy is unique to buccal graft surgery [23]. Injury to Stensen's duct is extremely rare and can be avoided by marking the buccal mucosa and careful closure of the donor site. When it is difficult to perform closure, some surgeons prefer to leave the harvest site open. One randomized study found that while there were no long-term differences, primary closure of the buccal mucosal graft bed decreased postoperative pain and improved oral intake [24]. Hampson et al. [25] describe the largest published series of 39 female patients with urethral stricture managed with dorsal onlay buccal mucosal graft. No reported graft donor site complications in any of the patients. Other authors, such as Kore et al. [26], reported pain and numbness in the graft donor site in 14% of the patients.

If a buccal mucosa graft is used ventrally and adequate periurethral tissue does not exist for coverage of the graft, it may be advisable to use well-vascularized tissue flaps to provide an adequate blood supply and prevent fistula formation. However, to our knowledge, tissue flaps have not been utilized in the dorsal approach.

Sharma has described the use of dorsal onlay lingual graft urethroplasty in 15 women with urethral stricture [27]. Lingual mucosa, harvested from lateral and ventral surfaces of the tongue, has similar tissue characteristics as buccal mucosa thick epithelium, high content of elastic fibers, thin lamina propria, and rich vascularization [28]. There were no functional limitations or intraoral complications at 1-year follow-up. Advantages reported of harvesting lingual mucosa graft instead of buccal mucosa graft are avoidance of injury to the parotid gland duct and facial nerve without risk of mouth deviation or lip retraction [27].

Intraoperative Complications

Intraoperative complications during urethral reconstructive surgery are rare, based on our review of the literature. One case of intraoperative hemorrhage has been reported in early series by Elkins on 20 women who underwent repair of a vesicovaginal fistula involving the urethra with the anterior bladder flap technique and Martius flap. During total urethral reconstruction, a patient developed hemorrhage in the space of Retzius and required postoperative blood transfusion [29]. However, there is no surgery that spares the patient from the potential risk of other anesthetic complications or injury to adjacent organs such as bladder, ureter, or rectum. For bleeding that occurs during the dissection for creating vaginal flaps, we believe it is best to simply apply pressure with a pack unless there is an obvious bleeding vessel that can be coagulated or ligated. Bleeding that occurs from the retropubic space after entry from the vagina is best handled with the same approach. If bleeding seems excessive, we advise against trying to explore from the vaginal wound; rather, one or two 4 × 4 sponges or a lap pad should be inserted into the retropubic space through the vagina to tamponade the bleeding while other parts of the operation are continued. In thousands of reconstructive surgeries, we have never found it necessary to explore the retropubic space from above to control bleeding. Another potential source of excessive bleeding is during the dissection for the Martius flap that is discussed in the section "Complications of Ancillary Procedures." It is theoretically possible to injure the distal ureter during a dissection for urethral reconstruction, but we have never seen this, nor has it been reported. On two occasions, though, the ureter has been transected or avulsed in the course of removing mesh to which the ureter was adherent. One should be alert to the possibility of this complication whenever the dissection extends to the vicinity of the ureter or when traction is exerted on the retropubic mesh. For that reason, it is always prudent to administer intravenous dye and check for ureteral patency by observing efflux of urine from each ureteral orifice through a cystoscope. If there is preoperative suspicion of ureteral involvement with mesh, ureteral stent placement prior to commencing surgery is helpful. If intraoperative concern exists about ureteral injury, retrograde pyelography should be done and a ureteral stent left in place if there appears to be an injury. In cases of avulsion or transaction of the ureter, immediate ureteroneocystotomy should be done.

Early Complications

All types of urethral reconstructive surgery share common complications like infection, flap necrosis, urinary retention, and postoperative bleeding, yet the overall incidence of major complications such as bleeding is very low. Complications related to the ancillary procedures, like graft, flap, or sling placement, are discussed below.

One of the earliest, but rare, complications of urethral reconstruction is wound infection and flap necrosis. Unrecognized infection may lead to the disruption of the suture lines, flap necrosis, and fistula formation; however, we could find no reports on this, and none has ever occurred in our series.

Sharma et al., in a case series of 15 patients who underwent dorsal onlay lingual mucosal graft urethroplasty for urethral stricture, reported one case of wound infection requiring antibiotics. The patient subsequently developed submeatal stenosis, treated with monthly dilation [27].

Another potential complication is inadvertent traction on the urethral catheter that occurred in one elderly patient in our series, completely disrupting the repair. To prevent that, we suture the Foley catheter to the anterior abdominal wall with a gentle loop in order to minimize tension on the urethra. Failure to maintain a correct position of the catheter may result in necrosis of the urethra. The urethral wound and the catheter should be checked frequently during postoperative care to ensure that there is no pressure on the suture line. Additionally, adequate bladder drainage should be maintained with the catheter until the patient undergoes a trial of voiding at 3 weeks postoperatively. If there is concern a voiding cystourethrogram (VCUG) can be done at that time to confirm the absence of contrast extravasation. We no longer routinely do VCUG after dorsal onlay buccal mucosal graft urethroplasty.

Another complication that may be encountered in the early postoperative period is urinary retention. If urinary retention were to occur, first check for meatal stenosis, and if present, a gentle attempt at urethral dilation should be done. If there is no obvious meatal stenosis, we recommend a gentle attempt at placement of a small Foley catheter followed by a trial of voiding after about 2 weeks. If placement of the catheter is unsuccessful, a suprapubic catheter should be placed. If the patient fails the second voiding trial, we recommend cystoscopy, and if there is no obvious cause of obstruction, videourodynamics should be done. One case has been reported in the literature [25] of stricture recurrence associated with urinary retention. Work-up with urodynamics confirmed hypocontractility, and the patient was managed with intermittent catheterization. If a urethral stricture is diagnosed, it should be dilated. Recurrent strictures may require repeat reconstruction.

Late Complications

Because of the relatively small number of case series reported in the literature, available data cannot provide a consensus for management of various complications of urethral reconstructive surgery. In general, when urethral reconstruction is properly performed, it is associated with high long-term anatomic success rate and low complication rates (Table 21.1). However, functional complications including overactive bladder and stress incontinence have been reported.

1. Postoperative Sphincteric Incontinence
   Postoperative stress urinary incontinence (SUI) is a result of unrecognized sphincteric incontinence before the procedure or a consequence of injury to the sphincter during dissection. In proximal urethral injuries, postoperative incontinence rates may range between 44% and 80% unless a concomitant anti-incontinence surgery is performed [36]. In the majority of studies, the criteria for incontinence following the reconstructive surgery are not specified, leading to a likely underestimation of incidence.

   In our previously published series of 74 patients who underwent vaginal flap urethroplasty, 62 women with preoperative incontinence underwent concomitant fascial pubovaginal sling placement. Successful anatomical repair was achieved in 93% patients, and 87% considered themselves cured or improved with respect to incontinence. All patients with persistent postoperative stress incontinence were successfully treated by secondary procedures [2].

   In a case series of nine women who underwent urethral stricture repair, five concomitant fascial slings were performed synchronously due to sphincteric incontinence. Postoperatively, no urinary incontinence was reported. Success or failure of anatomical repair and incontinence was assessed subjectively and objectively by vali-

Table 21.1 Complications after Urethroplasty for Stricture

Author (year)	Type of Urethral Reconstruction	# Patients	Median Follow-up Period, months	Complications
Prabhuswamy et al. [22]	Dorsal Onlay BMG	37	30	Stricture recurrence (10.8%) Clavien-Dindo Grade 1 (16.2%) Urinary Incontinence (0%)
Higgings et al. [30]	Dorsal Onlay BMG	23	23	Stricture recurrence (17%) Urinary Incontinence (8.7%)
Khawaja et al. [31]	Dorsal Onlay BMG	22	25	Stricture recurrence (8%) Urinary Incontinence (0%)
Kore et al. [26]	Dorsal Onlay BMG	21 BMG	26	Clavien–Dindo Grade 1 (23.8%)—Dysuria Clavien–Dindo Grade 2 (6%)—UTI Stricture recurrence (4.7%) BMG donor site complications—pain, numbness (14.2%)
	Vaginal Wall Graft	11VWG		Clavien–Dindo Grade 1–2 (45%) Dysuria, UTI, Dyspareunia Stricture recurrence (0%)
Manasa et al. [32]	Dorsal Onlay Vaginal Graft	13	8	Stricture recurrence (23%) Urinary Incontinence (0%)
Richard et al. [33]	Dorsal Onlay BMG	19	12	Stricture recurrence (5.3%) Urinary Incontinence (15.7% at 1–3 months) (9.1% at 1 year)
Ozlulerden et al. [34]	Ventral Onlay BMG	7	6	Stricture recurrence (0%) Urinary Incontinence (0%) BMG harvest site complication (0%) Sexual Dysfunction (0%)
Hampson et al. [25]	Dorsal Onlay BMG	39	32	Stricture recurrence (33%) Urinary Incontinence (0%)
Gomez et al. [35]	Dorsal Onlay BMG	17	15	Stricture recurrence (24%)

BMG Buccal Mucosal Graft, *UTI* Urinary Tract Infection, *VWG* Vaginal Wall Graft

dated questionnaires, physical examination, voiding diaries, and 24-hour pad tests. There was no recurrence at 1 year, but two women had stricture recurrence at 5.5 and 6 years, respectively [37].

In patients undergoing urethral reconstruction following mesh sling surgery, some authors suggest that extensive scarring may preclude the successful repair, and recommend a staged procedure to correct the incontinence [7]. Amundsen et al. reported persistent stress incontinence in 2 of 3 cases following synthetic sling removal, repair of the urethra, and Martius flap placement. All were treated with a second-stage pubovaginal sling placement and injection of transurethral collagen. Interestingly, none of the patients after excision of the nonsynthetic sling required further anti-incontinence procedures. Clemens et al. reported five cases of recurrent postoperative stress incontinence in six patients who underwent removal of an eroded sling from the urethra or vaginal mucosa [38]. In our view, documented preoperative sphincteric incontinence and compromised integrity of the sphincter during reconstruction are sufficient reasons to perform concomitant pubovaginal sling at the time of urethral reconstruction. First, harvesting of the fascial graft and placement of the sling around the urethra should be done, then the urethral reconstruction should be completed, and, when necessary, a Martius flap is interposed between the reconstructed urethra, followed by tensioning and tying the sling in place [39] (Fig. 21.6a–c).

When sphincteric incontinence develops after urethral reconstruction, treatment should

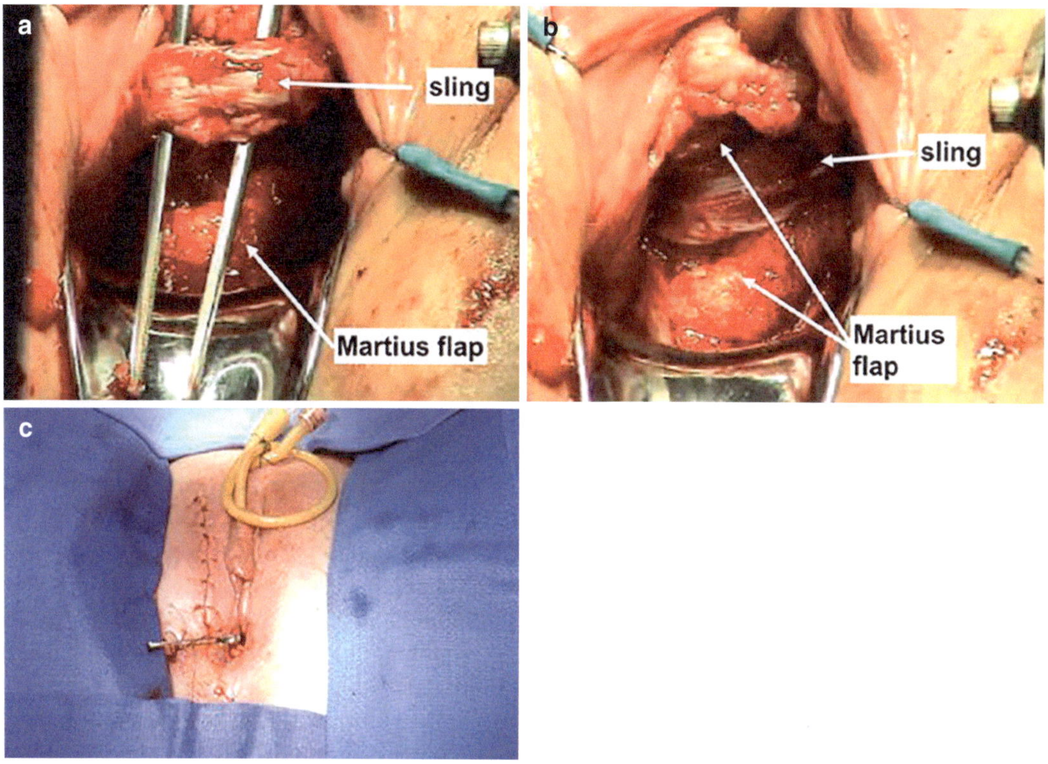

Fig 21.6 (**a, b**) After mobilization of the Martius flap, it is placed between the reconstructed urethra and the autologous fascial sling. (**c**) The completed repair with the Foley catheter sutured in place to prevent downward traction that could disrupt the wound. (Courtesy of J.G. Blaivas)

be tailored to the patient. Of course, any treatment at all is elective, and some patients are not bothered enough to want to consider further treatment. In our judgment, the patient should be evaluated just as would be done if she had not had prior urethral reconstruction, and, for us, that means a bladder questionnaire, diary, exam, uroflow, assessment of postvoid residual urine, videourodynamics, and cystoscopy. As a general rule, though, we defer this evaluation until about 3 months from the reconstructive surgery. If recurrent sphincteric incontinence is documented, we recommend a biologic sling, preferably with autologous fascia. Ideally, the sling should be placed at a virgin site at the bladder neck, or the mid or proximal urethra, proximal to the site of the reconstruction. If the entire mid and proximal urethra has been reconstructed, it is possible to place the sling at the reconstructed urethra, but special care should be taken not to injure the urethra during the surgery. To this end, we recommend that the plane of dissection around the urethra be accomplished sharply under direct vision with a scissor staying in a very superficial plane just beneath the vaginal epithelium. If there is any difficulty extending the dissection into the retropubic space, it should be opened from abdominal side and completed under direct vision. Depending on the nature of the prior reconstruction and the characteristics of the urethra, a Martius flap may be considered as well, placing it between the sling and reconstructed urethra. We believe a synthetic sling is contraindicated in these circumstances.

2. Overactive Bladder

   Persistent or de novo overactive bladder symptoms can be problematic postoperatively. In our series of 74 women after urethral reconstruction, 16% of patients had severe urinary urgency or urge incontinence postoperatively, including those who underwent concomitant autologous pubovaginal sling placement [2]. The series by Onol et al. reports two cases of persistent urge incontinence in 17 women who underwent urethral stricture repair [10]. Similarly, Gormley counted two cases of persistent urge incontinence and one de novo urge incontinence among 12 women who had repair for urethral stricture [4].

The assessment of OAB symptoms should commence within days to weeks after their occurrence to look for remediable causes such as urinary tract infection (UTI), urethral obstruction, and incomplete bladder emptying.

3. Urinary tract infection should be treated with culture-specific antibiotics and urethral obstruction and incomplete emptying ruled out by uroflow and measurement of postvoid residual urine. Women who preoperatively have a long-standing history of obstruction and high detrusor voiding pressure will often maintain a "normal" maximum flow rate but can still be significantly obstructed. One clue for recurrence of obstruction to consider in the uroflow is a flattening of the flow curve, even if maximum flow is normal. If obstructive symptoms persist after these conditions have been treated or excluded, empiric treatment can be tried, but if they prove unsuccessful after a month or so, we recommend cystoscopy and urodynamics to look for obstruction, foreign body, and stones. Patients with refractory OAB after 3 months or so, who underwent sling surgery as part of the reconstruction, are candidates for empiric sling incision or urethrolysis even if they appear unobstructed, but in our series this has not been necessary
4. Urethral Stricture
   Strictures have occurred after dorsal labia minora skin graft urethroplasty [12], dorsal lingual mucosa graft urethroplasty [27], ventral buccal mucosa graft urethroplasty [18], vaginal free grafts [32], and dorsal buccal mucosa graft urethroplasty [22, 25, 35]. In the first case, the patient reported recurrent urinary tract infections and lower urinary tract symptoms at 9 months after surgery. Meatal stenosis was diagnosed and treated with meatotomy, and she was asymptomatic thereafter [12]. In another series, 2 patients presented with obstructive voiding symptoms at 3 months and lower urinary tract symptoms at 5 months follow-up [18, 27]. Both were found to have submeatal stenosis requiring urethral dilations that resulted in complete resolution of symptoms at 12 months follow-up. The dorsal onlay buccal mucosal graft (BMG) urethroplasty series by Hampson et al. [25] reported a 77% success rate. This rate is slightly lower than other smaller series, likely due to their longer follow-up period of mean 33 months (7–106 months). They reported a recurrence rate of 23% (9 patients). Seven patients were managed with dilation or urethrotomy. Another patient was managed with vaginal flap urethroplasty. The last case had a urethral stricture recurrence with associated vesicovaginal fistula and persistent stress urinary incontinence, she underwent simple cystectomy with ileal conduit. In a more recent study by Prabhuswamy et al. [22], a total of 37 patients were included in the study. They had a similar follow-up period of 30 months, with a higher success rate of 89%. Recurrence in this group was managed with urethral dilation in three patients (who did not wish to undergo repeat surgery) and vaginal graft urethroplasty in the remaining fourth patient.

In our experience, late stricture recurrence of 5 years or more after surgery is possible. In two women from our series who underwent vaginal flap urethroplasty, urethral stricture recurrence was noted at 5 and 6 years. Subsequently, both patients underwent successful urethral repair using dorsal buccal mucosa graft and were stricture-free at 12 and 15 months follow-up [37]. Both of these patients developed the recurrent stricture at the time of menopause, so it is possible that hormonal influences played a role in their genesis.

To prevent recurrent strictures, we recommend that peri-menopausal and menopausal women be treated with topical vaginal estrogens. In a report by Gormley, who described follow-up on 12 patients after vaginal flap urethroplasty for female stricture disease, one patient underwent repeat dilation 3 weeks after the procedure due to narrowing of the bladder neck and another required cystoscopy with catheter insertion in the Operating Room 58 months postoperatively [4].

Although most studies report good short-term success, long-term follow-up of every patient is recommended to avoid complications of unrecognized urethral stricture recurrence.

Unfortunately, current data is too sparse to determine what factors predispose a patient to stricture recurrence. We hypothesize that failure to expose and incise the full proximal extent of the stricture during surgery, ischemic changes, and wound contracture might possibly lead to stricture recurrence.

5. Sexual Dysfunction
One of the possible adverse effects of urethral reconstruction is sexual dysfunction. From a theoretical standpoint, this is of particular concern after the dorsal dissection between the clitoris and urethra that is done for dorsal buccal mucosal graft urethroplasty, which could damage the corporal bodies or nerves. To date, though, we are unaware of any reports of this complication after reconstructive surgery and in many other cases using the same incision for take-down of Marshall-Marchietti-Krantz (MMK) or Burch procedures for urethral obstruction. Kore et al. [26] described dyspareunia in patients who underwent vaginal wall graft urethroplasty. Although we have not published this data, we have specifically queried all of our patients who underwent urethral reconstructive surgery about changes in sexual function, including orgasm and pain, and none have suffered any negative sequelae.

Complications of Ancillary Procedures

As discussed, after reconstruction of the severely damaged urethra, it is sometimes advisable to perform a concomitant pubovaginal sling and interpose a vascularized pedicle flap over the repair site. When an anti-incontinence procedure is deemed necessary, in the vast majority of cases, a Martius flap incorporating a labia majora fat pad can be successfully used. Other flaps include rectus abdominus muscle and gracilis myocutaneous flaps have never been necessary in our experience. Flaps improve vascularity of periurethral tissue bed, enhance granulation, separate the suture lines, and promote graft survival.

For construction of a Martius flaps, a vertical incision is made over the labia majora and is carried down through Scarpa's fascia. The fat pad is mobilized with attention to preserve the ventral blood supply from the external pudendal artery or dorsal from the internal pudendal artery. We almost always base the flap on the internal pudendal artery. To minimize blood loss, it is important to incise Scarpa's fascia and dissect between it and the fat pad to create a flap. The fat pad is tunneled underneath the vaginal epithelium and sewn in place over the suture lines of the reconstructed urethra. To the inexperienced surgeon, the plane between Scarpa's fascia and the skin looks like a better plane. However, there are multiple, broad, flat veins from which bleeding is difficult to control, so that plane should be avoided.

If a Martius flap is used, a Penrose drain is traditionally left in for 24–48 h. The overall incidence of major complications attributable to Martius flaps is low. In data by Elkins et al. on 35 women who underwent vesicovaginal and rectovaginal fistula repair with a Martius graft, two had blood loss of more than 350 mL from the harvest site, three experienced cellulitis, and two had dyspareunia due to narrowing of the vagina. However, in two circumstances of cellulitis and vaginal narrowing, closure of the vaginal mucosa over the flap was not possible, and it was left to heal by secondary intention [2]. Kasyan et al.

[40] reported on 37 patients who underwent vaginal reconstruction with Martius flap for management of genito-urinary fistulas: seven patients had bleeding from the flap bed, three had hematomas, five had lymphorrhea, and two had wound infection. In addition, 17% of patients complained of poor cosmesis, 8% had episodic mild pain, and 12% had decreased sensation or numbness of labia. Similar complications of the labial flap may include undesirable cosmetic effects, asymmetry, and impaired sensation at the harvest site have been reported in other series [41].

Serious hemorrhage can be prevented by careful dissection of the plane of fibroadipose tissue with avoidance of deep muscle tissue and attainment of meticulous hemostasis. Urinary retention, obstruction, urgency, and urge incontinence are well-known complications after pubovaginal sling. The American Urological Association (AUA) panel data reports a 5–8% urinary retention rate after pubovaginal fascial sling placement without concurrent repair of prolapse. The rates of de novo urge incontinence and postoperative urge incontinence in patients with preexisting incontinence were 9% and 33%, respectively [42]. In our retrospective review of more than 500 women who underwent pubovaginal fascial sling procedure for stress incontinence, de novo urge incontinence occurred in 3% patients. Other complications such as wound infections, incisional hernia, or long-term urethral obstruction requiring surgery or intermittent catheterization each occurred in 1% of patients [43].

Conclusions

Urethral reconstruction in women is an uncommon surgery, and such complications are not well described in the literature. Complications can be minimized by a thorough preoperative work-up and preoperative planning of the surgical approach. Intraoperative complications include hemorrhage and ureteral injury, though both are rare. Perioperative and postoperative complications include complications specific to the graft or flap site, recurrence, incontinence, urethral obstruction, or detrusor overactivity. In our experience, these complications are unusual and can be treated successfully. Because of the possibility of late recurrence of stricture, long-term follow-up is mandatory.

References

1. Tsivian A, Sidi A. Dorsal graft urethroplasty for female urethral stricture. J Urol. 2006;176(2):611–3.
2. Flisser AJ, Blaivas JG. Outcome of urethral reconstructive surgery in a series of 74 women. J Urol. 2003;169(6):2246–9.
3. Elkins TE, DeLancey JO, McGuire EJ. The use of modified Martius graft as an adjunctive technique in vesicovaginal and rectovaginal fistula repair. Obstet Gynecol. 1990;75(4):727–33.
4. Gormley EA. Vaginal flap urethroplasty for female urethral stricture disease. Neurourol Urodyn. 2010;29(Suppl 1):S42–5.
5. Tanello M, Frego E, Simeone C, Cosciani CS. Use of pedicle flap from the labia minora for the repair of female urethral strictures. Urol Int. 2002;69(2):95–8.
6. Blaivas JG, Purohit RS, Benedon MS, Mekel G, Stern M, Billah M, et al. Safety considerations for synthetic sling surgery. Nat Rev Urol. 2015;12(9):481–509.
7. Amundsen CL, Flynn BJ, Webster GD. Urethral erosion after synthetic and nonsynthetic pubovaginal slings: differences in management and continence outcome. J Urol. 2003;170(1):134–7; discussion 7.
8. Tsivian A, Sidi AA. Dorsal graft urethroplasty for female urethral stricture. J Urol. 2006;176(2):611–3; discussion 3.
9. Migliari R, Leone P, Berdondini E, De Angelis M, Barbagli G, Palminteri E. Dorsal buccal mucosa graft urethroplasty for female urethral strictures. J Urol. 2006;176(4 Pt 1):1473–6.
10. Onol FF, Antar B, Kose O, Erdem MR, Onol SY. Techniques and results of urethroplasty for female urethral strictures: our experience with 17 patients. Urology. 2011;77(6):1318–24.
11. Onol FF, Onol SY, Tahra A, Boylu U. Ventral inlay labia minora graft urethroplasty for the management of female urethral strictures. Urology. 2014;83(2):460–4.
12. Rehder P, Glodny B, Pichler R, Exeli L, Kerschbaumer A, Mitterberger MJ. Dorsal urethroplasty with labia minora skin graft for female urethral strictures. BJU Int. 2010;106(8):1211–4.
13. Montorsi F, Salonia A, Centemero A, Guazzoni G, Nava L, Da Pozzo LF, et al. Vestibular flap urethroplasty for strictures of the female urethra. Impact on symptoms and flow patterns. Urol Int. 2002;69(1):12–6.
14. O'Connell HE, DeLancey JO. Clitoral anatomy in nulliparous, healthy, premenopausal volunteers using unenhanced magnetic resonance imaging. J Urol. 2005;173(6):2060–3.

15. Mozafarpour S, Nwaoha N, Pucheril D, De E. Robotic assisted proximal dorsal urethral diverticulectomy. Int Urogynecol J. 2021;32:2863–6.
16. Sivarajan G, Glickman L, Faber K, Kim M, Fromer D, Munver R. Transabdominal robot-assisted laparoscopic urethral Diverticulectomy of a complex anterior horseshoe diverticulum of the proximal urethra. J Endourol Case Rep. 2015;1(1):33–5.
17. Park JM, Hendren WH. Construction of female urethra using buccal mucosa graft. J Urol. 2001;166(2):640–3.
18. Berglund RK, Vasavada S, Angermeier K, Rackley R. Buccal mucosa graft urethroplasty for recurrent stricture of female urethra. Urology. 2006;67(5):1069–71.
19. Bhargava S, Chapple CR. Buccal mucosal urethroplasty: is it the new gold standard? BJU Int. 2004;93(9):1191–3.
20. Souza GF, Calado AA, Delcelo R, Ortiz V, Macedo A Jr. Histopathological evaluation of urethroplasty with dorsal buccal mucosa: an experimental study in rabbits. Int Braz J Urol. 2008;34(3):345–51; discussion 51–4.
21. Dublin N, Stewart LH. Oral complications after buccal mucosal graft harvest for urethroplasty. BJU Int. 2004;94(6):867–9.
22. Prabhuswamy VK, Somashekarappa HH, Ganeshappa PM, Prabhu K, Krishnamoorthy V. Dorsal onlay buccal mucosal graft urethroplasty for female urethral stricture: techniques and outcomes. Asian J Urol. 2024;11:611–7.
23. Kamp S, Knoll T, Osman M, Hacker A, Michel MS, Alken P. Donor-site morbidity in buccal mucosa urethroplasty: lower lip or inner cheek? BJU Int. 2005;96(4):619–23.
24. Wong E, Fernando A, Alhasso A, Stewart L. Does closure of the buccal mucosal graft bed matter? Results from a randomized controlled trial. Urology. 2014;84(5):1223–7.
25. Hampson LA, Myers JB, Vanni AJ, Virasoro R, Smith TG 3rd, Capiel L, et al. Dorsal buccal graft urethroplasty in female urethral stricture disease: a multicenter experience. Transl Androl Urol. 2019;8(Suppl 1):S6–12.
26. Kore RN, Martins FE. Dorsal onlay urethroplasty using buccal mucosal graft and vaginal wall graft for female urethral stricture—outcome of two-institution study. Indian J Urol. 2022;38:140–5.
27. Sharma GK, Pandey A, Bansal H, Swain S, Das SK, Trivedi S, et al. Dorsal onlay lingual mucosal graft urethroplasty for urethral strictures in women. BJU Int. 2010;105(9):1309–12.
28. Simonato A, Gregori A, Lissiani A, Galli S, Ottaviani F, Rossi R, et al. The tongue as an alternative donor site for graft urethroplasty: a pilot study. J Urol. 2006;175(2):589–92.
29. Elkins TE, Ghosh TS, Tagoe GA, Stocker R. Transvaginal mobilization and utilization of the anterior bladder wall to repair vesicovaginal fistulas involving the urethra. Obstet Gynecol. 1992;79(3):455–60.
30. Higgins M, Oliver J, Flynn B. Female urethroplasty with dorsal onlay buccal mucosal graft: a single-institutional experience. Int Urol Nephrol. 2023;55(5):1149–54. https://doi.org/10.1007/s11255-023-03520-5. Epub 2023 Mar 1.
31. Khawaja AR, Dar YA, Bashir F, et al. Outcome of dorsal buccal graft urethroplasty in female urethral stricture disease (FUSD); our institutional experience. Int Urogynecol J. 2022;33:697–702.
32. Manasa T, Khattar N, Tripathi M, Varshney A, Goel H, Sood R. Dorsal onlay graft urethroplasty for female urethral stricture improves sexual function: short-term results of a prospective study using vaginal graft. Indian J Urol. 2019;35(4):267–72.
33. Richard C, Peyronnet B, Drain A, Rosenblum N, Hascoet J, Sussman R, Freton L, Zhao L, Nitti V, Brucker B. Dorsal onlay oral mucosa graft urethroplasty for female urethral stricture. Urology. 2021;158:215–21.
34. Ozlulerden Y, Celen S, Zumrutbas AE, Aybek Z. Female buccal mucosa graft urethroplasty: a new modified ventral onlay "AZ" technique. Int Urogynecol J. 2020;31:2543–50.
35. Gomez RG, Segura FJ, Saavedra A, Campos RA. Female urethral reconstruction: dorsal buccal mucosa graft onlay. World J Urol. 2020;38(12):3047–54. https://doi.org/10.1007/s00345-019-02958-6. Epub 2019 Sep 21. PMID: 31542825.
36. Blaivas JG, Sandhu J. Urethral reconstruction after erosion of slings in women. Curr Opin Urol. 2004;14(6):335–8.
37. Blaivas JG, Santos JA, Tsui JF, Deibert CM, Rutman MP, Purohit RS, et al. Management of urethral stricture in women. J Urol. 2012;188(5):1778–82.
38. Clemens JQ, DeLancey JO, Faerber GJ, Westney OL, McGuire EJ. Urinary tract erosions after synthetic pubovaginal slings: diagnosis and management strategy. Urology. 2000;56(4):589–94.
39. Blaivas JG, Heritz DM. Vaginal flap reconstruction of the urethra and vesical neck in women: a report of 49 cases. J Urol. 1996;155(3):1014–7.
40. Kasyan G, Tupikina N, Pushkar D. Use of Martius flap in the complex female urethral surgery. Cent European J Urol. 2014;67(2):202–7. https://doi.org/10.5173/ceju.2014.02.art20. Epub 2014 Jun 23. PMID: 25140241; PMCID: PMC4132599.
41. Petrou SP, Jones J, Parra RO. Martius flap harvest site: patient self-perception. J Urol. 2002;167(5):2098–9.
42. Dmochowski RR, Blaivas JM, Gormley EA, Juma S, Karram MM, Lightner DJ, et al. Update of AUA guideline on the surgical management of female stress urinary incontinence. J Urol. 2010;183(5):1906–14.
43. Blaivas JG, Chaikin DC. Pubovaginal fascial sling for the treatment of all types of stress urinary incontinence: surgical technique and long-term outcome. Urol Clin North Am. 2011;38(1):7–15.

Urethral Diverticulectomy

22

Emma Bacharach, Lindsey Cox,
Alienor S. Gilchrist, and Eric S. Rovner

Introduction

Urethral diverticulum (UD) is a rare condition and diagnosis can be challenging to the clinician [1]. Once the correct diagnosis is made, transvaginal surgical excision is the mainstay of definitive treatment [2]. Although options for the surgical treatment of urethral diverticula include marsupialization, which would be appropriate for some lesions with a distal ostium, this review will focus on complications from the transvaginal approach for mid- and proximal urethral diverticulum excision, as has been previously described [3]. A full discussion of urethral diverticulectomy surgical technique is beyond the scope of this chapter, but specific points will be discussed where appropriate.

Prevention of Complications

Although most complications of urethral diverticulectomy are treatable and reversible, it is optimal to prevent or minimize adverse outcomes. Prevention of complications begins in the preoperative period, during the diagnostic evaluation and work-up. The typical evaluation of patients with a suspected UD consists of a history, physical examination, cystourethroscopy, and appropriate imaging, including voiding cystourethrography and magnetic resonance imaging (MRI) as clinically indicated (Fig. 22.1). For patients with lower urinary tract symptoms or incontinence, videourodynamic studies may be utilized to evaluate for the presence of stress incontinence, detrusor overactivity, bladder outlet obstruction, and specifically for the presence of a closed, competent bladder neck at rest. Patients with stress incontinence or an incompetent bladder neck can be offered concomitant placement of an autologous fascial sling at the time of UD excision. Urine cytology, when positive, can assist in making the correct diagnosis of malignancy; however, negative cytology does not rule out malignancy. In all cases, UD specimens should be sent for permanent pathologic evaluation following excision to evaluate for malignant tissue. Preoperative urine cultures are obtained to appropriately tailor preoperative antibiotics and decrease the risks of perioperative and postoperative infection. The differential diagnosis of periurethral masses (Table 22.1) is extensive and includes Skene's gland cyst or abscess (Fig. 22.2), vaginal leiomyoma [4], and primary urethral malignancy. Therefore, the importance of a correct diagnosis prior to

E. Bacharach · L. Cox · E. S. Rovner (✉)
Department of Urology, Medical University of South Carolina, Charleston, SC, USA
e-mail: rovnere@musc.edu

A. S. Gilchrist
Department of Urology, Piedmont Hospital, Stockbridge, GA, USA

H. B. Goldman, J. Zillioux (eds.), *Complications of Urogynecology and Reconstructive Pelvic Surgery*, https://doi.org/10.1007/978-3-032-00339-3_22

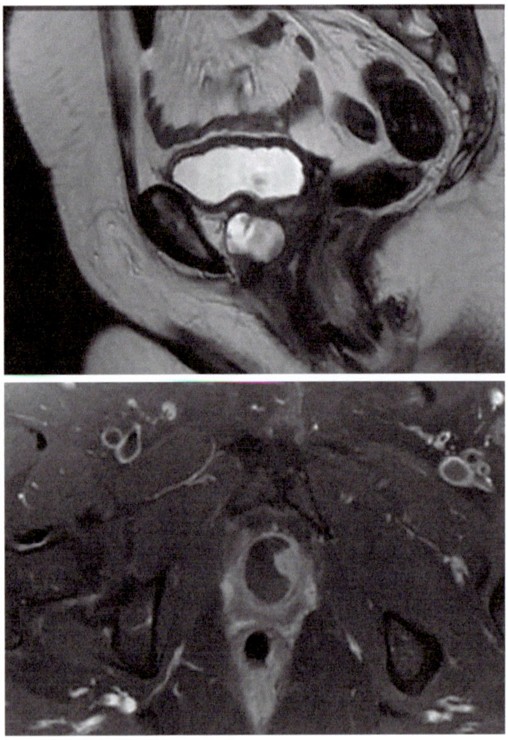

Fig. 22.1 (Top) Sagittal view T2 MRI demonstrating near circumferential configuration of urethral diverticulum (Bottom) Axial view T1 MRI showing lateral horseshoe urethral diverticulum

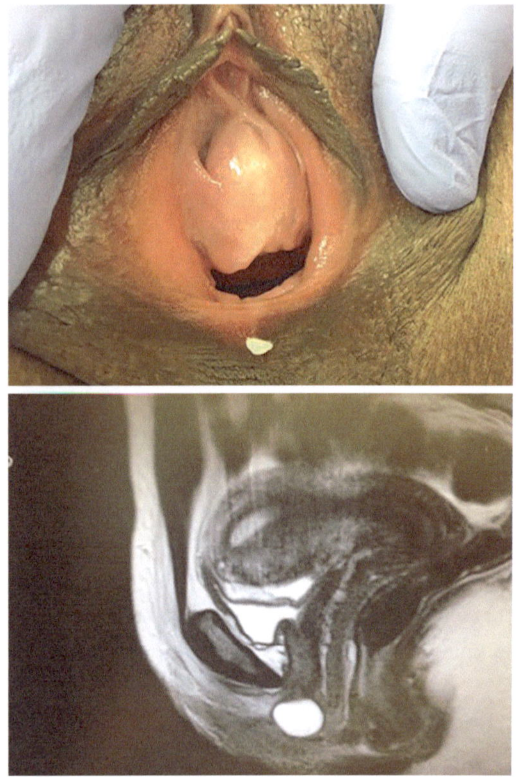

Fig. 22.2 Skene's gland abscess clinically (top) and on MRI (bottom)

Table 22.1 Differential diagnosis of periurethral masses

Leiomyoma
Skene's gland abnormalities
Gartner's duct abnormalities
Vaginal wall cysts
Urethral mucosal prolapse
Urethral caruncle
Periurethral bulking agents
Malignancy
Endometriosis

undertaking surgical excision cannot be overemphasized.

Preoperative topical estrogen replacement in those with postmenopausal vaginal atrophy can be helpful in improving tissue quality.

Intraoperative Complications

Intraoperative complications related to anterior compartment vaginal surgery have been previously described and include, but are not limited to, bleeding and injury to the urinary tract.

Bleeding

The risk of bleeding during surgery can be minimized, but not entirely eliminated, by good operative technique. Multiple blood vessels traverse the deep pelvis, including large venous channels in the retropubic space. Most of these vessels are not a risk during urethral diverticulectomy surgery, but if concomitant anti-incontinence or vaginal prolapse surgery is being considered, bleeding from these is a potential complication. Named vessels in the obturator fossa along the pelvic sidewall, including branches of the internal iliac, and those vessels within the vascular pedicle of the bladder are at risk for injury, particularly during passage of trocars or needles for concomitant pubovaginal sling. Major vascular injury can quickly lead to life-threatening hemorrhage if not recognized intraoperatively and may result in large retropubic hematomas postoperatively [5, 6]. Bleeding during the harvest of a concomitant Martius flap is usually easily visualized and controlled with a combination of cautery, suture ligature, and direct compression. Labial hematomas have been reported with postoperative bleeding [7].

Bleeding during UD surgery, however, can also be problematic. The initial dissection of the vaginal flap from the underlying periurethral fascia should be associated with minimal bleeding. Bleeding encountered during this early dissection may indicate an excessively deep and incorrect surgical plane. In this circumstance, immediate recognition and reevaluation are necessary to avoid inadvertent entry into the urethral diverticulum or urinary tract and to minimize bleeding. Following identification of this situation, dissection should proceed in the proper surgical plane; in reoperative surgery, however, this may be difficult to identify.

Another common site of bleeding during transvaginal UD surgery occurs when traversing the endopelvic fascia for placement of a pubovaginal sling, as noted previously. Entry into the retropubic space from the transvaginal side or placement of the suprapubic needles or trocars from the abdominal side may be associated with copious bleeding as the endopelvic fascia is perforated. If the bleeding continues and is brisk, the vagina can be packed. It can be very helpful to manually elevate the anterior vaginal wall and compress it anteriorly against the posterior symphysis pubis for several minutes using the surgeon's hand, sponge stick, or a retractor. These maneuvers will effectively tamponade bleeding in the retropubic space. Packing and compression will result in adequate control in the majority of cases; if not, the surgeon should expeditiously complete the procedure, close the incisions, and pack the vagina [8]. Additionally, absorbable sutures can be placed through and through the vaginal wall in the lateral fornices of the anterior vagina to ligate vessels that cannot be visualized in the operative field. Brisk bleeding that does not respond to manual compression for an extended period of time may suggest a major vessel injury and mandates retropubic exploration.

Urinary Tract Injury

Urethra

The Foley catheter is usually seen following complete excision of UD at the location of the entry of the ostium into the urethra. The urethra can be reconstructed over as small as a 14F Foley catheter without long-term risk of urethral stricture and should be closed in a watertight fashion with absorbable suture [9]. The closure should be tension-free. Uncommonly, an UD may extend circumferentially around the urethra and require transection of the involved portion of the urethra and complex reconstruction [10, 11].

Ureter

Ureteral injury during UD surgery is rare but may occur with a large or proximal UD extending beyond the bladder neck and posterior to the bladder trigone, especially in the setting of anterior vaginal wall prolapse. In these instances, cystoscopic placement of ureteric catheters prior to the dissection may aid in ureteral identification. Virtually all of these injuries can be identified by intraoperative cystoscopy. The administration of intravenous vital dyes such as indigo carmine permits obvious visualization of ureteral efflux, confirming ureteral patency. With limited availability of indigo carmine, preoperative oral phenazopyridine, 50% dextrose solution for bladder filling, or intraoperative intravenous 10% fluorescein can be used as alternatives [12, 13]. Suspected ureteral injuries are confirmed by retrograde pyeloureterography. Ureteral transection requires ureteroneocystostomy. Inadvertent ureteral obstruction by sutures can also be recognized with cystoscopic confirmation of ureteral patency. If obstruction is suspected, offending sutures can be identified and removed, and placement of a temporary indwelling ureteral stent can be considered.

Bladder

Intraoperative bladder injury may occur during dissection of a large UD extending proximal to the bladder neck and inferior to the bladder (Fig. 22.3), or alternatively, may occur with passage of a ligature carrier through the retropubic space if placing a pubovaginal sling.

Injury to the bladder during UD excision is diagnosed intraoperatively by careful endoscopic examination of the bladder and bladder neck with a 70° lens or a flexible cystoscope with retroflexion following UD dissection. The bladder should be filled and then examined to ensure that a small injury does not go unrecognized in a fold of the bladder wall.

If there is injury to the bladder during UD dissection, intravenous dyes should be administered to confirm ureteral integrity. Small cystotomies may be closed in layers with absorbable sutures transvaginally. More extensive injuries involving the trigone or more proximal bladder may require transabdominal repair. Postoperative drainage of the bladder with a Foley catheter will help avoid urinoma, fistula formation, and pelvic abscess.

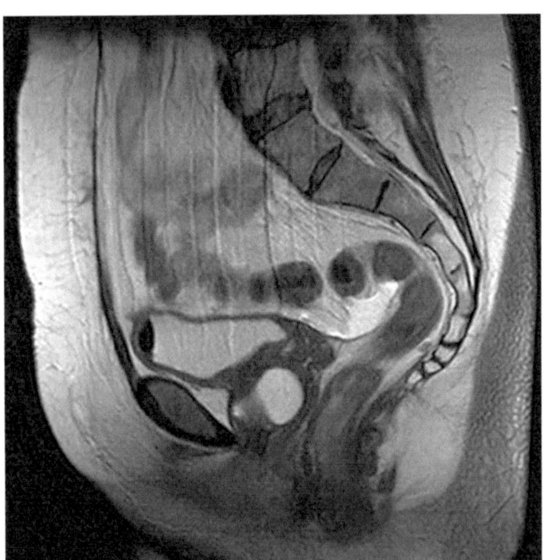

Fig. 22.3 Urethral diverticulum extending below the trigone

Postoperative Complications

Careful adherence to the principles of transvaginal urethral diverticulectomy should minimize postoperative complications (Table 22.2). Nevertheless, complications may arise (Table 22.3). One small series suggested that large diverticula (>4 cm) or those associated with a lateral or horseshoe configuration may be associated with a greater likelihood of postoperative complications, and risk factors for failure or poor functional outcome included horseshoe or circumferential configuration or a previous (failed) surgical intervention [14]. Large or more complex UD typically require greater dissection and more involved reconstruction.

Raup and coworkers described 30-day complications of diverticulectomy in the multi-institutional cohort derived from the National Surgical Quality Improvement Program user files. There were 122 female urethral diverticulectomy cases reported from the 2.3 million cases in the database. Minor complications occurred in 3.3% of cases, with urinary tract infection (UTI) being most common (four patients), and one each of superficial wound infection and hemorrhage requiring transfusion [15]. Bradley and colleagues reported a multi-

Table 22.2 Principles of transvaginal urethral diverticulectomy

Mobilization of a well-vascularized anterior vaginal wall flap(s)
Preservation of the periurethral fascia as a separate layer
Identification and excision of the neck of the UD or ostium
Removal of entire UD wall or sac (epithelium)
Watertight urethral closure
Multilayered, nonoverlapping closure with absorbable suture
Closure of dead space
Preservation or creation of continence

Data from Ref. Rovner [2]

Table 22.3 Complications of transvaginal urethral diverticulectomy

Complication (% range of reported incidence)
Urinary incontinence (1.7–16.1%)
Urethrovaginal fistula (0.9–8.3%)
Urethral stricture (0–5.2%)
Recurrent UD (1–25%)
Recurrent UTI (0–31.3%)
Other
Hypospadias/distal urethral necrosis
Bladder or ureteral injury
Vaginal scarring or narrowing: dyspareunia, etc.

Data from Ref. Dmochowski [51]

center cohort study of 389 patients undergoing diverticulectomy, with short-term complications including UTI in 61 (15.7%), urinary retention in 15 (3.9%), and wound infection in 4 (1.0%) [16]. Nickles and coworkers report a series of 43 patients who underwent urethral diverticulectomy with UTI rates of 3/11 (27%) for complex UD, and 1/32 (3%) for simple UD [17]. In a series of 38 patients undergoing autologous rectus fascial pubovaginal sling and UD repair, Enemchukwu and coworkers report a 5% (2/38) rate of wound infection, presumably at the sling harvest site [18].

Incontinence

Stress Urinary Incontinence

Patients with preoperative symptomatic stress urinary incontinence (SUI) in association with UD can be offered simultaneous anti-incontinence surgery. Preoperative videourodynamics may be helpful in evaluating the anatomy of the UD, assessing the competence of the bladder neck, and confirming the diagnosis of SUI. In patients with SUI and UD, Ganabathi and others have described excellent results with concomitant needle bladder neck suspension [9, 19], although such needle suspensions are rarely done in contemporary practice. More recently, pubovaginal autologous fascial slings have been utilized in patients with UD and SUI with satisfactory outcomes [1, 16, 18, 20–22]. The role of synthetic midurethral slings, however, has not been well defined in this population, and the current AUA Guideline recommends against using synthetic material contemporaneously at the time of urethral diverticulectomy [23]. Placement of synthetic material adjacent to a fresh suture line following diverticulectomy in the setting of potentially infected urine may place the patient at higher risk for subsequent urethral erosion and vaginal extrusion of the sling material, as well as urethrovaginal fistula formation and foreign body granuloma formation [23].

Significant postoperative de novo SUI may occur in between 7% and 19% of individuals undergoing urethral diverticulectomy surgery without a concomitant anti-incontinence surgery [7, 24–26]. However, Lee and colleagues noted at least minor de novo SUI in 49% of patients following urethral diverticulectomy, the majority of which was minor and did not require additional therapy [27]. Only 10% of these individuals underwent a subsequent SUI operation. Risk factors for de novo SUI may include the size of the diverticulum (>30 mm) and a more proximal location [25]. Ljungqvist and colleagues correlated de novo SUI with wide diverticulum excision in addition to size and location [7]. Malde and colleagues reported that of 33 patients, de novo SUI occurred in 0% with simple UD, 6% with horseshoe configuration, and 20% with circumferential configuration suggesting that a higher rate of de novo SUI occurs in complex UD [28]. Popat and Zimmern [29] reported long-term follow-up for 12 women with horseshoe diverticula who underwent diverticulectomy using a urethral preservation technique. Four patients had stress incontinence related to a more proximal UD location, which may compromise the urethral sphincter and bladder neck anatomical support and/or the sphincter mechanism [25, 29]. Alternatively, large UD at the bladder neck may cause obstruction [30], and occult SUI may be unmasked after removing the obstructing UD [31]. A more recent small study by Shaaf and colleagues found no evidence of association between UD complexity and postoperative SUI. In their cohort, de novo SUI occurred in 19%, and, conversely, 47% of preexisting SUI resolved with diverticulectomy [26].

Management of de novo postoperative SUI is undertaken after allowing postsurgical inflammation to subside. Autologous pubovaginal sling is a reasonable option in this setting. Synthetic materials such as midurethral polypropylene slings must be used judiciously in this setting; however, safety data are lacking. Repeat preoperative imaging may be helpful in excluding a recurrent or persistent UD, or urethrovaginal fistula prior to surgery for incontinence [7].

Urinary Urgency and Urgency Incontinence

Stav and colleagues reported that rates of urgency/frequency symptoms decreased significantly postoperatively from 60% to 16% and noted complete resolution of urgency incontinence in some [25]. Other series, however, have demonstrated rates of postoperative urgency of 54% [32] and de novo urgency incontinence in 36% of patients [7], including the recent series by Nickles and coworkers which showed urgency urinary incontinence in 3/11 (27.3%) patients undergoing complex diverticulectomy and 6/32 (24%) of patients undergoing simple UD repair [17].

Preoperative counseling should include a discussion of new-onset storage symptoms. These symptoms may be managed expectantly postoperatively; nonetheless, continued symptoms postoperatively may herald UD persistence, UD recurrence, or de novo urethral obstruction. Importantly, urinary incontinence following UD excision should be evaluated to rule out the presence of urethrovaginal or vesicovaginal fistula.

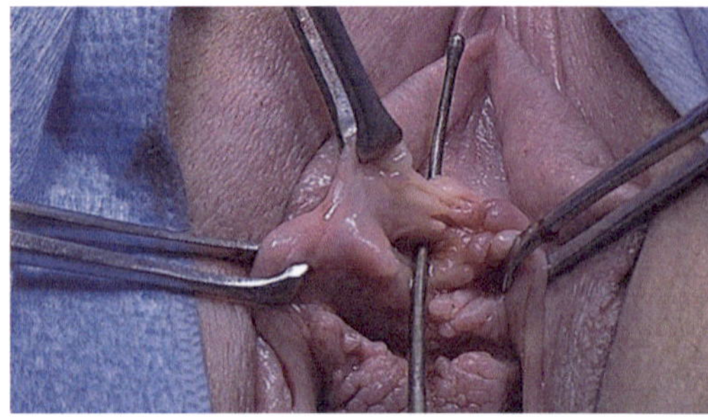

Fig. 22.4 Distal urethrovaginal fistula

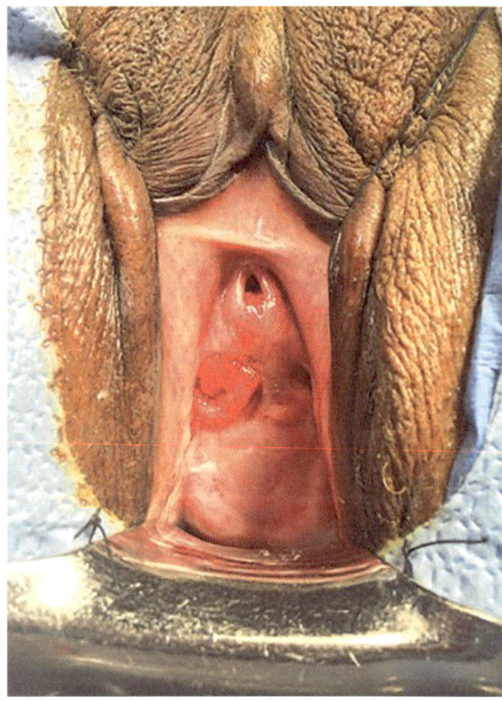

Fig. 22.5 Midurethral urethrovaginal fistula

Urethrovaginal Fistula

A urethrovaginal fistula located distal to the sphincteric mechanism (Fig. 22.4) should not be associated with symptoms other than perhaps a split urinary stream and/or vaginal voiding. As such, an asymptomatic distal urethrovaginal fistula may not require repair although some patients may request repair. A proximal urethrovaginal fistula located at the bladder neck, or at the midurethra in patients with an incompetent bladder neck will likely result in considerable symptomatic urinary leakage (Fig. 22.5). Fistula repair in these symptomatic cases can be undertaken transvaginally with consideration for the use of an adjuvant tissue flap such as a Martius flap to provide a well-vascularized additional tissue layer. The timing of urethrovaginal fistula repair relative to the initial diverticulectomy is controversial, but should allow for tissue inflammation to subside at 3–6 months postoperatively. Meticulous attention to surgical technique, good hemostasis, avoidance of infection, preservation of the periurethral fascia, and a well-vascularized anterior vaginal wall flap, combined with a multilayered closure and nonoverlapping suture lines, should minimize the potential for postoperative urethrovaginal fistula formation [31]. Urethrovaginal fistula rates in two recent publications combining diverticulectomy series showed 7/580 or 1.2% rate of fistula [33], and of the 42 studies with 1928 patients mentioning fistula outcomes, 38 fistulas were described, but the data were too heterogeneous to combine, giving a range of 1–8% [34].

Recurrent Symptoms

While complete resolution of obstructive and irritative urinary symptoms after UD excision may occur [25, 34], some patients will have persistence or recurrence of their preoperative symptoms postoperatively. Ljungqvist and colleagues noted reoperation (but not necessarily the extent of the primary operation) was the greatest clinical factor associated with residual symptoms postoperatively [7]. These symptoms may be a result of surgery itself, and, if so, may resolve over time. Such symptoms should be carefully investigated, as recurrent UD, new UD, or urethral stricture should be high on the differential diagnosis.

Recurrent Urethral Diverticulum

Recurrence of UD may be due to incomplete removal of the epithelialized UD sac, failure to recognize a second ostium, inadequate closure of the urethra, failure to close residual dead space, excessive tension on the repair, infection, or other technical factors [31, 35]. Lee noted recurrent UD in 8/85 patients at follow-up of between 2 and 15 years from the initial UD resection [36], while Ljungqvist and colleagues reported recurrence in 11/68 patients over a 26-year follow-up [7]. Vaidya reported a recurrence rate of 8% in 14/172 patients at a mean follow-up of 1.4 years [37]. The risk of recurrence of UD following transvaginal excision may be related to the complexity of the anatomical configuration. Han and coworkers reported no recurrent UD in 17 patients with simple UD, but of the 10 patients with circumferential UD, recurrence was noted in 6 (60%) [24]. Notably, in this series, secondary procedures were not as successful in completely removing the UD. Ockrim and coworkers similarly cured all 19 patients presenting with simple urethral diverticula on the first attempt, but the 11 patients with complex anatomical configurations required a total of 17 procedures for success [30]. Ingber reported a 10% reoperation rate for UD recurrence, which was associated with proximal UD location, multiplicity, and prior urethral vaginal surgery [32]. Zhou et al. reported UD recurrence in 13 of 66 patients, and risk factors for recurrence included prior urethral surgery, multiple diverticula, and proximal location [38]. Nickles reported one recurrent complex UD out of 11, and no recurrences in 32 simple UD [17]. Popat reported one recurrence in 12 patients with horseshoe UD [29]. In a series of 38 patients undergoing UD repair with rectus sheath pubovaginal sling, there were two UD recurrences [18]. Malde and associates reported that among women with predominantly complex UD and undergoing Martius flap interposition, the recurrence rate was 2 out of 70, suggesting a lower rate of recurrence with the Martius technique [39].

Recurrent UD after failed prior surgeries may lead to more complex, circumferential involvement [10]. Repeat urethral diverticulectomy surgery can be challenging due to altered anatomy, scarring, and the difficulty in identifying the proper anatomic planes. Prevention of recurrence, especially in reoperative UDs, includes the use of a Martius flap, while MRI remains invaluable in surgical planning to ensure complete excision [30, 40]. Complications such as fistula and recurrence of the UD are more common in reoperative cases [7].

Urethral Stricture

Urethral strictures are rare following UD excision; Rovner and Wein noted urethral stricture in 1/44 patients, Ljungqvist in 1/27 patients, and Bradley in 7/389 patients (1.8%) [7, 10, 16].

Stricture may result from closing the urethra too tightly or reconstructing it over too small a sound/catheter or, in one instance, postoperative catheter dislodgement [10]. Additionally, poorly vascularized periurethral tissues could result in ischemia and stricture formation postoperatively. A Martius flap should be considered intraoperatively if urethral reconstruction is complex to provide a healthy graft and assist in stricture prevention. A urethral stricture may be managed postoperatively initially with urethral dilation. Rarely is open reconstruction with urethroplasty using a vaginal flap or buccal mucosa graft necessary.

Recurrent Urinary Tract Infections

Frequent UTIs may persist following UD excision and may be due to the recurrence of the diverticulum or other etiologies. Ingber and coworkers found 23% of patients reported having three or more infections in the last year of follow-up after urethral diverticulectomy [32]. In a series of 389 patients, Bradley found the incidence of recurrent UTIs decreased from 33.4% to 2.6% [16]. Bodner-Adler report in their systematic review of the literature that 7–31% of patients have recurrent UTIs after diverticulectomy [34]. Recurrent UTI work-up can be undertaken once recurrent UD has been excluded.

Pain

Urethral pain and/or severe pelvic pain was significantly relieved or resolved in all patients following diverticulectomy in one series [10]. Romanzi found resolution of preoperative urethral pain in all but two patients postoperatively [1]. Nonetheless, urethral pain may persist despite surgical intervention. Ockrim and coworkers reported persistent pain in two patients, despite repeat diverticulectomy including extensive dissection of the urethra [30]. Bradley reported persistent vaginal pain in 24/389 (6.2%) of patients post op [16]. Persistent postoperative urethral and pelvic pain, in the absence of UD recurrence, may be secondary to postsurgical changes, chronic inflammation of the periurethral tissues from the prior UD, pelvic floor muscle disorders, or may be multifactorial in etiology and may ultimately require a multimodal treatment approach.

Dyspareunia

Dyspareunia is one of the classic presenting symptoms of UD. In two larger series of UD patients with preoperative dyspareunia rates of 54% and 56%, rates dropped to 10% and 8%, respectively, postoperatively [25, 30]. In another large series, preoperative dyspareunia was noted in 100/389 (25.7%) and dropped to 11/389 (2.8%) post diverticulectomy [16]. An additional study of 40 patients with UD indicated that female sexual function index (FSFI) scores at 12 months postoperatively improved in all domains, with the greatest improvements in pain and satisfaction [41]. Similarly, Sun and colleagues noted that for 83 patients undergoing urethral diverticulectomy, female sexual function index (FSFI) scores postoperatively at 12 months improved for all women, with the greatest score improvements in patients with complex UD (large, multiple, horseshoe configuration) [42].

Persistent or de novo dyspareunia postoperatively may result from postsurgical changes, including vaginal scarring and narrowing, especially in patients undergoing reoperative surgery. Vaginal narrowing can be prevented by harvesting a wide-based vaginal flap, thereby avoiding subsequent devascularization and contracture. Romanzi and coworkers reported dyspareunia resulting from the Martius flap and labial point tenderness on the harvest side [1]. Patients should be counseled appropriately regarding possible postoperative persistence of this symptom and be well informed of the possible sequelae of the Martius flap harvest. Similar to persistent urethral and pelvic pain, postoperative management of dyspareunia may require a multimodal approach.

Hypospadias/Distal Urethral Necrosis

Distal urethral tissue loss and hypospadias are possible complications of the Spence-Duckett marsupialization procedure. Changes in the distal urethra can cause a spraying stream or vaginal voiding.

Malignant Lesions

Malignant and benign neoplasms may be found in urethral diverticula at the time of permanent pathologic specimen. Approximately 10% of urethral diverticulectomy specimens may demonstrate histopathological abnormalities, including metaplasia, dysplasia, or frank carcinoma, which require long-term follow-up or additional therapy [43]. The rates of frank malignancy variations, however, are thought to be exceedingly low. A large retrospective study by Vaidya and colleagues reported a rate of malignancy of 1.2%, accounting for 2/172 patients undergoing diverticulectomy over 15 years [37]. The most common malignant pathology in UD is adenocarcinoma, followed by transitional cell and squamous cell carcinomas [43, 44]. In contrast, the most common histologic type of primary urethral carcinoma is squamous cell carcinoma. Non-excisional therapy of UD, such as marsupialization or endoscopic incision, can be combined with a biopsy to rule out malignancy [45].

It has not been conclusively demonstrated that any particular preoperative imaging modality, such as ultrasound or MRI, can reliably and prospectively diagnose a small malignancy arising in an UD [46]. Nonetheless, when concern for malignancy exists, the contemporary approach often involves gadolinium-enhanced MRI of the pelvis followed by transurethral or transvaginal biopsies for definitive diagnosis [47]. Urine cytology has been noted to be potentially useful as an initial screening test with a high sensitivity of 91% [47].

There is no consensus on proper treatment in cases where a malignancy is found in a diverticulectomy specimen, and recurrence rates are high with local treatment alone [44]. For both local and advanced disease, case report-based literature indicate that surgical management is the cornerstone of current treatment strategies and may include urethral diverticulectomy, urethrectomy in conjunction with cystectomy or anterior exenteration [47]. Multimodal therapy, including neoadjuvant or adjuvant chemotherapy and radiotherapy, is also employed, especially in more advanced cases [47, 48]. Major prognostic factors include local extent of tumor, histology, and lymph node involvement [48]. For adenocarcinoma, platinum-based chemotherapy is standard, and there is evidence that the neoadjuvant approach is superior to adjuvant [48]. Targeted therapies can be utilized in the setting of failure of platinum-based chemotherapy [48].

Stones

Calculi within UD are not uncommon and may be diagnosed in 4–10% of cases [1, 49, 50] and are most likely due to urinary stasis and/or infection. This may be suspected by physical exam findings or noted incidentally on preoperative imaging. The presence of a stone will not significantly alter the evaluation or surgical approach, and it can be removed with the UD specimen at the time of surgery.

References

1. Romanzi LJ, Groutz A, Blaivas JG. Urethral diverticulum in women: diverse presentations resulting in diagnostic delay and mismanagement. J Urol. 2000;164(2):428–33.
2. Rovner ES. Bladder and female urethral diverticula. In: Wein AJ, Kavoussi L, Novick A, Partin A, Peters C, editors. Campbell-Walsh urology. 10th ed. Philadelphia: Elsevier Saunders; 2012.
3. Leach GE, Schmidbauer CP, Hadley HR, Staskin DR, Zimmern P, Raz S. Surgical treatment of female urethral diverticulum. Semin Urol. 1986;4(1):33–42.
4. Shirvani AR, Winters JC. Vaginal leiomyoma presenting as a urethral diverticulum. J Urol. 2000;163(6):1869.
5. Rajan S, Kohli N. Retropubic hematoma after transobturator sling procedure. Obstet Gynecol. 2005;106(5 Pt 2):1199–202.

6. Walters MD, Tulikangas PK, LaSala C, Muir TW. Vascular injury during tension-free vaginal tape procedure for stress urinary incontinence. Obstet Gynecol. 2001;98:957–9.
7. Ljungqvist L, Peeker R, Fall M. Female urethral diverticulum: 26-year followup of a large series. J Urol. 2007;177(1):219–24; discussion 224
8. Ficazzola M, Nitti V. Complications of incontinence procedures in women. In: Taneja S, Smith R, Ehrlich R, editors. Complications of urologic surgery: prevention and management. 3rd ed. Philadelphia: WB Saunders; 2001. p. 482–98.
9. Ganabathi K, Leach GE, Zimmern PE, Dmochowski R. Experience with the management of urethral diverticulum in 63 women. J Urol. 1994;152:1445–52.
10. Rovner ES, Wein AJ. Diagnosis and reconstruction of the dorsal or circumferential urethral diverticulum. J Urol. 2003;170(1):82–6. discussion 86.
11. Tamada S, Iwai Y, Tanimoto Y, et al. Urethral diverticula surrounding the urethra in women: report of 2 cases. Hinyokika Kiyo. 2000;46(9):639–42.
12. Doyle PJ, Lipetskaia L, Duecy E, Buchsbaum G, Wood RW. Sodium fluorescein use during intraoperative cystoscopy. Obstet Gynecol. 2015;125(3):548–50.
13. Narasimhulu DM, Prabakar C, Tang N, Bral P. Use of 50% dextrose as the distension medium during cystoscopy for visualization of ureteric jets. Obstet Gynecol. 2016;127(1):78–80.
14. Porpiglia F, Destefanis P, Fiori C, Fontana D. Preoperative risk factors for surgery of female urethral diverticula. Urol Int. 2002;69:7–11.
15. Raup VT, Hess DS, Hanske J, et al. Patient characteristics and perioperative outcomes of female urethral diverticulectomy: analysis of a multi-institutional prospective database. Urology. 2015;86(4):712–5.
16. Bradley SE, Leach DA, Panza J, Sassani J, Escobar C, Ogorek J, Jackson E, et al. A multicenter retrospective cohort comparing urethral diverticulectomy with and without concomitant pubovaginal sling. Am J Obstet Gynecol. 2020;222(3):S772. Elsevier Inc.
17. Nickles SW, Ikwuezunma G, Maclachlan L, El-Zawahry A, Rames R, Rovner E. Simple vs complex urethral diverticulum: presentation and outcomes. Urology. 2014;84(6):1516–20.
18. Enemchukwu E, Lai C, Reynolds WS, Kaufman M, Dmochowski R. Autologous pubovaginal sling for the treatment of concomitant female urethral diverticula and stress urinary incontinence. Urology. 2015;85(6):1300–3.
19. Lockhart JL, Ellis GF, Helal M, Pow-Sang JM. Combined cystourethropexy for the treatment of type 3 and complicated female urinary incontinence. J Urol. 1990;143(4):722–5.
20. Faerber GJ. Urethral diverticulectomy and pubovaginal sling for simultaneous treatment of urethral diverticulum and intrinsic sphincter deficiency. Tech Urol. 1998;4(4):192–7.
21. Swierzewski SJ, McGuire EJ. Pubovaginal sling for treatment of female stress urinary incontinence complicated by urethral diverticulum. J Urol. 1993;149(5):1012–4.
22. Greiman A, Rittenberg L, Freilich D, Rames R, El-Zawahry A, Koski M, Rovner E. Outcomes of treatment of stress urinary incontinence associated with female urethral diverticula: a selective approach. Neurourol Urodyn. 2018;37(1):478–84. United States: Wiley Subscription Services, Inc.
23. Kobashi KC, Vasavada S, Bloschichak A, et al. Updates to surgical treatment of female stress urinary incontinence (SUI): AUA/SUFU guideline (2023). J Urol. 2023;209(6):1091–8.
24. Han DH, Jeong YS, Choo M-S, Lee K-S. Outcomes of surgery of female urethral diverticula classified using magnetic resonance imaging. Eur Urol. 2007;51(6):1664–70.
25. Stav K, Dwyer PL, Rosamilia A, Chao F. Urinary symptoms before and after female urethral diverticulectomy—can we predict de novo stress urinary incontinence? J Urol. 2008;180(5):2088–90.
26. Schaaf AL, Lee YS, Myers AA, Schommer J, Gonzalez G, Chen A, Petrou S. Complex urethral Diverticulectomy: is a synchronous prophylactic autologous fascial sling needed? Urogynecology (Phila). 2023;29(6):552–7. https://doi.org/10.1097/SPV.0000000000001311. Epub 2023 Feb 4
27. Lee UJ, Goldman H, Moore C, Daneshgari F, Rackley RR, Vasavada SP. Rate of de novo stress urinary incontinence after urethal diverticulum repair. Urology. 2008;71(5):849–53.
28. Malde S, Naaseri S, Kavia R, et al. Preliminary report on the effect of urethral diverticulum magnetic resonance imaging configuration on the incidence of new onset urodynamic stress urinary incontinence following excision. Urol Ann. 2017;9(4):321–3. https://doi.org/10.4103/UA.UA_13_17.
29. Popat S, Zimmern PE. Long-term outcomes after the excision of horseshoe urethral diverticulum. Int Urogynecol J. 2016;27(3):439–44.
30. Ockrim JL, Allen DJ, Shah PJ, Greenwell TJ. A tertiary experience of urethral diverticulectomy: diagnosis, imaging and surgical outcomes. BJU Int. 2009;103(11):1550–4.
31. Patel AK, Chapple CR. Female urethral diverticula. Curr Opin Urol. 2006;16(4):248–54.
32. Ingber MS, Firoozi F, Vasavada SP, et al. Surgically corrected urethral diverticula: long-term voiding dysfunction and reoperation rates. Urology. 2011;77(1):65–9.
33. Cameron AP. Urethral diverticulum in the female: a meta-analysis of modern series. Minerva Ginecol. 2016;68(2):186–210.
34. Bodner-Adler B, Halpern K, Hanzal E. Surgical management of urethral diverticula in women: a systematic review. Int Urogynecol J. 2016;27(7):993–1001.
35. Aspera AM, Rackley RR, Vasavada SP. Contemporary evaluation and management of the female urethral diverticulum. Urol Clin North Am. 2002;29(3):617–24.

36. Lee RA. Diverticulum of the female urethra: postoperative complications and results. Obstet Gynecol. 1983;61(1):52–8.
37. Vaidya R, Olson K, Wolter C, Khan A. Characterization of urethral diverticula in women. Female Pelvic Med Reconstr Surg. 2022;28(1):54–6. https://doi.org/10.1097/SPV.0000000000001060.
38. Zhou L, Luo DY, Feng SJ, Wei X, Liu Q, Lin YF, Jin T, et al. Risk factors for recurrence in female urethral diverticulectomy: a retrospective study of 66 patients. World J Urol. 2017;35(1):139–44. Berlin/Heidelberg: Springer Berlin Heidelberg.
39. Malde S, Sihra N, Naaseri S, Spilotros M, Solomon E, Pakzad M, Hamid R, et al. Urethral diverticulectomy with Martius labial fat pad interposition improves symptom resolution and reduces recurrence. BJU Int. 2017;119(1):158–63. England: Wiley Subscription Services, Inc.
40. Lorenzo AJ, Zimmern P, Lemack GE, Nurenberg P. Endorectal coil magnetic resonance imaging for diagnosis of urethral and periurethral pathologic findings in women. Urology. 2003;61(6):1129–33.
41. Hoehn D, Mohr S, Nowakowski Ł, Mueller MD, Kuhn A. A prospective cohort trial evaluating sexual function after urethral diverticulectomy. Eur J Obstet Gynecol Reprod Biol. 2022;272:144–9. Ireland: Elsevier B.V.
42. Sun Y, Tang C, Li N, Luo D, Peng L, Shen H, Wei Q. Risk factors of postoperative sexual function in patients with urethral diverticulum and their partners: a cohort study of 83 women. Int Br J Urol. 2019;45(6):1216–26. Sociedade Brasileira de Urologia.
43. Thomas AA, Rackley RR, Lee U, Goldman HB, Vasavada SP, Hansel DE. Urethral diverticula in 90 female patients: a study with emphasis on neoplastic alterations. J Urol. 2008;180(6):2463–7.
44. Rajan N, Tucci P, Mallouh C, Choudhury M. Carcinoma in female urethral diverticulum: case reports and review of management. J Urol. 1993;150(6):1911–4.
45. McLoughlin MG. Carcinoma in situ in urethral diverticulum: pitfalls of marsupialization alone. Urology. 1975;6(3):343.
46. Chung DE, Purohit RS, Girshman J, Blaivas JG. Urethral diverticula in women: discrepancies between magnetic resonance imaging and surgical findings. J Urol. 2010;183(6):2265–9.
47. O'Connor E, Iatropoulou D, Hashimoto S, Takahashi S, Ho DH, Greenwell T. Urethral diverticulum carcinoma in females-a case series and review of the English and Japanese literature. Transl Androl Urol. 2018 Aug;7(4):703–29.
48. Oluyadi F, Ramachandran P, Gotlieb V. A rare case of advanced urethral diverticular adenocarcinoma and a review of treatment modalities. JIM – High Impact Case Rep. 2019;7:2324709619828408. Los Angeles, CA: SAGE Publications
49. Ward JN, Draper JW, Tovell HM. Diagnosis and treatment of urethral diverticula in the female. Surg Gynecol Obstet. 1967;125(6):1293–300.
50. Ginesin Y, Bolkier M, Nachmias J, Levin DR. Primary giant calculus in urethral diverticulum. Urol Int. 1988;43(1):47–8.
51. Dmochowski R. Surgery for vesicovaginal fistula, urethrovaginal fistula, and urethral diverticulum. In: Walsh P, Retik A, Vaughn Jr E, Wein A, editors. Campbell's urology. 8th ed. Philadelphia: WB Saunders; 2002.

23 Vesicovaginal and Urethrovaginal Fistula Repair

Michael Ingber

Introduction

A fistula represents an abnormal connection between two body parts. In the case of a urogenital fistula, an abnormal communication between the urinary tract and the vagina develops that causes urine to leak into the vagina via a route other than the urethral meatus. Vesicovaginal fistulae represent the most common type of fistula encountered by pelvic surgeons today. In developed countries, the more common etiologies include pelvic surgeries for hysterectomy, incontinence, or pelvic reconstructive procedures [1]. In developing countries, pregnancy-related complications from obstructed labor result in ischemic injury to the bladder and vagina and can lead to very large fistulae that can be difficult to treat [2] (Table 23.1).

Regardless of the etiology, repair of vesicovaginal fistulae can be technically challenging, and complications can occur even when performed by expert surgeons. Patients with fistulae, by their nature, often have significant comorbidities that make them more prone to having complications. Furthermore, not only do tissue ischemia, inflammation, and devitalized tissue cause fistulae, but they also can be a limiting factor in proper management and cure. Controversies continue to exist with respect to the proper timing of treatment, route and method of surgery, and use of any adjuvant flaps. Nevertheless, several steps may be performed in order to minimize such perioperative issues. Herein, we describe complications related to vesicovaginal and urethrovaginal fistulae and ways to prevent adverse outcomes from surgical repair.

Preoperative Considerations

Timing of Repair

Obstetrical fistulae typically have significant tissue ischemia due to prolonged pressure from the fetal head on the bladder wall. Furthermore, fistulae from radiation damage may have surrounding ischemic tissue, which may take several months to a year to stabilize. As such, most experts agree that waiting several months to fix such fistulae increases the likelihood of success (Fig. 23.1) [3]. However, when to fix an iatrogenic fistula has been a subject of controversy for many years [4]. Each case should be managed individually, as both early repair and delayed repair may be successful in the appropriate circumstances [5–8]. In general, fistulae, which are recognized in the immediate postoperative period, can be immediately repaired. Delaying in cases of immediate

M. Ingber (✉)
Rutgers New Jersey Medical School, Newark, NJ, USA

Department of Urology, Atlantic Health System, Morristown Medical Center, Morristown, NJ, USA

H. B. Goldman, J. Zillioux (eds.), *Complications of Urogynecology and Reconstructive Pelvic Surgery*, https://doi.org/10.1007/978-3-032-00339-3_23

Table 23.1 Causes of urogenital fistulae

Congenital
Acquired
Iatrogenic
Postoperative
Hysterectomy
Abdominal
Transvaginal
Laparoscopic
Incontinence procedures
Transvaginal slings
Retropubic
Laparoscopic
Prolapse procedures
Anterior colporrhaphy
Mesh kits
Sacrospinous/uterosacral fixation
Sacral colpopexy
Urethral diverticulectomy
Endoscopic procedures
Bowel and vascular surgeries
Radiation injury
Noniatrogenic
Pelvic malignancy
Obstructed labor
Trauma
Sexual injury
Infection
Foreign body

recognition only causes additional psychological suffering, given the significant amount of leakage that patients will experience while waiting for repair. In cases where tissue edema and inflammation prevent successful repair, a waiting period of several weeks to months may be appropriate.

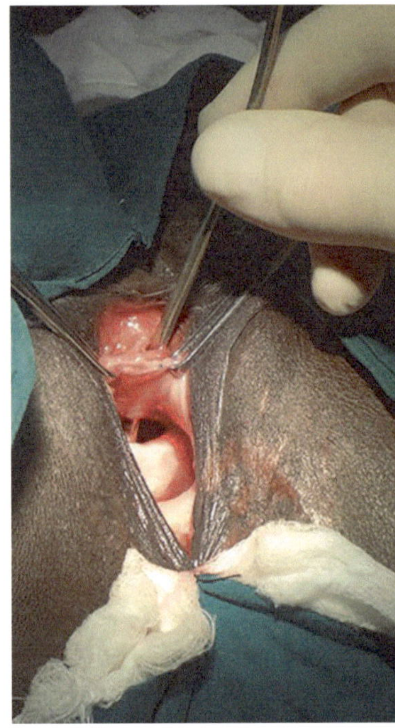

Fig. 23.1 Obstetric vesicovaginal fistulae are typically larger, due to prolonged tissue ischemia

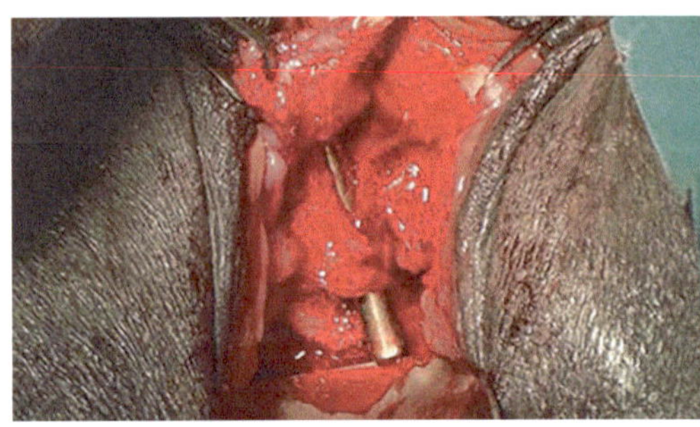

Fig. 23.2 Performing a careful examination is essential, as many patients have multiple fistulae, which should all be addressed simultaneously during surgical repair. This patient had both a vesicovaginal and a urethrovaginal fistula

Diagnostic Studies

Determining the location of a fistula in cases of severe vaginal urinary leakage is often the most challenging part of an incontinence evaluation. While voiding cystourethrograms and plain cystograms can often demonstrate the presence of a fistula, they often fail to demonstrate the exact location of vesicovaginal fistulae, as well as the presence of multiple fistulae (Fig. 23.2). Additionally, ureteral injury can be present in up to 12% of cases of vesicovaginal fistulae, and recognition of this preoperatively is essential [9]. CT urography has largely replaced intravenous pyelography as a diagnostic modality of choice when evaluating upper tract damage or fistula. Cystoscopy is an essential component in the evaluation of any woman with unexplained or continuous incontinence. Typically, cystoscopy can show a fistulous tract, or at least suggest a fistula due to severe inflammatory changes (Fig. 23.3). Retrograde pyelogram at the time of cystoscopy can usually demonstrate ureteral extravasation of contrast (Fig. 23.4). Alternatively, CT urography can show locations of urinary extravasation and often be diagnostic of ureterovaginal fistula (Fig. 23.5).

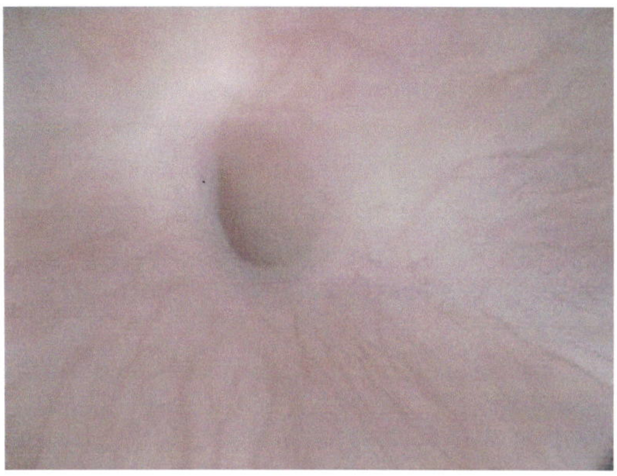

Fig. 23.3 Cystoscopic examination will often show a fistula tract, or area of inflammation suspicious for vesicovaginal fistula

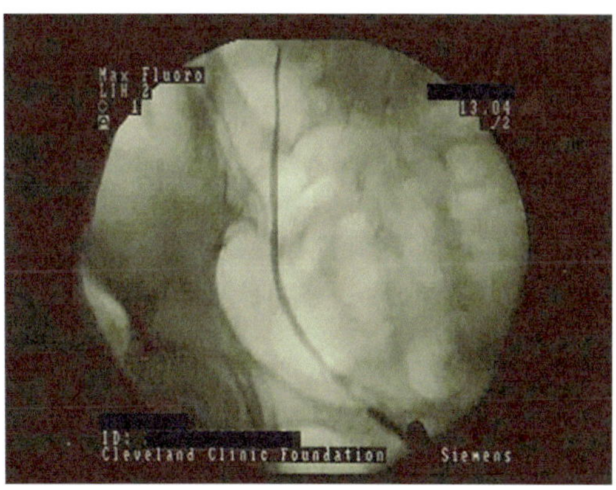

Fig. 23.4 Retrograde pyelogram demonstrating ureteral extravasation of contrast into the vagina. With ureterovaginal fistulae, early ureteral stenting may avert the need for ureteral reimplantation

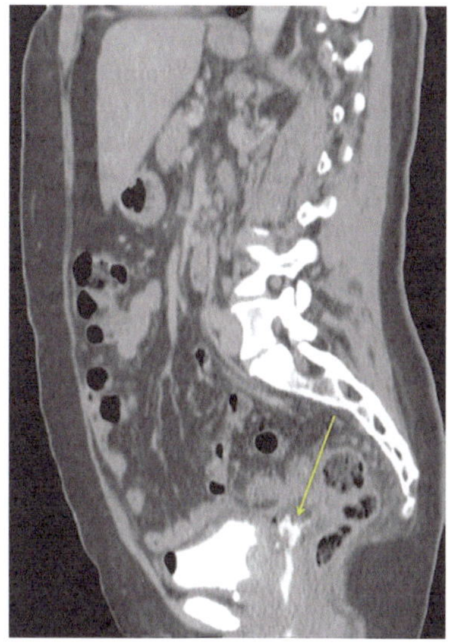

Fig. 23.5 CT urography can be an excellent imaging modality when evaluating for the presence of fistula. Here, a communication can be seen (*arrow*) between the distal ureter and vagina

Approaches to Fistula Repair

Determining which route to perform fistula repair is of utmost importance in order to prevent untoward complications. Most fistula experts agree that the first attempt at repair is the most important surgery which can provide the surgeon with the best opportunity to definitively repair the defect. Therefore, the first attempt should be the route which the surgeon feels most comfortable with. There are some benefits, however, to choosing specific methods based on the type of fistula.

Open Abdominal Repair

The abdominal route may be preferred in women who have poor vaginal access, ischemic tissue from radiation, or those in whom a laparoscopic approach is contraindicated. Women with multiple fistulae, including other organs (i.e., enterovaginal fistulae), are often better served with an open abdominal approach. Large, well-vascularized adjuvant tissue flaps are a major advantage available with open abdominal approaches and may decrease recurrence risk in such cases. Complications related to open repair include wound infection, incisional hernia, and increased bleeding risk.

Transvaginal Repair

Choosing a transvaginal route and avoiding intra-peritoneal access is often a preferred method in most fistulae, provided that the surgeon has access to the site. Specifically, for distally located fistulae, the transvaginal route is recommended, as fistula repair can be performed in an outpatient setting. Some practitioners prefer the Latzko partial colpocleisis to repair apical fistulae, as this method has rather high success rates [10–12]. Most women handle postoperative pain well with the transvaginal route. Complications specific to the transvaginal route include vaginal shortening and vaginal stenosis which may lead to dyspareunia.

Laparoscopic and Robotic-Assisted Laparoscopic Repair

Several authors have described laparoscopic and robotic-assisted laparoscopic repair of vesicovaginal fistulae [13–15]. The advantage of utilizing robotic technology is the ability to have excellent magnified views of the repair, along with the ability to suture for those surgeons not experienced in laparoscopic suturing techniques. Robotic and laparoscopic repairs are often a preferred route in apical fistulae that are unable to be reached vaginally, as they provide superior visualization to defects in this area when compared to the open route. One potential disadvantage that could lead to increased risk for recurrence is the difficulty in obtaining an interposed omental flap. Some recommend obtaining the omental flap utilizing a laparoscopic approach prior to docking of the robotic instruments [15], although in the author's experience, both omental and peritoneal flaps are typically easy to obtain during robotic-assisted laparoscopic repair.

With a laparoscopic or robotic-assisted laparoscopic approach, the fistula tract can be approached either transvesically, utilizing an incision into healthy bladder tissue anterior and superior to the fistula tract, or by direct dissection between the vaginal wall and the bladder. The author's preference is the former approach, which allows for prompt identification of the location of the fistula and easier dissection toward the necessary tissue planes. With robotic-assisted approaches, one may consider the use of a catheter within the fistula site, placed cystoscopically at the beginning of the procedure, for later irrigation or placement of indocyanine green (Akorn, Lake Forest IL, USA) [15].

Agrawal compared intraoperative data and outcomes of 12 robotic-assisted repairs with 20 open surgical repairs [16]. All subjects in the robotic group and 90% of those in the open cohort were managed successfully. Not surprisingly, mean blood loss was significantly less in the robotic group (88 mL vs. 170 mL, $p < 0.05$). Mean hospital stay was also shorter in the robotic group (3.1 vs. 5.6 days, $p < 0.05$). Another single-institution experience noted a mean operative time of 214 min and a median length of stay of 1 day [17]. In the author's experience, laparoscopic and robotic-assisted repaired patients can typically be discharged home after a 23 h stay. Neither group had a significant difference in complication rate. Complications relevant to laparoscopic repair include port-site hernias, bowel injury, and adjacent organ injury.

Intraoperative Considerations

Because of the already present poor tissue conditions that led to the development of a fistula in the first place, intraoperative complications can be relatively common during fistula surgery.

Complications During Dissection

Many fistulae are surrounded by significant inflammation, which can lead to excessive bleeding and poor visualization intraoperatively. Careful dissection is of utmost importance when performing repair, as the surgeon must obtain several layers of closure to prevent recurrence. Complications may occur if the initial dissection of the vaginal epithelium is too deep, and additional layers of closure are unattainable. Excess bleeding may result when improper tissue planes are entered. In cases where flaps are too thin for a good watertight closure, adjuvant tissue flaps utilizing omentum (in abdominal repair) or a Martius flap (in vaginal repair) are crucial.

The author does not routinely excise the entire fistula tract. Nevertheless, in cases of prior malignancy or in postradiation fistulae, one should obtain a biopsy to ensure that there is no malignancy at the site of the fistula. Any nonviable tissue should always be removed in order to obtain better healing. Avoidance of cautery is important, as excess cautery can compromise blood supply to tissue flaps and jeopardize healing. Hence, significant bleeding should be controlled with an interrupted suture.

Complications related to adjacent organ injury are relatively uncommon. If the ureters are close to the repair, they should be stented initially. Ureteral injury may be a result of cautery injury or sharp dissection and should be recognized immediately. A small ureteral defect may be repaired primarily. However, extensive cautery injury, or full transection, typically requires reimplantation in order to prevent ureteral leak or stricture formation. Injury to the bowel may occur during transperitoneal repair, either immediately from dissection injury, or 1–2 weeks following repair due to cautery injury. Patients with prior pelvic radiation may have more inflammation, resulting in additional adhesions, and can be more prone to such injuries.

Closure

Choosing the proper suture is extremely important in minimizing complications. Closure of the bladder or urethral defect should be performed with an absorbable suture such as 3-0 polygalactin or 3-0 chromic. If knots are tied on the intravesical side, a patient may be predisposed to developing calcifications or infections due to delayed absorption when exposed to urine. Nonabsorbable suture should never be used during fistula repair, as permanent suture material can lead to infections and stone formation within the bladder (Fig. 23.6). Additional layers such as a pubocervical fascial layer should also be closed with absorbable suture so that suture lines are nonoverlapping. Once fully closed, the repair should be tested for water-tightness by instilling saline. Any sites of leakage along the suture line should be oversewn with additional suture to ensure complete closure.

Adjuvant Flaps

Providing an additional layer of coverage should be considered when a three-layer closure is not able to be performed, or when tissue quality may compromise proper healing. Interposed tissue flaps should

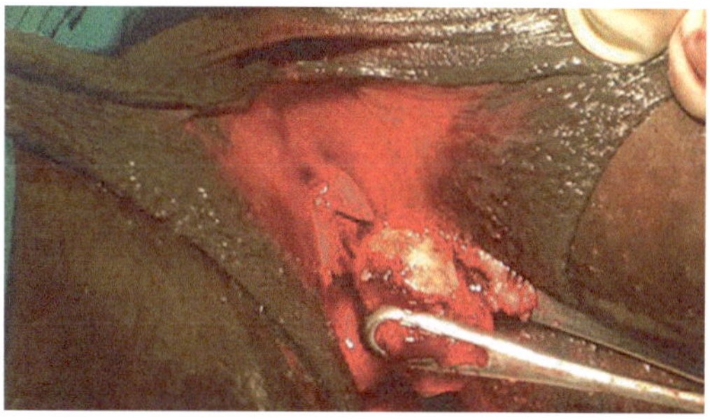

Fig. 23.6 Permanent sutures should never be used during fistula repair. Similarly, absorbable suture knots should be tied external to the bladder mucosa, in order to prevent fistula recurrence and stone formation, as in this patient. (Courtesy of Michael Breen, MD)

be secured with absorbable suture at least 1–2 cm beyond the site of repair. Complications related to harvesting flaps are relatively minimal and are typically limited to bleeding from the site where the flap was obtained. A Martius flap (labial fat pad flap) is often easily accessible during vaginal repair of fistula, and can provide aid in repair when there is significant tissue loss [18]. One study evaluated eight women who underwent Martius flap surgery and questioned subjects on the appearance of the harvest site and any postoperative complications [19]. Three (38%) women felt the appearance of the flap site was different from the contralateral labia. At 1 year after the procedure, one patient (13%) complained of dyspareunia, three (38%) patients had intermittent discomfort in the harvest area, and five patients (62%) complained of permanently decreased sensation or numbness at the harvest site. Another study evaluating mostly obstetrical urethrovaginal and vesicovaginal fistulae, however, showed decreased incidence of dyspareunia as well as recurrence after Martius interposition [20].

Larger defects may require thicker flaps, and the gracilis flap can be utilized in these cases. The gracilis muscle is found in the medial thigh, originating from the ischiopubic ramus. It can be transferred into the pelvis via the medial circumflex femoral artery and can be used in a wide variety of fistula repairs [21].

Omental flaps are an excellent source of adjuvant tissue during transabdominal repair and can occasionally be accessible during transvaginal repair in post-hysterectomy vesicovaginal fistulae. The blood supply to omental flaps is based on the right or left gastroepiploic artery, although the right gastroepiploic is both larger and more caudal, allowing for better reach distally during intra-abdominal fistula repair. Meta-analyses have demonstrated that omentum is readily available during both open and laparoscopic, robotic-assisted repairs, and complication rates of Dindo class I–II are 0–40% with recurrence rates quite low 0–6.7% [22]. Regardless, tissue interposition should be determined based on the quality of repair. All patients should be counseled about the potential use of flaps and the complications specific to the site of tissue interposition.

Lastly, utilizing tissue sealants has recently been shown to possibly lower recurrence rates, with some authors reporting 100% success rates in large fistulae using fibrin glue [23, 24]. While these items are relatively easy to use during repair, their cost may limit their use, especially in some regions where it is not widely available.

Postoperative Complications

Not unexpectedly, the most common complication encountered after vesicovaginal and urethrovaginal fistula repair is recurrence of the fistula. With a complete preoperative workup, attention to basic fistula principles, and careful surgical repair, recurrence rates can be minimal. Should a recurrence occur, management can be via any route.

To a woman suffering from continuous incontinence from a fistula, persistence of urinary incontinence despite a properly repaired fistula can be devastating. Stress incontinence may occur after both transvaginal and transabdominal fistula repair if the dissection disrupts the ligamentous support of the urethra or the sphincteric mechanism. In several series, the rate of stress incontinence after fistula repair ranges from 4 to 33% after surgery and are likely higher in obstetrical fistula [25, 26]. Risk factors of stress incontinence after fistula surgery include involvement of the urethra, small bladder capacity, large fistula, and need for extensive vaginal reconstruction [27]. In women with vesicovaginal fistula and concomitant stress incontinence, a polypropylene mesh midurethral sling may be performed, provided that the urethral dissection is well away from any fistula repair. Others prefer placement of an autologous fascial sling at the time of original fistula repair [28]. Utilizing a patient's own tissue has a far less likely chance of complications such as mesh erosion or exposure; however, it adds additional time and morbidity to the procedure. Nevertheless, in the setting of any periurethral dissection during fistula repair, it is the authors' preference that any therapy for stress incontinence wait until after total healing occurs after fistula surgery.

Urinary tract infection is a relatively common complication of fistula repair postoperatively, as instrumentation of the urinary bladder itself can predispose a woman to infection. Studies evaluating antibiotic use during and after fistula repair are limited to obstetric fistula. In a review of single-dose gentamicin vs. extended postoperative antibiotics during 722 obstetric fistula repairs in Ethiopia, Muleta and colleagues showed no difference in rates of postoperative infection [29]. Regardless of postoperative antibiotic use, sterilization of the urine prior to repair is of utmost importance, as preoperative urinary tract infection may increase the likelihood of fistula recurrence [30]. The author occasionally uses a low-dose antibiotic such as nitrofurantoin while patients await repair not only to prevent perioperative urinary tract infection but also to decrease tissue edema and inflammation, which allows for easier repair.

Urinary urgency may occur after any vaginal surgery that involves dissection around the urethra and the bladder. Rates of postoperative urinary urgency are difficult to determine due to the few studies that have used urinary urgency as an outcome. However, in one small study evaluating 20 genitourinary fistulae, seven (35%) developed urinary urgency postoperatively. Because de novo urgency can be an irritative complication, it should be discussed preoperatively with patients. It is the authors' preference to offer patients beta agonist or anticholinergic therapy during the healing phase when catheters are present to minimize uninhibited detrusor contractions. Rarely, patients may have persistent urinary urgency even several months after repair. When such a complication occurs, urodynamic investigation to ensure no evidence for bladder outlet obstruction is essential. Should conservative therapies fail to adequately address urinary urgency, frequency, or de novo urge urinary incontinence, long-term treatment of these symptoms may be required in some patients with third-line or advanced treatment options such as tibial nerve stimulation, onabotulinum toxin injection, or sacral neuromodulation.

Vaginal shortening is more common with apical fistulae when the Latzko partial colpocleisis is utilized. However, when done appropriately, only 1–2 cm of vaginal length is compromised, and this should not be an issue. Typically, women can remain sexually active without major problems with dyspareunia even when significant vaginal shortening occurs [31]. Nevertheless, vaginal shortening should be mentioned when counseling women who are sexually active, as women may recognize the change in anatomy with deep penetration of their partner.

Urethrovaginal Fistula

While vesicovaginal fistulae are relatively common, there is a paucity of information on the repair of urethrovaginal fistula. In developed countries, urethrovaginal fistulae are most commonly a result of previous vaginal surgery. Symptoms are variable, as are techniques for repair. Like vesicovaginal fistula, complications specific to urethrovaginal fistula most commonly involve recurrence, with 10% of primary repairs recurring in a recent series [32]. Knowing the location and number of the fistulae is extremely important.

Because of the proximity to the urethral sphincter, patients with urethrovaginal fistula that occur within the proximal and/or middle urethra are prone to development or worsening of stress urinary incontinence after repair (Fig. 23.7). In the aforementioned study, of 71 subjects undergoing repair, 37 (52.1%) developed stress incontinence after repair [32]. Some surgeons advocate the use of autologous fascia in order to correct stress incontinence during urethrovaginal fistula repair [33, 34], but the author typically prefers to wait until any fistula repair is complete. Once several months of healing has occurred, if the incontinence remains, it may be assessed, and a synthetic or autologous sling may be placed if necessary.

Like vesicovaginal fistula repair, reoperation after urethrovaginal fistula repair is relatively common. In a recent study with long-term follow-up, Lee and Zimmern published their results of 18 women who underwent urethrovaginal fistula repair [35]. At a mean follow-up of

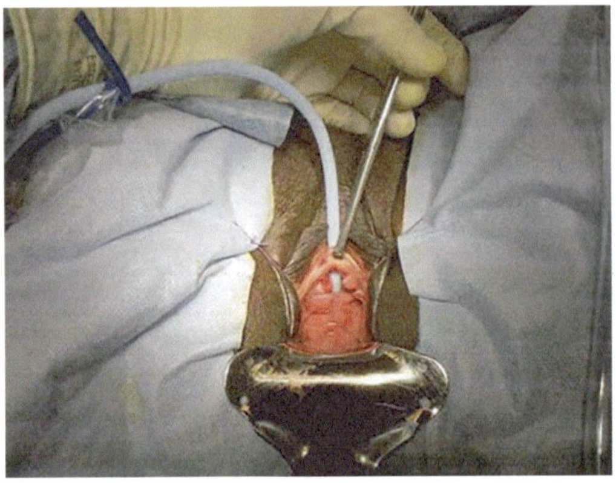

Fig. 23.7 Urethrovaginal fistula can affect the external sphincter and simple repair of the defect may still result in chronic incontinence. This patient required an autologous fascial sling to correct the resulting stress incontinence after fistula repair. (Courtesy of Howard B. Goldman, MD)

52 months (range 9–142), the success rate overall was 95%. Reoperation in this group was 33%, with three women requiring periurethral bulking agent injection, two requiring excision of additional mesh, and one requiring urethral dilation.

Conclusion

Vesicovaginal and urethrovaginal fistulae are conditions, which require extensive preoperative planning, experience-driven intraoperative judgment, and close outpatient follow-up. When basic principles of fistula repair are followed, complications may be minimized, and subsequently, chances of a successful repair can be maximized.

References

1. Lafay Pillet M, Leonard F, Chopin N, et al. Incidence and risk factors of bladder injuries during laparoscopic hysterectomy indicated for benign uterine pathologies: a 14.5 years experience in a continuous series of 1501 procedures. Hum Reprod. 2009;24(4):842–9.
2. Muleta M. Obstetric fistula in developing countries: a review article. J Obstet Gynaecol Can. 2006;28(11):962–6.
3. Breen M, Ingber M. Controversies in the management of vesicovaginal fistula. Best Pract Res Clin Obstet Gynaecol. 2019;54:61–72.
4. Blaivas J, Heritz D, Romanzi L. Early versus late repair of vesicovaginal fistulas: vaginal and abdominal approaches. J Urol. 1995;153(4):1110–2.
5. Shelbaia AM, Hashish NM. Limited experience in early management of genitourinary tract fistulas. Urology. 2007;69(3):572–4.
6. Badenoch D, Tiptaft R, Thakar D, et al. Early repair of accidental injury to the ureter or bladder following gynaecological surgery. Br J Urol. 1987;59(6):516–8.
7. Persky L, Herman G, Guerrier K. Non-delay in vesicovaginal fistula repair. Urology. 1979;13:273.
8. Blandy J, Badenoch D, Fowler C, et al. Early repair of iatrogenic injury to the ureter or bladder after gynecological surgery. J Urol. 1991;146(3):761–5.
9. Goodwin W, Scardino P. Vesicovaginal and ureterovaginal fistulas: a summary of 25 years of experience. J Urol. 1980;123:370–4.
10. Tancer M. The post-total hysterectomy (vault) vesicovaginal fistula. J Urol. 1980;123(6):839–40.
11. Ansquer Y, Mellier G, Santulli P, Bennis M, Mandelbrot L, Madelenat P, et al. Latzko operation for vault vesicovaginal fistula. Acta Obstet Gynecol Scand. 2006;85(10):1248–51.
12. Dorairajan L, Khattar N, Kumar S, et al. Latzko repair for vesicovaginal fistula revisited in the era of minimal- access surgery. Int Urol Nephrol. 2008;40(2):317–20.
13. Gellhaus P, Bhandari A, Monn M, Gardner T, Kanagarajah P, Reilly C, et al. Robotic management of genitourinary injuries from obstetric and gynaecological operations: a multi-institutional report of outcomes. BJU Int. 2015;115(3):430–6.
14. Hemal AK, Kolla SB, Wadhwa P. Robotic reconstruction for recurrent supratrigonal vesicovaginal fistulas. J Urol. 2008;180(3):981–5.
15. Medina L, Lee R, Celis V, Rodriguez V, Poncel J, Sayegh A, Sotelo R. Robotic management of urinary fistula. Asian J Urol. 2024;11:357–65.
16. Agrawal V, Kucherov V, Bendana E, Joseph J, Rashid H, Wu G. Robotic-assisted laparoscopic repair of vesicovaginal fistula: a single-center experience. Urology. 2015;86(2):276–81.
17. Gupta NP, Mishra S, Hemal AK, Mishra A, Seth A, Dogra PN. Comparative analysis of outcome between open and robotic surgical repair of recurrent supra- trigonalvesico-vaginal fistula. J Endourol. 2010;24(11):1779–82.
18. Kapriniotis K, Loufopoulos I, Gresty H, Greenwell T, Ockrim J. The utility of Martius fat pad in the repair of urogenital fistulae: review of current evidence. BJU Int. 2024;134(3):365–74.
19. Petrou SP, Jones J, Parra RO. Martius flap harvest site: patient self-perception. J Urol. 2002;167(5):2098–9.
20. Rangnekar NP, Imdad Ali N, Kaul SA, Pathak HR. Role of the martius procedure in the management

of urinary- vaginal fistulas. J Am Coll Surg. 2000;191(3):259–63.
21. Doersch K, Hines L, Ajay D. Narrative review of flaps and grafts in robotic reconstructive urologic surgery. Ann Laparosc Endosc Surg. 2024;9:5.
22. Anderson C, Spinos T, Liatsikos E, Kalidonis P, Tatanis V, Dietel A, Stolzenburg J. Use of omentum during robotic-assisted reconstructive urological surgery: a systematic review of the current literature. World J Urol. 2024;42(1):620.
23. Bouchard ME, Stairs J, Hickling D, Clancy A, Khalil H. The use of tissue adhesive in management of genitourinary fistulas: a systematic review and case report. Int Urogynecol J. 2023;34(2):445.
24. Choudhury S, Dutta A, Gupta N, Pal D. Interposing layer of fibrin glue: a new horizon in vesico-vaginal fistula repair. Urologia. 2022;89(3):484–7.
25. Holme A, Breen M, MacArthur C. Obstetric fistulae: a study of women managed at the Monze Mission Hospital. Zambia BJOG. 2007;114(8):1010–7.
26. Zambon JP, Batezini NS, Pinto ER, Skaff M, Girotti ME, Almeida FG. Do we need new surgical techniques to repair vesico-vaginal fistulas? Int Urogynecol J Pelvic Floor Dysfunct. 2010;21(3):337–42.
27. Browning A. Risk factors for developing residual urinary incontinence after obstetric fistula repair. BJOG. 2006;113(4):482–5.
28. Pope R, Browning A, Chipungu E, George J, Tamimu M, Wilkinson J. Prophylactic autologous slings at the time of obstetric fistula repair: a randomized clinical trial. Female Pelvic Med Reconstr Surg. 2021;27(2):78–84.
29. Muleta M, Tafesse B, Aytenfisu HG. Antibiotic use in obstetric fistula repair: single blinded randomized clinical trial. Ethiop Med J. 2010;48(3):211–7.
30. Ayed M, El Atat R, Hassine LB, Sfaxi M, Chebil M, Zmerli S. Prognostic factors of recurrence after vesicovaginal fistula repair. Int J Urol. 2006;13(4):345–9.
31. Occhino JA, Trabuco EC, Heisler CA, Klingele CJ, Gebhart JB. Changes in vaginal anatomy and sexual function after vaginal surgery. Int Urogynecol J Pelvic Floor Dysfunct. 2011;22(7):799–804.
32. Pushkar DY, Dyakov VV, Kosko JW, Kasyan GR. Management of urethrovaginal fistulas. Eur Urol. 2006;50(5):1000–5.
33. Blaivas JG, Purohit RS. Post-traumatic female urethral reconstruction. Curr Urol Rep. 2008;9(5):397–404.
34. Golomb J, Leibovitch I, Mor Y, Nadu A, Ramon J. Fascial patch technique for repair of complicated urethrovaginal fistula. Urology. 2006;68(5):1115–8.
35. Lee D, Zimmern P. Long-term functional outcomes following non-radiated urethrovaginal fistula repair. World J Urol. 2016;34(2):291–6.

Transvaginal Bladder Neck Closure

24

Mitchell G. Goldenberg and David A. Ginsberg

Indications

The primary indication for an adult woman to undergo a transvaginal bladder neck closure (BNC) is an eroded and destroyed bladder neck/urethra secondary to a chronic, indwelling catheter. While the indication for the initial catheter placement may be varied, the chain of events leading to this scenario is usually quite similar. The catheter is usually placed for refractory urinary incontinence or retention, usually of neurogenic etiology but not necessarily. With long-term catheter use, female patients may experience detrusor overactivity and urethral erosion, which often leads to urinary leakage around the catheter. This initial erosive reaction is often further exacerbated by the caregivers' decision to use a larger catheter size and inflate the balloon with larger volumes of water. The hope is that this will minimize leakage around the catheter; however, this often results in further urethral erosion. Erosion can be so severe that catheters cannot be maintained in the bladder and spontaneously fall out. In addition, a poorly secured catheter that is repeatedly pulled out can also contribute to urethral injury. If severe enough, the urethra becomes overly patulous and a urethral indwelling catheter cannot be maintained. The urethra can be wide enough and short enough that one or two fingers can be inserted directly into the bladder [1]. In addition, the erosion can be severe enough that when a finger is inserted into the urethra, the undersurface of the pubic symphysis is directly palpated as there is no remaining urethral tissue anteriorly. Because of the length of the urethra, this is rarely an issue in the male patient; the analogous reaction in the male to long-term catheter usage would be a traumatic hypospadias.

For these women, there are few options besides the use of pads/diapers. While external-type catheters exist (i.e., PureWick™), these are often challenging to fit correctly, leading to ongoing leakage and patient frustration. Many of these patients are not interested in or physically able to undergo lower urinary reconstruction due to their disability. Placement of a suprapubic catheter (SP) is a simple option for these patients, and by itself, may be sufficient to control leakage of urine per the eroded urethra [2]. However, depending on the degree of the erosion and damage to the urethral sphincteric mechanism, leakage may still occur through the urethra despite continuous drainage per the SP tube. For these patients who wish to continue with SP drainage, further options include placement of an obstructing sling or BNC. A potential advantage of sling placement is that it does not permanently close the bladder neck; however, these outlets are often

M. G. Goldenberg · D. A. Ginsberg (✉)
Department of Urology, Keck School of Medicine of USC, USC Institute of Urology,
Los Angeles, CA, USA
e-mail: Mitchell.goldenberg@med.usc.edu; ginsberg@med.usc.edu

H. B. Goldman, J. Zillioux (eds.), *Complications of Urogynecology and Reconstructive Pelvic Surgery*, https://doi.org/10.1007/978-3-032-00339-3_24

so damaged that there is an adequate amount of healthy urethral tissue to allow for sling placement.

Approaches for BNC include transvaginal and transabdominal. The transabdominal approach is often done in conjunction with some type of urinary reconstruction, is more invasive than a vaginal procedure, and has been reported to have a lower rate of post-op leak/fistula formation. The alternative is a transvaginal approach which is often done in conjunction with SP tube placement and is less invasive but may be a more challenging procedure for surgeons less experienced with vaginal surgery [3].

Complications

Short-term complications following transvaginal BNC are similar to those of other vaginal surgical procedures, including urinary tract infection, vaginal bleeding and wound breakdown, and urinoma from breakdown of the urinary tract suture line. There is essentially one primary long-term complication associated with BNC, which is continued leakage and formation of a vesicovaginal fistula (VVF) between the attempted closure site and the anterior vaginal wall. As reported in a limited number of case series, the fistula rate after the initial surgery ranges between 0 and 100% and is summarized in Table 24.1. The various surgical techniques described are similar and are based on several essential principals: (1) complete mobilization of the urethra/bladder neck off the supporting pelvic ligaments; (2) resection of necrotic tissue down to healthy, viable tissue before closure is attempted: (3) multilayered closure; (4) mobilization of a large anterior vaginal wall flap to advance over the BNC.

Depending on the degree of erosion, it is possible that BNC may occur in close proximity to the ureteral orifices. It is important that the ureteral orifices are identified prior to BNC to minimize the risk of damage. Placement of temporary ureteral catheters can be used to ensure patency is maintained during dissection and closure of the bladder mucosa. Certainly, there is a theoretical risk of ureteral injury at the time of transvaginal BNC, though that has not been previously described in the literature.

Table 24.1 Bladder neck closure fistula rate, transvaginal approach

References	Patients (n)	Fistula rate (%)
Zimmern et al. [1]	6	0
Nielsen and Bruskewitz [11]	5	20
Eckford et al. [12]	50	22
Levy et al. [3]	4	50
Andrews and Shah [2]	8	50
Stoffel and McGuire [13]	8	87.5
Ginger et al. [4]	2	100
Rovner et al. [6]	11	9
Willis et al. [5]	35	14

Table 24.2 Perioperative steps to minimize complication risk after transvaginal bladder neck closure

Pre-op factors	Appropriate patient selection
	Surgeon expertise
	Optimization of nutritional status
Intra-op factors	Complete mobilization of the urethra/bladder neck off supporting pelvic ligaments
	Resection of necrotic tissue down to healthy, viable tissue
	Multilayered closure
	Mobilization and advancement of the anterior vaginal wall flap over the bladder neck closure
Post-op factors	Optimize bladder drainage
	Minimize detrusor overactivity

The remainder of this chapter will focus on perioperative steps to minimize the risk of fistula formation after transvaginal BNC as well as how to manage the problem if a fistula does occur. These steps are summarized in Table 24.2.

Pre-op

There is unfortunately little that can be done preoperatively to enhance the postoperative success in these patients. One important decision the surgeon should make is whether or not to perform BNC at all, and if so, via which approach. Levy et al. reviewed their experience with 12 patients, all of whom underwent BNC for urethral injury secondary to long-term indwelling catheters [3].

The first four patients all underwent a primary transvaginal approach. Of those, two succeeded and the other two failed a total of five transvaginal attempts to close the bladder neck, resulting in a success rate of 50%. Both of these patients ultimately underwent successful BNC with a combined abdominal and vaginal approach. The next ten patients (eight new patients and the two that had failed the prior transvaginal attempts) underwent a combined abdominal and vaginal approach with 100% success. The authors' recommendation at the time was that a purely transvaginal approach may not be appropriate if the operating surgeon does not have extensive experience performing transvaginal surgery.

There are few studies that evaluated outcomes using multiple approaches. Ginger et al. revealed an 11% leakage rate in 26 patients undergoing a transabdominal BNC compared to a 100% leakage rate in the two patients in their study who underwent transvaginal BNC [4]. Willis et al. reviewed their experience with both approaches in 64 patients (35 transvaginal, 29 retropubic) and noted residual urethral leakage in five patients in both the transvaginal (5/35—14.3%) and retropubic (5/29—17.2%) cohorts [5].

Poor nutrition is one issue that can be addressed preoperatively. Rovner et al. correctly state that many of these patients often have multiple medical comorbidities and poor nutritional status at baseline [6]. Poor nutrition has been shown to impact wound healing, increase susceptibility to infection, and place the patient at increased risk for pulmonary complications, prolonged hospitalization, and mortality [7]. However, preoperative nutritional supplementation appears to only be valuable in severely malnourished patients; in all other patients, surgery does not need to be delayed [8].

Intra-op

To minimize the risk of postoperative failure and leak, there are several surgical steps that should be emphasized. Initially, two incisions are made. One is made circumferentially around the external urethral meatus. The other incision, more proximal and along the anterior vaginal wall, allows for the dissection of a wide, anterior vaginal wall flap when beginning the procedure. This flap is advanced once the BNC is complete past the area of repair, thus minimizing the presence of overlapping suture lines. Prior to closing the bladder neck, appropriate mobilization is necessary. This includes transection of the urethra completely off the pubourethral ligament dorsally and the urethropelvic ligaments and remaining attachments laterally. Optimal mobility of the bladder neck is extremely important. Without mobility, the closure of the bladder neck itself is very challenging. Prior to closing the urethra/bladder neck, all necrotic tissue should be resected down to viable tissue. This often results in resecting all, if not the entire urethra. Adequate mobility allows the surgeon to pull the bladder neck out with stays, thus making the actual closure of the bladder neck less challenging. In addition, with adequate mobility of the closed bladder neck, the repair itself can be mobilized anteriorly away from the vaginal wall closure. After closing the bladder neck in two layers, these same cystorrhaphy sutures can be brought through the undersurface of the pubic symphysis or even the anterior abdominal wall. This results in mobilization of the suture line of the BNC anterior, away from the vaginal wall closure. Theoretically, this will help minimize fistula formation if the initial repair is not watertight. This maneuver cannot be done if adequate mobility of the bladder neck has not been obtained.

Closure of the bladder neck with multiple layers is certainly an important step and several techniques have been described. Zimmern et al. used an initial vertical and anterior–posterior layer followed by a second layer placed transversely in the perivesical fascia and detrusor muscle superficially [1]. Rovner et al. described a modification of this technique using a posterior urethral flap (Fig. 24.1). Once the bladder neck has been fully mobilized, the dorsal urethra is bivalved into the anterior bladder wall for 2–3 cm. The bivalved posterior urethral flap is then rotated cephalad and secured to the anterior bladder wall. That suture line is subsequently rotated upward to the retropubic space, behind the pubic sym-

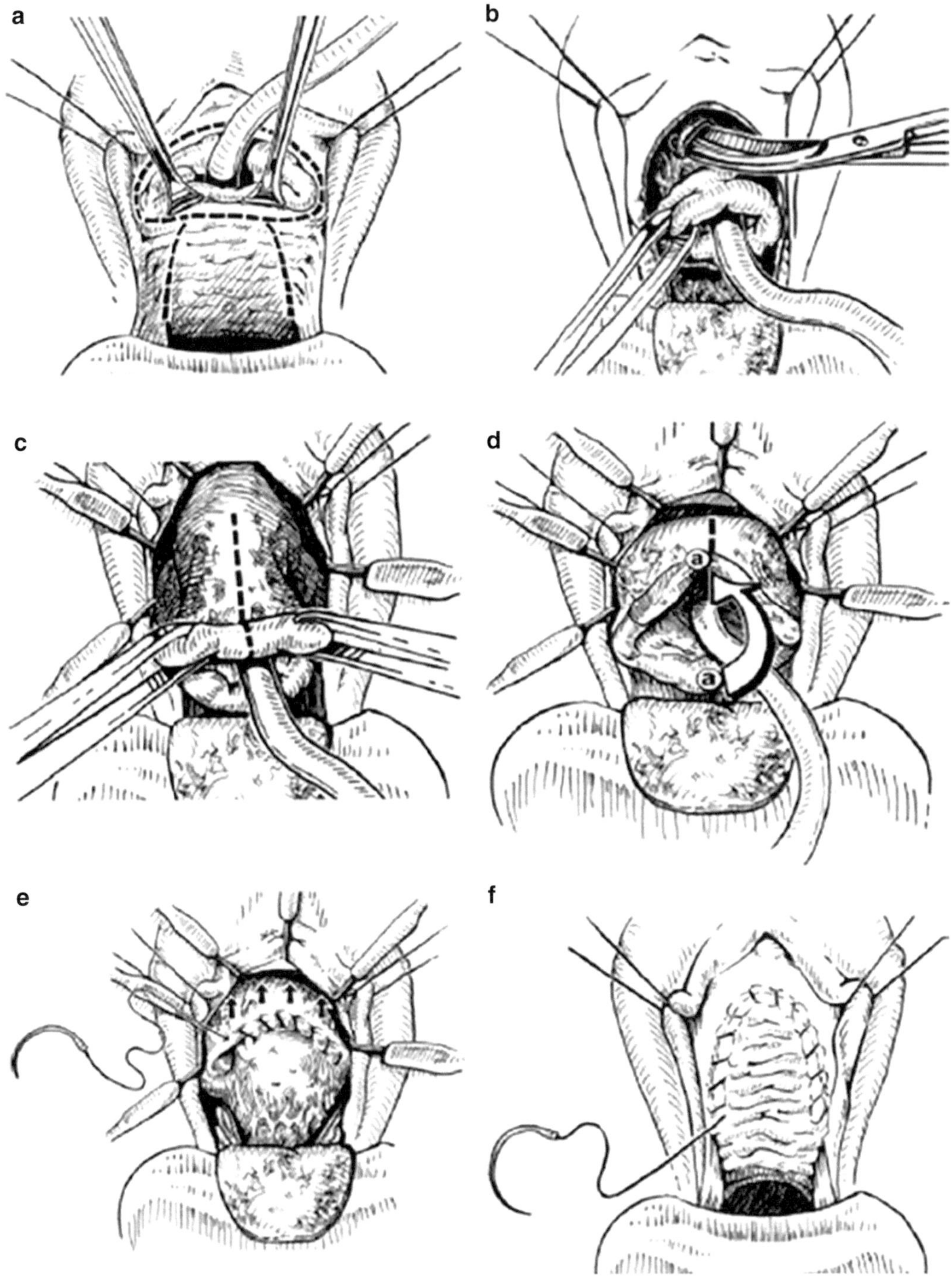

Fig. 24.1 (**a**) Incision made circumferentially around urethra with arms extending proximally to develop anterior vaginal wall flap. (**b**) Urethra is freed from its attachments as the urethropelvic and pubourethral ligaments are divided. (**c**) Dorsal urethra bivalved up to bladder neck. (**d**) Ventral urethra flap rotated up to edge of bivalved urethra. (**e**) Closure of bladder beck. With rotation of flap in a cephalad direction, the suture line rotates under the symphysis pubis. (**f**) Anterior vaginal wall advanced and vaginal wall closed with no overlapping suture lines

physis [6]. It should be noted that the use of an adjuvant flap or graft placement is not usually required for primary repairs; these techniques are more commonly seen for patients requiring redo surgery for postoperative fistula after failure of primary BNC [4].

Post-op

Without appropriate postoperative management even the best of repairs will break down, resulting in the formation of a VVF. The importance of optimal drainage post-op in these patients cannot be overemphasized. Ginger et al. noted a significant association between poor post-op catheter care and persistent leakage [4]. A total of 29 patients in their series underwent retropubic BNC, with eight of these patients continuing to have persistent urinary leakage postoperatively. This was directly attributable to catheter mismanagement in seven of eight patients. An appropriately sized suprapubic tube should be placed, secured, and optimally drained postoperatively to help ensure healing of the suture line along the closed bladder neck.

In addition to poor drainage, residual detrusor overactivity can negatively impact the healing process. Even with a catheter in place, allowing for continuous bladder drainage, patients can have residual detrusor overactivity. The bladder's natural response to a detrusor contraction is relaxation of the bladder neck and a spontaneous void. If the bladder neck has been surgically closed, this only leads to increased pressure on the suture line and a greater risk of postoperative failure. Bladder antispasmodics (i.e., anticholingerics or beta-3 adrenergic agonists) are thus an important part of the postoperative management of these patients and should be started immediately postoperatively. Theoretically, injection of botulinum toxin A into the detrusor muscle could be done at the time of BNC with the hope that minimization of postoperative detrusor overactivity would improve the likelihood of a successful repair [9].

Fistula Diagnosis

The diagnosis of a post-BNC fistula is straightforward and can be made clinically in most cases without radiographic investigation. A leak at the closure site may be suggested at the postoperative visit if the patient complains of continued urinary leakage vaginally. However, a lack of leakage does not necessarily mean that the BNC has adequately healed. All patients should have a cystogram 2–3 weeks postoperatively to adequately assess the quality of the repair. If a residual leak is noted, then catheter drainage should be continued. Experience with post-hysterectomy vesicovaginal fistula suggests if the patient is dry with the catheter in place, prolonged catheter drainage can be successful and lead to closure of the tract, but is unlikely to succeed if the patient continues to leak per the fistula site despite continuous catheter drainage. While this has not been evaluated in post-BNC leaks, it is likely that the theory and healing process is similar.

If the cystogram is equivocal or if the patient returns complaining of leakage despite a previously noted negative cystogram, then direct examination may be helpful in identifying a fistula. As opposed to most post-hysterectomy fistulae, which tend to be deep toward the vaginal vault and can be challenging to identify on examination, these fistulae are often easy to see on examination. A simple technique to easily evaluate for a leak is to perform a pelvic examination while an assistant fills the bladder through the suprapubic tube with normal saline colored with a dye such as methylene blue or indigo carmine. If a leak is present, it will be readily apparent when the blue-tinged fluid is noted leaking through the fistula site in the vagina. If the patient is concerned that a leak is present but cannot come to the office for immediate evaluation, another option would be for her to do a Pyridium (phenazopyridine) pad test at home. A pad that turns orange after taking Pyridium post-BNC is strongly suggestive of the presence of a fistula.

Fistula Management

If a VVF develops between the vagina and bladder neck closure site despite appropriate surgical technique and perioperative care, then several options are available. An attempt to maximize drainage with supravesical diversion using bilateral nephrostomy tubes could be attempted. This has primarily been used in the postoperative setting in patients with a urine leak at the ureteroileal anastomosis site after urinary diversion. With a mature fistula tract, it is unlikely this will allow for closure of the fistula, though this may theoretically help close a leak early in the postoperative period.

Once the fistula tract has matured, the patient is destined to undergo further surgery if repair is desired. Prior to returning to the operating room, it is important to realize that not all fistulas have to be repaired. At times, patients may have a fistula on cystogram but are dry when the catheter is left to drain. If this is the case and the patient is content, then further intervention is generally unnecessary.

For experienced vaginal surgeons, a second attempt at a transvaginal BNC could be considered. The technique is essentially the same as was attempted with the initial attempt at closure. However, use of an adjuvant flap or graft is highly recommended in a redo procedure, especially if one was not used in the initial procedure. Rotation of a Martius labial fibrofatty flap on its superior pedicle is a familiar technique for most vaginal surgeons. Alternatives would include the use of biological grafts, such as pericardium allograft (i.e., Tutoplast) or similar. If a graft/flap was used with the initial attempt at BNC, it is possible that it could be identified intraoperatively and reused if viable.

For those surgeons not experienced with transvaginal surgery, an abdominal approach should be considered after a failed prior attempt at BNC. If an abdominal BNC is performed, an omental flap can be harvested and placed at the closure site to add an extra layer of repair [10]. If further evaluation finds that the bladder is not salvageable or the BNC cannot be done, then the surgeon and patient should also be prepared for possible cystectomy and either continent or incontinent diversion to the skin. This is certainly a much larger undertaking than BNC and, if it is thought that this might be a possibility, appropriate preoperative preparation is required including patient counseling, stoma site marking, and obtaining of adequate informed consent.

References

1. Zimmern PE, Hadley RH, Leach GE, et al. Transvaginal closure of the bladder neck and placement of a suprapubic catheter for destroyed urethra after long-term indwelling catheterization. J Urol. 1985;134:554–6.
2. Andrews HO, Shah PJR. Surgical management of urethral damage in neurologically impaired female patients with chronic indwelling catheters. Br J Urol. 1998;82:820–4.
3. Levy JB, Jacobs JA, Wein AJ. Combined abdominal and vaginal approach for bladder neck closure and permanent suprapubic tube: urinary diversion in the neurologically impaired woman. J Urol. 1994;152:2081–2.
4. Ginger VA, Miller JL, Yang CC. Bladder neck closure and suprapubic tube placement in the debilitated patient population. Neurourol Urodyn. 2010;29:382–6.
5. Willis H, Safiano NA, Lloyd LK. Comparison of transvaginal and retropubic bladder neck closure in women. J Urol. 2015;193:196–202.
6. Rovner ES, Goudelocke CM, Gilchrist A, et al. Transvaginal bladder neck closure with posterior urethral flap for devastated urethra. Urology. 2011;78:208–12.
7. Detsky AS, Baker JP, O'Rourke K. Perioperative parenteral nutrition: a meta-analysis. Ann Intern Med. 1987;107:195–203.
8. Hebbar R, Harte B. Do preoperative nutritional interventions improve outcomes in malnourished patients undergoing elective surgery? Cleve Clin J Med. 2007;74(Suppl 1):8–10.
9. Smith CP, Somogyi GT, Chancellor MB. Emerging role of botulinum toxin in the treatment of neurogenic and non-neurogenic voiding dysfunction. Curr Urol Rep. 2002;3:382–7.

10. Shpall AI, Ginsberg DA. Bladder neck closure with lower urinary tract reconstruction: technique and long-term followup. J Urol. 2004;172:2296–9.
11. Nielsen KT, Bruskewitz RC. Female urinary incontinence treated by transvaginal urethral closure and suprapubic tube. Int Urol Nephrol. 1989;21:603–8.
12. Eckford SB, Kohler-Ockmore J, Feneley RCL. Long-term follow-up of transvaginal urethral closure and suprapubic cystostomy for urinary incontinence in women with multiple sclerosis. Br J Urol. 1994;74:319–21.
13. Stoffel JT, McGuire EJ. Outcome of urethral closure in patients with neurologic impairment and complete urethral destruction. Neurourol Urodyn. 2006;25:19–22.

25 Bladder Augmentation

Noah Stern and Sender Herschorn

Abbreviations

CIC Clean intermittent catheterization

Introduction

Bladder augmentation with an ileal patch was first described by Von Mickulicz in 1899 [1]. Subsequent reports detailed the use of different gastrointestinal (GI) segments: colon by Lemoine in 1912, sigmoid by Bisgard in 1943, cecum by Couvelaire in 1950, and stomach by Leong in 1978 [2–5]. Other attempts using organic tissues, such as peritoneum, omentum, human dura, skin, pericardium, placenta, gallbladder, free fascial grafts, and preserved bladder tissue, as well as synthetic materials, were unsuccessful [6]. The modern operative technique utilizing a detubularized ileal patch was described by Goodwin in 1959 [7]. These advancements marked significant progress in the field of bladder augmentation, laying the groundwork for current practices. Today, bladder augmentation continues to evolve, incorporating new techniques, materials, and approaches to improve patient outcomes.

Contemporarily, bladder augmentation has been utilized to treat patients with neurogenic detrusor overactivity secondary to multiple sclerosis, spinal cord injuries, and myelodysplasia, as well as other causes of reduced bladder capacity. It is also reserved as a surgical option for patients with bladder overactivity who have not responded to less invasive treatment options. The primary goal of augmentation cystoplasty is to create a low-pressure storage reservoir, thereby increasing bladder capacity and compliance, protecting against upper tract deterioration, improving urinary continence, and enhancing quality of life. Bladder augmentation is often performed alongside other surgical procedures, such as the creation of a continent stoma or bladder outlet procedures to reduce urinary incontinence. This chapter outlines the indications and techniques of bladder augmentation, emphasizing the management of short- and long-term complications.

Indications

In 1977, Smith et al. reviewed augmentation cystoplasty and suggested that the procedure was "a successful long-term solution for patients with small contracted bladders of almost any etiology." [8] Table 25.1 lists the current indications.

N. Stern
Department of Surgery Division of Urology, North York General Hospital, Toronto, ON, Canada

S. Herschorn (✉)
Division of Urology, Sunnybrook Health Science Centre, Toronto, ON, Canada
e-mail: s.herschorn@utoronto.ca

H. B. Goldman, J. Zillioux (eds.), *Complications of Urogynecology and Reconstructive Pelvic Surgery*, https://doi.org/10.1007/978-3-032-00339-3_25

Table 25.1 Indications for augmentation cystoplasty (usually with associated symptoms of urinary incontinence, high detrusor pressures, or renal dysfunction refractory to other management options)

	Indication
Congenital	Myelodysplasia Posterior urethral valves Exstrophy/epispadias complex
Acquired neurogenic bladder	Spinal cord injury Multiple sclerosis
Acquired non-neurogenic bladder	Overactive bladder
Infectious	Tuberculosis Schistosomiasis
Inflammatory	Radiation cystitis (interstitial cystitis/bladder pain syndrome)
Iatrogenic	Intraoperative loss of bladder wall Urinary undiversion

Congenital Conditions

Myelodysplasia, a form of spinal dysraphism, may lead to neurogenic bladder dysfunction. Approximately one-third of patients have sphincter dyssynergia, and the urodynamic pattern often changes as the child ages [9]. The failure of conservative or medical therapy to adequately treat urinary incontinence, high detrusor leak point pressures, and renal dysfunction is indication for bladder augmentation in these patients. It was previously estimated that 5–30% of patients with spina bifida may undergo an augmentation cystoplasty [10, 11]. However, with improved diagnostic and therapeutic techniques, along with more structured and standardized treatment protocols, there has been a 25% decrease in number of pediatric patients who have undergone cystoplasty [12–15]. Augmentation is often combined with other procedures such as a catheterizable abdominal stoma and bladder neck procedure or sling to increase urinary outlet resistance.

Posterior urethral valves in males can lead to bladder dysfunction and renal failure. Augmentation cystoplasty may be required prior to renal transplantation [16–20]. Patients with exstrophy/epispadias complex also require bladder augmentation when staged functional reconstruction is unsuccessful [21–25].

Other congenital anomalies that may lead to the need for bladder augmentation include sacral agenesis, cloacal exstrophy, imperforate anus, and persistent urogenital sinus [25, 26].

Acquired Neurogenic Bladder

Spinal cord injury can lead to severe detrusor overactivity, poor bladder compliance, and decreased capacity over time. The changes are frequently related to the level of injury. Suprasacral spinal cord lesions often lead to detrusor overactivity with sphincter dyssynergia. This antagonistic dysfunction of the bladder and the outlet can impair detrusor compliance, and over time lead to reduced bladder capacity [24]. Sacral spinal cord lesions often lead to detrusor areflexia with a fixed, nonrelaxing sphincter. Generally, the bladder has normal compliance; however, over time, decreased compliance and reduced capacity can develop [27].

Bladder augmentation may be indicated if incontinence, high detrusor leak point pressures, severe autonomic dysreflexia, or renal dysfunction occur due to failure of the bladder to store urine at a low pressure. Often augmentation is considered when other measures such as behavioral modifications, anticholinergics and/or beta 3 agonists, intravesical botulinum toxin, or rarely anterior nerve root stimulation are ineffective [28–31].

Multiple sclerosis is another cause of neurogenic bladder dysfunction that may result in detrusor overactivity with sphincter dyssynergia [32]. Bladder dysfunction can worsen over time, and progressive neuromuscular deterioration can make intermittent self-catheterization difficult [33]. Medical therapy with anticholinergics and/or beta 3 agonists and intravesical botulinum toxin is usually the preferred treatment. However, occasional cases may be amenable to augmentation cystoplasty [34].

Overactive Bladder

Overactive bladder (OAB) is a syndrome or symptom complex of urinary urgency with or without urgency incontinence, urinary frequency, and nocturia [35]. Bladder augmentation is a treatment of last resort for refractory symptoms associated with detrusor overactivity that cannot be controlled with behavioral therapy, anticholinergics and/or beta 3 agonists, intravesical botulinum toxin, or sacral/peripheral neuromodulation [36, 37]. The number of cystoplasty procedures for OAB fell in the United Kingdom in the years 2000–2010, possibly secondary to the advent of botulinum toxin and sacral neuromodulation [38].

Infection

Genitourinary tuberculosis occurs in 10–20% of patients with pulmonary tuberculosis [39]. Tuberculous cystitis causes velvety granulations, bladder ulceration, and bladder wall thickening, and can progress to a bladder with severely reduced capacity [33]. Tuberculosis, once a common indication for augmentation, is now a rarity due to improved and aggressive therapies and a decreased incidence in the developed world [40–42].

Schistosomiasis, an endemic parasitic infection found historically in the Middle East and still prevalent in sub-Saharan Africa, may cause bladder wall fibrosis due to granulomatous inflammation [43, 44]. Reduced bladder capacity may be improved by augmentation [45].

Inflammatory Causes

Radiation changes may follow external beam radiation therapy for the treatment of pelvic malignancy. Acute cystitis symptoms usually resolve within a few months; however, occasionally bladder wall fibrosis may occur and reduce bladder capacity and impair function [46].

Bladder augmentation has been used as treatment for interstitial cystitis in patients with contracted small capacity bladders [47]. However, augmentation has shown only modest success as treatment for pain associated with interstitial cystitis [33, 48]. Its use in this population is still controversial [33, 49–51].

Iatrogenic

Bladder augmentation also serves as a crucial intervention in cases where bladder function is compromised due to iatrogenic causes. In cases of extensive surgical resection, particularly for locally advanced non-urologic cancers or benign bladder conditions, there may be a significant loss of bladder tissue. This loss can compromise bladder capacity and function, necessitating augmentation cystoplasty to restore adequate bladder volume and compliance.

Additionally, radiation therapy, commonly employed in the treatment of pelvic cancers, such as prostate, cervical, or bladder cancers, can lead to radiation-induced cystitis. This condition involves chronic inflammation, fibrosis, and reduced bladder compliance, which may progress to severe bladder contracture or reduced capacity. Augmentation cystoplasty may be considered in such cases to alleviate symptoms and improve bladder capacity and storage function.

Augmentation cystoplasty may be required for patients with significant loss of bladder wall due to surgical resection, which can occur from the removal of locally advanced non-urologic cancer or benign bladder lesions. For patients with previous urinary diversions who did not undergo a cystectomy, redirecting the ureters to an augmentation cystoplasty can be a viable method of undiversion in certain cases [52].

Ketamine Cystitis

Ketamine cystitis is a challenging condition associated with chronic misuse of ketamine, a dissociative anesthetic and recreational drug. It manifests as severe bladder dysfunction, ranging from LUTS to significant bladder wall damage and dysfunction [53, 54]. The exact mechanisms underlying ketamine-induced bladder injury are multifactorial and not entirely understood. Chronic ketamine abuse is thought to lead to direct toxic effects on the bladder epithelium, resulting in inflammation, ulceration, fibrosis, and reduced bladder compliance. Additionally, ketamine metabolites may contribute to oxidative stress and apoptosis within bladder tissues, exacerbating the damage [54]. Deciding to proceed with augmentation cystoplasty in patients with ketamine cystitis requires careful consideration of the risks and benefits.

Chronic ketamine use predisposes patients to poor wound healing, potential recurrence of bladder dysfunction, and increased risk of major surgical complications [55]. Ensuring patients are abstinent is essential, as continued use increases the risk of further damage, including additional bladder wall fibrosis and ureteric stricturing [56, 57].

Contraindications

Relative contraindications to augmentation cystoplasty traditionally include bowel pathologies such as inflammatory bowel disease, post-abdominal radiation, or post-bowel resection, where there are concerns for the development of short gut syndrome due to increased postoperative risks and GI complications. Additionally, any concern for malignancy in either the bowel or bladder should be thoroughly evaluated before proceeding with augmentation [58, 59]. In patients with underlying short gut syndrome ileum and colon should not be used, although the stomach may be an alternative [60].

Poor baseline renal function may predispose patients to severe electrolyte abnormalities and worsening renal function, and is a relative contraindication [60, 61]. However, in patients with continuing renal dysfunction as a direct result of bladder dysfunction, augmentation may be appropriate and can slow the decline in renal function [60, 62]. Additionally, more contemporary studies have indicated that the risk of renal deterioration post augmentation may be overstated, with some studies showing no impact on renal function two years post augmentation [63].

In patients set to be augmented with a continent stoma or neobladder, one must ensure that either the patient or caregiver is able to perform clean intermittent catheterization (CIC). Therefore, compromised manual dexterity, cognitive function, or lack of access to skilled care remains an important contraindication [64].

Surgical Considerations

Preparing for bladder augmentation surgery requires a comprehensive preoperative evaluation to ensure optimal outcomes, minimize complications, and properly inform and manage patient expectations. This evaluation should include cross-sectional imaging to assess genitourinary and gastrointestinal anatomy, with a preference for cross-sectional imaging over ultrasound to thoroughly evaluate anatomy, detect obstructions, and identify stones or other pathologies. Videourodynamics is helpful for assessing the bladder neck and determining the need for concurrent bladder neck or incontinence surgery, while cystoscopy examines the lower urinary tract anatomy. Preoperative lab work, including a complete blood count, renal function assessment, and electrolyte levels, provides important baseline data. Additionally, a urine culture should be obtained preoperatively.

Although the necessity and safety of full preoperative bowel preparation have been debated, a large study involving 8442 patients from the National Surgical Quality Improvement Program (NSQIP) database found that preoperative oral antibiotics and mechanical bowel preparation significantly reduced postoperative incidences of surgical site infection, anastomotic leak, and ileus. These findings support the continued use of bowel preparation in elective colorectal surgeries, which can be relevant for patients undergoing bladder augmentation [65–67].

The bladder is usually exposed through a lower midline abdominal incision, and the bowel segment is assessed for its suitability for use. The surgeon assesses the ease of moving the segment down to the bladder, combined with the possible nutritional and metabolic consequences that will be discussed below. The bowel segment is usually detubularized to maximize the surface area (and therefore the resulting bladder volume) and reduce bowel contractions and postoperative detrusor pressure [68].

Ileum is often the preferred segment due to its familiarity among urologists, low complication rate, and tolerable metabolic profile [33, 61]. It may result in lower postoperative maximal detrusor pressures, and may reduce uninhibited contractions more effectively than sigmoid [69]. A 20–40 cm segment is selected (depending on the need), at least 20 cm proximal to the ileocecal valve. It is detubularized and used in various configurations for augmentation (Figs. 25.1 [70] and 25.2).

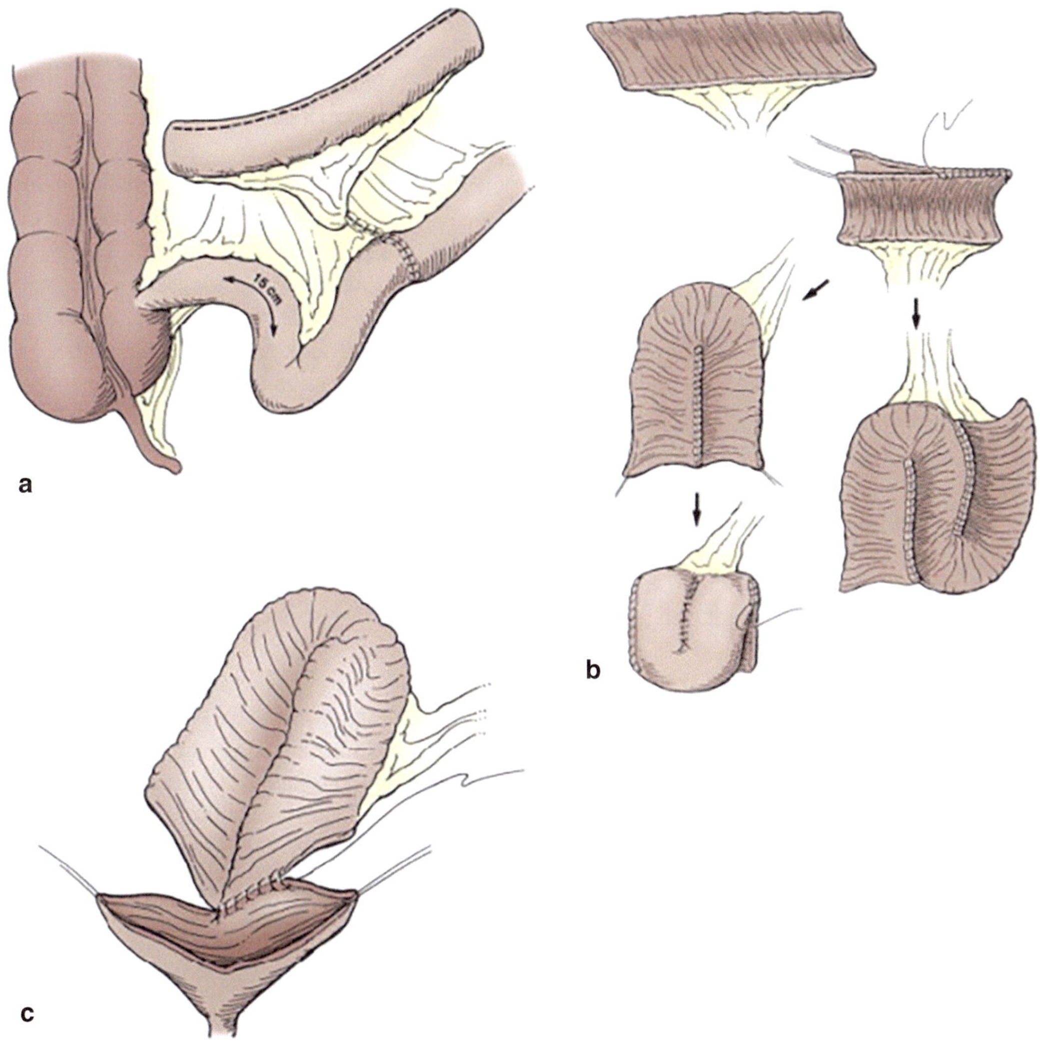

Fig. 25.1 (**a**) Ileocystoplasty. A 20–40 cm segment of ileum at least 15 cm from the ileocecal valve is removed and opened on its antimesenteric border. Ileoileostomy reconstitutes the bowel. (**b**) The opened ileal segment should be reconfigured. This can be done in a U, S, or W configuration. It can be further folded as a cup patch. (**c**) The reconfigured ileal segment is anastomosed widely to the native bladder. (From Adams and Joseph in Campbell-Walsh Urology [57])

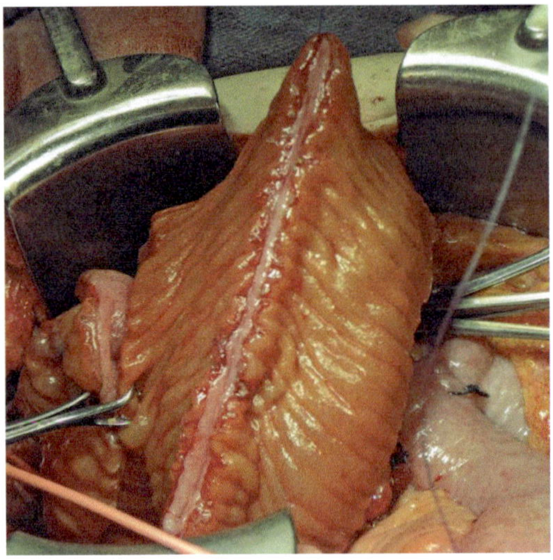

Fig. 25.2 A 40 cm length of ileum is shown. The segment has been isolated from the GI tract and reconfigured. The anti-mesenteric border was incised and the bowel segment was detubularized into an inverted U-shape. It will be anastomosed to the bladder

Sigmoid is an alternative and has been reported to have a lower rate of bowel obstruction [71, 72]. A 15–20 cm detubularized segment can be used.

Another alternative is the cecum and ascending colon that can be mobilized up to the hepatic flexure. Cecum can be detubularized and used alone or in conjunction with a 15–30 cm segment of detubularized ileum to form the augment. The ileal segment can also be used as a bladder "chimney" to reach resected or obstructed ureters for reimplantation if necessary.

If a continent catheterizing stoma is required, the ileum or appendix can be used as a continent catheterizable channel with the ileocecal valve (or intravesical tunneling of the appendix) providing the continence mechanism. Recently, we have reported on the use of an ileal continent catheterizable channel with a modified intussuscepted nipple valve along with the ileal augmentation cystoplasty [73].

Stomach is rarely used, and the jejunum should be avoided because of the high risk of associated metabolic complications, such as hyperchloremic, hyperkalemic metabolic acidosis, and hyponatremia, that have been reported with conduits [74].

Alternative procedures for bladder augmentation include ureterocystoplasty (which is an option in patients with megaureter and an ipsilateral nonfunctional kidney) and autoaugmentation. Autoaugmentation involves performing a detrusor myectomy to create a large, low-pressure bladder diverticulum [75, 76]. Autoaugmentation avoids the complications associated with bowel; however, it has poor long-term efficacy [77–81]. This was analyzed in a 2013 review of alternatives to enterocystoplasty [82].

Once the bowel segment has been selected, the bladder is opened with a sagittal incision and bivalved ("clamshell" cystoplasty) [83]. An alternative is a wide U-shaped anterior or posterior incision that effectively creates a large flap for a wide anastomosis [84]. Supratrigonal bladder excision can also be done [85]. The ureteric orifices are identified to avoid injury. The bowel segment is sutured to the bladder with a wide anastomosis to ensure good drainage of the augmentation. A pelvic drain, suprapubic tube, and Foley catheter may be placed for the postoperative period.

Postoperative care remains relatively unstandardized. There is growing evidence for the role of a structured enhanced recovery after surgery (ERAS) protocol, which has shown impressive results in adults following liver, gynecologic oncology, bariatric, vascular, pancreatic, colorectal, and urologic surgeries, among others. [86–91] ERAS has shown impressive results in high-income countries; however, many of the ERAS society recommendations remain cost-prohibitive in low- and middle-income countries, where subspecialists and multidisciplinary teams are less commonly available. The ERAS society therefore created a project aimed at less resource-rich environments with adapted guidelines that are more resource accessible [92].

Traditionally, augmentation cystoplasty has been performed open; however, there is growing popularity of minimally invasive approaches [93–96]. The first series comparing robotic total intracorporeal versus open cystoplasty in the pediatric population was a retrospective two surgeon, two center retrospective series published in 2016 by Cohen et al. showing significantly increased operative times in the robotic arm (623 min) as compared to the open arm (265 min) with no difference in length of stay observed (6 vs 7 days) [97]. A 2021 retrospective series involving 10 patients undergoing completely intracorporeal robot-assisted supratrigonal cystectomy and augmentation cystoplasty found a mean operative time of 250 minutes and a mean length of stay of 13 days. All patients reported to be continent with significantly improved bladder volumes. Postoperatively, two patients had postoperative ileus, two developed UTIs, and one had a trocar site bleed requiring embolization. Two urinary fistulas developed, one at 6 weeks and one at 9 months [98].

There is a growing body of literature and evolving surgical skills. Reports of completely intraperitoneal laparoscopic, robotic-assisted, and single-port augmentation cystoplasties in both adults and children have been published. These procedures require advanced laparoscopic skills and are not yet widely used.

The management of tubes, catheters, and drains is typically at the surgeon's discretion. Traditionally, a nasogastric tube was left in place until bowel function returned, but this practice has largely been abandoned, partly due to ERAS data and standardized protocols [91, 99]. Continuous bladder drainage via a suprapubic tube with or without a Foley catheter is recommended with standardized (often three times daily) flushing to prevent mucus plugging. An extravesical drain is often left and removed once outputs have slowed and no concern of urine leak is apparent. Some centers perform cystograms prior to discharge, while others prefer to assess the patient 3 weeks postoperatively with a cystogram prior to clamping the suprapubic tube. Once the suprapubic tube is clamped, patients should begin CIC up to 6–8 times daily with 1–2 overnight catheterizations until bladder volumes increase.

ERAS post bladder augmentation has been shown to be feasible and successful in the pediatric population; however, a relative paucity of data exists in the adult population [100, 101]. An adapted ERAS protocol for adult augmentation cystoplasty has been developed, aimed at low- and middle-income countries. The protocol remains multidisciplinary and requires the involvement of the urologist, a nutritionist, and nurses. Similar to the standard ERAS protocol, an emphasis is placed on limited perioperative fasting (8 hours), a high protein/low carbohydrate diet preoperatively, limited narcotics, early nasogastric tube removal, early ambulation and diet, and the use of metoclopramide and neostigmine to prevent postoperative nausea and ileus. The major deviations from the standard ERAS protocol are the lack of an epidural and alvimopan. In the study of 33 patients, all saw bowel function return by postoperative day 2 [102].

Follow-Up

Close follow-up is necessary in the immediate postoperative period until indwelling catheters are removed and the patient adjusts to CIC and bladder irrigation. The augmentation will often enlarge with time, and urinary incontinence will improve. A routine ultrasound is often performed to ensure no residual hydronephrosis, with some recommending ultrasounds at 6 weeks, 6 months, then annually. Lab work assessing renal function and electrolytes should be monitored at each visit. Some authors have advocated screening cystoscopy 5–10 years after augmentation to assess for bladder cancer; however, this is controversial, with many recommending against this practice [103, 104]. Urodynamics may be done if there is a change in symptoms, onset of new hydronephrosis, or worsening renal function.

The overall complication rates in various series range from 3 to 41% depending on the duration of follow-up and completeness of reporting and nearly one-third require further surgery [105–108].

Early Postoperative Complications

As with any major abdominal surgery, there are associated cardiovascular, respiratory, and gastrointestinal complications. Postoperative mortality rates range between 0 and 3.2%, generally due to postoperative myocardial infarction (0–2.7%) and pulmonary embolus/deep vein thrombosis (0–7%) [60, 105, 109–116]. There have been a few reports of severe complications such as major bleeding requiring reoperation and bowel segment necrosis [8, 116].

Small bowel obstruction requiring operative intervention may occur in 3–6% of patients, and approximately 5–6% of patients may develop a wound infection or dehiscence [60]. Anastomotic leak from the bladder occurs in 2–4% of patients. Postoperative ileus is common, and prolonged ileus occurs in approximately 5% of patients, though ERAS protocols may help alleviate this risk. Severe postoperative complications are less frequent in contemporary case series [60].

Continence and Urodynamic Outcomes

Several groups have reported long-term functional outcomes in adult and pediatric populations. Blavias et al. reported on 65 adult patients who underwent augmentation cystoplasty (primarily with an ileocecal segment) with or without creation of an abdominal stoma (and included an additional 11 patients who had a continent diversion) [84]. At a mean follow-up of 5 years, 70% considered themselves cured, and 18% considered themselves improved. Failures consisted almost exclusively of interstitial cystitis patients. Mean bladder capacity increased from 166 mL to 572 mL, and mean maximal detrusor pressure fell from 53cmH2O to 14 cmH2O. Flood et al. reported on 122 augmentation cystoplasties (67% ileocystoplasty, 30% ileocecocystoplasty) with a mean follow-up of 3 years [117]. They had a primarily adult population. They reported similar urodynamic improvements, a 75% cure rate, and a 20% improvement rate in incontinence.

Quek and Ginsberg reported durability of the urodynamic improvements and 96% patient satisfaction among 24 patients with a mean follow-up of 8 years (range 4–13) [118]. Herschorn and Hewitt performed a cross-sectional survey of 59 adults who underwent augmentation cystoplasty (usually with additional simultaneous reconstructive procedures) at a median follow-up of 6 years. In total, 67% of patients reported complete continence, and 30% reported only mild incontinence (requiring on average 1–2 pads per day). Almost all patients were very satisfied with their urologic management [105].

Results in the pediatric populations are similar, although the majority of patients require additional reconstructive procedures such as ureteral reimplantation, bladder neck procedures, and creation of catheterizable channels. Lopez Pereira et al. reported on 29 children with a mean follow-up of 11 years [119]. Mean postoperative bladder capacity increased from 90 mL to 521 mL, and mean maximal detrusor pressure fell from 45 cmH_2O to 10 cmH_2O. Shekarriz et al. reported a 95% continence rate among 133 pediatric patients at a mean follow-up of 5 years [71].

A number of authors have compared the outcomes of the ileum, ileocecal, and sigmoid segments, and have not shown any consistent advantages of any segment in terms of urinary continence or renal function [116, 120–122]. Urodynamically demonstrated contractions might persist postoperatively with colonic segments [69, 123]. Early contractions that generate high pressures may result in incontinence, reflux, and hydronephrosis, whereas low amplitude contractions that occur near capacity are of little clinical significance [99].

Long-Term Consequences

The possible long-term consequences of augmentation are listed in Table 25.2 and discussed below. Complications requiring intervention may occur years after the original surgery [105, 106]. This underscores the necessity of long-term follow-up.

Growth Retardation and Decreased bone mineral density

Small case series by Mundy and Nurse and Wagstaff et al. were the first to suggest there is a

Table 25.2 Long-term consequences of augmentation cystoplasty and potential management strategies

	Description	Management
Growth retardation and osteopenia	Conflicting evidence on the presence of linear growth reduction Chronic acidosis may lead to osteopenia.	Consider monitoring bone mineral density Treat acidosis
Electrolyte abnormalities *Ileum/Colon* *Stomach*	Hyperchloremic, metabolic acidosis ± hypokalemia Hypochloremic, hypokalemia, metabolic alkalosis ± hematuria-dysuria syndrome	Chloride restriction, bicarbonate, niacin, and chlorpromazine IV fluids, potassium supplementation, histamine antagonists, proton pump inhibitors
Renal insufficiency	May occur as a result of complications associated with augmentation cystoplasty, especially in patients with poor preoperative renal function	Postoperative monitoring of renal function
Vitamin B12 deficiency	Due to ileal resection	Postoperative monitoring of complete blood count B12 supplementation
Bladder Cancer	Increased risk of aggressive bladder cancer among patients with neurogenic bladder; controversial if the augmentation is an independent risk factor	Aggressive investigation of hematuria, frequent urinary infections, or penile/scrotal discharge
Bladder perforation	Consider any patient with peritonitis, septic shock, abdominal pain and distension, nausea and vomiting, fever, referred shoulder pain, or intraperitoneal fluid	In stable patients, a trial of conservative therapy may be attempted Standard treatment is laparotomy for surgical repair
Stone disease	Due to metabolic alterations, poor bladder emptying, mucus, and chronic infection	Endoscopic, percutaneous, or open surgical procedure Increased fluid intake and dietary modifications
Mucus	Produced by the bowel segment	Bladder irrigations Acetylcysteine/urea irrigations.
Urinary tract infection	Asymptomatic bacteriuria is common Symptomatic urinary infection requires treatment.	Antibiotic therapy for symptomatic infections Antibiotic prophylaxis or intravesical irrigations for frequent symptomatic infections
Bowel dysfunction	Due to alterations to bile acid metabolism, often exacerbates underlying neurogenic bowel or irritable bowel syndrome.	Low-fat diet Antidiarrheal medication Bile acid binders (cholestyramine)
Voiding dysfunction	Incomplete emptying or inability to void Incontinence may occur due to an incompetent outlet.	CIC is commonly required postoperatively Surgical treatment of incontinence is common.
Pregnancy		Vaginal delivery preferable. Urologic assistance is helpful during elective cesarean sections.

decrease in linear growth in children after augmentation cystoplasty [124, 125]. Since then, several additional studies have been published, of which two suggested there is approximately a 15% decrease in linear growth after augmentation, and six, which did not demonstrate a significant change in linear growth [126, 127]. There is also contradictory evidence as to whether decreased bone mineral density or osteopenia is a result of the augmentation [127]. In a case series of 24 children followed for an average of 9 years after augmentation, Hafez et al. reported a 20% incidence of significant osteopenia [128]. The osteopenia is likely a result of buffering of the acidosis by the skeletal system, which leads to changes in bone mineralization [129]. Correction of this acidosis may improve bone density [130]. Other mechanisms of osteopenia include reduced renal tubular reabsorption of calcium and intestinal malabsorption of calcium [131]. A more recent study by Haas et al. demonstrated that bone mineral density was significantly related to ambulatory status and secondarily to neurological level rather than to the presence or absence of augmentation cystoplasty [132]. The long-term impact of osteopenia and how it affects children as adults is still unknown; however, the loss of bone mineral density may not be due to the enterocystoplasty alone, with confounding risk factors including systemic acidosis and renal dysfunction potentially driving density loss [127, 133].

Management includes appropriate screening and treatment of postoperative metabolic acidosis. Patients with renal failure are more likely to have uncompensated acidosis and should be followed closely and treated for this complication. Some authors have advocated bone mineral density measurements and monitoring after augmentation [128].

Electrolyte Abnormalities

The expected pattern of metabolic abnormality is dependent on the segment of bowel used in the augmentation cystoplasty. Other factors that influence the severity of the electrolyte imbalance include the surface area of the augmentation, urine pH, and the urine contact time, as well as renal function and acid secretion [131].

Ileum and Colon

With an ileal or colonic augmentation, the classic electrolyte pattern is hyperchloremic metabolic acidosis. The symptoms associated with metabolic acidosis are fatigue, anorexia, weight loss, and polydipsia. There are several possible mechanisms: frequent pyelonephritis may lead to distal tubular acidification defect, urea in the urine may be metabolized by intestinal flora to ammonium which is then absorbed by the bowel, loss of bicarbonate from the bowel that lead to metabolic acidosis, or chloride that is actively transported from the bowel into the urine leads to reabsorption of ammonium or hydrogen ions [134]. The most likely mechanism is ammonium substitution for sodium in a sodium-hydrogen ion antiport; this antiport is coupled with a bicarbonate-chloride exchanger, leading to a net reabsorption of hydrogen ions, ammonium, and chloride [135]. Hypokalemia can occur during treatment of an acidosis, which unmasks low total body potassium, or as a result of renal potassium wasting (seen more frequently with colonic segments) [135, 136]. Associated hypocalcemia and hypomagnesemia (usually restricted to patients with renal insufficiency and more commonly seen in colonic augmentations) may be due to reduced renal reabsorption due to a high level of sulfate that is reabsorbed from the bowel, or due to chronic acidosis, causing calcium mobilization and subsequent activation of parathyroid hormone [136, 137].

Normal renal function can often compensate for this acidosis; the majority of patients will have a measurable abnormality; however, it will only be clinically relevant in approximately 10–20% of patients [60, 138, 139]. The absorptive properties of the bowel may be attenuated with time due to mucosal atrophy [140, 141]. Treatment of the acidosis is usually considered once the base excess falls below −2.5 mmol/L. [136, 139] Therapy consists of dietary chloride restriction, bicarbonate supplementation (sodium bicarbonate, potassium citrate), and maximal urinary drainage [137]. Niacin or chlorpromazine inhibits active chloride transportation in the intestine and may be useful, especially when the solute load of bicarbonate therapy is undesirable [128].

Stomach

In a gastric augment, the classic electrolyte pattern is hypochloremic, hypokalemic, and metabolic alkalosis. Associated clinical symptoms include pelvic pain, fatigue, mental status changes, seizures, or cardiac arrhythmias [136]. Treatment of the electrolyte disturbance involves maximal bladder drainage, normal saline fluid resuscitation, and potassium replacement when necessary [136, 142]. Long-term therapy with potassium chloride may be required. Acid secretion can be suppressed with histamine antagonists or proton pump inhibitors [136].

Hematuria-dysuria syndrome is characterized by excess acid secretion causing peptic ulcer disease, hematuria, and dysuria; it occurs in up to 25% of patients, and treatment with a proton pump inhibitor is required intermittently or continuously in a small proportion of patients [143].

Hyperammonemia

The liver is responsible for metabolizing ammonium (absorbed from an augmentation cystoplasty) into urea. Impaired hepatic function or sepsis can lead to the inability of the liver to cope with the hyperammonemia; symptomatically this presents as ammoniagenic encephalopathy [137]. Treatment is maximal urinary drainage, low protein diet, ammonium binders (such as lactulose or neomycin), and in severe cases, intravenous arginine glutamate [136].

Renal Insufficiency

Deterioration of renal function may occur in 0–15% of patients after augmentation [60]. It is unknown whether this is a direct result of the augmentation or due to associated complications [144]. Renal insufficiency occurs independent of the bowel segment selected [145, 146]. The etiology of renal dysfunction may be urinary stone disease, bacteriuria, high detrusor pressures, vesicoureteral reflux, unrecognized obstruction, and lack of compliance with catheterization [145]. One study suggests that approximately 5% of patients will have renal dysfunction after augmentation without a clear etiology [145]. Some authors have demonstrated that baseline renal function is a significant predictor of renal deterioration after augmentation cystoplasty, with an increased risk when creatinine clearance is <40 mL/min [8, 60, 147, 148]. Other studies in children and adults with baseline renal dysfunction did not appear to demonstrate that they have accelerated renal failure after augmentation cystoplasty [62, 105].

A contemporary review of 80 patients post-ileocystoplasty identified new renal scarring in 40%, with 38% of these patients going on to develop ≥ stage 3 chronic renal failure. Of the patients with renal scarring, 69% had been non-compliant with CIC. Of note, the onset of upper tract deterioration was clinically silent in one-third of the patients, further underscoring the need for careful and lifelong monitoring [149].

There is no consensus on the order of a staged augmentation cystoplasty and a renal transplant [62]. However, augmentation cystoplasty after renal transplantation is considered safe if performed concomitantly or concurrently, and while higher risks of urinary tract infections have been identified in these patients, similar patient and graft survival rates have been noted [150–152].

Postoperatively, patients should have renal imaging and serum creatinine measurements to screen for renal insufficiency [137]. Serum creatinine can be difficult to interpret in this population, due to a low muscle mass in neurogenic patients, and increased reabsorption of urine creatinine by the ileum. Nuclear renograms may be better for definitive measurement.

Vitamin B12 Deficiency

Vitamin B12 is bound to intrinsic factor in the duodenum which allows it to be absorbed in the terminal ileum. With ileocystoplasty, the most distal 15 cm of the ileum should be preserved to prevent this complication [137]. Vitamin B12 deficiency may cause megaloblastic anemia and neurologic changes. In nutritionally normal individuals, it takes up to 3 years for the liver's store of B12 to be depleted and the resulting deficiency to manifest. The incidence of B12 deficiency related to ileal resection is 3–20% [137, 153].

This complication may be treated prophylactically with B12 supplementation if more than 50 cm of ileum is used for the bladder augmentation [154]. Otherwise, patients should have complete blood counts in follow-up to screen for pernicious anemia.

Bladder Cancer

The overall incidence of bladder malignancy remains low (1–4.6%), and it is unclear whether augmentation itself is a risk factor for bladder cancers; however, cancers have been reported in young patients after augmentation [103, 106, 155–158]. It has also been reported that spinal cord injury patients and spina bifida patients develop bladder cancer at a young age (40–50 years), have an increased risk of locally advanced disease, an increased number of adenocarcinomas and squamous cell carcinomas, and a short median survival after diagnosis [104, 159]. In a matched cohort study from a registry of patients with bladder dysfunction due to neurologic abnormalities, exstrophy, and posterior urethral valves, Higuchi et al. did not find a significant difference in the incidence of bladder cancer among patients with augmentation cystoplasty (using ileum or colon) compared to patients managed with intermittent catheterization [103]. The authors demonstrated that the incidence of bladder cancer was higher in both groups with congenital bladder anomalies, independent of augmentation status, when compared to the SEER database. Possible reasons for a higher rate of bladder cancer in patients with neurogenic bladder may be recurrent urinary tract infections, reduced intracellular antioxidant activity (leading to increased rates of DNA mutation), impaired DNA repair in the bowel due to the hyperosmolar urine, and immunosuppressant use in patients after renal transplantation [103, 160, 161]. However, patients who have undergone a gastric augmentation may have a higher cancer risk compared to other bowel segments [103, 162, 163].

Urologists should have a particular awareness of the potential for aggressive bladder cancer in this population, whether or not they have had an augmentation cystoplasty. Symptoms such as hematuria, frequent urinary infections, or penile/scrotal discharge need to be aggressively investigated; visual changes in the bladder due to the augmentation, recent infections, or catheterization can make cystoscopy challenging, and biopsy or CT should be considered if there is any uncertainty [159].

Bladder Perforation

Bladder perforation is a potentially life-threatening complication that occurs in approximately 6–13% of patients [26, 151, 164–169]. Patients with neurogenic bladders, those with competent bladder necks, those without a catheterizable channel, and those who abuse alcohol appear to be at an increased risk [60, 106, 170, 171]. Perforation can occur at any time postoperatively, even years after surgery. It can present with fever, abdominal pain and distension with intraperitoneal fluid, nausea and vomiting, referred shoulder pain, peritonitis, and septic shock. Because of neurologic abnormalities of these patients, the presenting symptoms are often nonspecific, and perforation should be considered in all patients presenting with acute abdominal pain, peritonitis, or septic features [71, 166]. Diagnosis can be made with a CT cystogram; standard fluoroscopic cystography has a 10–20% false negative rate [71, 165, 172]. CT or US can demonstrate intraperitoneal fluid, which is an important sign that bladder perforation has occurred [173]. Due to the augmentation, extraperitoneal ruptures are rare [174]. The area of perforation is usually at the bowel-bladder anastomosis or within the weaker bowel wall [165]. The etiology of bladder perforation is thought to be from traumatic catheterization, acute overdistension, increased intravesical pressure, chronic overdistension (from CIC noncompliance), or infection leading to localized areas of ischemia and necrosis [172, 175].

The treatment of patients with large perforations and clinical instability is usually laparotomy for surgical repair. In patients that are stable (usually with a small perforation), a trial of conservative therapy (Foley catheter and antibiotics) may be considered [175, 176]. Mortality is high in patients with clinical instability on presentation and those with a delayed diagnosis; overall mortality has been estimated at up to 25% [164, 177, 178]. If clinical suspicion is high, and imaging is negative, the patient should still be treated as a possible bladder perforation [60]. There is a 25% rate of recurrence of bladder perforation after the initial episode [106, 172, 179].

Stone Disease

Patients are at increased risk for bladder and upper tract calculi, and urinary stones have been reported in 9–15% of patients after augmentation, and in some series as high as 50%. [60, 105, 180–183] Many of the risk factors for stones are present in patients who undergo augmentation and may not be directly related to the surgical procedure [184]. Patients with a continent catheterizable channel (which may not drain the bladder completely), those using urethral CIC (compared to those voiding spontaneously), and patients with urease-splitting bacteriuria are at increased risk [60, 181]. Possible reasons for stone formation include chronic bacteriuria (a significant risk factor in multivariable analysis), intravesical foreign bodies, elevated post-void residuals, and mucus secretion from the bowel segment [185, 186]. Similar to a typical stone-forming population, dietary choices and inadequate fluid intake increase the risk of stone disease [187]. Metabolic changes, such as hypercalciuria and hypocitraturia secondary to metabolic acidosis, water loss through the cystoplasty bowel segment, and mild enteric hyperoxaluria (from the bowel resection or antibiotic-related deficiency of oxalobacter formigenes), can predispose these patients to stone formation [183, 187, 188]. Most stones are struvite due to frequent bacteriuria, or calcium oxalate; they are usually mixed with calcium phosphate due to the alkaline urine [183, 187, 189].

Treatment of stones includes endoscopic, percutaneous, or open surgical procedures depending on the stone size, location, and patient factors [60, 180]. Prevention of stones consists of bladder irrigation, which may or may not be preventive, increased fluid intake, decreased salt, purine, and oxalate intake, and medical therapy directed by 24 h urine and stone analysis [190, 191].

Mucus

Ileal and colonic segments used in augmentations continue to produce mucus. Up to 40 g of mucus can be produced daily, and this continues over time despite villous atrophy [192]. Colonic bowel segments produce more mucus than the ileal segments [183]. The mucus is thought to help reduce malignant changes; however, it has been implicated as a causative factor in urinary tract infections, stone formation, poor bladder emptying, and bladder perforation [60, 193].

Problematic mucus secretion can be treated with daily bladder irrigations (>250 mL per day) [157]. These can be augmented with acetylcysteine or urea irrigations, which help dissolve mucus, or oral ranitidine, which may help to reduce mucus production [194, 195].

Urinary Tract Infection

Asymptomatic bacteriuria is nearly universal among augmentation enterocystoplasty patients and usually does not require treatment except in cases of urease-splitting organisms (such as Proteus and Klebsiella) [196]. Studies in ileal conduits have shown that bacteria freely adhere to bowel mucosa and do not incite an inflammatory reaction [197]. This chronic bacteriuria has been cited as a risk factor for stone disease, incontinence, and bladder cancer [60, 198]. The most common organism is *Escherichia Coli* [199].

Symptomatic urinary tract infection which occurs in 5–40% of patients requires antibiotic treatment [60, 116, 121]. Risk factors are similar to asymptomatic bacteriuria and include urinary stasis, mucus production, and intermittent catheterization [43]. Symptoms may be nonspecific if bladder sensation is absent and include incontinence, abdominal pain, hematuria, new onset foul-smelling urine, and lethargy.

Management of urinary tract infection consists of appropriate antibiotic therapy. In patients with frequent symptomatic infections despite oral antibiotic prophylaxis, intravesical irrigation with antibiotics may reduce symptomatic infections [200].. In a small pilot study of 15 patients after ileocystoplasty, cranberry extract reduced asymptomatic bacteriuria [201].

Bowel Dysfunction

Bowel dysfunction after bowel resection for augmentation or diversion occurs in approximately 20–50% of patients [105, 202, 203]. However, bowel dysfunction after bladder augmentation alone is rare unless the ileocecal valve is incorporated [99]. Bowel dysfunction is more common among patients with a neurologic diagnosis as a result of associated neurogenic bowel dysfunction and among patients with previous radiation or bowel resections [202, 203]. Approximately 30% of patients with irritable bowel syndrome have detrusor overactivity; this may be due to an intrinsic disorder of smooth muscle calcium metabolism [203].

Specific surgical factors may contribute to postoperative changes in bowel function that lead to diarrhea. Bile acids, generated in the liver and secreted into the small intestine, are necessary for fat absorption. Bile acids are reabsorbed in the distal ileum, enter the liver, and participate in the feedback mechanism for regeneration. Resection of long sections of the terminal ileum can lead to bile acid malabsorption. Bile acids entering the colon may cause diarrhea by inducing water and salt secretion and by promoting motility [204]. Ileal resection of more than 100 cm results in severe bile acid malabsorption that cannot be compensated for by increased hepatic synthesis. In such cases, steatorrhea results from impaired micelle formation due to decreased luminal concentrations of conjugated bile acids. In shorter ileal resections, bile acid malabsorption can usually be compensated for by an increase in hepatic synthesis, and malabsorbed bile acids cause diarrhea rather than steatorrhea [205, 206]. Resection of the ileocecal valve leads to bacterial colonization of the distal ileum that destroys the bile acids. The lack of bile acids, which leads to unabsorbed fatty acids in the large bowel, stimulates the colon to secrete more water and mucus, increase motility, and prompt defecation [207].

Treatment of this complication involves a low-fat diet and antidiarrheal medications. Bile acid-related diarrhea can be diagnosed with a selenium homocholic acid taurine test. A therapeutic trial of bile acid binders such as cholestyramine may be helpful [207].

Voiding Dysfunction and Incontinence

The interposition of bowel into the bladder usually prevents the efficient detrusor contractions that are necessary for voiding [208]. The urethral outlet resistance may be high due to neurologic disease or concomitant surgery to treat incontinence. Some patients are able to void spontaneously with abdominal straining.

If the patient is unable to void or has complications from incomplete emptying, they will need to use CIC to empty their bladder. This is necessary in 25–100% of neurogenic patients, and a lower proportion of neurologically intact patients [60].

Continence rates range from 60 to 100% [104, 118, 209]. Nocturnal incontinence can occur due to failure of the urethral sphincter to respond to contractions of the augmented bowel and increased urine output due to water loss from the augmented bowel segment. Daytime incontinence can be due to stress incontinence, detrusor overactivity, or phasic contractions of the augmented bowel segment [210, 211]. These phasic contractions are usually <40 cm H2O and occur at higher volumes [118].

Treatment of incontinence in these patients includes behavioral modification (such as more frequent CIC), anticholinergics, and surgical procedures such as midurethral slings, bladder neck slings or bladder neck reconstruction, and artificial urinary sphincters [60, 212].

A retrospective review of intravesical onabotulinumtoxinA in patients who failed augmentation saw 13/33 patients respond to the injection, with a higher peak DO pressure predictive of benefit. Rarely repeat augmentation is necessary [182].

Pregnancy

While not a postoperative complication, pregnancy after augmentation cystoplasty is becoming more common [172]. Complications such as premature labor (10%), urinary tract infection (60–100%), renal dysfunction, and urinary tract obstruction are more prevalent in this population [213–215]. Patients usually require antibiotic treatment of bacteriuria, as screening urinalysis for infection or proteinuria is not accurate due to mucus from the augmentation cystoplasty [216].

Vaginal delivery is preferable when safe due to concerns that a cesarean section has a risk of damaging the vascular pedicle. There is also controversy as to whether cesarean section is necessary for patients with artificial sphincters and bladder neck procedures. [198, 216, 217] If an elective cesarean section is scheduled for other reasons, urologic assistance during the surgery, and a high segment section may help avoid major intraabdominal adhesions and damage to the bladder augmentation [60, 216]. The bowel segment can survive inadvertent damage to the vascular pedicle; however, this may lead to eventual contraction of the bowel segment [218]. When an elective cesarean section is planned, preoperative imaging to define the anatomy is valuable.

Conclusion

Bladder augmentation with intestine has been successfully used to treat various conditions that result in small-capacity bladders. The surgical technique involves detubularization and reconfiguration of a segment of bowel (usually the ileum or colon) to create a patch. A successful clinical outcome is dependent upon creating a large capacity, low-pressure reservoir to store urine; additional procedures to aid in catheterization or continence are often necessary. Potential complications have been well described and are usually reported in case series. Medical and surgical treatments of complications are similarly well elucidated, although some are still controversial. Since complications may occur at any time after surgery, prolonged follow-up and monitoring are essential.

References

1. Mikulicz J. Zur Operation der angeborenen Blasenspalte. Zentralbl Chir. 1899;26:641–3.
2. Charghi A, Charbonneau J, Gauthier GE. Colocystoplasty for bladder enlargement and bladder substitution: a study of late results in 31 cases. J Urol. 1967;97:849–56.
3. Bisgard JD. Substitution of the urinary bladder with a segment of sigmoid: an experimental study. Ann Surg. 1943;117:106–9.
4. Couvelaire R. The "little bladder" of genito-urinary tuberculosis; classification, site and variants of bladder-intestine transplants. J Urol Medicale Chir 1950;56:381–434.
5. Leong CH. Use of the stomach for bladder replacement and urinary diversion. Ann R Coll Surg Engl. 1978;60:283–9.
6. Elbahnasy AM, Shalhav A, Hoenig DM, Figenshau R, Clayman RV. Bladder wall substitution with synthetic and non-intestinal organic materials. J Urol. 1998;159:628–37.
7. Goodwin WE, Winter CC, Barker WF. Cup-patch technique of ileocystoplasty for bladder enlargement or partial substitution. Surg Gynecol Obstet. 1959;108:240–4.
8. Smith RB, Cangh P, Skinner DG, Kaufman JJ, Goodwin WE. Augmentation enterocystoplasty: a critical review. J Urol. 1977;118:35–9.
9. Sidi AA, Dykstra DD, Gonzalez R. The value of urodynamic testing in the management of neonates with myelodysplasia: a prospective study. J Urol. 1986;135:90–3.
10. Lendvay TS, Cowan CA, Mitchell MM, Joyner BD, Grady RW. Augmentation cystoplasty rates at children's hospitals in the United States: a pediatric health information system database study. J Urol. 2006;176:1716–20.
11. Kaefer M, Pabby A, Kelly M, Darbey M, Bauer SB. Improved bladder function after prophylactic treatment of the high risk neurogenic bladder in newborns with myelomentingocele. J Urol. 1999;162:1068–71.
12. Schlomer BJ, Saperston K, Baskin L. National trends in augmentation cystoplasty in the 2000s and factors associated with patient outcomes. J Urol. 2013;190:1352–7.
13. Stein R, Bogaert G, Dogan HS, et al. EAU/ESPU guidelines on the management of neurogenic bladder in children and adolescent part I diagnostics and conservative treatment. Neurourol Urodyn.

2020;39(1):45–57. https://doi.org/10.1002/nau.24211.
14. Joseph DB, Baum MA, Tanaka ST, et al. Urologic guidelines for the care and management of people with spina bifida. Brei T, Castillo H, Castillo J, eds. PRM. 2020;13(4):479–89. https://doi.org/10.3233/PRM-200712.
15. Vasdev R, Softness K, Cahill D, et al. Intradetrusor botox injection and augmentation cystoplasty trends among spina bifida patients at US freestanding children's hospitals. J Pediatr Urol. 2024;20(3):482.e1–6. https://doi.org/10.1016/j.jpurol.2024.02.012.
16. Aki FT. Renal transplantation in children with augmentation enterocystoplasty. Transplant Proc. 2006;38:554–5.
17. Fisang C, Hauser S, Muller SC. Ureterocystoplasty: an ideal method for vesical augmentation in children. Aktuelle Urol. 2010;41(Suppl 1):50–2.
18. Kajbafzadeh AM, Quinn FM, Duffy PG, Ransley PG. Augmentation cystoplasty in boys with posterior urethral valves. J Urol. 1995;154:874–7.
19. Peters CA. The urodynamic consequences of posterior urethral valves. J Urol. 1990;144:122–6.
20. Pereira PL, Urrutia MJ, Lobato R, Jaureguizar E. Renal transplantation in augmented bladders. Curr Urol Rep. 2014;15:431.
21. Amirzargar MA. Reconstruction of bladder and urethra using ileocecal segment and appendix in patients with exstrophy-epispadias complex: the first report of a new surgical approach. Int Urol Nephrol. 2007;39:779–85.
22. Castro R, Pavanello P, Domini R. Indications for bladder augmentation in the exstrophy-epispadias complex. Br J Urol. 1994;73:303–7.
23. Gearhart JP, Peppas DS, Jeffs RD. The failed exstrophy closure: strategy for management. Br J Urol. 1993;71:217–20.
24. Lund DP, Hendren WH. Cloacal exstrophy: a 25-year experience with 50 cases. J Pediatr Surg. 2001;36:68–75.
25. Carrasco A Jr, Vemulakonda VM. Managing adult urinary incontinence from the congenitally incompetent bladder outlet. Curr Opin Urol. Published online 2016.
26. Metcalfe PD. Spontaneous bladder perforations: a report of 500 augmentations in children and analysis of risk. J Urol. 2006;175(1466–1470):1470–61.
27. Jeong SJ, Cho SY, Oh SJ. Spinal cord/brain injury and the neurogenic bladder. Urol Clin North Am. 2010;37:537–46.
28. Sidi A, Becher E, Reddy P, Dykstra D. Augmentation enterocystoplasty for the management of voiding dysfunction in spinal cord injury patients. J Urol. 1990;143:83–5.
29. Rey F, Heesakkers J. Applications of neurostimulation for urinary storage and voiding dysfunction in neurological patients. Urol Int. 2008;81:373–8.
30. Lewis J, Cheng E. Non-traditional management of the neurogenic bladder: tissue engineering and neuromodulation. Sci World J. 2007;7:1230–41.
31. Anquetil C, Abdelhamid S, Gelis A, Fattal C. Botulinum toxin therapy for neurogenic detrusor hyperactivity versus augmentation enterocystoplasty: impact on the quality of life of patients with SCI. Spinal Cord. Published online 2016.
32. Litwiller S, Frohman E, Zimmern P. Multiple sclerosis and the urologist. J Urol. 1999;161:743–57.
33. Reyblat P, Ginsberg D. Augmentation cystoplasty: what are the indications? Review. 2008;9:452–8.
34. Khavari R, Fletcher SG, Liu J, Boone TB. A modification to augmentation cystoplasty with catheterizable stoma for neurogenic patients: technique and long-term results. Urology. 2012;80:460–4.
35. Abrams P. The standardisation of terminology in lower urinary tract function: report from the standardisation sub-committee of the international continence society. Urology. 2003;61:37–49.
36. Reyblat P, Ginsberg D. Augmentation enterocystoplasty in overactive bladder: is there still a role? Curr Urol Rep. 2010;11:432–9.
37. Lightner DJ, Gomelsky A, Souter L, Vasavada SP. Diagnosis and treatment of overactive bladder (non-neurogenic) in adults: AUA/SUFU guideline amendment 2019. J Urol. 2019;202(3):558–63. https://doi.org/10.1097/JU.0000000000000309.
38. Shreck E, Gioia K, Lucioni A. Indications for augmentation cystoplasty in the era of OnabotulinumtoxinA. Curr Urol Rep. 2016;17:27.
39. Wise G, Shteynshlyuger A. An update on lower urinary tract tuberculosis. Curr Urol Rep. 2008;9:305–13.
40. Abel B, Gow J. Results of caecocystoplasty for tuberculous bladder contracture. Br J Urol. 1978;50:511–6.
41. Wesolowski S. Late resuls of cystoplasty in chronic tuberculous cystitis. Br J Urol. 1970;42:697–703.
42. Figueiredo A, Lucon A, Srougi M. Bladder augmentation for the treatment of chronic tuberculous cystitis. Clinical and urodynamic evaluation of 25 patients after long term follow-up. Neurourol Urodyn. 2006;25:433–40.
43. Kehinde E, Anim J, Hira P. Parasites of urological importance. Urol Int. 2008;81:1–13.
44. Wang XY, Li Q, Li YL, et al. Prevalence and correlations of schistosomiasis mansoni and schistosomiasis haematobium among humans and intermediate snail hosts: a systematic review and meta-analysis. Infect Dis Poverty. 2024;13(1):63. https://doi.org/10.1186/s40249-024-01233-0.
45. Badr M, Zaher M. Ileocystoplasty in the treatment of bilharzial contracted bladder. J Egypt Med Assoc. 1959;42:33–49.
46. Smit S, Heyns C. Management of radiation cystitis. Nat Rev Urol. 2010;7:206–14.
47. Webster G, Maggio M. The management of chronic interstitial cystitis by substitution cystoplasty. J Urol. 1989;141:287–91.
48. Nielsen K, Kromann-Andersen B, Steven K, Hald T. Failure of combined supratrigonal cystectomy and Mainz ileocecocystoplasty in intractable inter-

stitial cystitis: is histology and mast cell count a reliable predictor for the outcome of surgery? J Urol. 1990;144(255–258):258–9.
49. Worth P. The treatment of interstitial cystitis by cystolysis with observations on cystoplasty. A review after 7 years. Br J Urol. 1980;52:232.
50. Nurse D, Parry J, Mundy A. Problems in the surgical treatment of interstitial cystitis. Br J Urol. 1991;68:153–4.
51. MacDermott J, Charpied G, Tesluk H, Stone A. Recurrent interstitial cystitis following cystoplasty: fact or fiction? J Urol. 1990;144:37–40.
52. Herschorn S, Rangaswamy S, Radomski SB. Urinary undiversion in adults with myelodysplasia: long-term followup. J Urol. 1994;152:329–33.
53. Shahani R, Streutker C, Dickson B, Stewart RJ. Ketamine-associated ulcerative cystitis: a new clinical entity. Urology. 2007;69(5):810–2. https://doi.org/10.1016/j.urology.2007.01.038.
54. Jhang J, Hsu Y, Kuo H. Possible pathophysiology of ketamine-related cystitis and associated treatment strategies. Int J Urol. 2015;22(9):816–25. https://doi.org/10.1111/iju.12841.
55. Sihra N, Ockrim J, Wood D. The effects of recreational ketamine cystitis on urinary tract reconstruction - a surgical challenge. BJU Int. 2018;121(3):458–65. https://doi.org/10.1111/bju.14094.
56. Chung SD, Wang CC, Kuo HC. Augmentation enterocystoplasty is effective in relieving refractory ketamine-related bladder pain. Neurourol Urodyn. 2014;33(8):1207–11. https://doi.org/10.1002/nau.22477.
57. Ng CF, Chiu PKF, Li ML, et al. Clinical outcomes of augmentation cystoplasty in patients suffering from ketamine-related bladder contractures. Int Urol Nephrol. 2013;45(5):1245–51. https://doi.org/10.1007/s11255-013-0501-4.
58. Biers SM, Venn SN, Greenwell TJ. The past, present and future of augmentation cystoplasty. BJU Int. 2012;109(9):1280–93. https://doi.org/10.1111/j.1464-410X.2011.10650.x.
59. Çetinel B, Kocjancic E, Demirdağ Ç. Augmentation cystoplasty in neurogenic bladder. Investig Clin Urol. 2016;57(5):316–23. https://doi.org/10.4111/icu.2016.57.5.316.
60. Greenwell T, Venn S, Mundy A. Augmentation cystoplasty. Review. 2001;88:511–25.
61. Kilic N. Bladder augmentation: urodynamic findings and clinical outcome in different augmentation techniques. Eur J Pediatr Surg. 1999;9:29–32.
62. Ivancic V. Progression of renal insufficiency in children and adolescents with neuropathic bladder is not accelerated by lower urinary tract reconstruction. J Urol. 2010;184:1768–74.
63. Veeratterapillay R, Thorpe AC, Harding C. Augmentation cystoplasty: contemporary indications, techniques and complications. Indian J Urol. 2013;29(4):322–7. https://doi.org/10.4103/0970-1591.120114.
64. Cetinel B. Reconstructive surgery in neuropathic bladder. Adv Exp Med Biol. 2003;539(Pt A):509–33. https://doi.org/10.1007/978-1-4419-8889-8_35.
65. Matsou A. Mechanical bowel preparation before elective colorectal surgery: is it necessary? Tech Coloproctol. 2011;15(Suppl 1):59–62.
66. Wells T, Plante M, McAlpine JN. Preoperative bowel preparation in gynecologic oncology: a review of practice patterns and an impetus to change. Int J Gynecol Cancer. 2011;21:1135–42.
67. Kiran RP, Murray AC, Chiuzan C, Estrada D, Forde K. Combined preoperative mechanical bowel preparation with oral antibiotics significantly reduces surgical site infection, anastomotic leak, and ileus after colorectal surgery. Ann Surg. 2015;262(416–425):423–15.
68. Hinman FJ. Selection of intestinal segments for bladder substitution: physical and physiological characteristics. J Urol. 1988;139:519–23.
69. Radomski S, Herschorn S, Stone A. Urodynamic comparison of ileum vs. sigmoid in augmentation cystoplasty for neurogenic bladder dysfunction. Neurourol Urodyn. 1995;14:231–7.
70. Adams MC, Joseph DB. Urinary tract reconstruction in children. In: Wein A, Kavoussi LR, Novick AC, Partin AW, Peters CA, editors. Campbell-Walsh urology, vol. 4. Saunders Elsevier; 2007. p. 3656–702.
71. Shekarriz B, Upadhyay J, Demirbilek S, Barthold J, Gonzalez R. Surgical complications of bladder augmentation: comparison between various enterocystoplasties in 133 patients. Urology. 2000;55:123–8.
72. Gough DE. Enterocystoplasty. BJU Int. 2001;88:739–43.
73. Herschorn S, Locke J, Vigil H. Hemi-Kock continent stoma with augmentation Cystoplasty: modifications and outcomes. Urology. 2022;160:217–22. https://doi.org/10.1016/j.urology.2021.10.004.
74. Morales PA, Whitehead ED, editors. High jejunal conduit for supravesical urinary diversion. Report of 25 cases. Urology. 1973;1:426–31.
75. Hitchcock R, Duffy P, Malone P. Ureterocystoplasty: the "bladder" augmentation of choice. Br J Urol. 1994;73:575–9.
76. Anderson P, Dewan P. Ureterocystoplasty: an alternative reconstructive procedure to enterocystoplasty in suitable cases. J Pediatr Surg. 2001;36:962.
77. MacNeily A, Afshar K, Coleman G, Johnson H. Autoaugmentation by detrusor myotomy: its lack of effectiveness in the management of congenital neuropathic bladder. J Urol. 1646;170:1643–6.
78. Stohrer M. Bladder autoaugmentation in adult patients with neurogenic voiding dysfunction. Spinal Cord. 1997;35:456–62.
79. Skobejko-Wlodarska L, Strulak K, Nachulewicz P, Szymkiewicz C. Bladder autoaugmentation in myelodysplastic children. Br J Urol. 1998;81(Suppl 3):114–6.

80. Duel B, Gonzalez R, Barthold J. Alternative techniques for augmentation cystoplasty. J Urol. 1998;159:998–1005.
81. Cartwright P, Snow B. Bladder autoaugmentation: early clinical experience. J Urol. 1989;142:505–8.
82. Gonzalez R, Ludwikowski BM. Alternatives to conventional enterocystoplasty in children: a critical review of urodynamic outcomes. Front Pediatr. 2013;1:25.
83. Bramble F. The clam cystoplasty. Review. 1990;66:337–41.
84. Blaivas J. Long-term followup of augmentation enterocystoplasty and continent diversion in patients with benign disease. J Urol. 2005;173:1631–4.
85. Gil Vernet SG. Neurogenic bladder, neuromuscular bladder and intestinal bladder. Acta Urol Belg. 1962;30:405–20.
86. Joliat GR, Kobayashi K, Hasegawa K, et al. Guidelines for perioperative care for liver surgery: Enhanced Recovery After Surgery (ERAS) Society recommendations 2022. World J Surg. 2023;47(1):11–34. https://doi.org/10.1007/s00268-022-06732-5.
87. Nelson G, Fotopoulou C, Taylor J, et al. Enhanced recovery after surgery (ERAS®) society guidelines for gynecologic oncology: addressing implementation challenges - 2023 update. Gynecol Oncol. 2023;173:58–67. https://doi.org/10.1016/j.ygyno.2023.04.009.
88. Stenberg E, dos Reis Falcão LF, O'Kane M, et al. Guidelines for perioperative care in bariatric surgery: Enhanced Recovery After Surgery (ERAS) society recommendations: a 2021 update. World J Surg. 2022;46(4):729–51. https://doi.org/10.1007/s00268-021-06394-9.
89. McGinigle KL, Spangler EL, Pichel AC, et al. Perioperative care in open aortic vascular surgery: A consensus statement by the Enhanced Recovery After Surgery (ERAS) Society and Society for Vascular Surgery. J Vasc Surg. 2022;75(6):1796–820. https://doi.org/10.1016/j.jvs.2022.01.131.
90. Gustafsson UO, Scott MJ, Hubner M, et al. Guidelines for perioperative care in elective colorectal surgery: Enhanced Recovery After Surgery (ERAS®) society recommendations: 2018. World J Surg. 2019;43(3):659–95. https://doi.org/10.1007/s00268-018-4844-y.
91. Cerantola Y, Valerio M, Persson B, et al. Guidelines for perioperative care after radical cystectomy for bladder cancer: Enhanced Recovery After Surgery (ERAS®) society recommendations. Clin Nutr. 2013;32(6):879–87. https://doi.org/10.1016/j.clnu.2013.09.014.
92. Oodit R, Biccard BM, Panieri E, et al. Guidelines for perioperative care in elective abdominal and pelvic surgery at primary and secondary hospitals in low–middle-income countries (LMIC'S): Enhanced Recovery After Surgery (ERAS) society recommendation. World J Surg. 2022;46(8):1826–43. https://doi.org/10.1007/s00268-022-06587-w.
93. Traxel EJ, Minevich EA, Noh PH. A review: the application of minimally invasive surgery to pediatric urology: upper urinary tract procedures. Urology. 2010;76(1):122–33. https://doi.org/10.1016/j.urology.2009.11.072.
94. Noguera R. Laparoscopic augmentation enterocystoplasty through a single trocar. Urology. 2009;73:1371–4.
95. Challacombe B, Dasgupta P. Reconstruction of the lower urinary tract by laparoscopic and robotic surgery. Curr Opin Urol. 2007;17(6):390–5. https://doi.org/10.1097/MOU.0b013e3282f07488.
96. Flum AS. Completely intracorporeal robotic-assisted laparoscopic augmentation enterocystoplasty with continent catheterizable channel. Urology. 2014;84:1314–8.
97. Cohen AJ, Brodie K, Murthy P, Wilcox DT, Gundeti MS. Comparative outcomes and perioperative complications of robotic vs open cystoplasty and complex reconstructions. Urology. 2016;97:172–8. https://doi.org/10.1016/j.urology.2016.06.053.
98. Tsoi H, Elnasharty SF, Culha MG, et al. Current evidence of robotic-assisted surgery use in functional reconstructive and neuro-urology. Ther Adv Urol. 2023;15:17562872231213727. https://doi.org/10.1177/17562872231213727.
99. Wein AJ, Kavoussi LR, Partin AW, Peters CA. Campbell-Walsh urology. 11th ed. Elsevier Saunders; 2016.
100. Strine AC, Chu DI, Brockel MA, et al. Feasibility of enhanced recovery after surgery (ERAS) implementation in pediatric urology: pilot-phase outcomes of a prospective, multi-center study. J Pediatr Urol. 2024;20(2):256.e1–256.e11. https://doi.org/10.1016/j.jpurol.2023.12.017.
101. Strine AC, VanderBrink BA. Enhanced recovery after surgery (ERAS) for lower urinary tract reconstruction in children. Curr Treat Options Peds. 2022;8(3):174–91. https://doi.org/10.1007/s40746-022-00241-2.
102. Jahantabi E, Soleimanzadeh F, Salehi-Pourmehr H, Saadat MZ, Nouri M, Hajebrahimi S. An adapted enhanced recovery protocol for adult augmentation cystoplasty in limited sources countries: a pilot clinical trial. Turk J Urol. 2021;47(6):509–17. https://doi.org/10.5152/tud.2021.21108.
103. Higuchi T, Granberg C, Fox J, Husmann D. Augmentation cystoplasty and risk of neoplasia: fact, fiction and controversy. J Urol. 2010;184:2492–6.
104. Austin J. Long-term risks of bladder augmentation in pediatric patients. Curr Opin Urol. 2008;18:408–12.
105. Herschorn S, Hewitt R. Patient perspective of long-term outcome of augmentation cystoplasty for neurogenic bladder. Urology. 1998;52:672–8.
106. Metcalfe PD, Rink RC. Bladder augmentation: complications in the pediatric population. Curr Urol Rep. 2007;8:152–6.
107. Kispal Z, Balogh D, Erdei O, et al. Complications after bladder augmentation or substitution in chil-

dren: a prospective study of 86 patients. BJU Int. 2011;108(2):282–9.
108. Chang JW, Kuo FC, Lin TC, et al. Long-term complications and outcomes of augmentation cystoplasty in children with neurogenic bladder. Sci Rep. 2024;14(1):4214. https://doi.org/10.1038/s41598-024-54431-z.
109. Fontaine E. Combined modified rectus fascial sling and augmentation ileocystoplasty for neurogenic incontinence in women. J Urol. 1997;157:109–12.
110. Cheng C, Hendry W, Kirby R, Whitfield H. Detubularisation in cystoplasty: clinical review. Br J Urol. 1991;67:303–7.
111. Sethia KK, Webb RJ, Neal DE. Urodynamic study of ileocystoplasty in the treatment of idiopathic detrusor instability. Br J Urol. 1991;67:286–90.
112. Kockelbergh R. Clam enterocystoplasty in general urological practice. Br J Urol. 1991;68:38–41.
113. George V, Russell G, Shutt A, Gaches C, Ashken M. Clam ileocystoplasty. Br J Urol. 1991;68:487–9.
114. Gonzalez R, Sidi A, Zhang G. Urinary undiversion: indications, technique and results in 50 cases. J Urol. 1986;136:13–6.
115. Gearhart J, Albertsen P, Marshall F, Jeffs R. Pediatric applications of augmentation cystoplasty: the Johns Hopkins experience. J Urol. 1986;136:430–2.
116. Mitchell M, Kulb T, Backes D. Intestinocystoplasty in combination with clean intermittent catheterization in the management of vesical dysfunction. J Urol. 1986;136:288–91.
117. Flood H. Long-term results and complications using augmentation cystoplasty in reconstructive urology. Neurourol Urodyn. 1995;14:297–309.
118. Quek M, Ginsberg D. Long-term urodynamics followup of bladder augmentation for neurogenic bladder. J Urol. 2003;169:195–8.
119. Lopez Pereira P. Enterocystoplasty in children with neuropathic bladders: long-term follow-up. J Pediatr Urol. 2008;4:27–31.
120. Kreder K, Webster G. Management of the bladder outlet in patients requiring enterocystoplasty. J Urol. 1992;147:38–41.
121. Khoury J, Timmons S, Corbel L, Webster G. Complications of enterocystoplasty. Urology. 1992;40:9–14.
122. Lockhart J, Bejany D, Politano V. Augmentation cystoplasty in the management of neurogenic bladder disease and urinary incontinence. J Urol. 1986;135:969–71.
123. Goldwasser B, Barrett DM, Webster GD, Kramer SA. Cystometric properties of ileum and right colon after bladder augmentation, substitution or replacement. J Urol. 1987;138:1007–8.
124. Mundy A, Nurse D. Calcium balance, growth and skeletal mineralisation in patients with cystoplasties. Br J Urol. 1992;69:257–9.
125. Wagstaff K, Woodhouse C, Duffy P, Ransley P. Delayed linear growth in children with enterocystoplasties. Br J Urol. 1992;69:314–7.
126. Taskinen S, Makitie O, Fagerholm R. Intestinal bladder augmentation at school age has no adverse effects on growth. J Pediatr Urol. 2008;4:40–2.
127. Mingin G, Maroni P, Gerharz E, Woodhouse C, Baskin L. Linear growth after enterocystoplasty in children and adolescents: a review. World J Urol. 2004;22:196–9.
128. Hafez A. Long-term evaluation of metabolic profile and bone mineral density after ileocystoplasty in children. J Urol. 2003;170(1639–1641):1641–32.
129. Vajda P. Metabolic findings after colocystoplasty in children. Urology. 2003;62(542–546):546.
130. Abes M, Sarihan H, Madenci E. Evaluation of bone mineral density with dual x-ray absorptiometry for osteoporosis in children with bladder augmentation. J Pediatr Surg. 2003;38:230–2.
131. McDougal W. Metabolic complications of urinary intestinal diversion. J Urol. 1992;147:1199–208.
132. Haas RE. Lower extremity bone mineral density in children with congenital spinal dysfunction. Dev Med Child Neurol. 2012;54:1133–7.
133. Hensle TW, Reiley EA, Fam MM, Carpenter CP. Enterocystoplasty: the long-term effects on bone mineral density. J Pediatr Urol. 2016;12(4):245.e1–6. https://doi.org/10.1016/j.jpurol.2016.02.017.
134. Koch M, McDougal W, Reddy P, Lange P. Metabolic alterations following continent urinary diversion through colonic segments. J Urol. 1991;145:270–3.
135. Stein R, Schroder A, Thuroff J. Bladder augmentation and urinary diversion in patients with neurogenic bladder: non-surgical considerations.
136. Tanrikut C, McDougal W. Acid-base and electrolyte disorders after urinary diversion. World J Urol. 2004;22:168–71.
137. Gilbert S, Hensle T. Metabolic consequences and long-term complications of enterocystoplasty in children: a review. J Urol. 2005;173:1080–6.
138. Mitchell M, Piser J. Intestinocystoplasty and total bladder replacement in children and young adults: followup in 129 cases. J Urol. 1987;138:579–84.
139. Poulsen A, Steven K. Acid-base metabolism after bladder substitution with the ileal urethral Kock reservoir. Br J Urol. 1996;78:47–53.
140. Hall M, Koch M, Halter S, Dahlstedt S. Morphologic and functional alterations of intestinal segments following urinary diversion. J Urol. 1993;149:664–6.
141. Akerlund S, Forssell-Aronsson E, Jonsson O, Kock N. Decreased absorption of 22Na and 36Cl in ileal reservoirs after exposure to urine. An experimental study in patients with continent ileal reservoirs for urinary or fecal diversion. Urol Res. 1991;19:249–52.
142. Plawker M, Rabinowitz S, Etwaru D, Glassberg K. Hypergastrinemia, dysuria-hematuria and metabolic alkalosis: complications associated with gastrocystoplasty. J Urol. 1995;154:546–9.
143. Kurzrock E, Baskin L, Kogan B. Gastrocystoplasty: long-term followup. J Urol. 1998;160:2182–6.
144. Jonsson O, Olofsson G, Lindholm E, Tornqvist H. Long-time experience with the Kock ileal res-

ervoir for continent urinary diversion. Eur Urol. 2001;40:632–40.
145. Fontaine E, Leaver R, Woodhouse C. The effect of intestinal urinary reservoirs on renal function: a 10-year follow-up. BJU Int. 2000;86:195–8.
146. Whitmore WF 3rd, Gittes RF. Reconstruction of the urinary tract by cecal and ileocecal cystoplasty: review of a 15-year experience. J Urol. 1983;129:494–8.
147. Decter R, Bauer S, Mandell J, Colodny A, Retik A. Small bowel augmentation in children with neurogenic bladder: an initial report of urodynamic findings. J Urol. 1987;138:1014–6.
148. Kuss R, Bitker M, Camey M, Chatelain C, Lassau J. Indications and early and late results of intestino-cystoplasty: a review of 185 cases. J Urol. 1970;103:53–63.
149. Husmann DA. Long-term complications following bladder augmentations in patients with spina bifida: bladder calculi, perforation of the augmented bladder and upper tract deterioration. Transl Androl Urol. 2016;5(1):3–11. https://doi.org/10.3978/j.issn.2223-4683.2015.12.06.
150. Sutojo B, Irdam GA. Safety of augmentation cystoplasty in patients with bladder abnormalities undergoing renal transplantation: a systematic review. Med J Indonesia. 2021;30(3):198–206. https://doi.org/10.13181/mji.oa.204358.
151. Chertin B, Koucherov S, Shenfeld OZ. Augmentation cystoplasty. In: Puri P, editor. Pediatric surgery. Berlin Heidelberg: Springer; 2023. p. 507–24. https://doi.org/10.1007/978-3-662-43567-0_196.
152. Marchal S, Kalfa N, Iborra F, et al. Long-term outcome of renal transplantation in patients with congenital lower urinary tract malformations: a multicenter study. Transplantation. 2020;104(1):165. https://doi.org/10.1097/TP.0000000000002746.
153. Matsui U, Topoll B, Miller K, Hautmann R. Metabolic long-term follow-up of the ileal neobladder. Eur Urol. 1993;24:197–200.
154. Pannek J, Haupt G, Schulze H, Senge T. Influence of continent ileal urinary diversion on vitamin B12 absorption. J Urol. 1996;155:1206–8.
155. Shaw J, Lewis MA. Bladder augmentation surgery–what about the malignant risk? Eur J Pediatr Surg. 1999;9(Suppl 1):39–40.
156. Carr LK, Herschorn S. Early development of adenocarcinoma in a young woman following augmentation cystoplasty for undiversion. J Urol. 1997;157:2255–6.
157. Husmann DA. Mortality following augmentation cystoplasty: a transitional urologist's viewpoint. J Pediatr Urol. 2017;13(4):358–64. https://doi.org/10.1016/j.jpurol.2017.05.008.
158. Soergel TM, Cain MP, Misseri R, Gardner TA, Koch MO, Rink RC. Transitional cell carcinoma of the bladder following augmentation cystoplasty for the neuropathic bladder. J Urol. Published online October 2004. https://doi.org/10.1097/01.ju.0000140194.87974.56.
159. Kalisvaart J, Katsumi H, Ronningen L, Hovey R. Bladder cancer in spinal cord injury patients. Spinal Cord. 2010;48:257–61.
160. Barrington J, Jones A, James D, Smith S, Stephenson T. Antioxidant deficiency following clam enterocystoplasty. Br J Urol. 1997;80:238–42.
161. Dixon B, Chu A, Henry J, Kim R, Bissler J. Increased cancer risk of augmentation cystoplasty: possible role for hyperosmolal microenvironment on DNA damage recognition. Mutat Res. 2009;670:88–95.
162. Castellan M, Gosalbez R, Bar-Yosef Y, Labbie A. Complications after use of gastric segments for lower urinary tract reconstruction. J Urol. Published online May 2012. https://doi.org/10.1016/j.juro.2011.12.105.
163. Plaire JC, Snodgrass WT, Grady RW, Mitchell ME. Long-term followup of the hematuria-dysuria syndrome. J Urol. Published online September 2000. https://doi.org/10.1016/S0022-5347(05)67218-7.
164. Couillard D, Vapnek J, Rentzepis M, Stone A. Fatal perforation of augmentation cystoplasty in an adult. Urology. 1993;42:585–8.
165. Braverman R, Lebowitz R. Perforation of the augmented urinary bladder in nine children and adolescents: importance of cystography. AJR. 1991;157:1059–63.
166. Fontaine E, Leaver R, Woodhouse C. Diagnosis of perforated enterocystoplasty. J R Soc Med. 2003;96:393–4.
167. DeFoor W, Tackett L, Minevich E, Wacksman J, Sheldon C. Risk factors for spontaneous bladder perforation after augmentation cystoplasty. Urology. 2003;62:737–41.
168. Bauer S. Perforation of the augmented bladder. J Urol. 1992;148:699–703.
169. Taghavi K, O'Hagan LA, Bortagaray J, Bouty A, Hutson M, J, O'Brien M. Complication profile of augmentation cystoplasty in contemporary paediatric urology: a 20-year review. ANZ J Surg. 2021;91(5):1005–10. https://doi.org/10.1111/ans.16736.
170. Novak T, Salmasi A, Mathews R, Lakshmanan Y, Gearhart J. Complications of complex lower urinary tract reconstruction in patients with neurogenic versus nonneurogenic bladder–is there a difference? J Urol. 2008;180:2629–34.
171. Fox J, Husmann D. Continent urinary diversion in childhood: complications of alcohol abuse developing in adulthood. J Urol. 2010;183:2342–6.
172. Kurzrock E. Pediatric enterocystoplasty: long-term complications and controversies. World J Urol. 2009;27:69–73.
173. Malone T, Lisle D, McNabb C, Ryan G. Traumatic rupture of an augmented bladder: computed tomography appearances. J Trauma-Injury Infect Crit Care. 2009;67:85–7.
174. Glass R, Rushton H. Delayed spontaneous rupture of augmented bladder in children: diagnosis with sonography and CT. AJR. 1992;158:833–5.

175. Slaton J, Kropp K. Conservative management of suspected bladder rupture after augmentation enterocystoplasty. J Urol. 1994;152:713–5.
176. Wolff J, Boeckmann W, Jakse G. Spontaneous bladder rupture following enterocystoplasty can be treated conservatively. Urol Int. 1994;52:113–4.
177. Rushton H, Woodard J, Parrott T, Jeffs R, Gearhart J. Delayed bladder rupture after augmentation enterocystoplasty. J Urol. 1988;140:344–6.
178. Elder J, Snyder H, Hulbert W, Duckett J. Perforation of the augmented bladder in patients undergoing clean intermittent catheterization. J Urol. 1988;140:1159–62.
179. Rink R. Bladder augmentation. Options, outcomes, future. Urol Clin N Am. 1999;26:111–23.
180. Kronner K. Bladder calculi in the pediatric augmented bladder. J Urol. 1998;160:1096–8.
181. Nurse D, McInerney P, Thomas P, Mundy A. Stones in enterocystoplasties. Br J Urol. 1996;77:684–7.
182. Metcalfe P. What is the need for additional bladder surgery after bladder augmentation in childhood? J Urol. 2006;176:1801–5.
183. Palmer L. Urolithiasis in children following augmentation cystoplasty. J Urol. 1993;150:726–9.
184. Barroso U, Jednak R, Fleming P, Barthold J, Gonzalez R. Bladder calculi in children who perform clean intermittent catheterization. BJU Int. 2000;85:879–84.
185. DeFoor W. Bladder calculi after augmentation cystoplasty: risk factors and prevention strategies. J Urol. 2004;172:1964–6.
186. Khoury A. Stone formation after augmentation cystoplasty: the role of intestinal mucus. J Urol. 1997;158:1133–7.
187. Hamid R, Robertson W, Woodhouse C. Comparison of biochemistry and diet in patients with enterocystoplasty who do and do not form stones. BJU Int. 2008;101:1427–32.
188. Woodhouse C, Robertson W. Urolithiasis in enterocystoplasties. World J Urol. 2004;22:215–21.
189. Robertson W, Woodhouse C. Metabolic factors in the causation of urinary tract stones in patients with enterocystoplasties. Urol Res. 2006;34:231–8.
190. Hensle T, Bingham J, Lam J, Shabsigh A. Preventing reservoir calculi after augmentation cystoplasty and continent urinary diversion: the influence of an irrigation protocol. BJU Int. 2004;93:585–7.
191. Brough R, O'Flynn K, Fishwick J, Gough D. Bladder washout and stone formation in paediatric enterocystoplasty. Eur Urol. 1998;33:500–2.
192. Murray K, Nurse D, Mundy A. Secreto-motor function of intestinal segments used in lower urinary tract reconstruction. Br J Urol. 1987;60:532–5.
193. Iannoni C. Abnormal patterns of colorectal mucin secretion after urinary diversion of different types: histochemical and lectin binding studies. Hum Pathol. 1986;17:834–40.
194. Gillon G, Mundy A. The dissolution of urinary mucus after cystoplasty. Br J Urol. 1989;63:372–4.
195. George V. The effect of ranitidine on urine mucus concentration in patients with enterocystoplasty. Br J Urol. 1992;70:30–2.
196. Akerlund S, Campanello M, Kaijser B, Jonsson O. Bacteriuria in patients with a continent ileal reservoir for urinary diversion does not regularly require antibiotic treatment. Br J Urol. 1994;74:177–81.
197. Bruce A, Reid G, Chan R, Costerton J. Bacterial adherence in the human ileal conduit: a morphological and bacteriological study. J Urol. 1984;132:184–8.
198. Greenwell T, Woodhams S, Smalley T, Mundy A. Effect of antibiotics on enterocystoplasty urinary nitrosamine levels. Urology. 2001;58:660–4.
199. Wagstaff K, Woodhouse C, Rose G, Duffy P, Ransley P. Blood and urine analysis in patients with intestinal bladders. Br J Urol. 1991;68:311–6.
200. Nieuwkoop C, Exter P, Elzevier H, Hartigh J, Dissel J. Intravesical gentamicin for recurrent urinary tract infection in patients with intermittent bladder catheterisation. Int J Antimicrob Agents. 2010;36:485–90.
201. Botto H, Neuzillet Y. Effectiveness of a cranberry (Vaccinium macrocarpon) preparation in reducing asymptomatic bacteriuria in patients with an ileal enterocystoplasty. Scand J Urol Nephrol. 2010;44:165–8.
202. Singh G, Thomas D. Bowel problems after enterocystoplasty. Br J Urol. 1997;79:328–32.
203. N'Dow J, Leung H, Marshall C, Neal D. Bowel dysfunction after bladder reconstruction. J Urol. 1998;159:1470–1474, 1474–1475.
204. Jacobsen O. Effect of enterocoated cholestyramine on bowel habit after ileal resection: a double blind crossover study. Br Med J (Clin Res Ed). 1985;290:1315–8.
205. Hofmann AF, Poley JR. Role of bile acid malabsorption in pathogenesis of diarrhea and steatorrhea in patients with ileal resection. I. Response to cholestyramine or replacement of dietary long chain triglyceride by medium chain triglyceride. Gastroenterology. 1972;62:918–34.
206. Fromm H, Malavolti M. Bile acid-induced diarrhoea. Clin Gastroenterol. 1986;15:567–82.
207. Pattni S, Walters J. Recent advances in the understanding of bile acid malabsorption. Br Med Bull. 2009;92:79–93.
208. Strawbridge L, Kramer S, Castillo O, Barrett D. Augmentation cystoplasty and the artificial genitourinary sphincter. J Urol. 1989;142:297–301.
209. Athawale HR, Mane SB, Vagheriya N, More P, Daginawala T. Ten years' experience of augmentation cystoplasty for varied indications and its outcome. Int Surg J. 2020;7(4):1031–5. https://doi.org/10.18203/2349-2902.isj20200999.
210. Robertson A, Davies J, Webb R, Neal D. Bladder augmentation and replacement. Urodynamic and clinical review of 25 patients. Br J Urol. 1991;68:590–7.

211. McInerney PD, DeSouza N, Thomas PJ, Mundy AR. The role of urodynamic studies in the evaluation of patients with augmentation cystoplasties. Br J Urol. 1995;76:475–8.
212. Lopez Pereira P, Somoza Ariba I, Martinez Urrutia M, Lobato Romero R, Jaureguizar Monroe E. Artificial urinary sphincter: 11-year experience in adolescents with congenital neuropathic bladder. Eur Urol. 2006;50:1096–101.
213. Hill D, Kramer S. Management of pregnancy after augmentation cystoplasty. J Urol. 1990;144:457–9.
214. Creagh TA, McInerney PD, Thomas PJ, Mundy AR. Pregnancy after lower urinary tract reconstruction in women. J Urol. Published online October 1995. https://doi.org/10.1016/S0022-5347(01)66848-4.
215. Ruan J, Zhang L, Duan MF, Luo DY. Pregnancy and delivery after augmentation cystoplasty: a case report and review of literature. World J Clin Cases. 2022;10(13):4177–84. https://doi.org/10.12998/wjcc.v10.i13.4177.
216. Niknejad K, Atala A. Bladder augmentation techniques in women. Int Urogynecol J Pelvic Floor Dysfunct. 2000;11:156–69.
217. Fenn N, Barrington J, Stephenson T. Clam enterocystoplasty and pregnancy. Br J Urol. 1995;75:85–6.
218. Kearse WJ, Clair S, Hixson C, Ritchey M. Functional characteristics of enterocystoplasty after interruption of the mesenteric blood supply. J Urol. 1993;150:593–6.

Anal Sphincteroplasty

26

Rachel Kopkin, Lauren Wilson,
and Brooke Gurland

Introduction

Direct sphincter trauma or neuropathic injuries from vaginal deliveries are the principal causative factors in the development of fecal incontinence in women less than 40 years old [1]. In patients of any age, reasons for fecal incontinence in addition to obstetrical injuries include conditions that predispose the patient to diarrhea, neurologic conditions, chronic medical conditions such as diabetes, obesity, and COPD, iatrogenic injuries from anorectal operations, trauma, and anatomic conditions including rectal prolapse and congenital abnormalities [2]. In many cases, there may be an occult sphincter or pelvic floor defect from an obstetrical injury that becomes clinically relevant when present in combination with other conditions [1].

Treatment options for the incontinent patient include non-operative interventions such as medications to improve stool consistency and biofeedback as well as vaginal bowel control systems (Eclipse system), procedures including injection of bulking (Solesta) agents and controlled delivery of radio frequency energy (Secca). Operative interventions including anal sphincteroplasty, sacral nerve modulation (SNM), artificial bowel sphincter, posterior anal repair, dynamic graciloplasty, transobturator posterior anal sling (TOPAS) procedure, Fenix™ magnetic sphincter augmentation, or colostomy. THD Gatekeeper involving injection of self-absorbing material equipped with a shape memory has also been reported. Albeit, few of these therapies are currently available in the United States [3, 4]. Currently, a clinical trial involving Iltamiocel is underway, assessing the impact of stem cell injections into injured sphincter muscles [5].

Historically, anal sphincteroplasty has been the preferred surgical treatment for the symptomatic patient with an anatomically disrupted external anal sphincter (EAS) muscle. Short-term results report improved bowel continence as high as 90% [6] with decreasing continence (0–73%) in long-term follow-up studies [7–11]. Recent studies evaluating suture choice and augmentation with synthetic materials explore ways to improve the longevity of the repair [12, 13].

Over the past 20 years, SNM has been utilized as a treatment modality with good results for patients with fecal incontinence with or without an anal sphincter defect, but requires an

R. Kopkin
Department of Urology and Gynecology, Stanford University, Stanford, CA, USA
e-mail: rkopkin@stanford.edu

L. Wilson
Department of General Surgery, Dartmouth Hitchcock Medical Center, Lebanon, NH, USA
e-mail: Lauren.R.Wilson@hitchcock.org

B. Gurland (✉)
Department of Surgery, Stanford Pelvic Health Center, Stanford, CA, USA
e-mail: bgurland@stanford.edu

H. B. Goldman, J. Zillioux (eds.), *Complications of Urogynecology and Reconstructive Pelvic Surgery*, https://doi.org/10.1007/978-3-032-00339-3_26

implantable device usually placed over two separate procedures and the potential for future procedures for device maintenance. In the pivotal US multicenter trial including 133 patients undergoing SNM procedures for FI in 2010, 90% had a successful test stimulation and proceeded to the permanent implantation. At 12 months, 83% of the patients achieved therapeutic success, and 41% had complete continence. Incontinence episodes decreased from 9.4 episodes per week at baseline to 1.9 at 12 months, and 2.9 at 24 months [14] In a sample of patients from this trial, FI episodes per week remained low (1.7) at 5 years, with 89% of the subjects having greater than or equal to 50% symptomatic improvement and 36% achieving complete continence [15]. Sustained clinical benefit of up to 14 years has been demonstrated in more than 80% of SNM subjects [16]. Common device related adverse events including implant side pain (28%) and paresthesia (15%). Infection and explanation rates are relatively low (3–11% and 3–4%, respectively).

The artificial bowel sphincter, a silastic band surgically placed around the lower rectum, has been shown to improve bowel control but with high complication rates. Infection rates are reported up to 34% in multicenter studies with device erosion and malfunction being other common complications. Approximately 50% of patients undergoing reconstruction with an artificial bowel sphincter will require explantation of the device due to infection or erosion, but those who do have successful implantation, have good results with respect to control of continence [17, 18]. At the present time, the artificial bowel sphincter is not being manufactured for implantation in the USA.

Posterior anal repair is described for neuropathic incontinence. Studies on postanal repair have variable results with some studies showing improvement in up to 68% of patients [19]. Mackey et al., however, reported that only 26% of patients have minimal incontinence with 74% of patients having moderate to severe incontinence. Of note, in this study, quality of life and satisfaction scores were high despite high rates of incontinence [20].

Dynamic graciloplasty is a complex procedure that involves gracilious muscle transposition and stimulation with an implantable stimulator. This requires expertise, it is associated with a high morbidity [21], and it is expensive [22, 23]. This procedure is not an option in the United States since the stimulator used for muscle contraction is not commercially available.

The transobturator posterior anal sling (TOPAS) procedure shows good results with respect to continence and safety [24]. Mellgren et al. in a multicenter trial demonstrated that at one year almost 70% of patients had more than a 50% decrease in incontinent episodes per week and 19% were completely continent. Side effects were mainly pain, though 15% had infections. There were no organ perforations, extrusions, or erosions [25]. While this study demonstrates success and the device is FDA approved, at the present time the device is not being manufactured. Mesh litigation has made companies hesitant to provide mesh devices for implantation in the pelvis.

Magnetic sphincter augmentation, FENIX™ is currently being evaluated and has shown promising early results for improving continence with a low complication profile [26, 27]. However, a new RCT of FENIX™ versus SNM showed success of each arm was much lower than previously reported (12.5% vs 14.6%) with 30% of patients in the FENIX™ group having their device explanted due to complications. This study was terminated early, only recruiting approximately one third of the targeted sample size. Further studies are needed to evalute the efficacy and safety of the FENIX™ device [28].

The Gatekeeper anal implant prostheses has shown promising results for patients with fecal incontinence and internal sphincter defects of less than 60 degrees. A study of 54 patients demonstrated 56% of patients had at least a 75% improvement in symptoms with 13% reporting full continence at 1 year follow up [3]. In another study of 49 patients with sphincter injuries less than 120 degrees, 52% of patients reported greater than 50% improvement in symptoms based on Vaizey score at 1 year follow up [4].

Unlike many of the alternatives mentioned, anal sphincteroplasty does not require expensive devices or postoperative maintenance necessary with implantable devices and remains an important treatment modality to treat patients with fecal incontinence with a disrupted anal sphincter who do not want an implantable device or who live in communities in which postoperative maintenance is not available. Furthermore, anal sphincteroplasty plays an important role in the management of other anorectal pathology, specifically rectovaginal fistula. Sphincteroplasty can also be performed in conjunction with other pelvic organ prolapse and urinary incontinence procedures without additional morbidity and potentially some improvement in continence [29]. The complications associated with anal sphincteroplasty are minor and include wound complications, UTI, chronic pain or discomfort, and recurrence of fecal incontinence. Major complications are rare. This chapter will address the prevention of complications and further management should a complication occur.

Patient Evaluation

Preventing failure of the procedure and occurrence of complications begins with appropriate patient selection and improving modifiable conditions. A comprehensive history and physical exam is imperative to appropriate patient selection. The following considerations are important when evaluating a patient with fecal incontinence for sphincteroplasty:

1. *Bowel habits*: Loose or watery stools may result in fecal incontinence. Bulking agents such as fiber and antidiarrheals to thicken and decrease the frequency of bowel movements remain first-line therapies and must be used in conjunction with operative interventions. Sphincteroplasty will not be effective in patients with loose and irregular stools. Markland et al. compared psyllium to loperamide for treatment of fecal incontinence. Both medications were effective for improving fecal incontinence and quality of life, but loperamide had more side effects, specifically constipation [30].
2. *Age of the patient*: Aging tissues are less likely to recover and maintain good quality over time. Several retrospective analyses suggest that older women have anorectal function that deteriorates over time [9, 31]. Advancing age may be associated with other pelvic floor defects, including increased fibrosis and collagen deposition [32]. Several studies suggest poor continence outcomes in older patients [8, 9, 33, 34], while other studies have found that age does not affect outcomes [6, 35, 36]. Each case should individually take into consideration factors such as tissue quality and anal muscle contractility rather than biologic age alone.
3. *Obesity and other medical conditions*: A high body mass index has been associated with poorer outcomes after sphincteroplasty [31, 37]. Obese women may have other factors that can contribute to the incontinence such as excessive pelvic floor descent and diabetes. Control of diabetes and minimizing immunosuppression will decrease infectious and local wound healing complications.
4. *Severity of symptoms*: Patients should be counseled preoperatively regarding realistic postsurgical expectations. Nikiteas et al. found that patients with severe symptoms undergoing primary repair reported the best outcomes [31]. Measures of success in studies of sphincter repair are not standardized but include some measure of gas and stool incontinence as well as patient quality of life and satisfaction scores. In contrast, most studies of sacral nerve stimulation use a more standardized measure of success of the procedure if there is an improvement of more than 50% in occurrence of incontinent episodes per week [15]. It is rare for a previously incontinent patient to experience complete continence following sphincteroplasty or any other continence procedure i.e. some degree of gas and stool incontinence should be expected. Importantly, many women consider their operation a success while reporting high rates of fecal incontinence [8].

5. *Local physical findings*: Lax anal sphincter muscles or a patulous anus may be associated with mucosal or full-thickness rectal prolapse. Decreased or no anal sphincter contractility noted on physical examination is a poor prognostic sign for sphincter repair as it represents a poorly functioning anal sphincter. Patients should be asked about symptoms of other pelvic organ problems, including urinary incontinence and pelvic organ prolapse. Physical exam should also include a vaginal exam in the female patient, assessing for pelvic organ prolapse. This can be performed by the colorectal surgeon or in conjunction with a gynecologist or urologist if co-management of multiple problems is anticipated based on history.
6. *Anal physiologic testing* includes endoanal ultrasound and anal manometry. Low-squeeze pressure on anal manometry in conjunction with an anterior sphincter defect on endoanal ultrasound is the primary indication for sphincteroplasty. Other sonographic findings may include a variegated appearance of the EAS-indicating atrophic muscles, a very thin internal anal sphincter (IAS), and a size estimate of the defect of the EAS muscle. Pudendal nerve terminal latencies (PNTML) have also been used to evaluate the neurologic function of the anal sphincters, but the significance of prolonged PNTML is debated. Gilliand et al. in the largest series evaluating the role of PNTML, found that bilateral normal PNTMLs were the only factor predictive of long-term success of anterior overlapping sphincteroplasty [38]. MRI or Fluoroscopic defecography can be used to confirm high-grade internal rectal prolapse, which can result in mucus discharge and fecal leakage. Prolapse prevents the sphincter from completely closing and results in sphincter stretch and long-term sphincter dysfunction.

Preoperative Management

In addition to appropriate patient selection, setting realistic postoperative continence expectations, and optimizing stool consistency and other comorbid conditions, preoperative management includes mechanical bowel preparation and administration of a single dose of intravenous antibiotics administered prior to the surgery. Some groups advocate using a full bowel prep, while others use enemas in the preop area.

Fecal diversion prior to sphincteroplasty has not been shown to improve outcomes and is not recommended. Hasegawa et al. [39] demonstrated equivalent sphincter-related outcomes between groups randomized to sphincteroplasty with or without diverting stoma. Patients in the stoma group suffered stoma-related complications.

Operative Management

Operative Technique and Results

Depending on surgeon preference, sphincter repair can be performed in lithotomy or prone position. After the perineum is prepped and draped, an anterior 120° curvilinear incision is made along the perineum to allow dissection and mobilization of the sphincter muscle and scar. It is important to preserve all scar tissue in order to anchor the sutures.

A number of techniques have been described for sphincteroplasty, and the choice is operator-dependent. Repair techniques include end-to-end apposition versus overlapping repair, choice of suture material, and augmentation of the repair with a biologic material. The data to support these options is limited but it can affect the complication profile and thus should be considered by the surgeon prior to repair.

Primary repair of obstetric anal sphincter trauma is typically carried out by gynecologists around the time of delivery. Several randomized studies of end-to-end versus overlapping sphincter repairs have shown conflicting results, with studies showing no difference, better outcomes with overlapping repair, and better outcomes with end-to-end repair [40]. Secondary repairs are carried out months to years after the injury and are most frequently performed by colorectal surgeons, though occasionally by urogynecologists in a national practice survey, it was found that 89% of colorectal surgeons perform an overlapping technique versus only 50% of obstetricians [41].

Both end-to-end repair and overlapping sphincteroplasty for secondary repairs have been described in the literature, though the majority of large series employ the overlapping technique. In a randomized controlled trial comparing these two techniques for secondary sphincter repairs for incontinence, Tjandra et al. [42] studied 23 patients with fecal incontinence caused by obstetric injuries, 12 underwent direct repair and 11 overlapping sphincter repair. At a median follow-up of 18 months, the functional results were significantly improved in both groups, irrespective of the technique, with improvement in continence in 75% and 73%, respectively. A RCT by Farrell et al. of 174 patients comparing the two techniques showed that end-to-end repair was associated with significantly lower rates of anal incontinence at 12 months (flatal incontinence 31% vs 56%; fecal incontinence 7% vs 16%); however, this difference was not sustained over 3 years [40].

End-to-end repair is performed by isolating the IAS from EAS and repairing these separately. Overlapping sphincteroplasty can be performed *en bloc,* thus avoiding separating the internal and external sphincters, though many series describe isolating the internal and external sphincters with repair of the internal sphincter and overlap of the external sphincter, as well as anterior levatorplasty [33, 43]. Mattress sutures are used to approximate the sphincter (Figs. 26.1, 26.2, and 26.3). While some studies have reported improved outcomes with independent suturing of the IAS [44, 45], others have shown that separate dissection does not provide improved function postoperatively [14, 46].

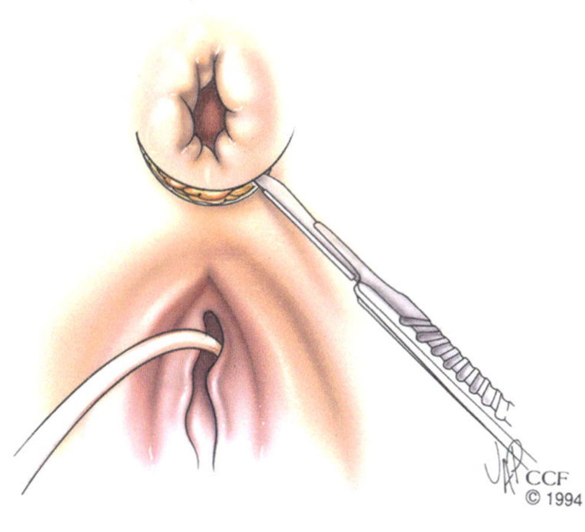

Fig. 26.1 A transverse incision along the perineum. Note the patient is positioned in the prone position with the anus superior and vagina inferior

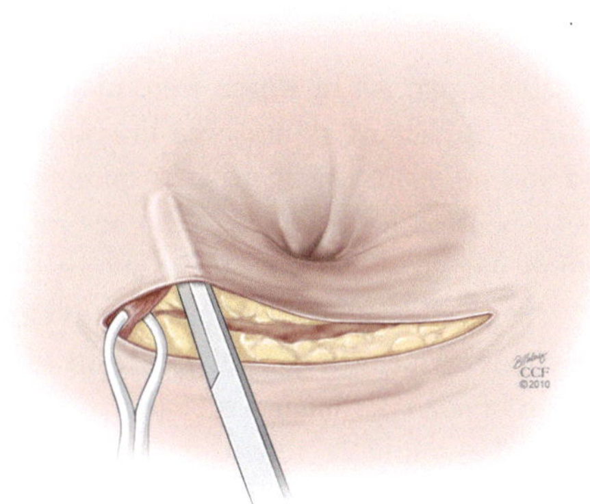

Fig. 26.2 The external sphincter is identified and grasped with the Allis clamp

There is a paucity of information on the choice of suture material. Parnell et al. [13] investigated the use of permanent versus absorbable sutures in overlapping anal sphincteroplasty specifically related to loss of solid stool and severity of incontinence symptoms. Four surgeons performed the overlapping technique with no separation of the IAS and EAS. Each surgeon used their preferred suture material. Permanent suture types included Gore-Tex, Nurulon, and Ethibond, while absorbable sutures were Vicryl and PDS. 40 patients were included in the study, with 20 in the permanent suture group and 20 in the absorbable group. The primary endpoint was loss of solid stool greater than 1–3 times per month. The groups had similar rates of overall incontinence to solid stool, but the use of permanent suture was associated with decreased severity of fecal incontinence and fewer social limitations. Complications of wound separation and wound infection occurred equally in both groups. 3 suture erosions occurred in the permanent suture group and one in the

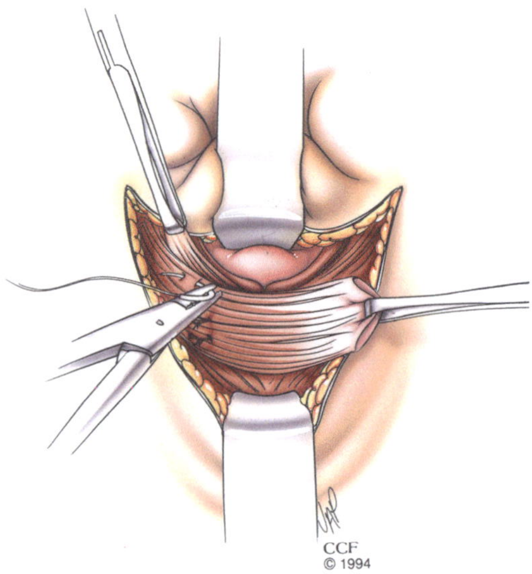

Fig. 26.3 The external sphincter is overlapped and sutured into place

absorbable group, all of which were managed in the clinic. Studies of suture type in sphincteroplasty and posterior repair or sacrospinous ligament suspension have indicated higher rates of infection with braided permanent sutures. This study suggests that permanent monofilament sutures may reduce the risk of infection associated with braided permanent sutures.

Once the sphincter repair is complete, the edges of the wound are approximated in a V shape or longitudinally with interrupted 3.0 Vicryl mattress sutures. The center of the wound can be left open, a small drain inserted, or the wound can be closed [37, 47].

Postoperative Management

Postoperative management requires keeping the stools soft, the area clean, and pain tolerable. In these author's practice, patients are usually kept overnight and discharged the following morning. With episioproctotomies, patients are kept overnight on bed rest with a clear diet and a foley until they have a bowel movement, at which time they are advanced to a regular diet and discharged home. There is no consensus on the routine administration of postoperative oral antibiotics at discharge. The patient is discharged on stool softeners with the goal of keeping the stool soft to avoid straining. The patient should be counseled to avoid liquid stools.

Warm soaks in a bathtub or sitz bath for 5–10 min help with pain relief by promoting relaxation of the pelvic floor muscles. Other surgeons instruct patients to avoid submerging the incision but rather directing a handheld shower or peri-bottle at the wound to facilitate hygiene and gently debride the perineum. Non-steroidal medications are encouraged over narcotics for pain relief to avoid the constipating side effects associated with narcotics.

Postoperative Complications

Complications that can occur in the early postoperative period include hematoma or seroma formation. These can be treated by opening the wound and evacuating the contents. Antibiotics with gram-positive, gram-negative, and anaerobic coverage are selectively prescribed in the setting of wound cellulitis.

Late complications include abscess formation, fistulas, and wound dehiscence. Abscesses and fistulas may require additional operative interventions, including debridement and, in rare cases, a stoma, while wound breakdown usually heals secondarily and rarely requires secondary suturing. In addition to prolonged healing and additional procedures for drainage, poor continence outcomes are more common in those patients with deep wound infections with an OR of 7.93 [33].

It is possible that wound infection may also adversely affect sexual function. Persistent dyspareunia is a possible longer-term complication. This has been reported to be up to six times more likely in those undergoing overlapping sphincteroplasty versus end-to-end anastomosis [48]; however, this could be confounded by higher rates of wound cellulitis in the former group. This finding was not reproduced in a subsequent study [49].

The patient's main complaint after surgery is pain from the perineal wound. Table 26.1 reports

Table 26.1 Complications and long-term outcomes after sphincteroplasty

References	*N*	Age at time of surgery, mean (ranges)	FU, mean (ranges)	Repair	Complications	Outcomes, good/ excellent *N* (%)
Huag et al. (2021) [50]	20	36 (29–59)	220 (183–278)	Anterior OSR with puborectal sling adaptation	6/20 (30%) 3/20 (15%) re-operation 3/20 (15%) wound infection	Excellent/improved 9/20 (45%) Fully continent 2/20 (10%) Improved 8/20 (40%) Unchanged/worse 10/20 (50%)
Berg et al. (2019) [44]	94	43 (25–77)	44.5 (25–84)	Internal sphincter end-to-end anastomosis, external sphincter OSR	27/94 (29%) 27 (28.7%) Wound infection 20 (25.6%) persistent dehiscence of anal sphincters on post operative ultrasound	Improvement at least 3 point on St Mark's score 60/94 (63%) Gas incontinence 32/94 (34%) Daily stool incontinence 6/94 (6%); weekly 14/9415%
Lamblin et al. (2014) [7]	20	46 (31–62)	NR	OSR	5/20 patients (25%) Skin hematoma (no drainage): 1 Delayed skin healing: 1 Severe pain: 3 (2 resolved spontaneously in 1 week, 1 pudendal neuropathy)	NR
Lehto et al. (2013) [51]	56	51 (30–79)	NR	OSR or end-to-end if overlap not possible	10/56 patients (26%): Postop superficial wound rupture and/or wound infection treated with antibiotics	NR
Johnson et al. (2010) [52]	33	36 (22–75)[a]	103 (62–162)[a]	OSR	6/33 patients (18%): Wound infection	Excellent/good 19/33 (58%) Fully continent 3/33 (9%) Improved 16/33 (49%) Unchanged/worse 14/33 (42%)

(continued)

Table 26.1 (continued)

References	*N*	Age at time of surgery, mean (ranges)	FU, mean (ranges)	Repair	Complications	Outcomes, good/ excellent *N* (%)
Oom et al. (2009) [33]	160	58 (30–85)[a]	111 (12–207)	OSR	39/160 patients (23%) Wound infection: 35 21 of these were abscesses requiring further surgery with fistula formation in 15 Ileus: 2 DVT: 1 Lung embolism: 1	Excellent/good 44/120 (37%) Moderate 28/120 (23%) Poor 48/120 (40%)–<50% reduction of incontinent episodes; not satisfied with their situation
Zutshi et al. (2009) [9]	31	44 (22–80)	129 (113–208)	OSR	NR	No patients completely continent No patients continent to liquid or solid stool
Riss et al. (2009) [53]	25	56 (32–82)	105 (71–138)	OSR	Wound infection 2/25 (8%)	Fully continent 3/21 (14%) Incontinent liquid stool 11/21 (52%) Incontinent solid stool 7/21 (33%)
Mevik et al. (2009) [49]	25	45 (6–77)	85 (74–185)	Anterior external sphincter end to end (prior to 1994); OSR + separate internal sphincter direct suture (after 1994)	725 (28%) 2/25 (8%) wound dehiscence 1/25 (4%) wound infection 1/25 (4%) abscess 2/25 (8%) UTI 1/25 (4%) pudendal nerve damage	Fully continent 9/25 (36%) Incontinent gas only 4/25 (16%) Subsequent stoma 4/25 (16%)
Maslekar et al. (2007) [54]	64	48 (36–67)	84 (72–120)	OSR + separate end-to-end internal sphincter direct suture	20/64 (31%) 4 (6.25%) Wound infection 4 (6.25%) Wound dehiscence 6 (9.4%) Hematoma 10 (15.6%) Perianal pain	Fully continent 14/64 (20%) Incontinent gas oonly 26/64 (40%) Incontinent liquid stool 15/64 (24%) Incontinent solid stool 10/64 (15%) No longer requiring pad use 33/52 (63%)

(continued)

Table 26.1 (continued)

References	*N*	Age at time of surgery, mean (ranges)	FU, mean (ranges)	Repair	Complications	Outcomes, good/ excellent *N* (%)
Grey et al. (2007) [43]	85	46 (22–80)	60+ (mean NR)	OSR	26/85 patients (31%) Wound infection: 11 UTI: 5 Hematoma: 3 Urinary retention: 2 Pain: 2 Fecal impaction: 2 Pneumonia: 1	Improved 28/47 (60%) Initial improvement, but since deteriorated 17/47 (36%) Unchanged 2/47 (4%)
Trowbridge et al. (2006) [48]	59	42 (NR)	67 (62–70)	OSR (44%) End to end (56%)	13/59 (22%) Wound cellulitis 10/59 (16.7%) Wound breakdown 3/59 (5.1%)	Fully continent 6/59 (10%) Incontinent gas only 8/59 (14%) Incontinent liquid or solid stool 41/59 (69%)
Barisic et al. (2006) [55]	56	35.9 (18–64)	80.1 (26–154)	OSR + puborectal muscle plasty	NR	Excellent 15/56 (27%) Good 12 (21%) Satisfactory 30 (48%) Fair 7(12%) Poor 22 (39%)
Zorcolo et al. (2005) [56]	93	56 (27–80)	62 (13–111)	OSR reinforced with levatoroplasty or IAS plication	Wound complication 24/93 (26%)	Excellent 6/62 (10%) Good 28/62 (44%) Fair 14/62 (23%) Poor 10/62 (16%)
Gutierrez et al. (2004) [8]	130	37	120 (84–192)	OSR	NR	Fully continent 8/130 (6%) Incontinent gas only 21/130 (16%) Soiling 25/130 (19%) Incontinent solid stool 74/130 (57%)
Vaizey et al. (2004) [47]	21	47 (27–66)	60 (48–86)	Repeat OSR	NR	Fully continent 1/21 (5%) Improved a lot 10/21 (48%) Improved a little 2/21 (10%) Unchanged 4/21 (19%) Worse 4/21 (19%)

(continued)

Table 26.1 (continued)

References	*N*	Age at time of surgery, mean (ranges)	FU, mean (ranges)	Repair	Complications	Outcomes, good/excellent *N* (%)
Halverson and Hull, (2002) [57]	44	38.5 (22–80)[a]	62.5 (47–141)[a]	OSR	4/44 patients (9%): All wound infection	Fully continent 6/44 (14%) Continent to liquid and solid stool 18/44 (41%) Best possible QoL score 16/44 (36%)
Buie et al. (2001) [58]	191	36 (20–74)	43 (6–120)	OSR	12/191 patients (8%) Urinary retention: 6 Hemorrhage not requiring transfusion: 2 Abscess: 2 UTI: 1 Fecal impaction: 1	Fully continent 36/158 (23%) Excellent/good 97/158 (61%) Incontinent to gas only 61/158 (39%) Pad or incontinence less than once a month 42/158 (26%) Incontinence greater than once a month 19/158 (12%)
Malouf et al. (2000) [59]	46	43 (26–67)	77 (60–96)	OSR	NR	Fully continent 0/46 (0%) Either no or monthly or less frequent urge FI 23/46 (50%)
Karoui et al. (2000) [10]	74	52.9 (21–85)	40 (range NR)	OSR	NR	Fully continent 21/74 (28%) Incontinent to gas only 17/74 (23%) Incontinent to solid or liquid stool 36/74 (49%)
London-Schimmer et al. (1994) [60]	128	43 (16–77)	58.5 (range NR)	OSR	Early complication (<30 days post op) 32 (25%) Wound infection 20 (15.6%) Wound dehiscence 3 (2.3%) Fecal impaction 9 (7%) Hematoma 2 (1.6%) Late complications 12 (9.3%) Recurrence of fistula-in-ano 4 (3.1%) Stricture 3 (2.3%) Formation of sinus 3 (2.3%) SBO 1 (0.8%)	Excellent 13/94 (14%) Good 34/94 (36%) Fair 24/94 (26%) Poor 23/94 (25%) Permanent colostomy 11/94 (9%)

(continued)

Table 26.1 (continued)

References	*N*	Age at time of surgery, mean (ranges)	FU, mean (ranges)	Repair	Complications	Outcomes, good/ excellent *N* (%)
Gibbs and Hooks (1993) [11]	36	47 (20–74)	43 (4–114)	OSR	11/36 patients (31%) Temporary voiding issues: 5 UTI: 3 Anal stenosis: 3 Colostomy for wound sepsis: 2 Congestive heart failure: 1 Perianal sinus tract: 1	Good/excellent 24/33 (73%) Reliable control solid and liquid stool 10/33 (30%) Occasional loss of liquid stool or gas 14/33 (42%)

OSR overlapping sphincter repair, *UTI* urinary tract infection
[a]Results reported as median

complications after sphincteroplasty. Among the studies analyzed, the overall complication rate ranged from 8% to 31%.

Long-Term Outcomes

Early symptom improvement is noted after sphincteroplasty [6, 43, 57, 58], however, long-term follow-up reveals a decline in continence and increasing fecal accidents [7]. Multiple randomized controlled trials have found no association between overlapping versus end-to-end sphincteroplasty with regard to continent status [42, 61–63]. Regardless of surgical technique, there is a deterioration of fecal continence over time with return to baseline by 10 years [8–10]. Johnson et al. reported improved results in 55% of patients but excellent results in just 9% of patients after 8.6 years [52]. A study follow-up in this group at 18 years post-repair showed that the degree of incontinence reached the preoperative level. The majority of symptom deterioration occurred between the short and long term follow-up, with less severe decline in continence status between the long and very long term follow-up [50]. Halverson and Hull reported 14% of patients were totally continent after 5 years and 41% continent to liquid and solid stools [57], but among the same cohort at 10 years, no patients were totally continent, and no patient was continent to liquid and solid stools [9]. Similarly, Buie et al. reported 23% total continence at 3 years and 39% with continence to liquid and solid stool [58]. The same cohort of patients showed worsened continence rates at 10 years, with only 6% with total continence and 16% incontinent to gas only [8]. Patient-specific factors such as the mechanism of injury, the presence of neuropathy, menopausal status at the time of repair, the time between injury and repair, concomitant procedures, and preoperative fecal incontinence score can also play a role in continence outcomes [44, 50, 55, 57, 64]. In general, the results of post-obstetric injury sphincteroplasty are considered worse than those with other surgery indications [54, 64]. The reporting of outcomes between studies can vary, making group comparison difficult. The inclusion of fecal urgency in the evaluation of outcome success is important as the ability to defer defecation has been described as the single most important determinant of patient satisfaction [56]. This parameter is not included in every scoring system; thereby a fully continent patient may be classified as a successful outcome, even if patient satisfaction is low. Grading systems and questionnaires that include subjective reports on quality of life in addition to objective data are useful as well. The outcomes are reported using different endpoints, making comparisons between study groups difficult. Overall, continence to solid stool in the long term is the most consistent improvement, with continence to liquid and/or flatus seen less commonly. Table 26.1 summarizes studies with long-term follow-up.

For patients with recurrent fecal incontinence after sphincteroplasty, reevaluation and repeat repair can be considered. The rate of acceptance of the repeat sphincter repair is the same as that after a primary repair [37, 47] and hence should be considered for selected patients with failed primary repairs.

Conclusion

Despite criticism regarding long-term functional results, sphincteroplasty is a viable option for women with sphincter trauma and associated fecal incontinence. Improvement in continence after sphincteroplasty is noted, but it is not to the level that it was before the sphincter injury and declines considerably over time. Complication rates are low, and this procedure can be offered with limited morbidity as well as low cost. While SNM is increasingly used in the United States and worldwide with promising results particularly with regard to durability of response, anal sphincteroplasty remains an important procedure for colorectal surgeons to be familiar with as it is a good option for patients who do not want or cannot have an implantable device and can also be combined with other procedures for treatment of fecal incontinence, pelvic organ prolapse, and rectovaginal fistula.

References

1. Bharucha AE, Fletcher JG, Melton LJ 3rd, Zinsmeister AR. Obstetric trauma, pelvic floor injury and fecal incontinence: a population-based case-control study. Am J Gastroenterol. 2012;107(6):902–11.
2. Varma MG, Brown JS, Creasman JM, Thom DH, Van Den Eeden SK, Beattie MS, et al. Fecal incontinence in females older than aged 40 years: who is at risk? Dis Colon Rectum. 2006;49(6):841–51.
3. Ratto C, Buntzen S, et al. Multicentre observational study of the Gatekeeper™ for faecal incontinence. BJS. 2016;103:290–9.
4. Trenti L, Biondo S, Noguerales F, Nomdedeu J, et al. Outcomes of GateKeeper TM prosthesis implantation for the treatment of fecal incontinence: a multicenter observational study. Tech Coloproctol. 2017;21:963–70.
5. https://fdaaa.trialstracker.net/trial/NCT05776277/.
6. Simmang C, Birnbaum EH, Kodner IJ, Fry RD, Fleshman JW. Anal sphincter reconstruction in the elderly: does advancing age affect outcome? Dis Colon Rectum. 1994;37(11):1065–9.
7. Lamblin G, Bouvier P, Damon H, Chabert P, Moret S, Chene G, et al. Long-term outcome after overlapping anterior anal sphincter repair for fecal incontinence. Int J Color Dis. 2014;29(11):1377–83.
8. Bravo Gutierrez A, Madoff RD, Lowry AC, Parker SC, Buie WD, Baxter NN. Long-term results of anterior sphincteroplasty. Dis Colon Rectum. 2004;47(5):727–31; discussion 731–2.
9. Zutshi M, Tracey TH, Bast J, Halverson A, Na J. Ten-year outcome after anal sphincter repair for fecal incontinence. Dis Colon Rectum. 2009;52(6):1089–94.
10. Karoui S, Leroi AM, Koning E, Menard JF, Michot F, Denis P. Results of sphincteroplasty in 86 patients with anal incontinence. Dis Colon Rectum. 2000;43(6):813–20.
11. Gibbs DH, Hooks VH 3rd. Overlapping sphincteroplasty for acquired anal incontinence. South Med J. 1993;86(12):1376–80.
12. Ayan F, Zengin K, Ulualp K. A new technique: prolene mesh sphincteroplasty for the treatment of fecal incontinence. Minerva Chir. 2008;63(4):315–7.
13. Parnell BA, Whitehead WE, Geller EJ, Jannelli ML, Connolly A. Overlapping anal sphincteroplasty: impact of suture selection on bowel symptoms. J Reprod Med. 2011;56(5–6):187–91.
14. Wexner SD, Marchetti F, Jagelman DG. The role of sphincteroplasty for fecal incontinence reevaluated: a prospective physiologic and functional review. Dis Colon Rectum. 1991;34:22–30.
15. Hull T, Giese C, Wexner SD, Mellgren A, Devroede G, Madoff RD, et al. Long-term durability of sacral nerve stimulation therapy for chronic fecal incontinence. Dis Colon Rectum. 2013;56(2):234–45.
16. Matzel KE, Lux P, Heuer S, et al. Sacral nerve stimulation for faecal incontinence: long-term outcome. Color Dis. 2009;11:636–41.
17. Wong WD, Congliosi SM, Spencer MP, Corman ML, Tan P, Opelka FG, et al. The safety and efficacy of the artificial bowel sphincter for fecal incontinence: results from a multicenter cohort study. Dis Colon Rectum. 2002;45(9):1139–53.
18. Parker SC, Spencer MP, Madoff RD, Jensen LL, Wong WD, Rothenberger DA. Artificial bowel sphincter: long-term experience at a single institution. Dis Colon Rectum. 2003;46(6):722–9.
19. Abbas SM, Bissett IP, Neill ME, Parry BR. Long-term outcome of postanal repair in the treatment of faecal incontinence. ANZ J Surg. 2005;75(9):783–6.
20. Mackey P, Mackey L, Kennedy ML, King DW, Newstead GL, Douglas PR, et al. Postanal repair–do

the long-term results justify the procedure? Color Dis. 2010;12(4):367–72.
21. Thornton MJ, Kennedy ML, Lubowski DZ, King DW. Long-term follow-up of dynamic graciloplasty for faecal incontinence. Color Dis. 2004;6(6):470–6.
22. Hetzer FH, Bieler A, Hahnloser D, Lohlein F, Clavien PA, Demartines N. Outcome and cost analysis of sacral nerve stimulation for faecal incontinence. Br J Surg. 2006;93(11):1411–7.
23. Adang EM, Engel GL, Rutten FF, Geerdes BP, Baeten CG. Cost-effectiveness of dynamic graciloplasty in patients with fecal incontinence. Dis Colon Rectum. 1998;41(6):725–33; discussion 733–4.
24. Yamana T, Takahashi T, Iwadare J. Perineal puborectalis sling operation for fecal incontinence: preliminary report. Dis Colon Rectum. 2004;47(11):1982–9.
25. Mellgren A, Zutshi M, Lucente VR, Culligan P, Fenner DE, TOPAS Study Group. A posterior anal sling for fecal incontinence: results of a 152-patient prospective multicenter study. Am J Obstet Gynecol. 2016;214(3):349.e1–8.
26. Pakravan F, Helmes C. Magnetic anal sphincter augmentation in patients with severe fecal incontinence. Dis Colon Rectum. 2015;58(1):109–14.
27. Lehur PA, McNevin S, Buntzen S, Mellgren AF, Laurberg S, Madoff RD. Magnetic anal sphincter augmentation for the treatment of fecal incontinence: a preliminary report from a feasibility study. Dis Colon Rectum. 2010;53(12):1604–10.
28. Jayne DG, Williams AE, Corrigan N, Croft J, Pullan A, Napp V, Kelly R, Meads D, Vargas-Palacios A, Martin A, Hulme C, Brown SR, Nugent K, Lodge J, Protheroe D, Maslekar S, Clarke A, Nisar P, Brown JM. Sacral nerve stimulation versus the magnetic sphincter augmentation device for adult faecal incontinence: the SaFaRI RCT. Health Technol Assess. 2021;25(18):1–96. https://doi.org/10.3310/hta25180. PMID: 33752794; PMCID: PMC8020198.
29. Steele SR, Lee P, Mullenix PS, Martin MJ, Sullivan ES. Is there a role for concomitant pelvic floor repair in patients with sphincter defects in the treatment of fecal incontinence? Int J Color Dis. 2006;21(6):508–14.
30. Markland AD, Burgio KL, Whitehead WE, Richter HE, Wilcox CM, Redden DT, et al. Loperamide versus psyllium fiber for treatment of fecal incontinence: the fecal incontinence prescription (Rx) management (FIRM) randomized clinical trial. Dis Colon Rectum. 2015;58(10):983–93.
31. Nikiteas N, Korsgen S, Kumar D, Keighley MR. Audit of sphincter repair. Factors associated with poor outcome. Dis Colon Rectum. 1996;39(10):1164–70.
32. Klosterhalfen B, Offner F, Topf N, Vogel P, Mittermayer C. Sclerosis of the internal anal sphincter–a process of aging. Dis Colon Rectum. 1990;33(7):606–9.
33. Oom DM, Gosselink MP, Schouten WR. Anterior sphincteroplasty for fecal incontinence: a single center experience in the era of sacral neuromodulation. Dis Colon Rectum. 2009;52(10):1681–7.
34. Warner MW, Jones OM, Lindsey I, Cunningham C, Mortensen NJ. Long-term follow-up after anterior sphincter repair: influence of age on functional outcome. Color Dis. 2012;14(11):1380–8.
35. Evans C, Davis K, Kumar D. Overlapping anal sphincter repair and anterior levatorplasty: effect of patient's age and duration of follow-up. Int J Color Dis. 2006;21(8):795–801.
36. El-Gazzaz G, Zutshi M, Hannaway C, Gurland B, Hull T. Overlapping sphincter repair: does age matter? Dis Colon Rectum. 2012;55(3):256–61.
37. Hong KD, DaSilva G, Dollerschell JT, Wexner SD. Suboptimal results after sphincteroplasty: another hazard of obesity. Tech Coloproctol. 2014;18(11):1055–9.
38. Gilliland R, Altomare DF, Moreira H Jr, Oliveira L, Gilliland JE, Wexner SD. Pudendal neuropathy is predictive of failure following anterior overlapping sphincteroplasty. Dis Colon Rectum. 1998;41(12):1516–22.
39. Hasegawa H, Yoshioka K, Keighley MR. Randomized trial of fecal diversion for sphincter repair. Dis Colon Rectum. 2000;43(7):961–4; discussion 964–5.
40. Farrell SA, Flowerdew G, Gilmour D, Turnbull GK, Schmidt MH, Baskett TF, et al. Overlapping compared with end-to-end repair of complete third-degree or fourth-degree obstetric tears: three-year follow-up of a randomized controlled trial. Obstet Gynecol. 2012;120(4):803–8.
41. Fernando RJ, Sultan AH, Radley S, Jones PW, Johanson RB. Management of obstetric anal sphincter injury: a systematic review & national practice survey. BMC Health Serv Res. 2002;2(1):9. https://doi.org/10.1186/1472-6963-2-9. PMID: 12006105; PMCID: PMC116576.
42. Tjandra JJ, Han WR, Goh J, Carey M, Dwyer P. Direct repair vs. overlapping sphincter repair: a randomized, controlled trial. Dis Colon Rectum. 2003;46(7):937–42; discussion 942–3.
43. Grey BR, Sheldon RR, Telford KJ, Kiff ES. Anterior anal sphincter repair can be of long term benefit: a 12-year case cohort from a single surgeon. BMC Surg. 2007;7:1.
44. Berg MR, Gregussen H, Sahlin Y. Long-term outcome of sphincteroplasty with separate suturing of the internal and the external anal sphincter. Tech Coloproctol. 2019;23(12):1163–72.
45. Sultan AH, Kamm MA, Hudson CN, Bartram CI. Third degree obstetric anal sphincter tears: risk factors and outcome of primary repair. BMJ. 1994;308:887–91.
46. Oberwalder M, Dinnewitzer A, Baig MK, et al. Do internal anal sphincter defects decrease the success rate of anal sphincter repair? Tech Coloproctol. 2006;10:94–7.
47. Vaizey CJ, Norton C, Thornton MJ, Nicholls RJ, Kamm MA. Long-term results of repeat anterior anal sphincter repair. Dis Colon Rectum. 2004;47(6):858–63.

48. Trowbridge ER, Morgan D, Trowbridge MJ, Delancey JO, Fenner DE. Sexual function, quality of life, and severity of anal incontinence after anal sphincteroplasty. Am J Obstet Gynecol. 2006;195:1753–7.
49. Mevik K, Norderval S, Kileng H, Johansen M, Vonen B. Long-term results after anterior sphincteroplasty for anal incontinence. Scand J Surg. 2009;98(4):234–8.
50. Haug HM, Carlsen E, Johannessen HO, Johnson E. Short-, long-, and very long-term results of secondary anterior sphincteroplasty in 20 patients with obstetric injury. Int J Color Dis. 2021;36(12):2775–8.
51. Lehto K, Hyoty M, Collin P, Huhtala H, Aitola P. Seven-year follow-up after anterior sphincter reconstruction for faecal incontinence. Int J Color Dis. 2013;28(5):653–8.
52. Johnson E, Carlsen E, Steen TB, Backer Hjorthaug JO, Eriksen MT, Johannessen HO. Short- and long-term results of secondary anterior sphincteroplasty in 33 patients with obstetric injury. Acta Obstet Gynecol Scand. 2010;89(11):1466–72.
53. Riss S, Stift A, Teleky B, et al. Long-term anorectal and sexual function after overlapping anterior anal sphincter repair: a case- match study. Dis Colon Rectum. 2009;52:1095–100.
54. Maslekar S, Gardiner AB, Duthie GS. Anterior anal sphincter repair for fecal incontinence: good longterm results are possible. J Am Coll Surg. 2007;204(1):40–6.
55. Barisic GI, Krivokapic ZV, Markovic VA, Popovic MA. Outcome of overlapping anal sphincter repair after 3 months and after a mean of 80 months. Int J Color Dis. 2006;21(1):52–6.
56. Zorcolo L, Covotta L, Bartolo DC. Outcome of anterior sphincter repair for obstetric injury: comparison of early and late results. Dis Colon Rectum. 2005;48:524–31.
57. Halverson AL, Hull TL. Long-term outcome of overlapping anal sphincter repair. Dis Colon Rectum. 2002;45(3):345–8.
58. Buie WD, Lowry AC, Rothenberger DA, Madoff RD. Clinical rather than laboratory assessment predicts continence after anterior sphincteroplasty. Dis Colon Rectum. 2001;44(9):1255–60.
59. Malouf AJ, Norton CS, Engel AF, Nicholls RJ, Kamm MA. Long-term results of overlapping anterior anal-sphincter repair for obstetric trauma. Lancet. 2000;355(9200):260–5.
60. Londono-Schimmer EE, Garcia-Duperly R, Nicholls RJ, Ritchie JK, Hawley PR, Thomson JP. Overlapping anal sphincter repair for faecal incontinence due to sphincter trauma: five year follow-up functional results. Int J Color Dis. 1994;9:110–3.
61. Williams A, Adams EJ, Tincello DG, Alfirevic Z, Walkinshaw SA, Richmond DH. How to repair an anal sphincter injury after vaginal delivery: results of a randomised controlled trial. BJOG. 2006;113:201–7.
62. Garcia V, Rogers RG, Kim SS, Hall RJ, Kammerer-Doak DN. Primary repair of obstetric anal sphincter laceration: a randomized trial of two surgical techniques. Am J Obstet Gynecol. 2005;192:1697–701.
63. Fitzpatrick M, Behan M, O'Connell PR, O'Herlihy C. A randomized clinical trial comparing primary overlap with approximation repair of third-degree obstetric tears. Am J Obstet Gynecol. 2000;183:1220–4.
64. Rothbarth J, Bemelman WA, Meijerink WJHJ, Buyze-Westerweel ME, van Dijk JG, Delemarre JBVM. Long-term results of anterior anal sphincter repair for fecal incontinence due to obstetric injury / with invited commentaries. Dig Surg. 2000;17(4):390–4.

Cosmetic Gynecologic Surgery 27

Dani Zoorob and Mickey Karram

Labioplasty

Labioplasty, also known as labial rejuvenation, is a term used to indicate surgical enhancement of the labia minora.

The documented origin of labioplasty dates back to the Pharaohs in Egypt [1]. This practice, although modified, has persisted in the African continent with variations as minor as modification of the labia minora up to extensive resection of all external female genital organs, including both labia majora and minora, as well as the clitoris.

Amongst the earliest modern medical references discussing labioplasty is that of Hodgkinson and Hait [2], where they discuss the functional and aesthetic standpoints. Over the years, multiple procedures by Alter [3], Rouzier [4], Choi [5], and others were devised with varied outcomes and complications inherent to the different techniques used. Most reviews focus on labial reduction [6], although less commonly, the term labioplasty may encompass the augmentation of the labia.

A common non-aesthetic indication for labioplasty is dyspareunia, often observed in women with labial hypertrophy, where inward displacement of the labia during coitus precipitates pain. Additional indications include vulvar irritation and discomfort associated with undergarment use, ambulation, or exercise. Moreover, some patients report detrimental effects on personal hygiene, particularly during menstruation. The negative psychological impact stemming from perceptions of the labia being "unnatural" or abnormal—although inherently subjective—frequently motivates patients to seek surgical consultation.

When performing a labioplasty, the essential goals [7, 8] should include the reduction of the hypertrophied labia minora with maintenance of the neurovascular supply, preservation of the introitus, optimal color/texture match, and minimal invasiveness.

While many systems to stage the severity of this condition exist, there is still no consensus on how best to define and classify labial hypertrophy. One system divides the classification into three stages: none (no edges protruding beyond the labia majora), mild (1–3 cm beyond the labia majora edges), severe (>3 cm). Another system described by Felicio [9] divides labial hypertrophy into four stages: I (<2 cm), II (2–4 cm), III

D. Zoorob
Division of Urogynecology and Pelvic Reconstructive Surgery, Department of Obstetrics and Gynecology, Louisiana State University Health Sciences Center in Shreveport, Shreveport, LA, USA

M. Karram (✉)
Division of Urogynecology and Pelvic Reconstructive Surgery, The Christ Hospital, University of Cincinnati, Cincinnati, OH, USA

Department of Obstetrics/Gynecology, University of Cincinnati, Cincinnati, OH, USA
e-mail: mickey.karram@thechristhospital.com

H. B. Goldman, J. Zillioux (eds.), *Complications of Urogynecology and Reconstructive Pelvic Surgery*, https://doi.org/10.1007/978-3-032-00339-3_27

(4–6 cm), IV (>6 cm). Franco and Franco [10] describe a similar classification. However, Rouzier et al. [4] considered that the normal maximal length of the labia minora should not exceed 4 cm whereas Radman [11] considers it to be 5 cm (Fig. 27.1).

A myriad of surgical techniques have been reported in the literature, including simple resection, wedge resection with modification of excisions, VY and Z-plasties, and de-epithelialization (Figs. 27.2 and 27.3).

In simple resection, the excess or protuberant labial tissue is removed using scissors, a scalpel, or even a laser [12], in an elliptical or straight line. The edges are thereafter reapproximated with sutures, preferably simple interrupted, to ensure appropriate healing while maintaining the new contour. Depending on the defect or abnormality, the resection is preferably made while preserving a regular labia minora edge. Hodgkinson and Hait [2] and Maas and Hage [13] suggested a remnant minimal depth/length of 1 cm of labia minora. A novel technique called "Lazy S" reported by Ellsworth [14] is reported to assist in reducing the likelihood of contractures and phimosis of the labia minora. This technique involves marking the area to be resected in an S shape—rather than an ellipse or straight line—prior to infiltration with local anesthetic and then resecting along the broadly wavy tract. It is reported that once healing occurs, the wavy line would take a relaxed appearance with little tension at the periphery of the tissue, giving a more "natural" and esthetic look.

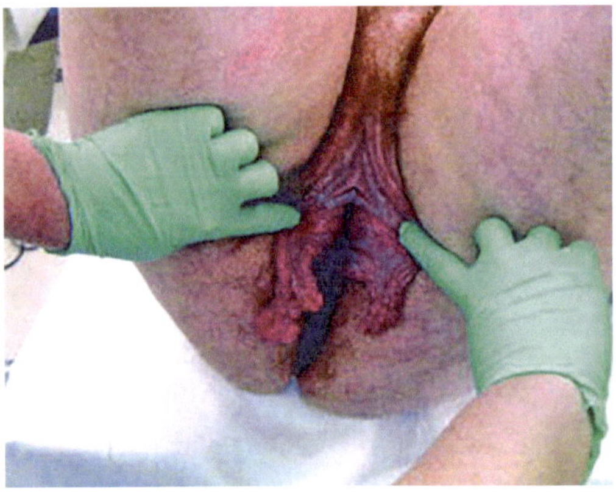

Fig. 27.1 Massive hypertrophy of the labia minor in a young woman with cerebral palsy

Another technique is wedge resection, which is reported to reduce hypersensitivity and contour irregularities upon healing. The wedge system targets the most hypertrophied region in the labia minora and resects it all the way to its base in a V or wedge form. This, in turn, allows for a smaller exposed healing area; however, depending on the resection required, it might be deep enough that it reaches the proximity of the labia majora. Multiple variants of this procedure have been devised, including Z-plasty and VY and the Matarasso modification/Star wedge resection [7]. The initial description of the technique was by Alter [3]. It involved a V-shaped wedge resection of the area with the most excess tissue identifiable. Maas and Hage [13] reported the wedge technique to strictly involve a W-shaped resection margin in the labia minora with no involvement of the clitoral dorsal hood, prepuce, or fourchette. The advantage of this technique (also known as the Zig-Zag technique) was reported to be less likelihood of dyspareunia and introital obliteration. This technique is reported by some to induce loss of pigmentation along the border of the labia minora despite the more natural contour being generated. In 2008, Alter [15] published the extended central wedge technique, a modification of his previous wedge resection, producing a more esthetic look, with the possibility of resection of excess tissue in the clitoral hood. This was based on the follow-up of previously operated patients. Among the modifications was one reported by Munhoz et al. [16] where the wedge is resected from the inferior aspect of the labia minora and a superior pedicle flap is developed. This is reported to provide a better esthetic look due to a more homogenous tinting of the labia.

In 2000, a novel technique devised by Choi and Kim [5] was reported to preserve tint, texture, sensation, and the neurovascular supply to the labia minora. This technique involved the central de-epithelialization of both labia minora on both sides, with suturing of the new edges together.

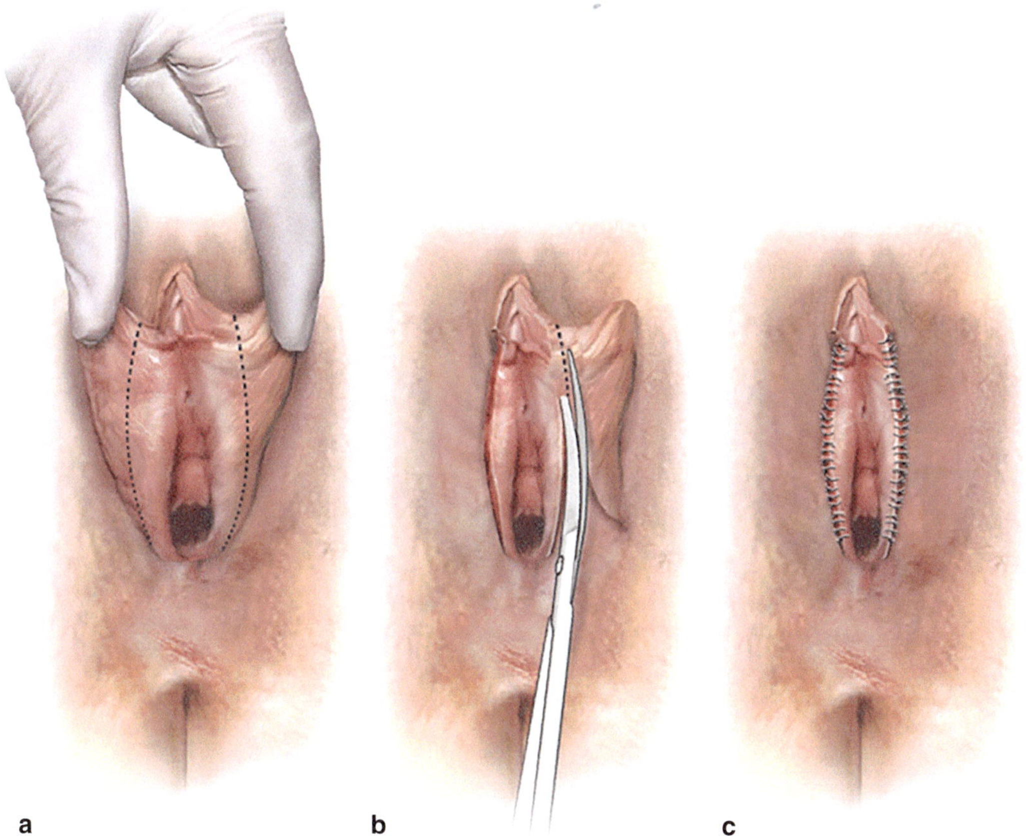

Fig. 27.2 The technique for simple excision of enlarged or hypertrophied labial skin. (**a**) Excess skin to be removed is marked. (**b**) Skin is excised. (**c**) Interrupted sutures reap proximate the edges of the labia

In 2011, Alter [15] described the use of YV advancement flaps for the reconstruction of either absent, abruptly terminated, distorted, or scalloped labial edges. Being the closest match to labial tissue, clitoral hood tissue is mobilized in such a manner as to release two parallel folds—including the Dartos fascia and blood supply—from around the clitoris and rotating them on each side to form the labia minora.

Relative to the labia majora, Salgado et al. [17] reported that grafts of fat pads as well as fat injections could improve the atrophied look in some patients. Felicio [9] reported up to a maximum of 60 mL of fat injected into each labia majora per session, while requiring a drain if more is to be implanted or a continuation of the procedure 6 months later. Labia minora injections are also possible. Labia majora augmentation is reported to assist in increased comfort and sexual satisfaction, possibly due to acting as a shock absorber and possibly due to increased fullness and firmness of the labial tissues. Relative to hypertrophied labia majora, the option of resection in an elliptical or S-shaped incision may be necessary. However, the closer the final incisional edge to the labia minora, the more inconspicuous the scar is. Miklos and Moore [18] reported the use of a semilunar incision on the medial border of the labia majora. The possibility of lipoplasty could assist in avoiding large incisions and shorten the recovery period, and reduce postoperative pain; however, the need for repeat or touch-up surgery may be required.

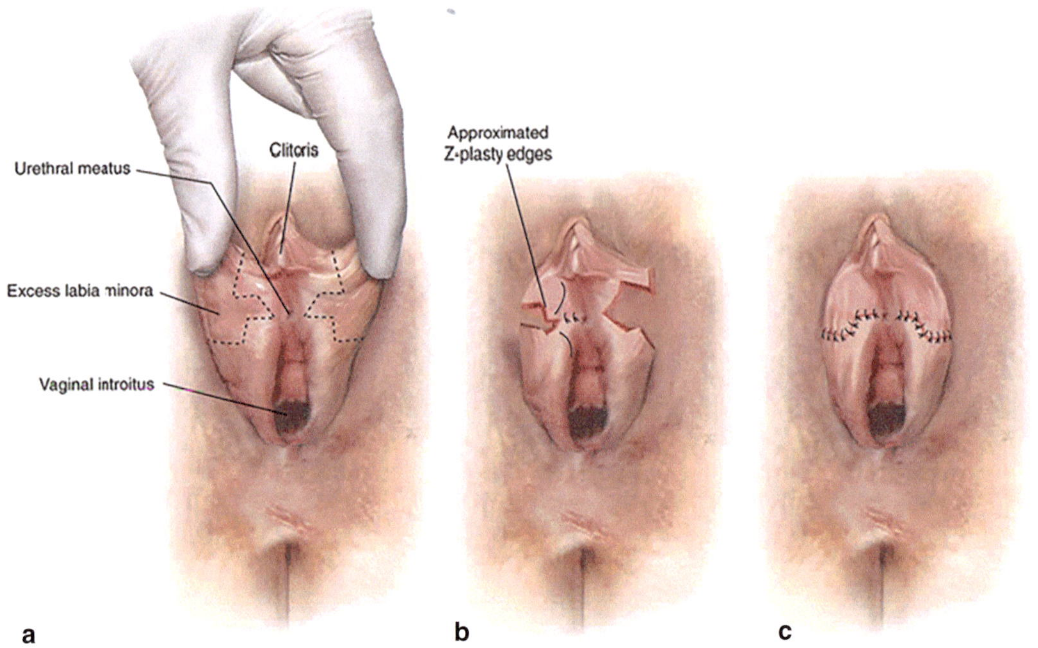

Fig. 27.3 Technique for Z-plasty. (**a**) Skin is to be excised. (**b**) Skin is excised and to be reapproximated transversely with fine interrupted sutures. (**c**) Completed repair

Labioplasty Complications

A variety of complications have been reported with labioplasty surgery. As a multitude of different techniques and modifications have been described, it is essential that the surgeon undertaking these procedures be intimately familiar with the anatomy of the external genitalia and its surrounding structures. A review of 110 women who underwent labia minora reduction suggested that complications arose in 76% of patients undergoing significant amputation of labial tissue, 21% in those undergoing wedge resection, and 3% in those undergoing de-epithelialization [19]. The rates of complications vary, however, as one study assessing 258 patients suggested that 8.5% of patients had complications requiring further management [20], whereas another reported it at 2.7% [21]. The variations in rates correlate with the techniques used, perioperative care, and surgeon skill and management.

Infection The perineal area seems less susceptible to infection compared to other regions of the body, but the potential for abscess formation does exist, and it is mandatory to follow the universal guidelines for surgical site cleansing prior to initiating surgery. Although no definitive recommendations for labioplasty have been set by any society, the routine gynecologic surgical antibiotic prophylaxis is advisable.

Surgical Site Breakdown The possibility of contractures, tissue breakdown along the suture line, flap necrosis, edge necrosis, irregular resorption, phimosis of the clitoral hood, new onset of dyspareunia, loss of sensation or hyperalgesia may occur in the resection areas.

Care following surgery, whether immediately postoperatively or few weeks out, is mandatory. No set criteria are available in the literature denoting particular postoperative wound care. However, it is advisable that postoperative patients should observe pelvic rest for a minimum of 4–6 weeks to ensure adequate healing with time and avoid trauma to the surgical site. Felicio [9] reports that ice packs and NSAIDs are ideal for postoperative edema and swelling. He also recommends ensuring that labioplasty is not concurrently performed with perineoplasty due to the intense swelling resulting in prolonged discomfort persisting up to 6 months. In addition to the discomfort, the likelihood of suture-line breakdown is much higher with the swelling. Thus staging the enhancement procedure would be advisable for both patient care and outcome.

Whether preceded by a wound hematoma or not, the development of a wound dehiscence is particularly ominous. Generalized flap degeneration or necrosis is more commonly seen in patients with sutures that have been placed tightly across the edges or when there is excessive traction on the attached tissue or flaps. It is crucial that when a flap is to be mobilized, the surgeon needs to ensure the persistence of the blood supply to allow the flap to survive as well as incorporate appropriately into the transposition site. Distal flap necrosis and subsequent gap formation in the labia may ensue if the vascular supply is not preserved. Additionally, in YV advancement flaps, the de-vascularization due to extensive undermining or extreme skinning prior to mobilization particularly endangers the survival of the transposed flap. Thus, ensuring minimal vessel distortion when mobilizing tissue with the least possible rotation/torque applied allows for better tissue survival. Tissue ischemia has been reported when using the wedge resection technique, requiring multiple revisions to reestablish esthetics and resolution of pain at the site of the procedure [6]. A meta-analysis of 43 studies referenced the preference of surgeons for the use of lasers to reduce postoperative edema, hematoma, and bleeding. However, it did stress the increased breakdown associated with such a technique [22].

Bleeding Hemorrhage and the possibility of hematomas may be encountered based on the vessels severed. Arterial blood vessels usually require active control by cautery or suture ligation, whereas venous bleeders may need less aggressive management, including pressure applied to the area involved or simple application of hemostatic agents.

The acute worsening of pain postoperatively may indicate the expansion of a hematoma, specifically if the labioplasty involved the labia majora. In addition to the psychological impact on a patient, the formation of a hematoma could potentially require drainage as well as prolonged courses of antibiotics, and ultimately, exploration to control the bleeding vessel. This can be attempted initially by freeing the suture line and then evacuating the hematoma. Since not all hematomas are associated with arterial bleeding, the use of fibrin clotting agents could be useful at times when persistent minimal venous oozing is noted. While multiple agents exist, there are no studies identifying the benefit of one vs. another in the setting of labial hematomas.

Dyspareunia Postoperative dyspareunia is known to occur more with wedge excisions as well as simple resection due to the newly formed exposed labial edge. Multiple studies [23–25] have been conducted to assess the innervations in hypertrophied labia compared to normal-sized ones with no evidence of variability relative to size. However, postoperative hyperalgesia has been noted to occur, especially with associated infection, severe inflammation, or severe edema ensuing postoperatively. If swelling occurs and the tissue perfusion is impacted, the possibility of labial retraction and contracture (called phimosis if involving the clitoral hood) may occur as the healing process continues. This contracture may, in turn, cause severe dyspareunia that may require reoperation due to inability to achieve penetration.

Suture Granulomas and Scarring The use of running sutures may predispose to contracture formation. Compared to simple interrupted sutures, the use of running locked sutures at the edges may predispose to a rugged or irregular labial edge due to localized necrosis or skin retraction. The use of simple interrupted sutures is preferred in simple excision procedures. The various studies available in the literature report the use of a variety of suture materials with none proven to be superior to the other. When using absorbable sutures, the use of Vicryl and Monocryl would be ideal, although the use of chromic sutures in the study by Choi and Kim [5] also had good outcomes. Use of nonabsorbable sutures is theoretically associated with the least reaction at the suture site, with possibly better cosmesis; however, it is less convenient to use due to the discomfort endured by the patient upon removal of the sutures. To ensure better outcomes, it is advisable to inquire preoperatively about any history of Vicryl-associated suture granulomas. The removal of any permanent sutures should be carried out within 1 week of surgery to assist in healing while ensuring the pressure on the incision site is lower, since the edema will have partially receded by then. When left too long, the sutures can potentially develop epithelialized tracts, and this may have an unsightly appearance. These tracts are often referred to as "railroad" tracks and related to surgeon's tying skillset, suture placement, and timing of suture removal [6].

Maas and Hage [13] reported that simple amputation of the protuberant labium will generate a stiff and weakly healed edge along which irritation and potential retraction. The stiff edge formation is mostly due to extensive local fibrosis developing when healing. A technique called "Lazy S" reported by [14] is reported to assist in reducing the likelihood of contractures and phimosis. This technique involves marking the area to be resected in an S shape. With healing, the wavy line takes a relaxed appearance with little tension at the margin. The homogenous or gradual labial pigmentary changes need to be preserved to ensure esthetic outcomes. The sudden change from dark pigmented folds to lightly pigmented labial folds is not advisable. The de-epithelialization and zig-zag techniques preserve this best.

Postoperative Labial Asymmetry A reported concern when performing labioplasty is the inability to accurately gauge the length of labial tissue to be excised once local anesthetic has been infiltrated. The distortion caused by the injected solution can render the tissue margins irregular and difficult to discern. To mitigate this risk, it is essential to mark the area for excision before administering the local anesthetic. This precaution helps prevent over-resection and ensures an aesthetically pleasing outcome. It is advisable to perform this marking immediately prior to surgery while the patient is awake, ideally during the preoperative consultation, which may also offer an opportunity to align the medically recommended labial size with the patient's expectations.

Vaginoplasty

Vaginoplasty refers to modifications in the vagina to incur visual, sexual, or functional improvement. Its indications remain vague but usually include the desire for enhancement of vaginal aesthetics and improvement and augmentation of the sexual experience. Ostrzenski [19] considers it a transformation involving both anatomy and function to allow for heightened sensation in intercourse. Typically, aesthetic vaginoplasty is primarily a perineoplasty. It involves restoring the normal visual anatomy of the region of the perineum/and posterior fourchette.

At all times, the vaginal canal should have a perpendicular relationship relative to the perineum. Having had an episiotomy or laceration during parturition, many women have been inadequately repaired and end up with an introitus that has a large membranous portion covering the posterior fourchette. This membrane often causes dyspareunia due to friction and stretching. This is usually due to an iatrogenic mal-approximation of musculature and overlying skin resulting in the perineum not having sufficient support and thus dyspareunia develops due to

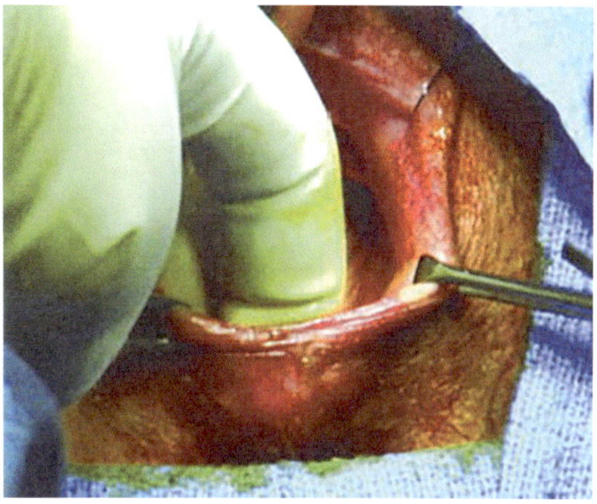

Fig. 27.4 The skin of the labia minor has been previously sewn across the midline, most likely at the time of the repair of a midline episiotomy

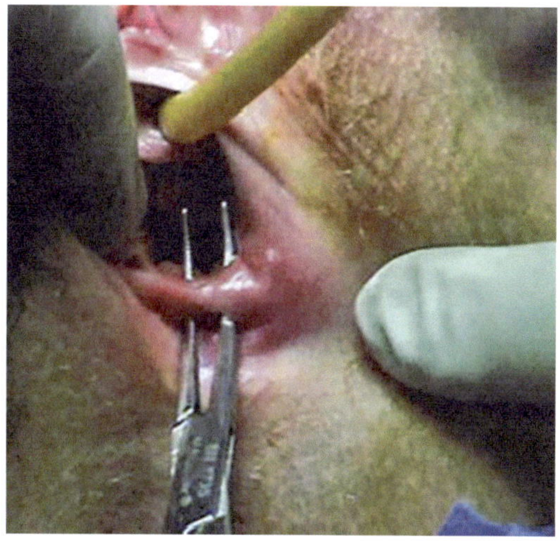

Fig. 27.5 Band of perineal scar tissue in a young patient following the repair of a perineal laceration

significant stretching and pulling of the thinned-out portion of this vulvovaginal structure (Fig. 27.4). The "membrane" itself does not have any physiologic purpose and thus it is advisable to have the "membrane" resected when restoring normal anatomy to the perineum.

Moving deeper into the vagina, the presence of significantly redundant tissue inside, whether following any surgical procedure or even if present naturally, could be reported as unappealing to the sexual partner. In rejuvenation and vaginoplasties, this may be considered as a potential repair site, where excess rugae may be excised, cauterized, or lasered. Certain areas to be targeted while resurfacing are episiotomy skin/mucosal tags or laceration repair sites, areas of previous colporrhaphies where dog-ears/tags have developed, as well as possible breakdowns in the repairs.

Another form of rejuvenation, called mucosal tightening/lateral colporrhaphy, involves excision of a wedge of vaginal mucosa, after which the raw edges are sutured together. A case series by Adamo and Corvi [26] showed a 95% improvement in sensation after such a procedure.

At times, band-like adhesions may be noted extending across the vagina due to varied resorption and healing after any kind of repair (Fig. 27.5). Sometimes, strictures may be seen across the vagina. Severing these adhesion bands may be accomplished by using a cautery that is allowed to go deep into the vaginal wall—releasing the adhesion at its base if possible.

This typically allows for restoration of the normal vaginal caliber. Healing in such cases may require secondary intention closure rather than surgical mucosal overlay. Recent studies have aimed at the regeneration of vaginal rugae to effect the augmentation of sensory-coital pleasure. Loss of this rugation may occur with age as estrogen production dwindles, as well as in areas with site-specific defects. Studies have also shown that the anterior vaginal wall has denser innervation relative to the posterior wall [27–29], particularly distally. Attempts at regenerating rugae using linear laser stratification with vaporization up to the vaginal fascia were noted to improve sexual satisfaction in a prospective observational study, but in only 20% of the test subjects [19].

Typically occurring postpartum, many women develop a widened genital hiatus as well as vaginal laxity. Prior to surgical repair aimed at tightening of the vagina itself, pelvic floor rehabilitation should be initiated to ensure adequate muscular toning of the vagina. In general, only a perineoplasty is required for tightening the genital hiatus, but some may consider doing a posterior colporrhaphy (Fig. 27.6). Studies done

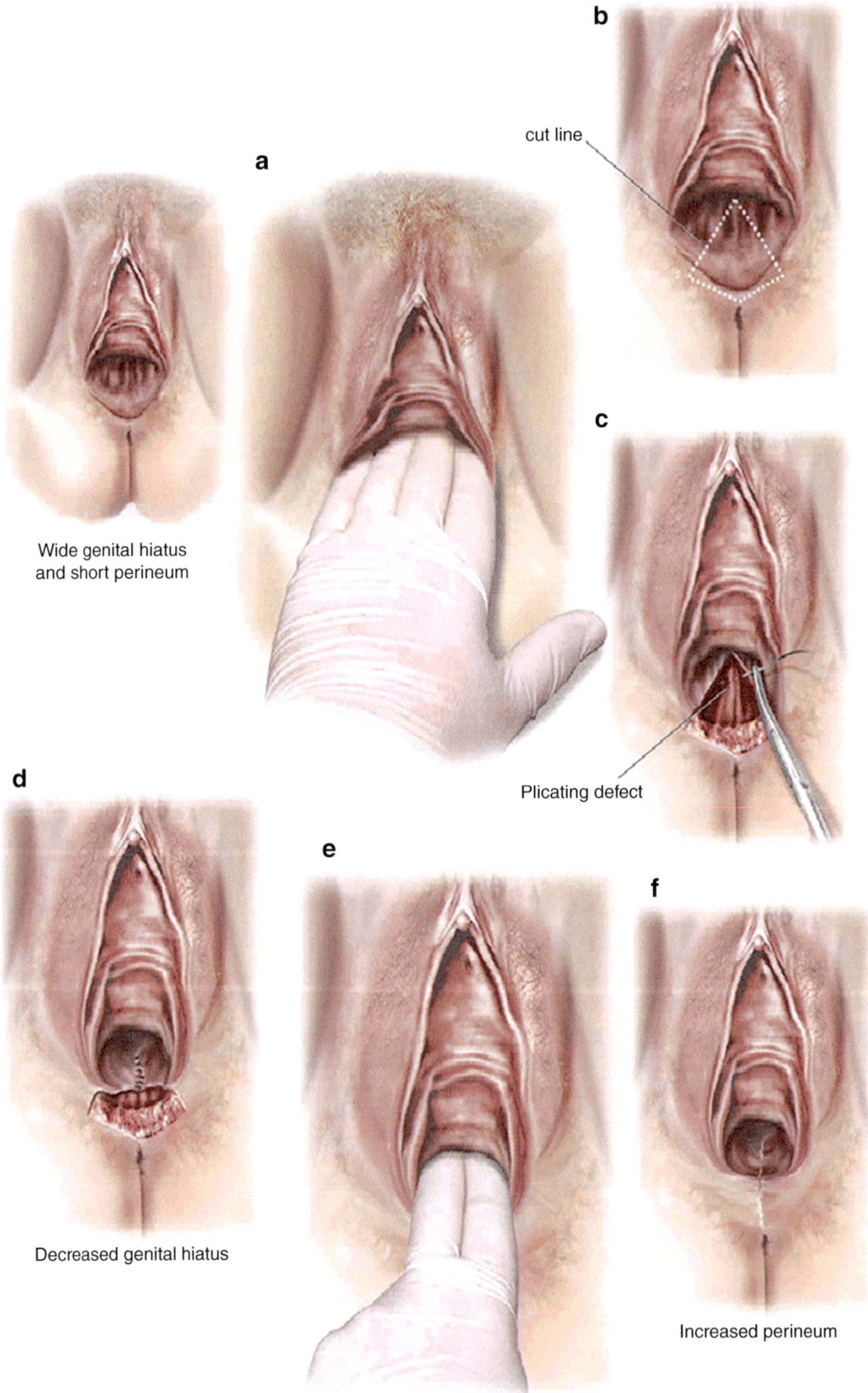

Fig. 27.6 The technique of vaginoplasty and reconstruction with the sole aim of tightening the vaginal introits. (**a**) Note the wide genital hiatus, which easily allows the insertion of four fingers. (**b**) A diamond-shaped piece of tissue to be excised is marked. (**c**) The tissue has been removed, and deep stitches are taken through the perirectal fascia and levitator muscles to build up the posterior vaginal wall. Great care is taken to avoid the creation of a posterior vaginal wall ridge. (**d**) The upper portion of the posterior vaginal wall is closed in preparation for perineal reconstruction. (**e**) After perineal reconstruction, the introits allows the insertion of only two fingers. (**f**) Completed repair; note the perpendicular relationship between the posterior vaginal wall and the perineum

to assess dyspareunia following colporrhaphy show that it is less frequent if perineorrhaphy involving the levators is avoided.

Complications of Vaginoplasty

Depending on the procedure used for vaginoplasty, a myriad of complications may occur.

Laser and Cautery-Related Complications If the laser is used to create rugae, the avoidance of damage to the fascial layers is important. Currently, there are no recommendations for the depth of vaporization, but it is best to avoid reaching the glistening fascial layer so as to avoid iatrogenic development of site-specific defects. The laser vaporization, if not used judiciously, may incur damage to any of the underlying tissues, including the bowels, bladder, and urethra. Furthermore, it is advisable to avoid prolonged tissue exposure—of the same spot—to avoid peripheral damage by heat conduction. As with the laser and due to significant peripheral heating of adjacent tissues, caution is advised with extensive use of monopolar cautery. In procedures of resurfacing where the extra rugae or skin tags in the vagina are removed, it is best to brush rather than attempt to cut or shave the rugae. The brushing technique, as its name implies, involves rapid and superficial back-and-forth cautery tip motion. This modality will result in the removal of only the necessary tissue, particularly since the extent of the cautery is well visualized and controlled. If the cautery tip is placed on the vaginal mucosal tag and activated continuously until the tag shrivels, the underlying tissue may be damaged by the heat generated from the tag degeneration, and accordingly, may result in a potential area of necrosis that could impact the integrity of vaginal walls. This, in turn, may predispose to vesicovaginal or rectovaginal fistulas. If reporting new onset of fluid leakage or foul odor on intercourse, then a detailed pelvic exam with assessment for fistulas should ensue. Furthermore, it is important to inform the patient of the significant discharge that will develop after surgery, which could last for weeks as the sloughing occurs. Pain should be absent to minimal with this type of procedure, and the patient should recover rapidly. If the patient develops worsening pain or if pain develops days after surgery, then the likelihood of damage to an adjacent structure is very high. The development of fever is unlikely unless an infection has occurred. The use of the cautery to create relaxing incisions when vaginal strictures exist is highly successful in resolving the constrictions as long as bleeding is controlled and vessels are avoided. Being familiar with the vascular anatomy of the vagina prior to any surgery is crucial. It is advisable to use simple interrupted sutures to control hemorrhage of actively bleeding tissues since cautery may sometimes make further suturing difficult, especially if retraction of the vessel occurs with unsuccessful cautery. The sutures applied should preferably be placed perpendicular to the band that was released so as to maintain the newly developed caliber. The use of any form of energy in the vagina increases the risk of stricture and fibrotic band formation, even if the initial surgery was for the release of strictures.

Persistent Postoperative Dyspareunia The vaginal innervation is densest anteriorly and distally. If colporrhaphy is primarily performed for rejuvenation and not defect repair, then the risk of dyspareunia is lower but is lowest when a perineoplasty is not performed. Severe superficial dyspareunia has been reported when the perineoplasty involved levator muscle plication. The discomfort classically occurs when the introitus is tightened significantly. The pain is muscular and not neurogenic in nature but the dyspareunia can be quite significant at times, resulting in abstinence instead of enhancement of the sexual experience.

Pelvic Muscle Dyssynergia The use of Botox described by some for alleviation of Levator ani spasm, has been reported in the literature with notable results. It has been described for the rejuvenation process as well; however, the associated complications, although rarely encountered, can potentially last for a few months until the medication wears off. Judicious injection could help avoid the development of retroperitoneal hematomas and internal bleeding, pelvic muscle dyssynergia, urinary and fecal incontinence and obstruction, pelvic abscess formation, permanent neural damage, leg and pelvic weakness, and new onset of referred pain. Careful assessment and application of Botox are necessary while ensuring an injection that is not too deeply placed.

Site-Specific Augmentation Complications To increase sensation to both partners, injections of fat or fillers into the vagina, and even grafts, have been described. The placement of grafts is potentially associated with erosions and dyspareunia as well as bowel and bladder perforation. Despite it being typically injected into the labia majora in vaginal rejuvenation, some have used fat to create ring formations within the vagina with the hope of providing an enhanced sexual experience. The complication that may ensue is severe edema that could potentially impact urination as well as abscess formation and vaginal mucosal wall breakdown with ulcer formation—with the breakdown developing immediately postoperatively or potentially during intercourse. Another potentially injectable and often topical form of treatment for vaginal rejuvenation is mesotherapy, which uses herbs and chemicals to induce lipolysis or change tissue consistency and thus theoretically enhance vaginal sensation. Since these compounds have not been tested adequately for vaginal use, they should be avoided as they may create irritative and potentially damaging effects, resulting in sclerosis and significant sloughing of the epithelium, causing pain and copious discharge.

Clitoroplasty

The first well-documented corrective clitoral surgery dates back to 1934 when Young [30] described a clitoridectomy. As time passed, studies in the mid- to late-1960s ascertained the need for and importance of the clitoris in the sexual experience.

Clitoroplasty can involve the increased exposure of clitoral tissue, which may augment sexual enjoyment. It may also involve the removal of tissues to assist in an enhanced visual genital appearance, especially when combined with labioplasty and possibly vaginoplasty. Furthermore, clitoroplasty may involve the repositioning and resizing of the clitoris, especially in women with evidence of hypertrophy—particularly if afflicted with hyperandrogenism.

Various techniques have been described to surgically manage clitoromegaly. One technique involves resecting the excess tissue from the clitoral hood and then reapproximating the edges with concurrent reduction in the clitoral size by resecting part of its corpora, then attaching it to the periosteum [31].

With the desire for increased sexual pleasure, a procedure for exposing the clitoris has been devised. Clitoral unhooding involves resection of tissue covering the clitoral tip, at times circumferentially, thus exposing it more, much like circumcision in males. A similar procedure is the reduction of the clitoral hood, which involves repositioning of the tissues overlying the clitoris with the help of sutures rather than actual tissue resection. This usually allows for increased stimulation during intercourse and accordingly, heightened sexual pleasure.

Complications of Clitoroplasty

Hemorrhage and Necrosis of the Clitoris When performing procedures that involve reducing, advancing, or repositioning the clitoris, there is a considerable risk of compromising its vascular supply. If unrecognized, such disruption may result in ischemia and necrosis of the reattached clitoral tip. Furthermore, partial clitoral resection—commonly observed in certain forms of female genital mutilation (often mischaracterized as "circumcision")—is associated with significant hemorrhage and can markedly impair sexual function.

The vascular supply to both the labia minora and the clitoris derives primarily from the posterior labial, perineal, and dorsal clitoral branches of the pudendal artery. The dorsal neurovascular bundle is situated on the clitoral surface, protected by an adipose cushion, with the suspensory ligament located immediately beneath. Consequently, meticulous surgical dissection is imperative to preserve these structures and mitigate the risk of adverse outcomes.

New-Onset Clitoral Pain When clitoral reduction procedures involve resection or repositioning, it is imperative to preserve the neurovascular connection between the clitoral tip and its body [30]. Disruption of this neural pathway can render the clitoris insensitive and eliminate its contribution to sexual function, underscoring the necessity of employing nerve-sparing techniques.

The posterior labial and perineal branches of the pudendal nerve (S2–S4) primarily mediate sensation to the labia minora, while the clitoris benefits from additional autonomic innervation provided by the hypogastric and pelvic plexuses. Moreover, there have been anecdotal reports of persistent postoperative pain localized to the periosteal clitoral insertion site, as well as diffuse clitoral discomfort during arousal.

Contractures Around the Clitoris Contracture of the incision line may result in phimosis and theoretically strangulation of the clitoral tip, especially if multiple gynecoplasty procedures are done simultaneously. Due to the edema that develops postoperatively, it is advisable to avoid using a running suture line and use widely spaced interrupted sutures instead.

In cases of clitoral reduction, development of contractures along the suture lines as well as long-standing pain are risks the patient needs to know about preoperatively—these develop more often in association with infection and hematomas. In clitoral unhooding, both the amount of tissue excised as well as the closure techniques are crucial. The complete exposure of the clitoris, causing hypersensitivity, could become bothersome due to the continuous friction with the patient's clothes. Furthermore, the appearance of the clitoris, if excessively unhooded, might be unsightly.

Conclusion

As women become increasingly aware of the discrepancy between their own genital appearance and prevailing standards of aesthetic normalcy, a growing number are electing to pursue surgical interventions for cosmetic enhancement and perceived improvements in sexual function. Cosmetogynecology is a rapidly evolving discipline, with innovative techniques continually emerging to optimize outcomes while mitigating associated risks. Given that the primary objective of cosmetogynecology is to enhance quality of life, it is imperative that any procedural modifications should align with the patient's individual desires and adhere to rigorous standards of surgical safety. Consequently, patients considering these interventions should be comprehensively informed about the potential complications, as delineated in this chapter.

References

1. Hosken FP. The epidemiology of female genital mutilations. Trop Dr. 1978;8(3):150–6.
2. Hodgkinson DJ, Hait G. Aesthetic vaginal labioplasty. Plast Reconstr Surg. 1984;74(3):414–6.
3. Alter GJ, Alter G. A new technique for aesthetic labia minora reduction. Ann Plast Surg. 1998;40(3):287–90.
4. Rouzier R, Louis-Sylvestre C, Paniel B-J, Haddad B. Hypertrophy of labia minora: experience with 163 reductions. Am J Obstet Gynecol. 2000;182(1):35–40.
5. Choi HY, Kim KT. A new method for aesthetic reduction of labia minora (the deepithelialized reduction labioplasty). Plast Reconstr Surg. 2000;105(1):419–22.
6. Oranges CM, Sisti A, Sisti G. Labia minora reduction techniques: a comprehensive literature review. Aesthet Surg J. 2015;35(4):419–31.
7. Tepper OM, Wulkan M, Matarasso A. Labioplasty: anatomy, etiology, and a new surgical approach. Aesthet Surg J. 2011;31(5):511–8.

8. Assaad MB. Female circumcision in Egypt: social implications, current research, and prospects for change. Stud Fam Plan. 1980;11(1):3–16.
9. Felicio Y. Intime chirurgie. La Rev Chir Esth Lang Franc XVII. 1992;67:37–43.
10. Franco T, Franco D. Hipertrofia de ninfas. J Bras Ginecol. 1993:163–8.
11. Radman HM. Hypertrophy of the labia minora. Obstet Gynecol. 1976;48(1 Part 2):78s–80s.
12. Pardo J, Sola V, Ricci P, Guilloff E. Laser labioplasty of labia minora. Int J Gynecol Obstet. 2006;93(1):38–43.
13. Maas SM, Hage JJ. Functional and aesthetic labia minora reduction. Plast Reconstr Surg. 2000;105(4):1453–6.
14. Ellsworth WA, Rizvi M, Lypka M, et al. Techniques for labia minora reduction: an algorithmic approach. Aesth Plast Surg. 2010;34:105–10.
15. Alter GJ. Labia minora reconstruction using clitoral hood flaps, wedge excisions, and YV advancement flaps. Plast Reconstr Surg. 2011;127(6):2356–63.
16. Munhoz AM, Filassi JR, Ricci MD, et al. Aesthetic labia minora reduction with inferior wedge resection and superior pedicle flap reconstruction. Plast Reconstr Surg. 2006;118(5):1237–47.
17. Salgado CJ, Tang JC, Desrosiers AE III. Use of dermal fat graft for augmentation of the labia majora. J Plast Reconstr Aesthet Surg. 2012;65(2):267–70.
18. Miklos JR, Moore RD. Simultaneous labia minora and majora reduction: a case report. J Minim Invasive Gynecol. 2011;18(3):378–80.
19. Ostrzenski A. Vaginal rugation rejuvenation (restoration): a new surgical technique for an acquired sensation of wide/smooth vagina. Gynecol Obstet Investig. 2012;73(1):48–52.
20. Goodman MP, Placik OJ, Benson RH III, et al. A large multicenter outcome study of female genital plastic surgery. J Sex Med. 2010;7(4_Part_1):1565–77.
21. Lista F, Mistry BD, Singh Y, Ahmad J. The safety of aesthetic labiaplasty: a plastic surgery experience. Aesthet Surg J. 2015;35(6):689–95.
22. Escandón JM, Duarte-Bateman D, Bustos VP, et al. Maximizing safety and optimizing outcomes of labiaplasty: a systematic review and meta-analysis. Plast Reconstr Surg. 2022;150(4):776e–88e.
23. Sommerova J, Malinovský L, Martincik J. Sensory nerve endings in hypertrophy of the human labium minus pudendi. Folia Morphol (Warsz). 1974;22(3):266–7.
24. Malinovský L, Sommerova J. Sensory nerve endings in the human labia minora pudendi and their variability. Folia Morphol (Warsz). 1973;21(4):351–3.
25. Malinovský L, Sommerova J, Martincik J. Quantitative evaluation of sensory nerve endings in hypertrophy of labia minora pudendi in women. Acta Anat. 1975;92(1):129–44.
26. Adamo C, Corvi M. Cosmetic mucosal vaginal tightening (lateral colporrhaphy): improving sexual sensitivity in women with a sensation of wide vagina. Plast Reconstr Surg. 2009;123(6):212e–3e.
27. Hilliges M, Falconer C, Ekman-Ordeberg G, Johansson O. Innervation of the human vaginal mucosa as revealed by PGP 9.5 immunohistochemistry. Cells Tissues Organs. 1995;153(2):119–26.
28. Alzate H, Londono ML. Vaginal erotic sensitivity. J Sex Marital Ther. 1984;10(1):49–56.
29. Hoch Z. Vaginal erotic sensitivity by sexological examination. Acta Obstet Gynecol Scand. 1986;65(7):767–73.
30. Young H. Genital abnormalities, hermaphroditism & related adrenal diseases. Baltimore: Williams & Wilkins; 1937.
31. Sayer RA, Deutsch A, Hoffman MS. Clitoroplasty. Obstet Gynecol. 2007;110(2 Part 2):523–5.

Vaginal Laser Treatment

28

Mikolaj Przydacz and Howard B. Goldman

Introduction

In recent years, lasers have gained popularity as a treatment option for urogynecological and gynecological conditions such as stress urinary incontinence, genitourinary syndrome of menopause, vaginal prolapse, and more. Because of growing concerns about the risks and complications associated with mesh use in treating stress urinary incontinence and pelvic organ prolapse, urologists have focused increased scrutiny and discussion on the adoption of new technologies and treatments within the field.

In 2018, the U.S. Food and Drug Administration issued a caution regarding the use of energy-based devices, including lasers, for "vaginal rejuvenation" or cosmetic vaginal procedures [1]. In several review articles and editorials, clinicians have since called for more robust evidence of the effectiveness and safety of vaginal laser treatments. Furthermore, prominent global scientific organizations such as the International Continence Society [2], the International Urogynecological Association [3], the International Society for the Study of Vulvovaginal Disease [4], and the European Association of Urology [5], have established international multidisciplinary expert panels. These panels have developed best practice consensus documents and recommendations, which primarily highlight the limitations of vaginal laser treatments [2–5]. In this chapter, we summarize the current evidence for and against the use of lasers in the treatment of gynecological and urogynecological conditions.

M. Przydacz (✉)
Department of Urology, Jagiellonian University Medical College, Krakow, Poland

Glickman Urological Institute, Cleveland Clinic, Cleveland, OH, USA

H. B. Goldman
Glickman Urological & Kidney Institute, Cleveland Clinic, Cleveland, OH, USA

Laser Techniques and Their Mechanisms of Action on Tissues

Lasers have traditionally been used in gynecology and urology for incision, excision, ablation, vaporization, coagulation, and hemostasis of various soft tissues [6]. Lasers are also used to stimulate tissue and collagen restructuring. Lasers can induce collagen contraction, followed by remodeling of the dermal connective tissue [7, 8]. This process can significantly improve conditions such as fine lines and scarring, particularly when used for aesthetic and dermatological treatments.

Because patients report positive results with minimal recovery time or complications following laser treatments for aesthetic and dermatological issues, laser use has become widespread. Consequently, clinicians and companies began

H. B. Goldman, J. Zillioux (eds.), *Complications of Urogynecology and Reconstructive Pelvic Surgery*, https://doi.org/10.1007/978-3-032-00339-3_28

investigating whether the tissue remodeling effects observed in the dermis could be applied to the vaginal epithelium and subepithelial fascia. This assessment was aimed at eventually offering a nonsurgical option for treating gynecological and urogynecological conditions associated with damaged or weakened connective tissues.

The two primary categories of lasers used for tissue remodeling in gynecology and urogynecology are distinguished on the basis of the medium that produces the laser energy: CO_2 lasers and Erbium YAG lasers. These two types of lasers have different effects on tissue, primarily classified as "ablative" or "non-ablative" collagen remodeling of the subepithelial connective tissue [1].

Ablative lasers, which include both CO_2 and Erbium YAG, deliver short pulses with high peak power, performing rapid, focused micro-ablation on the epithelium and subepithelial tissue. This process creates microscopic columns of thermal injury in deeper tissues while sparing the superficial layers. Consequently, this action triggers fibroblast activation and promotes collagen production without leading to fibrosis [7].

A non-ablative effect on tissues generates a gradual thermal response. A gradual response results in controlled heating of the subepithelial connective tissue, which is water-rich, leading to the breakdown of collagen crosslinks and a reduction in collagen fiber length. Following this shortening of collagen fibrils, thermo-mechanical interactions with the deeper tissues induce tissue shrinkage and retraction, ultimately resulting in new collagen fiber formation with time [8–10].

Importantly, different laser types exhibit varying degrees of tissue penetration and can induce distinct levels of collateral thermal injury and tissue fibrosis in the epithelial layer. As a result, there is no standardized protocol for laser therapy [1]. Various clinical trials have employed differing energy levels, treatment parameters, session counts, and intervals between treatments. Typically, laser procedures are conducted in outpatient settings, sometimes requiring pre-treatment with topical analgesics. Sessions generally last 15–20 min for the Erbium YAG laser and 5–10 min for the CO_2 laser. Treatments are usually scheduled 4–6 weeks apart, with a total of 3–4 sessions recommended. Side effects are generally minimal and temporary, often consisting of mild discomfort during the procedure (which is typically well tolerated), transient urgency, slight tissue edema and swelling lasting a few days, and a temporary increase in vaginal discharge [1].

Stress Urinary Incontinence

Stress urinary incontinence is characterized by the involuntary leakage of urine triggered by an increase in intra-abdominal pressure, occurring without a contraction of the detrusor muscle [11]. Various factors contribute to stress urinary incontinence, with childbirth and aging being the primary risk factors. These conditions can weaken the pelvic floor muscles and damage the connective tissues that support the bladder and urethra [12, 13]. The connective tissue in the endopelvic fascia contains a high concentration of collagen, about 80% of the fascia's protein, which serves as the main structural element. During childbirth, the sub-urethral fascial hammock is particularly susceptible to injury, which can lead to incontinence. Additionally, aging impairs the production of new collagen, further compromising the integrity of the sub-urethral collagen within the endopelvic fascia. In women experiencing incontinence, the pubocervical fascia has a reduced collagen content, which may weaken the support structures at the bladder neck and sub-urethral tissues [14, 15].

The goal of laser therapy for stress urinary incontinence is to enhance the connective tissue in the sub-urethral hammock and the supporting fascia of the paracolpium. In a recent systematic review, Alsulihem and Corcos evaluated the safety, efficacy, and outcomes of laser treatments for female stress urinary incontinence [16]. The authors highlighted the overall poor quality of the available studies, with most reports consisting of case series. The Erbium YAG laser demonstrated a modest reduction in mild stress urinary incontinence, with effects lasting no longer than 13–16 months. Although fractional CO_2 laser treatment showed some improvement in mild stress urinary incontinence in a few studies, there was a lack of long-term data. Reported adverse events were minimal, and they were not systematically documented. Further, the reviewed literature on vaginal lasers had several limitations, including significant variations in laser settings and protocols, short follow-up periods, and a lack of urodynamic evaluations and appropriate objective measures. Consequently, Alsulihem and Corcos concluded that, on the basis of the existing literature, lasers cannot be recommended as a treatment option for stress urinary incontinence [16].

In support of the aforementioned findings, a review by Phillips et al. indicated that overall outcomes showed improvement in symptom scores and pad weight at 6–12 months [1] but there was a decline in these results after 18–36 months unless additional treatments were administered. The data suggested that patients with mild stress urinary incontinence experienced better outcomes compared with patients who had moderate to severe stress urinary incontinence, as assessed by validated questionnaires [1].

Finally, Mortensen et al. reviewed the only two existing randomized controlled trials that assessed the effect of lasers on stress urinary incontinence [17]. In the first trial, CO_2 laser therapy showed similar improvements to intravaginal promestriene at a 2-week follow-up. The second trial demonstrated greater improvement in the Erbium YAG group compared with the sham group in a study of 114 women at a 3-month follow-up. However, trial heterogeneity complicates direct comparisons between the two trials.

Genitourinary Syndrome of Menopause

Genitourinary syndrome of menopause refers to a collection of vulvovaginal and urinary symptoms, such as vaginal pain, dryness, itching, dyspareunia, and tissue friability, as well as urinary issues like frequency, urgency, incontinence, hematuria, recurrent urinary tract infections, and sexual dysfunction [18]. Clinical signs include atrophic changes in the external and internal genitalia, including labial thinning, introital retraction, and a more prominent urethral meatus [19]. Histologically, genitourinary syndrome of menopause involves thinning of the stratified squamous epithelium, reduced glycogen in epithelial cells, and diminished vascularity and dermal papillae [19]. These symptoms can significantly impair sexual function and quality of life in postmenopausal women. Traditionally, genitourinary syndrome of menopause has been treated with non-hormonal options such as vaginal lubricants, moisturizers, or herbal remedies, with low-dose vaginal estrogen remaining the gold standard. Other alternatives include vaginal DHEA and oral SERMs like ospemifene [19].

Laser therapy is proposed as a promising alternative for managing symptoms of genitourinary syndrome of menopause, particularly as a "non-hormonal" option. This proposal is particularly appealing for women in whom hormonal treatments are either unsuitable or undesirable because of medical contraindications or personal preferences. Several studies have demonstrated the benefits of laser therapy for breast cancer survivors for whom hormonal therapy is contraindicated [20]. The mechanism of laser therapy for genitourinary syndrome involves stimulating tissue repair processes, leading to increased capillary density and collagen remodeling that helps restore and rejuvenate the affected tissues.

Many investigators have evaluated the effectiveness of CO_2 and Erbium YAG lasers, particularly the Mona Lisa Touch and Fotona lasers, in treating genitourinary syndrome of menopause symptoms. Most of the available research consists of short-term observational studies or case series, there being only one study in which the Erbium YAG ablative laser was used [1]. In their review, Phillips et al. included 1780 women treated across various trials. Most of the studies were prospective observational designs, with follow-up durations generally from 3 to 6 months, although 8 studies had follow-ups extending from 12 to 24 months. Primary outcome measures in most studies focused on improvements in vaginal symptom scores, which assess dryness, dyspareunia, irritation, and leukorrhea, as well as the vaginal health index score. Across all studies, there was a consistent improvement in symptom scores, with some benefits lasting up to 12 months, and in certain cases, extending to 18 months. In one study, Athanasiou et al. examined the effect of repeated laser treatments [21]. Notably, some studies were specifically focused on breast cancer survivors, who are often hesitant to use hormonal treatments, demonstrating the broader applicability of laser therapy in this population. In addition, Phillips et al. identified three randomized controlled trials that evaluated the use of lasers in treating genitourinary syndrome of menopause. Two studies compared the ablative CO_2 Mona Lisa laser with vaginal oestriol, and a third trial compared the CO_2 laser with either prometriene cream or a vaginal lubricant [22–24]. The follow-up periods for these trials were from 14 weeks to 6 months post-treatment. All trials demonstrated significant improvements in both vaginal symptom scores and vaginal health index scores for patients treated with the laser.

Therefore, current evidence indicates that laser therapy could serve as a promising non-hormonal alternative for treating genitourinary syndrome of menopause. However, the optimal treatment protocol, including the ideal number of sessions or intervals between treatments, has not been determined. Additionally, the potential function of vaginal estrogens, whether used prior to or alongside laser therapy, has yet to be established [1]. Furthermore, most of the studies have been short-term, and a significant limitation of these studies is that they do not address the potential risks of long-term complications, such as scarring [3].

Other Conditions

There are only a few studies in which investigators assessed lasers for managing other gynecological and urogynecological conditions. Excluding cosmetic applications, these studies primarily focus on three areas: overactive bladder, lichen sclerosis/vulvodynia, and prolapse. Another area often mentioned is "vaginal relaxation syndrome." However, "vaginal relaxation syndrome" is not recognized as a medical condition, and it lacks standardized terminology and definition; thus, any claims regarding laser efficacy for this "syndrome" should be viewed with caution.

Alsulihem and Corcos found that the clinical experience with Erbium YAG laser in the treatment of overactive bladder was limited to just one prospective cohort study and two retrospective studies [16]. These studies showed conflicting results, albeit with a trend to improve overactive bladder symptoms for up to 12 months. The effects of fractional CO_2 laser for patients with vaginal atrophy and overactive bladder symptoms have been addressed in only three case series and one non-blinded randomized control trial [16]. The CO_2 laser demonstrated minimal improvement in these short-term studies. Alsulihem and Corcos emphasized that all studies of lasers for OAB were of low quality, characterized by a high risk of bias, short follow-up durations, and a limited number of participants [16].

For lichen sclerosis, Phillips et al. identified only two papers describing laser efficacy [1, 25, 26]. One study demonstrated an improvement in patient symptoms at the one-month follow-up after treatment [26]. The other study was a randomized controlled trial that compared vaginal Erbium laser (Fotona Smooth) with topical corticosteroid therapy for lichen sclerosus [25]. Investigators were blinded to the assigned treatment groups, and both the laser and topical corticosteroid therapies showed improvements in clinical assessments of lichen sclerosis, histological analysis, and patient-reported symptoms.

Phillips et al. also found four studies that assessed the efficacy of the Erbium YAG smooth laser to treat women with "vaginal relaxation" or prolapse [1]. The four studies were prospective cohort studies, most with short-term follow-ups of only 3–6 months. In one study with a longer follow-up, investigators examined a cohort of 83 women with prolapse and reported significant improvement and satisfaction in prolapse symptoms at 6, 12, 24, and 36 months. The main outcome measures were patient symptom scores and prolapse assessment using the Baden-Walker Classification, instead of the POPQ classification.

Adverse Effects and Complications

Outpatient laser therapy is generally well tolerated, with most studies showing low pain scores on the visual analogue scale. Side effects tend to be mild and transient, including mild vaginal and vulvar edema, vaginal irritation, and urinary urgency or frequency. These symptoms typically resolve within 2 weeks. However, the Food and Drug Administration and independent experts have emphasized that women considering energy-based vaginal procedures utilizing lasers may also experience serious adverse events [6]. Potential complications include vaginal hematomas, acute bleeding, persistent burns, dryness, infection, altered sensation, dyspareunia, adhesions, scarring, chronic pain, or vaginal stenosis over time [27]. Vaginal fibrosis has also been reported and could contribute to sexual dysfunction, ultimately affecting quality of life [28]. The exact frequency of all these complications is often not systematically reported, even in the short term [16]. Long-term data, in particular, are lacking, so complications like scarring may not have been fully identified [2]. Further, an analysis of the MAUDE database and published case series indicate that overly vigorous use of the laser may lead to potential long-term complications, particularly persistent pain, dyspareunia, and vaginal fibrosis [28, 29]. In summary, the full extent of the risks remains unknown [6].

Conclusions

Energy-based devices for treating gynecological and urogynecological conditions are becoming increasingly popular. We note that most studies of the efficacy of lasers for these conditions are single-center, either prospective or retrospective cohort studies, often involving small patient populations and relatively short follow-up periods, with no placebo or control groups for comparison. Lasers have also not been adequately compared with standard treatments, and many studies are industry-sponsored. Furthermore, most of the available research lacks objective (or validated) outcome measures. A few large studies do exist, with longer follow-ups from 12 to 36 months, as well as some randomized controlled trials. Some of these studies indicate that vaginal laser therapy could be a viable treatment option, but mainly for genitourinary syndrome of menopause. However, the duration of its effectiveness appears modest, typically lasting between 12 and 18 months, suggesting that repeat treatments may be necessary for sustained benefits. The impact of repeated treatments is still uncertain and requires further investigation. Several multi-center randomized controlled trials are in progress, and their results will be crucial for establishing reliable recommendations. To further complicate matters, the mechanisms of action of lasers in treating gynecological and urogynecological conditions remain poorly understood and require thorough investigation [2]. Moreover, the effect of lasers on the vaginal microbiome needs to be evaluated.

Clinicians must recognize the distinctions between the types of lasers and the research surrounding the safety and effectiveness of each type. This recognition includes understanding the specific clinical indications, target tissues (such as skin, epithelium, or mucosa), energy levels, and treatment parameters associated with each laser. Most of the existing studies focus on the CO_2 Mona Lisa Touch (Italy) and the Erbium YAG Smooth Fotona (Slovenia). Insights gained from past controversies surrounding the use of mesh highlight the necessity for manufacturers to provide concrete evidence demonstrating the efficacy and safety of their products, instead of merely asserting that their devices are comparable to others.

Healthcare providers must recognize the limitations, risks, and potential outcomes associated with laser therapy, as well as the importance of thorough patient evaluations for proper selection. It is essential to set realistic expectations for patients regarding treatment results. A lack of comprehensive assessment and counseling can lead to low satisfaction rates and increased complications. At this stage, promoting the widespread use of laser therapy in gynecology and urogynecology outside of clinical trials is premature until larger, multicenter, and randomized studies yield conclusive results. Furthermore, it is advisable that any effective laser treatments be administered by practitioners who possess the necessary expertise in evaluating and managing the relevant conditions. Currently, lasers are being used by the aesthetic industry that often claims to address issues like vaginal atrophy and stress incontinence, but the claims lack adequate evaluation, which can result in poor outcomes and potential complications due to inappropriate application [1]. Future trials should concentrate on the precise function of lasers within the treatment algorithm. These studies must ensure sufficient sample sizes, long-term follow-up, thorough documentation of adverse events, and a detailed description of the equipment used. Finally, while generally safe, there are a number of serious adverse events that have been reported with vaginal laser therapy.

References

1. Phillips C, Hillard T, Salvatore S, Toozs-Hobson P, Cardozo L. Lasers in gynaecology. Eur J Obstet Gynecol Reprod Biol. 2020;251:146–55.
2. Preti M, Vieira-Baptista P, Digesu GA, et al. The clinical role of LASER for vulvar and vaginal treatments in gynecology and female urology: an ICS/ISSVD best practice consensus document. Neurourol Urodyn. 2019;38:1009–23.
3. Shobeiri SA, Kerkhof MH, Minassian VA, et al. IUGA committee opinion: laser-based vaginal devices for treatment of stress urinary incontinence, genitourinary syndrome of menopause, and vaginal laxity. Int Urogynecol J. 2019;30:371–6.
4. Preti M, Vieira-Baptista P, Digesu GA, et al. The clinical role of LASER for vulvar and vaginal treatments in gynecology and female urology: an ICS/ISSVD best practice consensus document. J Low Genit Tract Dis. 2019;23:151–60.
5. European Association of Urology (EAU), Non-Oncology Guidelines [Internet]; Non-neurogenic Female LUTS, Publicated: 2023 [Cited: 2023 December]. Available from: https://uroweb.org/guidelines/non-neurogenic-female-luts.
6. Digesu GA, Tailor V, Preti M, et al. The energy based devices for vaginal "rejuvenation," urinary incontinence, vaginal cosmetic procedures, and other vulvo-vaginal disorders: an international multidisciplinary expert panel opinion. Neurourol Urodyn. 2019;38:1005–8.
7. Niemz MN. Laser-tissue interactions: fundamentals and applications. Berlin/Heidelberg/New York: Springer; 2007.
8. Kulick MI. Lasers in aesthetic surgery. Springer; 2012.
9. Tadir Y, Gaspar A, Lev-Sagie A, et al. Light and energy based therapeutics for genitourinary syndrome of menopause: consensus and controversies. Lasers Surg Med. 2017;49:137–59.
10. Arunkalaivanan A, Kaur H, Onuma O. Laser therapy as a treatment modality for genitourinary syndrome of menopause: a critical appraisal of evidence. Int Urogynecol J. 2017;28:681–5.
11. Abrams P, Cardozo L, Fall M, et al. The standardisation of terminology of lower urinary tract function: report from the Standardisation Sub-committee of the International Continence Society. Neurourol Urodyn. 2002;21:167–78.
12. Bump RC, Norton PA. Epidemiology and natural history of pelvic floor dysfunction. Obstet Gynecol Clin N Am. 1998;25:723–46.
13. Leijonhufvud A, Lundholm C, Cnattingius S, et al. Risks of stress urinary incontinence and pelvic organ prolapse surgery in relation to mode of childbirth. Am J Obstet Gynecol. 2011;204(70):e71–7.
14. Rechberger T, Postawski K, Jakowicki JA, Gunja-Smith Z, Woessner JF Jr. Role of fascial collagen in stress urinary incontinence. Am J Obstet Gynecol. 1998;179:1511–4.
15. Keane DP, Sims TJ, Abrams P, Bailey AJ. Analysis of collagen status in premenopausal nulliparous women with genuine stress incontinence. Br J Obstet Gynaecol. 1997;104:994–8.
16. Alsulihem A, Corcos J. The use of vaginal lasers in the treatment of urinary incontinence and overactive bladder, systematic review. Int Urogynecol J. 2021;32:553–72.
17. Mortensen OE, Christensen SE, Lokkegaard E. The evidence behind the use of LASER for genitourinary syndrome of menopause, vulvovaginal atrophy, urinary incontinence and lichen sclerosus: a state-of-the-art review. Acta Obstet Gynecol Scand. 2022;101:657–92.
18. Portman DJ, Gass ML. Genitourinary syndrome of menopause: new terminology for vulvovaginal atrophy from the International Society for the Study of Women's Sexual Health and the North American Menopause Society. Maturitas. 2014;79:349–54.
19. Gandhi J, Chen A, Dagur G, et al. Genitourinary syndrome of menopause: an overview of clinical manifestations, pathophysiology, etiology, evaluation, and management. Am J Obstet Gynecol. 2016;215:704–11.

20. Jha S, Wyld L, Krishnaswamy PH. The impact of vaginal laser treatment for genitourinary syndrome of menopause in breast cancer survivors: a systematic review and meta-analysis. Clin Breast Cancer. 2019;19:e556–62.
21. Athanasiou S, Pitsouni E, Grigoriadis T, et al. Microablative fractional CO2 laser for the genitourinary syndrome of menopause: up to 12-month results. Menopause. 2019;26:248–55.
22. Cruz VL, Steiner ML, Pompei LM, et al. Randomized, double-blind, placebo-controlled clinical trial for evaluating the efficacy of fractional CO2 laser compared with topical estriol in the treatment of vaginal atrophy in postmenopausal women. Menopause. 2018;25:21–8.
23. Politano CA, Costa-Paiva L, Aguiar LB, Machado HC, Baccaro LF. Fractional CO2 laser versus promestriene and lubricant in genitourinary syndrome of menopause: a randomized clinical trial. Menopause. 2019;26:833–40.
24. Paraiso MFR, Ferrando CA, Sokol ER, et al. A randomized clinical trial comparing vaginal laser therapy to vaginal estrogen therapy in women with genitourinary syndrome of menopause: the VeLVET Trial. Menopause. 2020;27:50–6.
25. Bizjak Ogrinc U, Sencar S, Luzar B, Lukanovic A. Efficacy of non-ablative laser therapy for lichen sclerosus: a randomized controlled trial. J Obstet Gynaecol Can. 2019;41:1717–25.
26. Gomez-Frieiro M, Laynez-Herrero E. Use of Er:YAG laser in the treatment of vulvar lichen sclerosus. Int J Womens Dermatol. 2019;5:340–4.
27. ACOG Committee Opinion No. 378: Vaginal "rejuvenation" and cosmetic vaginal procedures. Obstet Gynecol. 2007;110:737–8.
28. Gordon C, Gonzales S, Krychman ML. Rethinking the techno vagina: a case series of patient complications following vaginal laser treatment for atrophy. Menopause. 2019;26:423–7.
29. Ahluwalia J, Avram MM, Ortiz AE. Lasers and energy-based devices marketed for vaginal rejuvenation: a cross-sectional analysis of the MAUDE database. Lasers Surg Med. 2019;51:671–7.

Martius Labial Fat Pad Procedure 29

Sonia Guérin, Dominic Lee,
and Philippe E. Zimmern

Introduction

The Martius labial fat pad (MLFP) is a modified version of the Martius flap as described by Heinrich Martius in 1928. The original technique used the bulbocavernosus muscle with fatty tissue harvested from the labia majora. MLFP consists solely of a pedicle graft of adipose tissue without the muscle. The procedure is rather simple, takes typically 15′ or so, and produces a well vascularized fat pad of variable length based on where it will ultimately be positioned. This fat pad can be used as an interposition layer during a variety of vaginal procedures. We describe a typical indication for MLFP, then the technical steps at length. Our outcome knowledge is based on a limited literature consisting of 18 series of more than 5 patients each and 30 case reports since 2000. Success rates are high and complications infrequent.

S. Guérin · P. E. Zimmern (✉)
University of Texas Southwestern Medical Center, Dallas, TX, USA
e-mail: sonia.guerin@chu-rennes.fr; Philippe.Zimmern@UTSouthwestern.edu

D. Lee
Department of Urology, ST George Hospital, Kogarah, NSW, Australia

Case Presentation

A 62-year-old woman presents with a history of chronic retention requiring daily use of intermittent catheterization and recurrent urinary tract infections after a Burch suspension. Urethral obstruction was confirmed by urodynamics and voiding cystourethrogram. A transvaginal urethrolysis with MLFP was discussed to decrease the risk of secondary scarring in the retropubic space.

Surgical Technique with Film [1]

The patient was placed in a low lithotomy position, and after completion of the transvaginal urethrolysis, we proceeded to wrap an MFLP around the urethra to prevent recurrent retropubic scarring. There are times when the MFLP is harvested first to avoid additional retropubic or vaginal bleeding during the time of harvesting. The prompt placement of the MFLP can fill the space where the bleeding takes place. This logistical detail needs to be discussed for each case individually.

Step 1. A vertical incision (6–8 cm) is made over the labia majora from the level of the mons pubis down towards the level of the fourchette (Fig. 29.1). The harvest side depends on the defect location and the preference of the sur-

H. B. Goldman, J. Zillioux (eds.), *Complications of Urogynecology and Reconstructive Pelvic Surgery*, https://doi.org/10.1007/978-3-032-00339-3_29

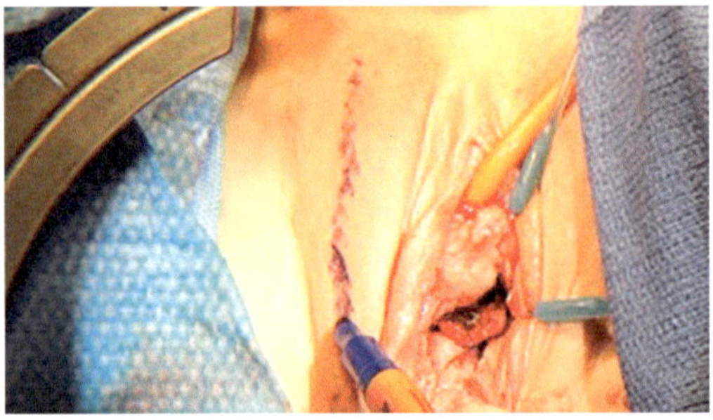

Fig. 29.1 A vertical incision (6–8 cm) is made over the labia majora from the level of the mons pubis down towards the level of the fourchette

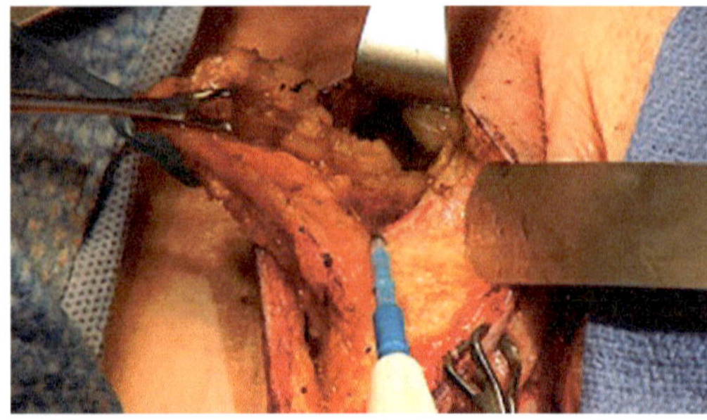

Fig. 29.2 The labial fat pad can be gently grasped with a Babcock clamp

geon. The length of the incision depends on the length of the fat pad required. It can always be extended upwards towards the mons pubis to gain more length.

A LoneStar® retractor can be placed to hold the skin edges open. The dissection is started on each side to separate the labial fat pad in the center of the incision from the skin edges. It is important to leave enough fat underneath the skin on each side to avoid labial distortion, especially medially.

Step 2. The labial fat pad can be gently grasped with a Babcock clamp (Fig. 29.2) and mobilized on an inferior pedicle supplied by a postero-inferior branch from the external pudendal artery. Although not our preference, a superior blood supply can also be considered. The dissection is continued medially first, with attention to keep sufficient fat attached underneath the medial labial edge; then it proceeds superiorly, aided by a small retractor, which exposes the tip of the fat pad at the mons pubis. When a sufficient length has been freed, the fat pad is divided superiorly. This can be done by using the bovie cautery or suture ligating the pedicle when larger blood vessels are present.

Step 3. Once divided at its extremity, the fat pad needs to be freely mobilized. To achieve this goal, the dissection then extends in depth until reaching the white shiny fascia covering the underlying ischiocavernosus and bulbocavernosus muscles. Next, the dissection of the back side of the fat pad allows its gradual freeing and elongation. While progressing, one must keep in mind to preserve a broad base inferiorly and avoid damaging the lateral branch of the obturator artery to preserve the fat pad vascularity.

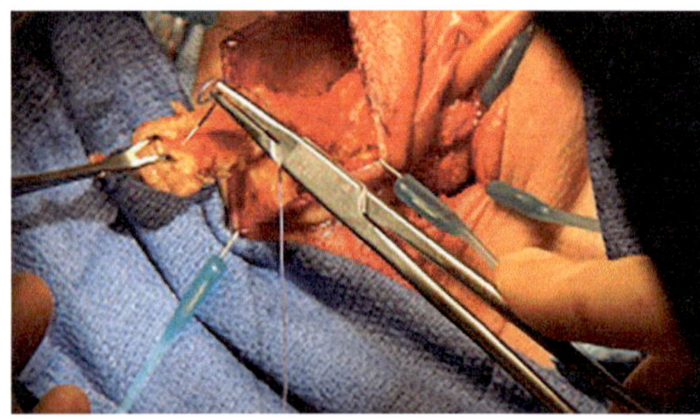

Fig. 29.3 After completing the fat pad mobilization, the extremity of the flap is secured with a figure of eight absorbable suture, which will allow its transfer alongside the vaginal wall and then anteriorly around the urethra

Step 4. After completing the fat pad mobilization, the extremity of the flap is secured with a figure-of-eight absorbable suture, which will allow its transfer alongside the vaginal wall and then anteriorly around the urethra (Fig. 29.3). The MFLP can be measured (Fig. 29.4). Then, a vaginal tunnel is created with long Metzenbaum scissors and/or a ring forceps beneath the ipsilateral vaginal wall. This tract is widened to accept at least two fingers to avoid compressing the fat pad and compromising its blood supply. Once tunnelled, the suture at the end of the fat pad graft is grasped and the MFLP is delivered in the vagina. Next, with a curved short Satinsky

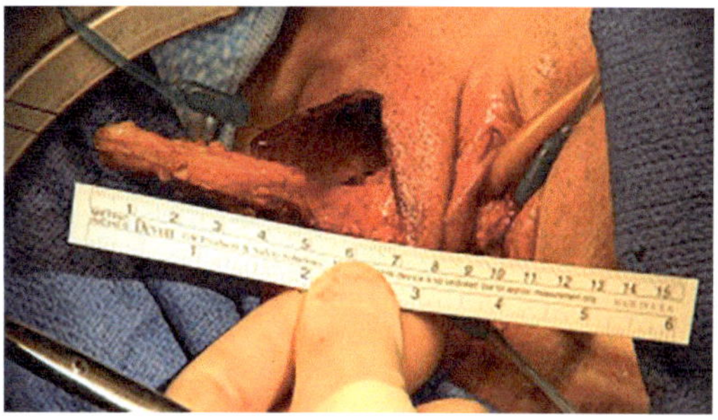

Fig. 29.4 The flap length can be measured

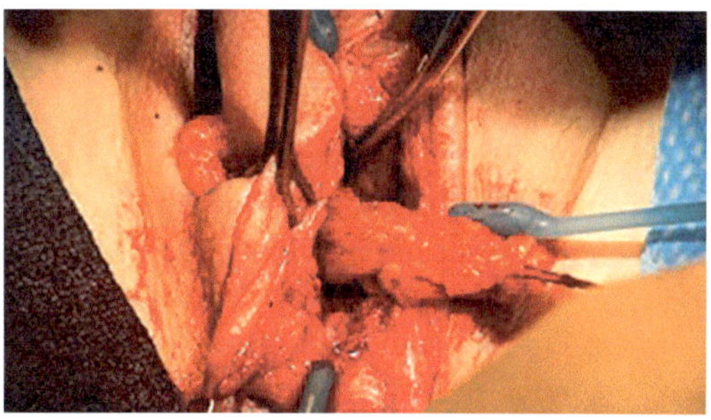

Fig. 29.5 With a curved short Satinsky clamp, the suture at the end of the Martius labial fat pad is grasped and is pulled from right to left in front of the urethra and bladder neck area

clamp, the suture at the end of the MFLP is grasped and the MFLP is pulled from right to left in front of the urethra and bladder neck area (Fig. 29.5) to serve as an interposition layer so that the urethra does not get attracted back by scar tissue to the back of the pubic bone.

Step 5. The labial incision is closed with interrupted absorbable sutures, over a small labial drain to prevent a secondary hematoma. This small drain is usually removed within 24 hours postoperatively. The vaginal incision is now closed with running sutures and the vagina is packed at the end (Fig. 29.6). A tight dressing is placed over the labia to avoid labial swelling post-operatively. We usually cover the skin incision with a vaseline gauze covered by fluffs and an ABD dressing secured with paper or silk tape over the fluffs to maintain them in place. Ice packs can be used as well.

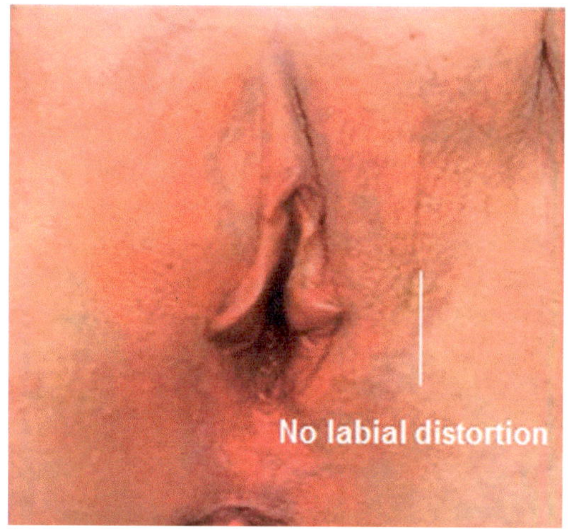

Fig. 29.6 Healed labia 1 year later

Antibiotic prophylaxis is usually administered and some publications mention antibiotics for a few days without giving any details on duration or antibiotic class.

Indications

MFLP has been used in the repair of uro-genital fistulae (vesico-vaginal fistulae [2, 3] and urethrovaginal fistulae [4–6] or after the closure of a recto-vaginal fistula, especially after obstetrics trauma [7–9]. It has also been used for filling large defects after mesh sling [10] or prolapse mesh removal procedures [11] or after an iatrogenic bladder injury, especially after hysterectomy [3, 6]. Other indications are for the prevention of a secondary fistula. For example, MFLP has been used after extensive urethral diverticulum repair [12, 13], after a trans-vaginal bladder neck closure in neurogenic patients with a completely destroyed outlet to reinforce the bladder neck closure [13], and after transvaginal urethrolysis [14, 15]. Rare indications have also been reported, such as after a vaginally placed artificial urinary sphincter to avoid a secondary exposure, after a neobladder-vaginal fistula repair [16, 17], after postcystectomy peritoneovaginal fistulae [18], or for vaginal reconstruction with skin attachment in case of a narrow vagina or a vaginal wall closure defect [19, 20].

Results from Reported Series and Case Reports

Malde et al. published the largest series of MLCP, including 159 patients over 10 years. They found a success rate of 95% for vulvovaginal repair ($n = 43$), 100% for female urethroplasty ($n = 12$), 100% for urethral diverticulectomy ($n = 74$), 100% urethral erosion of tape ($n = 24$), and 100% for vaginal closure of bladder neck ($n = 4$) [12]. MFLP has also been used for treating female stricture. Gul et al. reported a 100% cure rate after buccal mucosa graft urethroplasty [21], whereas Oliver et al. reported 2/11 urethrolysis failures [15]. The success rate of repairing a rectovaginal fistula was between 83.3% and 93.3% [9, 22, 23]. Taking all studies together, i.e., studies and case reports, there were 33/653 failures of surgeries combined with a Martius flap. Of course, case reports included a major bias because the surgery was always successful.

MFLP seems to increase the success rate of an ano-rectovaginal fistula with obstetrical anal sphincter injury repair compared to an endorectal advancement flap [24]. In the only prospective and randomized study reported so far, flap versus no flap for rectovaginal repair, the Martius flap did not demonstrate superiority. Success rate was 96.1% vs 96% without flap [23]. Another study compared MFLP to fibrin glue for vesicovaginal repair and did not find a significant difference in dryness rate (13/19 patients dry with the glue vs 11/19 with MFLP). Of note, more than 60% had a previous fistula repair [25].

Complications

Hematoma or Seroma

One of the benefits of the MFLP as a tissue interposition is its vascularity, but this contributes to the post-operative risk of bleeding and hematoma formation. Hematoma or seroma is a rare event. It has been reported in 3 series and affected 6 patients [12, 23, 26]. Kasyan et al. also reported lymphorrea in 5/37 patients [26].

Ensuring adequate hemostasis at the site of harvest as well as on the pedicle graft itself is of utmost importance in preventing hematoma formation. The use of a drain (Penrose or Jackson-Pratt) postoperatively may also decrease the likelihood of hematoma formation.

Typically, seromas and hematomas, when they occur, will resolve on their own over time without any intervention.

Infection

The incidence of infection after MFLP is rarely reported. A wound infection has been reported in 11 patients, a urinary tract infection in 1 patient, and a vaginal infection in 1 patient [12, 15, 26–28]. Prescription of antibiotics has been noted in some series and may decrease this risk [24, 27]. Practices are heterogeneous, and most series do not provide any details. Trompetto et al. administered an antibiotic prophylaxis with metronidazole and cephalosporin to all patients [9]. Local bactericidal use has also been used by Singh et al.; they packed the vagina with loose sterile cotton gauze soaked in 0.3% povidone iodine and removed it after 24 hours [23].

In case of labial erythema and/or purulent drainage from the incision, prompt drainage is indicated.

Pain

Some pain is expected in the immediate postoperative period and will usually last a few days, especially if a drain has been placed, and in case of swelling. Ice packs and loose underwear are suggested initially. In only one prospective randomized study, 4/29 MLFP patients operated for a vesicovaginal fistula complained of pain [23]. Chronic pain from a possible nerve injury during the MFLP, resulting in discomfort all the time or with intercourse, and/or excessive labial sensitivity, is a rare complication as well, but can be very debilitating [13, 26]

Sexual Dysfunction and Vulvar Sensitivity [13, 23, 26, 29]

Sexual dysfunction secondary to an MFLP is a complex matter because this interposition is used in re-operative situations where the vaginal wall can already be compromised by scar and some element of pre-existing denervation. Dyspareunia has been reported in two series in 6/24 patients [29, 30]. Sexual function is rarely assessed. However, in a series of 13 patients operated for urethral stricture, sexual function improved after surgery, with a median total FSFI score increased by 17.40 [21]. Lee D et al. described a post-operative median FSFI score between 24–29/36 according to the MFLP indication. Decreased sensation or numbness is more frequent and has been reported in 12.5 to 62% of patients [23, 26, 29, 30].

Wound Dehiscence

Wound dehiscence is a frequent complication of vulvar surgery, especially for vulvar cancer [31, 32]. However, it is rare with MFLP because the labia majora is soft and not under tension. Wound dehiscence has been reported in 4 patients. In the Hadi et al. case report, a wound dehiscence happened at D12 and resolved after 8 weeks. In Kavalious et al., the dehiscence happened at D7 and resolved by 5 weeks. Topical oestrogen may improve the quality of tissue [21, 33].

Labial Distortion

The removal of this fat pad from the labia majora can result in labial asymmetry or distortion later on. The incision should be slightly lateral to avoid distorting the medial aspect of the labia majora and to preserve sufficient fat under the skin edges. Two studies interviewed patients by telephone about their self-perception of labial appearance. Seventeen percent of patients (4/24) reported an aesthetic problem in the study by Kasyan et al., while 2/8 considered the change to be minor in the Perou et al. study; In 1/8, the change was reported to be major compared to the contralateral side [26, 30]. In the Study of Malde et al., the majority of patients (127 or 79%) found the post-operative appearance of their labia "as good or excellent" [12].

Conclusion

Harvesting an MFLP is part of the armamentarium of the pelvic reconstructive surgeon. It is a very traditional procedure that has a multitude of indications. In our experience, the morbidity, both early and late, is very limited, with rare labial distortion, permanent pain, or impact on sexual function. However, although uncommon, these complications should be clearly explained and discussed pre-operatively with the patient. Despite these recognized limitations, MFLP remains a very versatile and useful native tissue interposition graft that merits consideration in several specific instances.

References

1. Lee D, Dillon BE, Zimmern PE. Martius labial fat pad procedure: technique and long-term outcomes. Int Urogynecol J. 2015;26:1395–6.
2. Eilber KS, Kavaler E, Rodríguez LV, Rosenblum N, Raz S. Ten-year experience with transvaginal vesicovaginal fistula repair using tissue interposition. J Urol. 2003;169:1033–6.
3. Rangnekar NP, Imdad Ali N, Kaul SA, Pathak HR. Role of the martius procedure in the management of urinary-vaginal fistulas. J Am Coll Surg. 2000;191:259–63.
4. Patil U, Waterhouse K, Laungani G. Management of 18 difficult vesicovaginal and urethrovaginal fistulas with modified Ingelman-Sundberg and Martius operations. J Urol. 1980;123:653–6.
5. Kołodyńska A, Streit-Ciećkiewicz D, Kot A, Kuliniec I, Futyma K. Radiation-induced recurrent Vesicovaginal fistula-treatment with adjuvant platelet-rich plasma injection and Martius flap placement-case report and review of literature. Int J Environ Res Public Health. 2021;18:4867.
6. Chodisetti S, Boddepalli Y, Kota MR. Concomitant repair of stress urinary incontinence with proximal urethrovaginal fistula: our experience. Indian J Urol. 2016;32:229–31.
7. Elkins TE, DeLancey JO, McGuire EJ. The use of modified Martius graft as an adjunctive technique in

vesicovaginal and rectovaginal fistula repair. Obstet Gynecol. 1990;75:727–33.
8. Lee D, Zimmern PE. Long-term functional outcomes following non-radiated urethrovaginal fistula repair. World J Urol. 2016;34:291–6.
9. Trompetto M, et al. Use of the Martius advancement flap for low rectovaginal fistulas. Colorectal Dis. 2019;21:1421–8.
10. Mishra VV, Tanvir T, Choudhary S, Goraniya N. A transvaginal removal and repair of vesicovaginal fistula due to mesh erosion. J Life Health. 2016;7:97–9.
11. Al-Badr A. Martius graft for management of exposed vaginal prolapse mesh. J Minim Invasive Gynecol. 2013;20:227–9.
12. Malde S, et al. The uses and outcomes of the Martius fat pad in female urology. World J Urol. 2017;35:473–8.
13. Lee D, Dillon BE, Zimmern PE. Long-term morbidity of Martius labial fat pad graft in vaginal reconstruction surgery. Urology. 2013;82:1261–6.
14. Martius flap harvest site: patient self-perception - PubMed. https://pubmed.ncbi.nlm.nih.gov/11956448/.
15. Oliver JL, Raz S. Suprameatal urethrolysis with Martius flap for refractory bladder outflow obstruction following stress incontinence surgery in females. Neurourol Urodyn. 2018;37:449–57.
16. Okada Y, et al. Anterior enterocele immediately after cystectomy: a case report. J Obstet Gynaecol Res. 2020;46:2446–9.
17. Carmel ME, Goldman HB, Moore CK, Rackley RR, Vasavada SP. Transvaginal neobladder vaginal fistula repair after radical cystectomy with orthotopic urinary diversion in women. Neurourol Urodyn. 2016;35:90–4.
18. Blander DS, Zimmern PE, Lemack GE, Sagalowsky AI. Transvaginal repair of postcystectomy peritoneovaginal fistulae. Urology. 2000;56:320–1.
19. Carr LK, Webster GD. Full-thickness cutaneous martius flaps: a useful technique in female reconstructive urology. Urology. 1996;48:461–3.
20. The Martius flap neovagina revisited - PubMed. https://pubmed.ncbi.nlm.nih.gov/16174252/.
21. Gul D, et al. Ventral onlay buccal mucosa graft urethroplasty for female urethral stricture improves female sexual functions. Int J Impot Res. 2023; https://doi.org/10.1038/s41443-023-00743-z.
22. Dobrovodsky A, Pechan J, Duffek M, Skuta R, Hustak R. Modified Martius graft - a renaissance of surgical procedure. Bratisl Lek Listy. 2022;123:389–94.
23. Singh V, Mehrotra S, Bansal A, Akhtar A, Sinha RJ. Prospective randomized comparison of repairing vesicovaginal fistula with or without the interposition flap: result from a tertiary care Institute in Northern India. Turk J Urol. 2019;45:377–83.
24. Venara A, et al. Ano-rectovaginal fistula after obstetrical anal sphincter injury: diverting stoma does not improve the surgical results. Color Dis. 2022;24:1371–8.
25. Safan A, Shaker H, Abdelaal A, Mourad MS, Albaz M. Fibrin glue versus martius flap interpositioning in the repair of complicated obstetric vesicovaginal fistula. A prospective multi-institution randomized trial. Neurourol Urodyn. 2009;28:438–41.
26. Kasyan G, Tupikina N, Pushkar D. Use of Martius flap in the complex female urethral surgery. Cent Eur J Urol. 2014;67:202–7.
27. Osman NI, et al. The modified prone Jack-knife position for the excision of female urethral diverticula. Eur Urol. 2021;79:290–7.
28. Shaker H, Saafan A, Yassin M, Idrissa A, Mourad MS. Obstetric vesico-vaginal fistula repair: should we trim the fistula edges? A randomized prospective study. Neurourol Urodyn. 2011;30:302–5.
29. McNevin MS, Lee PYH, Bax TW. Martius flap: an adjunct for repair of complex, low rectovaginal fistula. Am J Surg. 2007;193:597–9; discussion 599.
30. Petrou SP, Jones J, Parra RO. Martius flap harvest site: patient self-perception. J Urol. 2002;167:2098–9.
31. Sinnott CJ, Glickman LT, Natoli NB, Dobryansky M, Veeramachaneni HB. Outcomes, techniques, and risk factors for dehiscence in central wedge Labiaplasty. Ann Plast Surg. 2020;85:S68.
32. Senn B, Mueller MD, Cignacco EL, Eicher M. Period prevalence and risk factors for postoperative short-term wound complications in vulvar cancer: a cross-sectional study. Int J Gynecol Cancer. 2010;20:646–54.
33. Karp DR, et al. A randomized clinical trial of the impact of local estrogen on postoperative tissue quality after vaginal reconstructive surgery. Urogynecology. 2012;18:211.

30 Autologous Graft Harvest Complications

Ava A. Delu, Lacey Hart, Joel T. Funk, and Christian O. Twiss

Introduction

The use of autologous fascia has been well-established in the graft-augmented treatment of stress urinary incontinence (SUI) and pelvic organ prolapse (POP). In 1942, Aldridge described the use of the external oblique aponeurosis as an autologous pubovaginal sling [1]. The autologous rectus fascia pubovaginal sling was popularized by McGuire et al. in 1978; this served as a treatment option for patients with SUI and low urethral closure pressure or a fixed, scarred urethra due to prior surgical interventions [2]. In 2001, Foley et al. described a minimally invasive technique for the harvest of fascia lata of the lower limb for use as a pubovaginal sling [3]. In addition to their use as autologous pubovaginal slings, both rectus fascia and fascia lata grafts serve as alternatives to synthetic mesh in sacrocolpopexy. Abraham et al. highlighted a rectus fascia graft harvest for use in a transabdominal sacrocolpopexy procedure to mitigate the risks of extrusion and infection associated with synthetic mesh [4]. In 2004, Latini et al. reported their experience with the use of fascia lata in abdominal sacrocolpopexy, highlighting similar efficacy compared to other graft materials and no significant morbidity [5]. While rectus fascia is the more commonly used autologous graft in pelvic surgery, fascia lata has been shown to be an acceptable and efficacious alternative, particularly in patients with poor quality rectus fascia due to prior abdominal surgeries, significant central obesity, or in instances in which a larger graft harvest is required [5].

The Food and Drug Administration's (FDA) reclassification of transvaginal mesh as a high-risk device has created a resurgence in the use of autologous grafts for stress incontinence and a renaissance in the application of autologous grafts in the surgical management of pelvic organ prolapse [6, 7]. Synthetic mesh is frequently used in urogynecologic procedures, but it carries the risk of mesh-related complications [8]. Although xenograft and allograft may be considered options in graft augmented procedures, these tissues have variable biomechanical durability and the potential for disease transmission [9]. While rectus fascia and fascia lata offer a biocompatible graft-augmented approach in the treatment of POP and SUI, complications do exist. The aim of this chapter is to highlight potential morbidities associated with autologous rectus and fascia lata grafts and strategies to prevent and treat potential complications.

A. A. Delu · L. Hart · J. T. Funk · C. O. Twiss (✉)
Department of Urology, University of Arizona College of Medicine, Tucson, AZ, USA
e-mail: ctwiss@urology.arizona.edu

H. B. Goldman, J. Zillioux (eds.), *Complications of Urogynecology and Reconstructive Pelvic Surgery*, https://doi.org/10.1007/978-3-032-00339-3_30

Rectus Fascia Graft Harvest Complications

Hernia

Abdominal wall hernia at the incision site is a known complication of autologous rectus fascia harvest, and larger harvests are generally associated with a higher risk of hernia formation [10, 11]. Chai et al. reviewed complications reported in the Stress Incontinence Surgical Efficacy Trial, a randomized trial that compared Burch colposuspension to the autologous rectus fascia sling, and found a 1.2% rate of hernias in patients who underwent a recuts fascia harvest for pubovaginal sling placement [12]. A systematic review by Matak et al. reported a 5% rate of ventral hernia and a 15% rate of dehiscence of the abdominal wall in patients undergoing rectus fascia colpopexy [13].

Evaluation of incisional hernias after rectus fascia harvest initially involves history and physical exam at the postoperative visit [14]. An abdominal wall protrusion that is more prominent with increased abdominal pressure is often present. Patients may be asymptomatic or report an abdominal bulge, pain, activity limitations, or additional symptoms if obstruction of intra-abdominal organs is present. Gomelsky et al. reported a case of an incisional bladder hernia after a rectus fascia sling harvest in which the patient presented with suprapubic fullness and worsening urinary incontinence [10]. Abdominal palpation can often reveal the presence and dimensions of the defect and may allow for palpation of the contents. Imaging may be necessary, especially when the physical exam is limited by patient body habitus or in complex cases [15]. Computed tomography (CT) scan is the most commonly used imaging modality utilized in the evaluation of incisional hernias and planning a repair [16]. Ultrasound and magnetic resonance imaging are less frequently used [17].

Management of ventral hernias involves conservative management vs surgical repair (open, robotic, or laparoscopic); surgical repair often involves mesh and may require referral to a general surgeon [18]. Symptomatic and large hernias are typically repaired, while asymptomatic and small hernias may be safely observed [19].

Prevention of hernias associated with rectus fascia harvest begins with patient selection. Some patients presenting for procedures involving rectus fascia harvest may have central obesity or a prior history of abdominal surgery, including prior Pfannenstiel incisions, abdominoplasty, Cesarean section, or prior ventral hernia repairs. Patients with this history who undergo rectus fascia harvest are at increased risk for wound complications, including incisional hernias, and may not be appropriate candidates [20]. In these cases, or in situations in which a larger graft is needed, a fascia lata harvest may be indicated. Comorbid conditions (diabetes, chronic steroid use, active tobacco consumption, etc.) that are associated with poor wound healing should be optimized before harvest. Intraoperatively, the closure should ensure proper re-approximation of the rectus fascia with slow-absorbing monofilament suture [21].

Infection

All surgical procedures convey a risk of operative site infection, affecting up to 2–5% of all inpatient surgeries [22]. Minimizing this complication should be of utmost importance to all members of the care team, as surgical site infection adds an average of 7–11 days to a patient's hospitalization [22]. Infection increases a patient's risk of mortality up to 11-fold, and represents a burden of up to $10 billion on the US healthcare system [20]. Like all surgeries, autologous harvests carry a risk of infection or cellulitis, although rates of this morbidity are low in the literature.

Peng et al. noted that four of 84 patients in the rectus fascia harvest group experienced wound complications, of which one required surgical drainage [23]. Cardenas-Trowers et al. compared the perioperative outcomes of autologous bladder neck slings with rectus fascia vs. fascia lata using the American College of Surgeons National Surgical Quality Improvement Program database. Of the 126 patients who underwent rectus fascia harvest, two experienced superficial wound infection, and none experienced a deep tissue infection. This represented a non-statistically significant difference between the rectus fascia and fascia lata groups [24].

Onset of infection may take days to weeks, and patients may endorse fever, worsening pain, or discharge from the operative site. Physical exam findings may include erythema or induration of the incision or surrounding tissue, purulent or non-purulent drainage, and dehiscence or a sinus tract [22].

Management of harvest site infection follows the same principles as those of other incision site infections, such as use of intravenous vs. oral antibiotics, drainage of fluid collections, and debridement of infected or necrotic tissue as necessary.

It is preferable to take appropriate steps to avoid infection altogether. In the preoperative period, data support avoiding operative site hair removal where possible, and using clippers instead of razors when necessary. This should ideally be done before the patient's arrival in the operating room. The operative site should be prepared with an antiseptic agent to reduce the skin flora burden prior to incision, and the patient should receive prophylactic antibiotics no more than 60 minutes prior to incision. Antibiotics should be re-dosed throughout the procedure as appropriate, with cessation of prophylactic antibiotics at wound closure [22].

Nerve Injury: Harvest Site Pain, Paresthesia, or Numbness

Nerve injury after rectus fascia harvest presents as postoperative pain, paresthesia, or numbness at the incision site. Some patients may report unilateral discomfort on one side of the Pfannenstiel incision and this may last for several weeks. This may be secondary to irritation from dissection or pain from sling sutures in the case of an autologous pubovaginal sling [25]. Cardenas-Trowers et al. determined a "safety zone" for autologous rectus fascia harvests based on dissections of the ilioinguinal and iliohypogastric nerves: 5.4 cm superior to the pubic symphysis and an inferior graft border measuring 9.4 cm in length [26]. These dimensions represented the largest safety zone that would avoid nerve injury. Ducic et al. performed a systematic review investigating abdominoplasty-related nerve injuries and found a rate of 1.46% (30/2061) for incisional nerve injury, with the most common deficits involving decreased sensation (hypesthesia or anesthesia) on the abdominal wall and pain or neuroma [27]. The most commonly injured nerves are the lateral femoral cutaneous (LFCN) and iliohypogastric nerves [27].

Evaluation of nerve injury after rectus fascia harvest involves a thorough history and physical exam to rule out other potential causes, including hernia, seroma, or infection. Patients may report burning pain, numbness, paresthesia, or allodynia located near the incision or within the sensory distribution of the affected nerve [27]. Neuropathic pain may be elicited with pinching or pressure over the affected area and may include a positive Tinel's sign [27]. If the diagnosis remains unclear, a nerve block utilizing local anesthetic may be used to confirm injury of the suspected nerve [27].

Conservative treatment serves as the initial management of nerve injury associated with the recuts fascia harvest. Physical therapy or patient-driven therapy with scar massage and desensitization techniques represent first-line treatments given that associated symptoms may resolve over time [27]. It is recommended to limit opioid medications, but multimodal pain control (nonopioids, antidepressants, anticonvulsants) and nerve blocks or steroid injections may provide relief [27]. Patients with bothersome symptoms, particularly pain that does not resolve within 6 months, may be candidates for referral for surgical decompression of the involved nerve [28].

Nerve injuries in this setting can best be avoided with a thorough understanding of the necessary anatomy, restricting dissection near susceptible areas (e.g., anterior superior iliac spine), avoiding wide dissection planes, and an awareness of anatomic variants, such as the relationship between the lateral femoral cutaneous nerve and anterior superior iliac spine [27]. To manage and avoid significant pain in the initial postoperative setting, a primed pain pump catheter may be placed subcutaneously in the rectus fascia site prior to closure with removal prior to discharge [29].

Seroma

Seroma is the accumulation of serous fluid within a potential space containing lymphatic fluid and plasma [30]. The typical rectus fascia harvest procedure parallels that of abdominoplasty, which has a 10–15% incidence rate of seroma formation [31]. Peng et al. investigated the perioperative outcomes of autologous fascia lata versus rectus fascia in pubovaginal slings [23]. Seroma formation occurred in 9 of the 84 women who underwent rectus fascia harvest.

Patients experiencing seroma formation at the rectus fascia harvest site are typically diagnosed via physical exam in the postoperative period. A fluctuant bulge or swelling at the incision site is noted. This may be asymptomatic or associated with pain, drainage, wound dehiscence, or functional limitations [30]. Ultrasonography (US) is not typically indicated to make a diagnosis; however, US imaging may be helpful in cases of uncertain diagnosis or failed treatment [32].

Management of seromas is based on size and associated symptoms. Small volume seromas that are not associated with wound closure strain, pain, or functional limitations will typically respond to conservative management and reabsorb over time [30]. Larger seromas (>75–100 cc) may present with pain, infection, or functional deficits of the associated area [33]. Aspiration is often indicated in these cases and may be carried out at the bedside or in the clinic [34]. Multiple aspirations may be indicated in cases of recollection with consideration for ultrasound-guided aspiration [32]. Rarely, open drainage and debridement are indicated for encapsulated pseudocysts or infectious cases [33]. Aspirated fluid may be sent for analysis as indicated [35].

To avoid seromas at the rectus fascia harvest site, patients are advised to refrain from activities that place strain on the incision for 4–6 weeks. Literature investigating seromas in the setting of abdominoplasty highlights other prevention techniques. Patients deemed to be at higher risk for seroma formation may be advised to wear an abdominal binder for several weeks postoperatively [36]. A Jackson-Pratt drain may also be placed subcutaneously to evacuate residual fluid and blood at the surgical site [36]. In a systematic review, Seretis et al. reported additional techniques including progressive tension sutures, preservation of Scarpa's fascia, and utilization of adhesives or fibrin sealants [37]. It is also recommended to avoid excessive cautery dissection of soft tissue, to close incisional dead space, and to ligate blood and lymph vessels as they are encountered during the dissection [38].

Vascular Complications

Rectus fascia harvest may lead to hematoma formation near the harvest site due to excessive retraction, inadvertent vessel laceration, or poor hemostasis [39]. A study by Peng et al. highlighted the perioperative outcomes of autologous fascia lata versus rectus fascia in pubovaginal slings. They reported a higher incidence of wound complications, such as hematoma and higher blood loss in the rectus fascia group compared to the fascia lata group [23]. Conversely, in a similar comparative study, Cardenas-Trowers et al. reported that the blood transfusion rate in patients undergoing the rectus fascia harvest was low and not statistically significantly different from that in the fascia lata harvest group [24].

Physical exam typically reveals a tender bulge near the harvest site with possible serosanguinous drainage, and patients may report incisional pain [39]. Hernia, seroma, and infection need to be ruled out. US or CT may be utilized for further hematoma characterization [40]. Conservative management with activity limitation and compressive wraps for small and largely asymptomatic hematomas (no skin breakdown, wound dehiscence, etc.) is a reasonable treatment [41]. Symptomatic hematomas may require management with drainage or debridement as indicated, and fascial re-approximation [39]. Early treatment may help prevent wound dehiscence or fascial disruption [39].

Anticoagulation medications should be held for an appropriate period of time preoperatively. Intraoperatively, it is recommended to avoid (1) excessive retraction, (2) inclusion of muscle in the fascial closure, (3) laceration of epigastric vessels, and (4) inadequate hemostasis [39]. A Jackson-Pratt suction drainage may be utilized in the early postoperative period to prevent hematoma, and patients should also be advised to avoid activities that place strain on the harvest site for 4–6 weeks and may be encouraged to wear a compressive dressing [29].

Deep Venous Thrombosis (DVT)

Studies suggest that the rates of DVT after rectus fascia harvest are low. A study by Cardenas-Trowers et al. comparing perioperative outcomes of rectus fascia vs. fascia lata slings in a group of 161 women found no significant difference in the rate of DVT between the groups (0.8% for the rectus fascia cohort and 0% for the fascia lata cohort) [24].

Femoropopliteal, iliofemoral, or isolated distal calf vein represent the three most frequent distributions of DVT [42]. Patients with acute DVT may be asymptomatic [43]. Postoperatively, small, distal, non-occlusive thrombi are more common [42]. Patients may report pain, edema, redness, erythema of the lower extremity, and fever [42]. Patients should also be questioned regarding chest pain and shortness of breath. Physical exam may reveal an edematous lower calf, a palpable" cord", erythematous skin, and tenderness [42, 44].

The National Institute for Clinical Excellence (NICE) guidelines outline the evaluation of DVT, which includes the following: D-dimers, coagulation profile, and lower extremity ultrasound [45]. DVT risk for individual patients is based on the Wells scoring system, which assesses the clinical probability of a DVT [46]. Anticoagulation remains the mainstay of treatment for DVT [44].

In the post operative period, sequential compression devices (SCDs) and subcutaneous heparin or enoxaparin are recommended for DVT prophylaxis according to risk [47]. Patients should also be encouraged to begin early ambulation within 24 hours after surgery.

Cosmesis

Little data exists on the cosmesis of rectus fascia harvest sites. In the absence of specific data, a more generalized approach may be adopted. It is important to recognize that there exists a general discrepancy in attitude towards surgical scars between patients and physicians. Among physicians, the importance of postoperative cosmesis varies among specialties and the circumstances of the surgery [48]. Patients, meanwhile, overwhelmingly report that they are dissatisfied with the appearance of their scars and would value even small improvements thereof, as discussed by Young et al. [49]

One option is to employ the use of validated tools and questionnaires such as the SCAR (Scar Cosmesis Assessment and Rating) scale. Use of this tool involves a series of clinician questions regarding scar spread, erythema, dyspigmentation, track marks or suture marks, and hypertrophy/atrophy, as well as patient questions regarding itch or pain associated with the scar. This scale has shown high reliability even when using photographs to evaluate a scar [50]. To address patient satisfaction, tools such as the Patient Attitudes to Scarring Scale (PASS) or Patient Scar Assessment Questionnaire may be used [51, 52]. A thorough evaluation should include asking the patient about pain and itching of the operative site, as these factors impact postoperative scarring [51].

Addressing scar cosmesis depends on the stage of healing of the operative site, as well as dual decision-making with the patient regarding the appropriate invasiveness of treatment. Topical treatments include silicone gel sheets or corticosteroids, pressure garments, or tension may be utilized in both scar management and prevention [53–56]. Invasive treatments or preventative options that may be used in conjunction with or after failure of topical options include laser therapy, microneedling, steroid injections, botulinum toxin injection, or surgical revision [57–61].

Techniques for minimizing surgical scarring start before the patient arrives in the operating room, including optimizing the patient's nutrition, smoking cessation, and appropriate blood glucose control in diabetic patients. In the operating room, time should be spent planning the incision; where possible, incisions should follow the relaxed skin tension lines [62, 63]. Once an incision is made, it is preferable to handle the deep dermal or subcutaneous layers instead of the superficial skin wherever possible and to be gentle when handling the skin surface. Care should be taken when closing the incision to minimize tension on the skin, and less reactive sutures used for patients who are prone to hypertrophic scarring [63]. In the immediate postoperative period, proper wound dressing assists with optimal healing. This includes choosing dressings that maintain moisture, prevent infection, and minimize inflammation [63, 64]. Table 30.1 summarizes the management and prevention strategies for complications of autologous fascial harvest.

Table 30.1 Summary of autologous fascia harvest complicatons, management, and prevention

Complication	Management	Preventative techniques
Hernia	Observation (rest, compressive garments) for small/asymptomatic defects Surgical repair with mesh for larger or symptomatic rectus fascia hernias Many surgical techniques available for lower extremity muscle hernias	Careful patient selection (e.g., severe obesity or multiple prior abdominal incisions) Optimize preoperative comorbidities (diabetes, chronic steroid use, smoking, etc.) Meticulous fascial closure with slow-absorbing monofilament suture Compressive bandage Activity limitations Proximal harvest site near the hip (fascia lata)
Infection	Local wound care Appropriate antibiotics (IV vs. PO) Drainage/debridement if indicated	Standard surgical site precautions Appropriate skin prep Prophylactic antibiotic administration with 60 minutes of incision
Nerve injury	Conservative measures (physical therapy, scar massage, non-opioid medications, nerve blocks, steroid injections) Surgery (decompression or neurectomy) rarely needed	Harvest graft within "safety zone" avoid wide dissection planes and excessive cautery Use of primed pain pump catheter in the postoperative period
Seroma	Conservative management if small and asymptomatic Aspiration or surgical drainage if larger and symptomatic	Refrain from strenuous activities for 4–6 weeks Avoid excessive cautery dissection of soft tissue Meticulous hemostasis Closure of dead space Use of closed-suction drainage Compressive bandage (abdominal binder or thigh wrap)
Vascular complications (hematoma)	Conservative management (compression, activity limitations) for small hematomas Larger or expanding hematomas may require drainage or debridement	Hold anticoagulants preoperatively Avoid excessive retraction Appropriate hemostasis Closed-suction drain Compressive bandage
Deep venous thrombosis (DVT)	Evaluation includes: D-dimers, coagulation profile, and lower extremity ultrasound Anticoagulation as mainstay of treatment	Sequential compression devices (SCDs) Heparin or enoxaparin for DVT prophylaxis Early ambulation
Cosmesis	Silicone gel pads, topical corticosteroids, pressure garments More invasive options include laser therapy, microneedling, steroid injections, botulinum toxin injection, or surgical revision	Optimization of preoperative comorbidities (nutrition, smoking cessation, blood glucose control) Gentle tissue handing Less reactive closure sutures (monofilament, synthetic) Proximal harvest site (fascia lata)

Fascia Lata Graft Complications

Hernia

Herniation, or muscle belly bulging of the vastus lateralis and biceps femoris, represents a known complication of fascia lata harvest. Although studies have documented a lower risk of wound complications, including hernias, with fascia lata harvests, the risk of muscle hernia is still present [23]. As the weakest fascial point in the lower extremity, the tibilais anterior is the most frequently reported muscle involved in hernias of the leg [65]. While herniation of muscle belly in the thigh is less common due to deeper fascia, iatrogenic hernias of the vastus lateralis and rectus femoris have been reported after fascia lata harvest. Burg et al. highlighted a case of muscle hernia after the fascia lata harvest was utilized in cruciate ligament repair [66]. Delu et al. reported nonpainful thigh bulges in 16 of 108 patients who underwent a large fascia lata harvest for pelvic organ prolapse repair [67]. Other studies have reported muscle herniation at the fascia lata defect at rates of 36% in patients undergoing ptosis surgery and 17% in patients undergoing pelvic reconstructive surgery [68, 69].

Patients with a muscle hernia may report a palpable bulge, soft tissue mass, or nodule near the fascia lata incision site. Patient cosmesis concerns often prompt the initial presentation [65]. The bulge may be asymptomatic or associated with pain, cramping, paresthesia, or weakness, often exacerbated by standing or physical activity. Herniation may be elicited with limb movements that cause muscle contraction; Chaus et al. reported identification of the vastus lateralis muscle bulge with knee extension during physical exam [29]. Hernia dimensions, reducibility, tenderness, lower extremity sensation, motor strength, and reflexes should also be elucidated. Diagnosis confirmation beyond physical exam involves ultrasonography (US) and, if equivocal, MRI of the affected limb. Although three-dimensional dynamic US provides visualization of fascial planes and muscle protrusion, MRI allows for greater musculofascial demarcation [70, 71]. Both imaging modalities are improved with dynamic techniques involving muscle movements [65].

Symptomatic muscle hernias are often amenable to conservative treatment (rest, activity restrictions, and compression garments) [72, 73]. Asymptomatic bulges do not require treatment. With conservative management, Delu et al. reported resolution in 50% (8 of 16) of patients presumably due to scar contraction over the fascial defect [67]. Patients who have failed conservative management with moderate to severe symptoms may be considered for operative repair. Many surgical techniques have been utilized in the repair of lower extremity muscle hernias with no absolute recommendations; these include decompressive fasciotomy, primary fascial repair, graft of fascial patch, augmentation with synthetic mesh, partial muscle excision, and injection of sclerosing agents, local anesthetics, or botulinum toxin [65].

Several techniques have been described to mitigate the development of muscle herniation at the fascia lata harvest site. Vitali et al. highlighted the use of bovine allograft in the repair of the fascia lata harvest site. In this retrospective review of 11 patients, there were no cases of muscle herniation [74]. Naugle et al. described a fascia lata harvest involving a proximal lateral leg incision (near the hip) vs. a few centimeters proximal to the knee. In their series of 23 patients, no patients developed muscle herniation, likely due to the deeper location of the fascia vs. that in the lower leg [75]. Patients should be counseled on the risk of hernia at the harvest site and advised to avoid activities that place excessive strain on the incision for 4–6 weeks after surgery. We recommend patients wear a mildly compressive bandage during this time for additional support.

Infection

Surgical site infections increase a patient's risk of morbidity and mortality and impose a burden on healthcare resources. The rate of wound infection in fascia lata harvest is lower than that of rectus fascia harvest. In their study of pubovaginal slings, Peng et al. and Govier et al.

reported no infections in a group of 21 patients and 32 patients, respectively, who underwent fascia lata harvest for sling surgery [23, 76]. Walter et al. reported five cases (7%) of incisional cellulitis that required oral antibiotics in a cohort of 71 patients who underwent autologous fascia lata harvest [69]. In a study of 108 large fascia lata harvests for pelvic organ prolapse repair, Delu et al. reported one patient who experienced a wound infection requiring IV antibiotics [67].

It is important to educate patients on the signs and symptoms of infection prior to discharge from the hospital, including fever, worsening pain at the incision site, and increased drainage. Physical exam findings may include erythema or induration of the incision or surrounding tissue, purulent or non-purulent drainage, wound dehiscence, or a sinus tract [22].

Patients who experience harvest site infection should receive appropriate local wound care, including debridement and intravenous vs. oral antibiotics as appropriate.

Validated infection prevention techniques are discussed above under the rectus fascia section.

Nerve Injury: Harvest Site Pain, Paresthesia, or Numbness

Cutaneous nerve injury after fascia lata harvest is a common complication and often presents with pain, paresthesia, or numbness. Injury may involve nerves of the lumbosacral plexus, including the ilioinguinal nerve, femoral branch of the genitofemoral nerve, lateral femoral cutaneous nerve, and cutaneous branch of the obturator nerve [77]. These nerves provide cutaneous innervation to the skin and penetrate the fascia lata [77].

Multiple studies report findings highlighting nerve disturbances after fascia lata harvest. In the study by Delu et al., which included large fascia lata harvests in 108 patients, the mean Visual Analog Pain (VAP) score was 1 (range: 0–10). In this study, all patients except for one (who later required a hip replacement ipsilateral to the harvest site) ultimately reported resolution of pain symptoms. Mild, non-bothersome paresthesia was the most common harvest site complication, occurring in 59 patients (53%) of whom 24 ultimately experienced resolution [67]. In a study by Govier et al., among 32 patients who underwent fascia lata autologous pubovaginal sling, one patient required 8 weeks to return to work and underwent physical therapy due to persistent pain near the knee, which ultimately resolved after 3 months [76]. In a study by Walter et al., subjective complaints were evaluated by questionnaire in 55 patients who underwent fascia lata harvest: 10 patients (19%) reported some amount of persistent numbness at the harvest site, and all patients noted that their discomfort level was mild [69]. Johnson et al. also highlighted patient-centered outcomes after fascia lata harvest for autologous pubovaginal sling, with 24% reporting leg discomfort, 17% reporting incision pain, 15% reporting incision numbness, and 17% reporting paresthesia at the harvest site. Nearly 83% of patients reported that these symptoms were non-bothersome [78].

Evaluation of pain, paresthesia, or numbness at the fascia lata harvest incision site should assess the degree of bother and impact on quality of life. Physical exam should include assessment of lower extremity motor strength and reflexes. Presence of a hematoma, seroma, hernia, or infection should be ruled out. Pinching or applying pressure over the affected area may elicit pain and a positive Tinel's sign in the distribution of the affected nerve [27]. A nerve block may be indicated in cases of unclear diagnosis [27].

Overall, the literature suggests that most neuropathic symptoms after fascia lata harvest are mild and do not cause significant bother or impact patients' quality of life. Moreover, many of these symptoms are self-limited and resolve without intervention. As such, conservative management is the mainstay of treatment, typically in the form of observation or physical therapy. If patients fail this approach, additional therapy with pain control, steroid injections, nerve blocks, and, if necessary, peripheral nerve surgery may be indicated [28].

Appropriate knowledge of the landmarks involved in fascia lata harvest is important to avoid nerve injury [79, 80]. Also, avoiding excessive dissection and use of cautery may aid in mitigating neuropathic symptoms in the postoperative setting. To manage pain in the initial postoperative setting, a primed pain pump catheter may be placed subcutaneously in the fascia lata harvest site prior to closure [29].

Seroma

Seromas represent a common postoperative complication at surgical incision sites and may occur at the site of fascia lata harvest. In the study by Peng et al., seroma formation occurred in 9 of the 84 women who underwent rectus fascia harvest and zero of the 21 women who underwent fascia lata harvest for pubovaginal slings [23]. Walter et al. reported 3% rate of seroma formation in their series of 71 fascia lata harvests [69], and Delu et al. reported that harvest site seroma occurred in 14% of patients undergoing large fascia lata harvest for pelvic organ prolapse repair [67].

Seromas of the lower extremity associated with fascia lata harvest are typically diagnosed by physical exam with or without associated pain, drainage, significant swelling, or activity limitations. A study by Chaus et al. investigating transvaginal repair of pelvic organ prolapse using autologous fascia lata reported the use of physical exam alone to diagnose thigh seromas, as additional testing has little effect on the management. Seromas in this study were identified as a fluid-filled bulge at the harvest site [29]. Other authors have reported on the use of imaging to diagnose lower extremity seromas using ultrasound, CT, and MRI [81, 82]. In cases of diagnostic uncertainty or treatment failure, these imaging modalities may be utilized.

Management of fascia lata harvest site seromas, similar to those occurring at the rectus fascia harvest site, is based on volume and associated symptoms. Most seromas of the lower extremity resolve spontaneously with conservative management. Seromas requiring intervention are typically managed with aspiration. In a study of large fascia lata harvests by Delu et al., patients proceeded through a treatment algorithm that involved expectant management alone or in-office seroma aspiration [67]. With these interventions, resolution occurred in 88% of patients. If a seroma is persistent or associated with infection, an indwelling drain or surgical excision and debridement may be needed [81].

Principles of seroma prevention involve placement of closed-suction drains at the time of surgery, ligation of vessels, and avoidance of activities that strain the harvest site [38]. Delu et al. noted a decrease in seroma formation with intraoperative placement of a Jackson-Pratt drain, which was removed prior to discharge [67]. Mild compression wraps are also recommended for 4–6 weeks postoperatively to aid in seroma prevention [29].

Vascular Complications

A hematoma may occur at the site of fascia lata harvest due to excessive retraction, rupture, or damage of blood vessels during the surgical procedure or poor hemostasis technique. Walter et al. reported that one patient (1%) experienced a hematoma that required drainage in the postoperative period in their review of 71 patients undergoing fascia lata harvest [69]. Delu et al. reported no cases of hematoma or blood transfusion in their investigation of a large fascia lata harvest in 108 patients [67]. A study by Bock et al. compared robotic sacrocolpopexy using autologous fascia lata vs. mesh and revealed one case of a hematoma requiring transfusion [83]. Cardenas-Trowers et al. compared the perioperative outcomes of autologous bladder neck fascia slings using rectus fascia vs. fascia lata grafts. Blood transfusion rates were low in the fascia lata group and not statistically different from those in the rectus fascia group [24]. In a study by Latini et al. evaluating the use of fascia lata in abdominal sacrocolpopexy, the mean blood loss was 107.5 cc, and no transfusions were required [5].

Physical exam of a hematoma associated with fascia lata harvest may demonstrate pain, tenderness, edema, erythema, or ecchymosis, and a bulge near the harvest site. Hernia, seroma, and infection at the harvest site should be ruled out. The incision should also be assessed for wound opening and signs of active bleeding [84]. Patients presenting with these signs in the early postoperative period are at a greater risk for tissue compromise, necrosis, and deep dissecting hematoma [84].

Patients without open wounds or evidence of deep hematoma may be managed conservatively with compression dressings, elevation, and activity limitation [84]. Local evacuation and drainage should be performed for patients without signs of compromised skin but with an open wound and active bleeding [84]. Hematoma extent may be determined with US or MRI [84]. Patients with signs of skin necrosis or deep dissecting hematoma should be managed surgically [84].

Preoperatively, the medical history should be reviewed for the use of anticoagulation medications, which should be held for an appropriate duration in the perioperative timeframe. Intraoperative management involves obtaining appropriate hemostasis and placement of a Jackson-Pratt drain until the patient is discharged. Naugle et al. highlighted a more proximal fascia lata harvest near the thigh compared to above the lateral knee, and they reported no instances of hematoma formation in this proximal harvest cohort [75]. Chibber et al. described a minimally invasive technique of fascia lata harvest involving the use of a fascial stripper with no reports of hematoma formation [85]. Patients should be encouraged to wear a mild compression bandage for 4–6 weeks postoperatively. While ambulation in the early postoperative period is encouraged to prevent DVT, patients should also be advised to avoid heavy physical activities that may place excessive strain on the harvest site.

Deep Venous Thrombosis (DVT)

Any form of pelvic surgery carries a risk of DVT, and there may be concern regarding increased rates of DVT after fascia lata harvest due to decreased mobility of the lower extremity in the postoperative setting. However, there is currently no compelling evidence to suggest that fascia lata graft harvests increase the risk of DVT. A study by Cardenas-Trowers et al. comparing perioperative outcomes of autologous bladder neck fascial slings (rectus fascia vs. fascia lata) in a group of 161 women found no significant difference in the rate of DVT between the groups (0.8% for the rectus fascia cohort and 0% for the fascia lata cohort) [24]. Bock et al. compared robotic sacrocolpopexy (RSC) utilizing autologous fascia lata to RSC using mesh; this study reported one case of DVT in the fascia lata group, but also highlighted that the rate of DVT in the fascia lata group was not statistically different from the mesh group [83]. In a cohort of 108 patients who underwent a large fascia lata harvest for use in POP repair, Delu et al. reported no instances of postoperative DVT [67].

The principles of diagnosis and management of DVT are the same as discussed above under the rectus fascia section. Additionally, in the case of fascia lata harvest, a compressive dressing should be maintained over the harvest site to support early ambulation; however, care should be taken to ensure that the dressing is not overly tight to the point that it is impairing circulation.

Compartment Syndrome

Compartment syndrome occurs when the pressure within a tissue space rises to a level that exceeds perfusion pressure, causing decreased perfusion to the involved tissue that may progress to necrosis without intervention. The mechanism by which compartment syndrome occurs involves either a decrease in the size of the tissue compartment, an increase in the contents within the compartment, or both [86, 87].

Harvesting of the fascia lata potentially decreases the compartment volume if the edges of the remaining fascial defect are reapproximated, and an increase of the compartment volume may occur secondary to edema or hemorrhage. Review of the literature on complications following fascia lata harvest rarely mentions compartment syndrome; while this complication is possible, it is rare. Rodriguez et al retrospectively analyzed 88 fascia lata harvests; of these, 64 patients had closure or imbrication of the fascia lata. Closure was not performed when the defect was >5 cm in size. None of these patients experienced compartment syndrome, though one required immediate fascial release prior to leaving the operating room due to loss of perfusion distally [63].

The diagnosis of compartment syndrome is crucial to make as early as possible to prevent irreversible tissue loss. The patient may provide the earliest indications; frequent patient complaints include pain that is severe, worsening, and out of proportion to their overall clinical appearance and the procedure performed. Physical exam, especially performed serially, is the primary means of diagnosis with findings classically described as the "five Ps": pain, paresthesia, pallor, paralysis, and pulselessness [86, 88].

Intracompartment pressure may be measured when uncertainty exists, though significant differences in measurement between observers have been noted, and differences in technique frequently result in measurements that do not accurately reflect the true pressure [86]. Additionally, the threshold pressure for diagnosing compartment syndrome is controversial. While some sources use 30- or 45-mm Hg as a threshold, it has also been noted that patients may be able to tolerate periods of a couple of hours at higher pressures without significant tissue ischemia [88]. As the exact pressure at which ischemia occurs varies among patients, the diagnosis of compartment syndrome should be made using all available clinical information and the judgment of the treating physician.

Once the diagnosis of compartment syndrome has been reached, the treatment is fasciotomy. The timeline of irreversible tissue damage differs depending on the patient, but in general, patients who undergo fasciotomy earlier have less irreversible ischemia than those who have delayed fasciotomy [89, 90].

Given the potentially devastating consequences of compartment syndrome, it is critical to avoid it wherever possible. One solution to this problem is to not close the defect in the fascia lata, as described by Chaus et al, who instead place a drain, then close the subcutaneous and cutaneous layers [29].

Activity Limitations

There are concerns that fascia lata harvests, particularly large harvests like those utilized in POP repair, may negatively impact functional outcomes and activity limitations. A study by Angelo et al. investigated the functional outcomes associated with the fascia lata harvest utilized in arthroscopic superior capsular reconstruction. In this cohort of 15 patients, no individual required postoperative physical therapy. The proportion of patients reporting daily activity limitation decreased from 20% at 1 week to 7% at 18 months. From 6 to 18 months, there was an increase in functional outcomes of the ipsilateral thigh that more closely paralleled that of the contralateral thigh [91]. Johnson et al. reported patient-centered outcomes of fascia lata harvest utilized in autologous pubovaginal sling placement, with approximately 10% of patients reporting leg weakness [78]. In a study by Amir et al., 43 patients underwent fascia lata harvest with no reported significant functional deficit [92].

Postoperative physical exam should include assessment of lower extremity motor function, sensation, and reflexes. The mainstay of treatment is physical therapy, and no further intervention is typically needed. Delu et al. reported that 5% of patients underwent physical therapy for leg weakness and harvest site pain after large fascia lata harvest, with all but one patient experiencing resolution of symptoms [67]. Referral to orthopedic surgery may be recommended for patients who fail physical therapy.

Utilizing the landmarks defined by Tay et al., Chaus et al. describe a technique for a large fascia lata harvest utilized in autologous pelvic organ prolapse repair and, if indicated, concurrent autologous pubovaginal sling placement [29, 79]. Destabilization of the knee and lateral thigh is prevented with a thorough understanding of harvest landmarks: the superior limit of harvest is the tensor fascia lata muscle (roughly 15 cm inferior to the anterior superior iliac spine), and the inferior limit of the harvest is 10 cm proximal to the lateral femoral condyle [29]. In the postoperative period, patients are advised to wear a compressive dressing around the harvest site for 4–6 weeks to support early ambulation. Avoidance of excessive use of the ipsilateral lower limb is also recommended [91].

Cosmesis

Cosmesis outcomes of the fascia lata harvest site represent a potential postoperative complication. Studies investigating patient-centered perspectives on leg incision cosmesis are largely derived from questionnaires and are often limited in quantity. Walter et al. investigated the harvest of autologous fascia lata for pelvic reconstructive surgery and included patient perceptions of outcome through the administration of a mailed questionnaire. Unacceptable cosmesis was reported by 8 of 55 patients (15%) [69]. Johnson et al. investigated patients' perspectives of the cosmesis of the fascia lata harvest in patients who underwent autologous pubovaginal sling placement. Twenty-nine patients met the inclusion criteria, with 72.4% reporting they were very or somewhat satisfied and 13.7% reporting they were dissatisfied or very dissatisfied regarding the look and feel of the leg incision [78]. Although limited, these studies suggest that patient counseling regarding cosmesis of the leg incision is necessary in the preoperative setting.

Evaluation and management of cosmesis related to the fascia lata harvest are the same as those discussed in the rectus fascia section above. Regarding intraoperative prevention, Naugle et al. also described the use of a high incision for fascia lata harvesting [75]. We recommended attempting to achieve as proximal of a leg incision as possible without risk of destabilization of the knee and lateral thigh. This will allow for more clothing coverage and less excision exposure. While staples facilitate a faster wound closure, a subcuticular closure provides a better cosmetic approach [93].

References

1. Aldridge AH. Transplantation of fascia for relief of urinary stress incontinence. Am J Obstet Gynecol. 1942;44(3):398–411. https://doi.org/10.1016/S0002-9378(42)90477-0.
2. McGuire EJ, Lytton B. Pubovaginal sling procedure for stress incontinence. J Urol. 1978;119(1):82–4. https://doi.org/10.1016/S0022-5347(17)57390-5.
3. Foley SJ, Adamson AS. Minimally invasive harvesting of fascia lata for use in the pubovaginal sling procedure. BJU Int. 2001;88(3):293–4. https://doi.org/10.1046/J.1464-410X.2001.02327.X.
4. Abraham N, Quirouet A, Goldman HB. Transabdominal sacrocolpopexy with autologous rectus fascia graft. Int Urogynecol J. 2016;27(8):1273–5. https://doi.org/10.1007/S00192-016-2987-7/METRICS.
5. Latini JM, Brown JA, Kreder KJ. Abdominal sacral colpopexy using autologous fascia lata. J Urol. 2004;171(3):1176–9. https://doi.org/10.1097/01.JU.0000103925.56765.BC.
6. Pelvic Organ Prolapse (POP): Surgical mesh considerations and recommendations | FDA. Accessed August 10, 2024. https://www.fda.gov/medical-devices/urogynecologic-surgical-mesh-implants/pelvic-organ-prolapse-pop-surgical-mesh-considerations-and-recommendations
7. Rac G, Younger A, Clemens JQ, et al. Stress urinary incontinence surgery trends in academic female pelvic medicine and reconstructive surgery urology practice in the setting of the food and drug administration public health notifications. Neurourol Urodyn. 2017;36(4):1155–60. https://doi.org/10.1002/NAU.23080.
8. Shah HN, Badlani GH. Mesh complications in female pelvic floor reconstructive surgery and their management: a systematic review. Indian J Urol. 2012;28(2):129–53. https://doi.org/10.4103/0970-1591.98453.
9. Claerhout F, De RD, Van BD, et al. Sacrocolpopexy using xenogenic acellular collagen in patients at increased risk for graft-related complications. Neurourol Urodyn. 2010;29(4):563–7. https://doi.org/10.1002/NAU.20805.
10. Gomelsky A, Dmochowski RR. Incisional bladder hernia after rectus fascial sling. J Urol. 2003;169(6):2299. https://doi.org/10.1097/01.JU.0000056728.52215.D7.
11. Flynn BJ, Yap WT. Pubovaginal sling using allograft fascia lata versus autograft fascia for all types of stress urinary incontinence: 2-year minimum followup. J Urol. 2002;167(2 Part 1):608–12. https://doi.org/10.1016/S0022-5347(01)69095-5.
12. Chai TC, Albo ME, Richter HE, et al. Complications in women undergoing burch colposuspension versus autologous rectus fascial sling for stress urinary incontinence. J Urol. 2009;181(5):2192–7. https://doi.org/10.1016/J.JURO.2009.01.019.

13. Matak L, Baekelandt J, Šimičević M, Matak M, Mikuš M, Orešković S. Comparison between fascia lata and rectus fascia in treatment of pelvic organ prolapse: a systematic review. Arch Gynecol Obstet. 2024;309(6):2395–400. https://doi.org/10.1007/S00404-024-07531-0.
14. Cherla DV, Bernardi K, Blair KJ, et al. Importance of the physical exam: double-blind randomized controlled trial of radiologic interpretation of ventral hernias after selective clinical information. Hernia. 2019;23(5):987–94. https://doi.org/10.1007/S10029-018-1856-3.
15. Halligan S, Parker SG, Plumb AA, Windsor ACJ. Imaging complex ventral hernias, their surgical repair, and their complications. Eur Radiol. 2018;28(8):3560–9. https://doi.org/10.1007/S00330-018-5328-Z.
16. Holihan JL, Karanjawala B, Ko A, et al. Use of computed tomography in diagnosing ventral hernia recurrence: a blinded, prospective, multispecialty evaluation. JAMA Surg. 2016;151(1):7–13. https://doi.org/10.1001/JAMASURG.2015.2580.
17. Hope W, Tuma F. Incisional hernia – StatPearls – NCBI Bookshelf. StatPearls [Internet]. Published June 12, 2023. Accessed August 10, 2024. https://www.ncbi.nlm.nih.gov/books/NBK435995/?report=reader
18. de Vries HS, Smeeing D, Lourens H, Kruyt PM, Mollen RMHG. Long-term clinical experience with laparoscopic ventral hernia repair using a ParietexTM composite mesh in severely obese and non-severe obese patients: a single center cohort study. Minim Invasive Ther Allied Technol. 2019;28(5):304–8. https://doi.org/10.1080/13645706.2018.1521431.
19. Dai W, Chen Z, Zuo J, Tan J, Tan M, Yuan Y. Risk factors of postoperative complications after emergency repair of incarcerated groin hernia for adult patients: a retrospective cohort study. Hernia. 2019;23(2):267. https://doi.org/10.1007/S10029-018-1854-5.
20. Ban KA, Minei JP, Laronga C, et al. American College of Surgeons and Surgical Infection Society: Surgical Site Infection Guidelines, 2016 Update. J Am Coll Surg. 2017;224(1):59–74. https://doi.org/10.1016/J.JAMCOLLSURG.2016.10.029.
21. Zucker BE, Simillis C, Tekkis P, Kontovounisios C. Suture choice to reduce occurrence of surgical site infection, hernia, wound dehiscence and sinus/fistula: a network meta-analysis. Ann R Coll Surg Engl. 2019;101(3):150–61. https://doi.org/10.1308/RCSANN.2018.0170.
22. Seidelman JL, Mantyh CR, Anderson DJ. Surgical site infection prevention: a review. JAMA. 2023;329(3):244–52. https://doi.org/10.1001/JAMA.2022.24075.
23. Peng M, Sussman RD, Escobar C, et al. Rectus fascia versus fascia lata for autologous fascial pubovaginal sling: a single-center comparison of perioperative and functional outcomes. Female Pelvic Med Reconstr Surg. 2020;26(8):493–7. https://doi.org/10.1097/SPV.0000000000000761.
24. Cardenas-Trowers OO, Stewart R, Meriwether KV, Francis S, Gupta A. Comparison of perioperative outcomes of autologous bladder neck fascial slings based on fascial harvest site: a secondary analysis of the National Surgical Quality Improvement Program Database. Female Pelvic Med Reconstr Surg. 2020;26(8):526–9. https://doi.org/10.1097/SPV.0000000000000773.
25. Goldman H. In: Goldman HB, editor. Complications of female incontinence and pelvic reconstructive surgery. Springer; 2017. https://doi.org/10.1007/978-3-319-49855-3.
26. Cardenas-Trowers OO, Bergden JS, Gaskins JT, Gupta AS, Francis SL, Herring NR. Development of a safety zone for rectus abdominis fascia graft harvest based on dissections of the ilioinguinal and iliohypogastric nerves. Am J Obstet Gynecol. 2020;222(5):480.e1–7. https://doi.org/10.1016/J.AJOG.2019.12.009.
27. Ducic I, Zakaria HM, Felder JM, Arnspiger S. Abdominoplasty-related nerve jnjuries: systematic review and treatment options. Aesthetic Surg J. 2014;34(2):284–97. https://doi.org/10.1177/1090820X13516341.
28. Ducic I, Dellon AL, Taylor NS. Decompression of the lateral femoral cutaneous nerve in the treatment of meralgia paresthetica. J Reconstr Microsurg. 2006;22(2):113–7. https://doi.org/10.1055/S-2006-932505.
29. Chaus FM, Funk JT, Pangilinan J, Lin FC, Twiss CO. Total autologous fascia lata anterior and apical pelvic organ prolapse repair: a new technique and initial experience. Urology. 2020;137:190–5. https://doi.org/10.1016/J.UROLOGY.2019.12.015.
30. Kazzam ME, Ng P. Postoperative seroma management. StatPearls Publishing; 2023. Accessed August 11, 2024. https://www.ncbi.nlm.nih.gov/books/NBK585101/
31. Hafezi F, Nouhi AH. Abdominoplasty and seroma. Ann Plast Surg. 2002;48(1):109–10. https://doi.org/10.1097/00000637-200201000-00022.
32. Goldman A, Wollina U, França K, Tchernev G, Lotti T. Chronic encapsulated seroma persisting for three years after abdominoplasty and a successful surgical solution. Open Access Maced J Med Sci. 2018;6(1):82–4. https://doi.org/10.3889/OAMJMS.2018.051.
33. H Turner EJ, Benson JR, Winters ZE. Techniques in the prevention and management of seromas after breast surgery. Future Oncol. 2014;10(6):1049–63. https://doi.org/10.2217/FON.13.257.
34. Warren M. Collaboration in developing a protocol for nurse-led seroma aspiration. Br J Nurs. 2008;17(15):956–60. https://doi.org/10.12968/BJON.2008.17.15.30697.
35. Klink CD, Binnebösel M, Lucas AH, et al. Do drainage liquid characteristics serve as predictors for seroma formation after incisional hernia repair? Hernia. 2010;14(2):175–9. https://doi.org/10.1007/S10029-009-0603-1.

36. Teimourian B. Management of seroma in abdominoplasty. Aesthetic Surg J. 2005;25(5):510–1. https://doi.org/10.1016/J.ASJ.2005.07.001/2/10.1016_J.ASJ.2005.07.001-FIG1.JPEG.
37. Seretis K, Goulis D, Demiri EC, Lykoudis EG. Prevention of seroma formation following abdominoplasty: a systematic review and meta-analysis. Aesthetic Surg J. 2017;37(3):316–23. https://doi.org/10.1093/ASJ/SJW192.
38. Janis JE, Khansa L, Khansa I. Strategies for postoperative seroma prevention: a systematic review. Plast Reconstr Surg. 2016;138(1):240–52. https://doi.org/10.1097/PRS.0000000000002245.
39. Henzel JH, Stephenson HE. Postoperative rectus hematoma: a preventable cause of wound dehiscence? Am J Surg. 1968;116(6):882–6. https://doi.org/10.1016/0002-9610(68)90459-5.
40. Pierro A, Cilla S, Modugno P, Centritto EM, De Filippo CM, Sallustio G. Spontaneous rectus sheath hematoma: the utility of CT angiography. Radiol Case Rep. 2018;13(2):328–32. https://doi.org/10.1016/J.RADCR.2018.01.016.
41. Teske JM. Hematoma of the rectus abdominis muscle; report of a case and analysis of 100 cases from the literature. Am J Surg. 1946;71(5):689–95. https://doi.org/10.1016/0002-9610(46)90453-9.
42. Waheed SM, Kudaravalli P, Hotwagner DT. Deep vein thrombosis. StatPearls Publishing; 2023. Accessed August 11, 2024. https://www.ncbi.nlm.nih.gov/books/NBK507708/
43. Naringrekar H, Sun J, Ko C, Rodgers SK. It's not all deep vein thrombosis: sonography of the painful lower extremity with multimodality correlation. J Ultrasound Med. 2019;38(4):1075–89. https://doi.org/10.1002/JUM.14776.
44. Schick MA, Pacifico L. Deep venous thrombosis of the lower extremity. StatPearls Publishing; 2022. Accessed August 11, 2024. https://www.ncbi.nlm.nih.gov/books/NBK470381/
45. National Institute for Health and Care Excellence (NICE). Venous thromboembolism in over 16s. NICE Guid. 2018;2(March):44. Accessed August 11, 2024. https://www.ncbi.nlm.nih.gov/books/NBK493720/
46. Modi S, Deisler R, Gozel K, et al. Wells criteria for DVT is a reliable clinical tool to assess the risk of deep venous thrombosis in trauma patients. World J Emerg Surg. 2016;11(1) https://doi.org/10.1186/S13017-016-0078-1.
47. Forrest JB, Clemens JQ, Finamore P, et al. AUA best practice statement for the prevention of deep vein thrombosis in patients undergoing urologic surgery. J Urol. 2009;181(3):1170–7. https://doi.org/10.1016/J.JURO.2008.12.027.
48. Lari A, Alherz M, Hussain S, et al. The importance of scar cosmesis across the surgical specialties: factors, perceptions, and predispositions. Plast Reconstr Surgery Glob Open. 2022;10(3):E4219. https://doi.org/10.1097/GOX.0000000000004219.
49. Young VL, Hutchison J. Insights into patient and clinician concerns about scar appearance: semi-quantitative structured surveys. Plast Reconstr Surg. 2009;124(1):256–65. https://doi.org/10.1097/PRS.0B013E3181A80747.
50. Kantor J. The SCAR (Scar Cosmesis Assessment and Rating) scale: development and validation of a new outcome measure for postoperative scar assessment. Br J Dermatol. 2016;175(6):1394–6. https://doi.org/10.1111/BJD.14812.
51. Kantor J. Utilizing the Patient Attitudes to Scarring Scale (PASS) to develop an outcome measure for postoperative scarring: a study in 430 patients. J Am Acad Dermatol. 2016;74(6):1280–1281.e2. https://doi.org/10.1016/j.jaad.2016.01.026.
52. Durani P, McGrouther DA, Ferguson MW. The Patient Scar Assessment Questionnaire: a reliable and valid patient-reported outcomes measure for linear scars. Plast Reconstr Surg. 2009;123(5):1481–9. https://doi.org/10.1097/PRS.0B013E3181A205DE.
53. MustoeTA.Siliconegelforscarprevention.In:Textbook on scar management. Springer; 2020. p. 203–8. https://doi.org/10.1007/978-3-030-44766-3_23.
54. Sheng M, Chen Y, Li H, Zhang Y, Zhang Z. The application of corticosteroids for pathological scar prevention and treatment: current review and update. Burn Trauma. 2023:11. https://doi.org/10.1093/BURNST/TKAD009.
55. Atkinson JAM, McKenna KT, Barnett AG, McGrath DJ, Rudd M. A randomized, controlled trial to determine the efficacy of paper tape in preventing hypertrophic sear formation in surgical incisions that traverse langer's skin tension lines. Plast Reconstr Surg. 2005;116(6):1648–56. https://doi.org/10.1097/01.PRS.0000187147.73963.A5.
56. Monstrey S, Middelkoop E, Vranckx JJ, et al. Updated scar management practical guidelines: non-invasive and invasive measures. J Plast Reconstr Aesthet Surg. 2014;67(8):1017–25. https://doi.org/10.1016/J.BJPS.2014.04.011.
57. Togsverd-Bo K. Early laser intervention for improved appearance of surgical scars. Br J Dermatol. 2019;180(1):25. https://doi.org/10.1111/BJD.17358.
58. Juhasz MLW, Cohen JL. Microneedling for the treatment of scars: an update for clinicians. Clin Cosmet Investig Dermatol. 2020;13:997–1003. https://doi.org/10.2147/CCID.S267192.
59. Chen MA, Davidson TM. Scar management: prevention and treatment strategies. Curr Opin Otolaryngol Head Neck Surg. 2005;13(4):242–7. https://doi.org/10.1097/01.MOO.0000170525.74264.F8.
60. Chen S, Yang Y, Zhang D, Liu Y, Li Y. Local injection of botulinum toxin type A to prevent postoperative scar. J Craniofac Surg. 2020;31(2):440–3. https://doi.org/10.1097/SCS.0000000000006144.
61. Garg S, Dahiya N, Gupta S. Surgical scar revision: an overview. J Cutan Aesthet Surg. 2014;7(1):3. https://doi.org/10.4103/0974-2077.129959.
62. Căiță GA, Lascu CF, Bodog FD, Buhaș CL, Voiță-Mekeres F, Voiță GF. Surgical scar management – an evaluation of surgical techniques. Med Pharm

Rep. 2024;97(2):149–53. https://doi.org/10.15386/MPR-2701.
63. Rodriguez ED, Bluebond-Langner R, Park J, You X, Rosson G, Singh N. Does fascia lata repair facilitate closure and does it affect compartment pressures of the anterolateral thigh flap donor site? Plast Reconstr Surg. 2007;120(5):1300–4. https://doi.org/10.1097/01.PRS.0000279347.40506.C6.
64. Liu A, Moy RL, Ozog DM. Current methods employed in the prevention and minimization of surgical scars. Dermatologic Surg. 2011;37(12):1740–6. https://doi.org/10.1111/J.1524-4725.2011.02166.X.
65. Nguyen JT, Nguyen JL, Wheatley MJ, Nguyen TA. Muscle hernias of the leg: a case report and comprehensive review of the literature. Can J Plast Surg. 2013;21(4):243. https://doi.org/10.1177/229255031302100408.
66. Burg D, Schnyder H, Buchmann R, Meyer VE. Effective treatment of a large muscle hernia by local botulinum toxin administration. Handchir Mikrochir Plast Chir. 1999;31(2):75–8. https://doi.org/10.1055/S-1999-13497.
67. Delu AA, Terrani KF, Funk JT, Twiss CO. Harvest of large fascia lata autograft: outcomes in 108 patients. Neurourol Urodyn. 2024;43(5):1179–84. https://doi.org/10.1002/NAU.25464.
68. Wheatcroft SM, Vardy SJ, Tyers AG. Complications of fascia lata harvesting for ptosis surgery. Br J Ophthalmol. 1997;81(7):581–3. https://doi.org/10.1136/BJO.81.7.581.
69. Walter AJ, Hentz JG, Magrina JF, Cornella JL. Harvesting autologous fascia lata for pelvic reconstructive surgery: techniques and morbidity. Am J Obstet Gynecol. 2001;185(6):1354–9. https://doi.org/10.1067/mob.2001.119074.
70. Gokhale S. Three-dimensional sonography of muscle hernias. J Ultrasound Med. 2007;26(2):239–42. https://doi.org/10.7863/JUM.2007.26.2.239.
71. Zeiss J, Ebraheim NA, Woldenberg LS. Magnetic resonance imaging in the diagnosis of anterior tibialis muscle herniation. Clin Orthop Relat Res. 1989;244:249–53.
72. Berglund HT, Stocks GW. Muscle hernia in a recreational athlete. Orthop Rev. 1993;22(11):1246–8.
73. Lane JE, Woody CM, Lesher JLJR. Tibialis anterior muscle herniation. Dermatologic Surg. 2002;28(7) https://journals.lww.com/dermatologicsurgery/fulltext/2002/07000/tibialis_anterior_muscle_herniation.27.aspx
74. Vitali M, Canevari FR, Cattalani A, Grasso V, Somma T, Barbanera A. Direct fascia lata reconstruction to reduce donor site morbidity in endoscopic endonasal extended surgery: a pilot study. Clin Neurol Neurosurg. 2016;144:59–63. https://doi.org/10.1016/J.CLINEURO.2016.03.003.
75. Naugle J, Fry CL, Sabatier RE, Elliott LF. High leg incision fascia lata harvesting. Ophthalmology. 1997;104(9):1480–8. https://doi.org/10.1016/S0161-6420(97)30107-9.
76. Govier FE, Gibbons RP, Correa RJ, Weissman RM, Pritchett TR, Hefty TR. Pubovaginal slings using fascia lata for the treatment of intrinsic sphincter deficiency. J Urol. 1997;157(1):117–21.
77. Peabody T, Bordoni B. Anatomy, bony pelvis and lower limb: fascia lata. StatPearls Publishing; 2023. Accessed August 11, 2024. https://www.ncbi.nlm.nih.gov/books/NBK557497/
78. Johnson C, Vollstedt A, Nakatsuka H, Orzel J, Takacs EB. Cosmetic and functional impact of fascia lata harvest for use in surgery for stress urinary incontinence. Neurourol Urodyn. 2024;43(5):1185–91. https://doi.org/10.1002/NAU.25462.
79. Tay VSL, Tan KS, Loh ICY. Minimally invasive fascia lata harvest: a new method. Plast Reconstr Surg Glob Open. 2013;1(1) https://doi.org/10.1097/GOX.0B013E31828C4406.
80. Patel S, Chaus FM, Funk JT, Twiss CO. Total autologous fascia lata sacrocolpopexy for treatment of pelvic organ prolapse: experience in thirty-four patients. Urology. 2022;170:73–7. https://doi.org/10.1016/J.UROLOGY.2022.08.038.
81. Andryk LM, Neilson JC, Wooldridge AN, et al. Outcomes and complications of postoperative seroma cavities following soft-tissue sarcoma resection. Front Oncologia. 2024:14. https://doi.org/10.3389/FONC.2024.1250069.
82. Adedigba JA, Volk AS, Roach HM. Periprosthetic seroma occurrence after femoropopliteal bypass grafting: surgical management after failure of non-surgical measures in relieving symptoms. Vascular. 2021;29(2):244–7. https://doi.org/10.1177/1708538120946546.
83. Bock ME, Nagle R, Soyster M, et al. Robotic sacral colpopexy using autologous fascia lata compared with mesh. J Endourol. 2021;35(6):801–7. https://doi.org/10.1089/END.2020.0537.
84. Study Results from Kent State University in the Area of Hematoma Reported (A Proposed Algorithm To Diagnose and Treat Lower Extremity Hematomas Br). Health & Medicine Week. https://link.gale.com/apps/doc/A716871871/AONE?u=oregon_oweb&sid=sitemap&xid=3f514549. Published August 11, 2022.
85. Chibber PJ, Shah HN, Jain P. A minimally invasive technique for harvesting autologous fascia lata for pubo-vaginal sling suspension. Int Urol Nephrol. 2005;37(1):43–6. https://doi.org/10.1007/S11255-004-6080-7/METRICS.
86. Guo J, Yin Y, Jin L, Zhang R, Hou Z, Zhang Y. Acute compartment syndrome: cause, diagnosis, and new viewpoint. Medicine. 2019;98(27) https://doi.org/10.1097/MD.0000000000016260.
87. Tillinghast CM, Gary JL. Compartment syndrome of the lower extremity. In: Mauffrey C, Hak D, Martin III M, editors. Compartment syndrome. Cham: Springer; 2019. p. 67–81. https://doi.org/10.1007/978-3-030-22331-1_8.
88. Taylor RM, Sullivan MP, Mehta S. Acute compartment syndrome: obtaining diagnosis, providing treat-

ment, and minimizing medicolegal risk. Curr Rev Musculoskelet Med. 2012;5(3):206–13. https://doi.org/10.1007/S12178-012-9126-Y/TABLES/3.
89. Rothenberg KA, George EL, Trickey AW, Chandra V, Stern JR. Delayed fasciotomy is associated with higher risk of major amputation in patients with acute limb ischemia. Ann Vasc Surg. 2019;59:195–201. https://doi.org/10.1016/j.avsg.2019.01.028.
90. Lin JH, Humphries MD, Hasegawa J, Saroya J, Mell MW. Outcomes after selective fasciotomy for revascularization of nontraumatic acute lower limb ischemia. Vasc Endovascular Surg. 2021;56(1):18–23. https://doi.org/10.1177/15385744211045493.
91. Ângelo ACLPG, de Campos Azevedo CI. Minimally invasive fascia lata harvesting in ASCR does not produce significant donor site morbidity. Knee Surg Sports Traumatol Arthrosc. 2019;27(1):245–50. https://doi.org/10.1007/S00167-018-5085-1.
92. Amir A, Gatot A, Zucker G, Sagi A, Fliss DM. Harvesting large fascia lata sheaths: a rational approach. Skull Base Surg. 2000;10(1):29–34.
93. Altman AD, Allen VM, McNeil SA, Dempster J. Pfannenstiel incision closure: a review of current skin closure techniques. J Obstet Gynaecol Can. 2009;31(6):514–20. https://doi.org/10.1016/S1701-2163(16)34213-X.

Periurethral Bulking Agent Injection

31

Austin J. Martin and Brian J. Linder

Introduction

Stress urinary incontinence is a common condition, impacting up to 50% of women in the United States over the age of 40 [1]. For many women, stress urinary incontinence has a significant impact on quality of life [2]. Secondary to this, up to 14% of women in the United States ultimately undergo a surgical procedure during their lifetime to treat stress urinary incontinence [3]. Furthermore, as the population ages and the incidence of urinary incontinence increases, the portion of women with stress urinary incontinence is expected to rise [4].

Current management of stress urinary incontinence includes conservative/behavioral measures (e.g. weight loss, etc), pelvic floor muscle exercises, vaginal insert use (e.g. continence pessary, Poise Impressa®, etc.), or procedural interventions in the form of urethral bulking agent injection, urethral slings (synthetic or autologous), or Burch colposuspension [5, 6]. Urethral bulking agent injection aims to improve sphincter coaptation during the filling phase of micturition, thereby increasing urethral pressure and reducing urine leakage during periods of increased intrabdominal pressure [7]. Historically, urethral bulking was limited to patients with intrinsic sphincter deficiency; however, urethral bulking has been increasingly utilized in patients with urethral hypermobility as well [8]. Some results suggest that outcomes are not different based on the underlying etiology of leakage [9].

While mid-urethral slings are the most utilized procedure for female stress urinary incontinence, urethral bulking remains an option in the index female with stress urinary incontinence [5]. Urethral bulking injection has traditionally represented a minority of the procedures performed, despite being less invasive than slings, secondary to limited long-term durability. Of note, in a randomized trial the most recently FDA approved agent in the United States (approved 2020), polyacrylamide hydrogel (Bulkamid®, Axonics, International A/S, Soeberg, Denmark) was reported to have a negative cough stress test rate of 78% at 3 years follow-up (compared to TVT, 95.7%) [10]. Likewise, most participants were subjectively 'cured or improved' with polyacrylamide injection (88.5% vs TVT 100%) [10]. Additional studies suggest durability with success rates between 43% and 67% with 7–8 years follow-up [11, 12]. The advantage of urethral bulking injection for the primary treatment of female stress urinary incontinence is reduced morbidity and recovery compared to urethral sling procedures.

Additional roles for urethral bulking agent injection include the treatment of recurrent stress incontinence following synthetic midurethral sling placement, those with prior pelvic radia-

A. J. Martin · B. J. Linder (✉)
Department of Urology, Mayo Clinic, Rochester, MN, USA
e-mail: Linder.Brian@mayo.edu

H. B. Goldman, J. Zillioux (eds.), *Complications of Urogynecology and Reconstructive Pelvic Surgery*, https://doi.org/10.1007/978-3-032-00339-3_31

tion, and for patients with surgically altered anatomy [13, 14]. For instance, a pooled analysis reported a roughly 80% success rate for bulking agent injection for managing recurrent stress incontinence following a midurethral sling [13]. In those with prior pelvic radiation, bulking agent injection may be preferable compared to synthetic sling placement due to concerns related to issues with wound healing and mesh-related complications [5, 14]. Additionally, urethral bulking agent injection has been utilized in patients with stress urinary incontinence following radical cystectomy with orthotopic neobladder [15] or after partial urethrectomy [16].

Available Periurethral Bulking Injection Agents

Since originally reported in 1938, with periurethral injection of sodium morrhuate, a sclerosing agent synthesized from cod liver oil [17], the agents used for urethral bulking for stress urinary incontinence have evolved. The currently available commercial agents are potentially more durable, generally safe, induce minimal local inflammatory reaction, and have a low prevalence of significant adverse events [8, 18].

The discussion herein will concentrate on the currently available FDA-approved bulking agents for periurethral use and can be grouped by particulate and non-particulate agents. Particulate agents are microparticles within a carrier that are injected and induce an inflammatory response [19, 20]. Particulate agents include: calcium hydroxylapatite (Coaptite™, Boston Scientific Corporation, Marlborough MA, USA), pyrolytic carbon coated zirconium beads (Durasphere® EXP, Coloplast Corporation, Minneapolis, MN, USA), and cross-linked polydimethysiloxane (Macroplastique®, Laborie, Portsmouth, NH, USA). Polyacrylamide hydrogel (Bulkamid®, Axonics, International A/S, Soeberg, Denmark) is a nonparticulate material (2.5% cross-linked polyacrylamide and 97.5% non-pyrogenic water), which relies on the volume of the injected agent [19].

The discontinuation of several older injected materials, including tetrafluoroethylene, autologous fat, and ethylene vinyl alcohol copolymer resulted from safety concerns, as well as limited efficacy [21–24]. As such, these agents should not be used in contemporary practice. Likewise, outside of the commercially available agents, stem cell periurethral injections have been described and are currently considered experimental [5, 25]. Current guidelines note that these treatments should not be offered outside of investigative trials [5]. Of note, one of the historic injection agents that was widely studied, glutaraldehyde cross-linked collagen (Contigen, Bard™, Covington, GA, USA), was discontinued in 2011 secondary to lack of a primary supplier of the bovine product, not because of lack of efficacy or safety concerns.

Of note, the complications related to bulking agent injection seen in one surgical discipline may provide insights for injection in other subspecialties. For example, polytetrafluoroethylene was associated with granuloma formation in multiple specialties [22, 26–28]. Likewise, local migration with radio-opaque carbon-coated zirconium beads has been reported in the colorectal literature [29], although without clinical consequences. Thus, when evaluating new injectable agents, complications reported in other specialties should be considered, as similar adverse events may be encountered in alternative applications. Notably, polyacrylamide hydrogel has been utilized in plastic surgery in other countries, with reports of little or minimal tissue reaction, without fibrosis or calcification up to 8 years following injection [30].

Complications

Complications from periurethral bulking agent injection will be divided into groupings of local early or delayed presentation or systemic presentation. It should be noted that the currently available bulking agents have a low overall complication rate, with most complications being related to transient voiding dysfunction, and major adverse events being rare and limited to case reports [8, 18, 31].

Early Onset Local Complications

The most common early-onset complications include urinary tract infection, transient urinary retention, urinary frequency, nocturia, dysuria, and hematuria [18]. The incidence of urinary tract infection is between 9% and 11% [32]. Anecdotally, we recommend obtaining a preoperative urine culture prior and treating with culture-appropriate antibiotics prior to surgery. Between 5% and 10% of women will experience transient dysuria following the procedure, which can be managed conservatively [32]. There does not appear to be a difference in post-operative urinary tract infection based on the type of bulking agent.

Urinary retention requiring clean intermittent catheterization or indwelling catheter occurs in 7–10% of patients [33]. This typically resolves within a week of intermittent catheterization with a 10-12Fr catheter [34]. If intermittent catheterization is not feasible, a small diameter (10-12Fr) indwelling catheter can be placed with subsequent voiding trial in the short term. Among the available agents, Coaptite® has been associated with a higher rate of transient retention (up to 34%) [8]. Transient postoperative retention is likely due to urethral edema, pain, and/or underlying detrusor underactivity. Given the theoretical risk of deformation of the bulking agent, we favor using a small catheter for the shortest duration possible; however, data regarding the risk of post-operative catheterization and bulking failure is scarce.

Rarely, patients may develop persistent urinary retention or de-novo urgency/urge incontinence. In one series, chronic retention seven days after injection occurred in 9% of patients following transurethral injection with Urolastic® (cross-linked polydimethysiloxane) [35]. Treatment involved endoscopic unroofing or aspiration of the bulking agent, with the resolution of retention in all patients. While subsequent rates of recurrent stress urinary incontinence were not reported in the series, patients undergoing aspiration/unroofing of bulking material should be counseled that their stress urinary incontinence is likely to recur.

While urethral bulking is generally safe for patients on therapeutic anticoagulation, at least one series has reported two patients with periurethral hematoma [36, 37]. Figure 31.1 Both patients presented with abdominal pain and urinary retention following urethral injection and were successfully managed conservatively with a foley catheter placement. In addition, at least one case of urethrovaginal fistula, potentially secondary to periurethral hematoma and acute urinary retention, has been reported [36].

Late-Onset Local Complications

For many of the available FDA-approved agents on the market, there does not appear to be significant differences in the incidence of long-term complications, although data is limited, and no comparative studies are sufficiently powered to detect meaningful differences between types of injectables. The most common late-onset local complications include urethral and bladder erosion, granuloma formation/sterile abscess, and chronic urethral pain. Notably, pseudoabscess formation has not been reported in studies involving Bulkamid® injection [10, 31, 34].

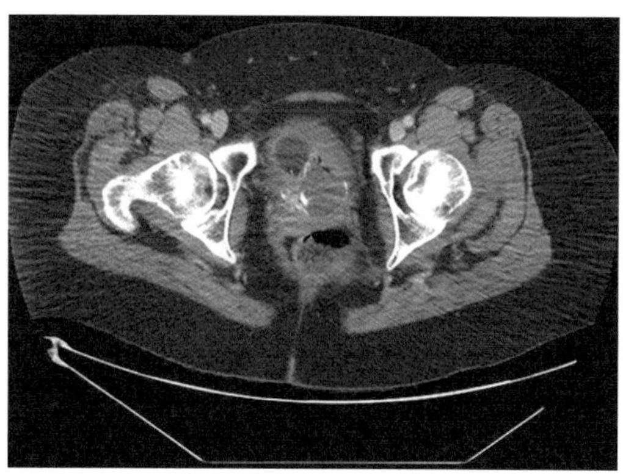

Fig. 31.1 Pelvic CT imaging demonstrates a large periurethral hematoma in a patient on warfarin presenting for pelvic pain and acute urinary retention following transurethral bulking agent injection. The hematoma is seen displacing the bladder neck and Foley catheter laterally

Erosion of injected material either through the anterior vaginal wall or transurethrally may occur in a delayed fashion. Patients with erosion of the material into the urethral lumen may present with recurrent urinary tract infections, overactive bladder symptoms, urge or stress urinary incontinence, or obstructive urinary symptoms [38, 39]. Figure 31.2 Implant erosion through the anterior vaginal wall can lead to chronic pain and dyspareunia [35, 40]. In a series of 65 patients undergoing transurethral bulking with Urolastic®, 26.2% of patients developed implant erosion, and 21.5% required surgical removal after two years, most commonly through an inverted U-shaped vaginal incision [35]. In addition, two patients in this study developed transurethral erosions, which were removed cystoscopically [35]. Of the patients who experienced transurethral erosion, one had a history of prior pelvic radiation, and the other had a history of previous failed mid-urethral sling and performed clean intermittent catheterization at baseline for chronic urinary retention. As is the case with any injectable, these results suggest that poor tissue perfusion, either from prior radiation or scarring from previous surgery, may be exacerbated by the injection of foreign material, leading to decreased blood flow and increased likelihood of implant erosion. In addition to Urolastic®, urethral erosions have been reported in patients following Macroplastique® and Coaptite® [8, 34, 38, 39].

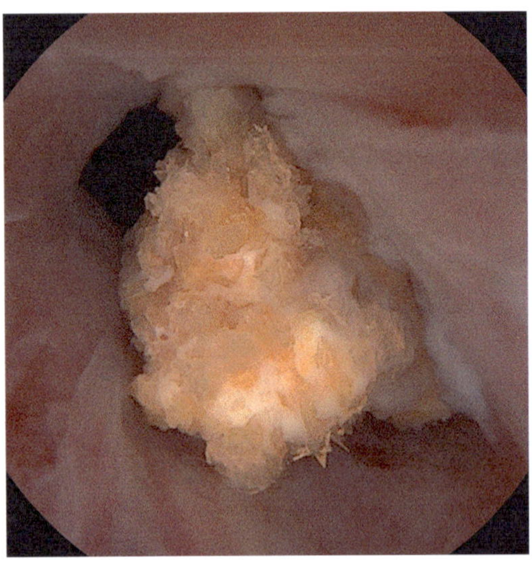

Fig. 31.2 Cystoscopy demonstrating urethral erosion of Macroplastique with associated stone formation

Periurethral pseudoabscess/granuloma may present with dysuria, obstructive urinary symptoms, or urinary retention 5–120 weeks following injection [34]. Figure 31.3 Diagnosis is primarily clinical with characteristic physical exam including a variably tender, well-circumscribed anterior vaginal wall mass. In most cases, treatment consists of transvaginal unroofing and antibiotics, although tissue cultures from surgery are usually negative [24, 31, 41, 42]. Rarely, complicated abscesses have been reported in patients following injection with Coaptite®, Durasphere®, and Macroplastique® [34]. While reports of pseudo-abscess/granuloma are limited to case reports and the true incidence of postoperative abscess is unknown, it should be noted that a survey among urologists in the UK found that granuloma formation/sterile abscess was the most commonly treated long-term sequela of urethral bulking [43].

In rare instances, urethrovaginal fistula has been reported following Zuidex™ (non-animal stabilized hyaluronic acid/dextranomer) and collagen injections [36, 42, 44]. Treatment involved transvaginal excision and Martius flap or autologous sling placement. In at least one instance, the fistula was suspected to develop following periurethral hematoma [44]. Fistulas have also been reported following collagen injections in women with previous cystectomy and neobladder formation [44]. While Zuidex™ and collagen injectables are no longer available in the USA, readers should be aware of potential fistula formation in patients with post-operative hematoma, altered anatomy, or previous radiation.

Chronic urethral pain has also been reported in 4% of patients following urethral bulking with Urolastic® [35]. After ruling out other causes, including sterile abscess and implant erosion, the etiology of pain was determined to be due to displacement of the injectable under the urethra, leading to pressure on the anterior vaginal wall and dyspareunia. In all cases, patients underwent transvaginal removal of bulking material with improvement in pain. In 12 out of 14 patients,

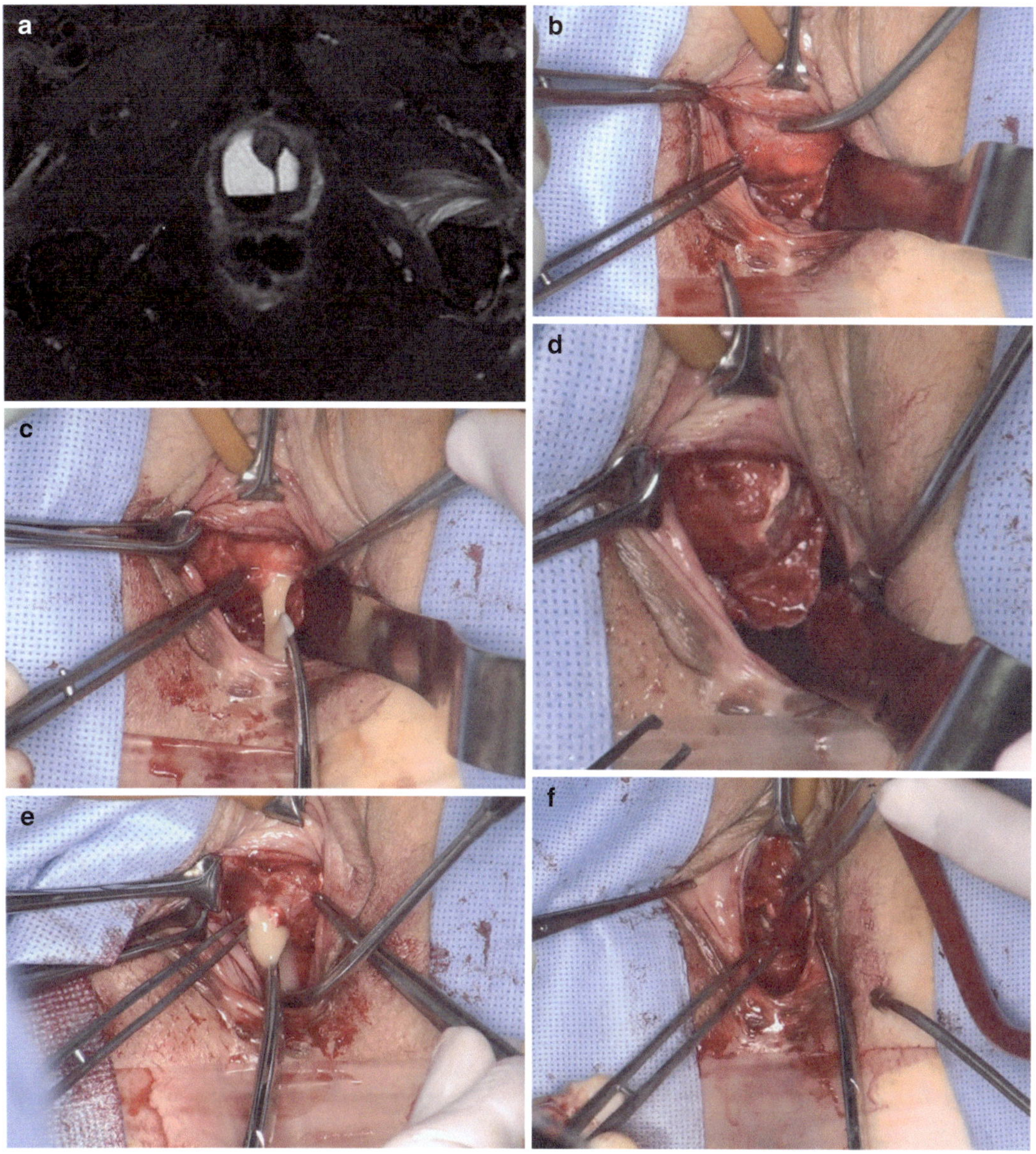

Fig. 31.3 Pseudoabscess from prior Coaptite injection. (**a**) MRI image with two periurethral pseudoabscesses with stone material, (**b**) an inverted-U incision for transvaginal drainage of the pseudo-abscess, (**c**) unroofing the left-sided cavity, (**d**) completed drainage on the left side, (**e**) unroofing the right-sided cavity, (**f**) completed drainage on the right side. No connection to the urethra was identified. A concomitant autologous pubovaginal sling was placed during the procedure (not shown)

transvaginal removal of bulking material led to recurrence of stress incontinence.

Another long-term sequela of urethral bulking includes delayed onset urinary retention, suspected to be due to de novo detrusor underactivity. In these instances, women experience resolution of their stress urinary incontinence and are initially able to void spontaneously, however, later develop worsening obstructive urinary symptoms. We typically would treat these women for incomplete bladder emptying without resection of the bulking agent itself.

Finally, bulking materials may lead to misdiagnosis of an incidental anterior vaginal wall or periurethral mass on pelvic imaging [45, 46]. Pelvic imaging with Computed Tomography (CT) does not reliably distinguish periurethral bulking material from other urethral pathology, including urethral diverticula, periurethral cyst, and periurethral masses [46]. Figure 31.4 Magnetic resonance imaging can differentiate between most injectable agents and urethral diverticula or cysts [47]. However, given the high percentage of water in the Bulkamid® agent (97.5% water), it may have a similar appearance to urethral diverticula or periurethral cyst on magnetic resonance imaging [48]. In one study, a non-contrast CT followed by voiding cystourethrogram, followed by repeat non-contrast CT was required to reliably differentiate between Bulkamid material and urethral diverticulum [48]. When an accurate history is not available, readers should be aware that women with previous bulking procedures are at risk for unnecessary and sometimes invasive diagnostic procedures, which may precipitate a return of their stress urinary incontinence when diagnosis relies on imaging alone.

Systemic Complications

Systemic complications following urethral bulking are primarily of historic interest. Contigen (bovine collagen) was associated with allergic reactions, and patients were recommended to undergo allergen testing prior to use [49]. All of the currently available FDA products are non-immunogenic, and none have been associated with allergic reactions.

Previous cases of particle migration into the lymphatics or pelvic vessels have been reported

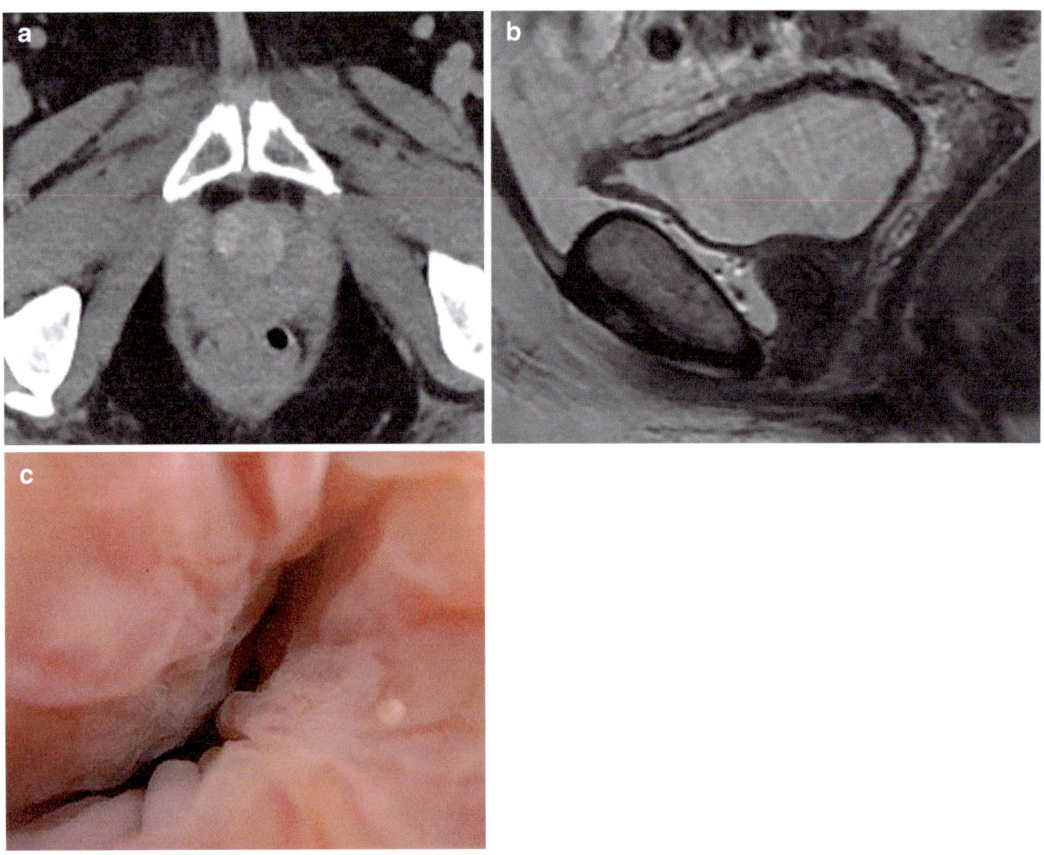

Fig. 31.4 Patient with a history of Macroplastique® injection who underwent work-up of a suspected solid periurethral mass. (**a**) CT Urogram, axial image of nephrographic phase, (**b**) MRI, Sagittal image of T2 phase, (**c**) cystoscopy

in patients following Durasphere® injection, although this was an incidental finding with unclear clinical significance [50]. In theory, particle migration places patients at risk of systemic emboli, and there has been one reported instance of pulmonary embolism following periurethral autologous fat injection [24]. Except Durasphere®, none of the current injectable agents have been associated with clinically systemic complications or embolic risk.

Conclusions

In summary, the use of the currently FDA-approved bulking agents (Bulkamid®, Coaptite™, Durasphere®, Macroplastique®) for the treatment of female stress incontinence is associated with a low incidence of complications, most of which are transient and amenable to conservative management. The most serious complications occur in a delayed fashion and consist of pseudoabscess formation and implant erosion. The treatment of these two complications typically requires procedural intervention and may be associated with the recurrence of stress urinary incontinence. The reader should also be cautioned that bulking agents may not be easily distinguishable from other urethral pathologies on pelvic imaging, which may lead to inaccurate diagnosis and unnecessary intervention. Despite this, urethral bulking remains a safe procedure with low morbidity that can be utilized in women with stress urinary incontinence.

References

1. Lee UJ, Feinstein L, Ward JB, et al. Prevalence of urinary incontinence among a nationally representative sample of women, 2005–2016: findings from the urologic diseases in America project. J Urol. 2021;205(6):1718–24.
2. Pizzol D, Demurtas J, Celotto S, et al. Urinary incontinence and quality of life: a systematic review and meta-analysis. Aging Clin Exp Res. 2021;33:25–35.
3. Wu JM, Matthews CA, Conover MM, Pate V, Funk MJ. Lifetime risk of stress incontinence or pelvic organ prolapse surgery. Obstet Gynecol. 2014;123(6):1201.
4. Wu JM, Hundley AF, Fulton RG, Myers ER. Forecasting the prevalence of pelvic floor disorders in US Women: 2010 to 2050. Obstet Gynecol. 2009;114(6):1278–83.
5. Kobashi KC, Vasavada S, Bloschichak A, et al. Updates to surgical treatment of female stress urinary incontinence (SUI): AUA/SUFU guideline (2023). J Urol. 2023;209(6):1091–8.
6. Bretschneider CE, Geynisman-Tan J, Mueller MG, Collins SA, Lewicky-Gaupp C, Kenton K. Rates of sling procedures and revisions—a National Surgical Quality Improvement Program Database Study. Urogynecology. 2021;27(6):e559–62.
7. Ismail MB, Al-Timimi HF, Al-Hamadani HF, Nassiri UA. The safety and efficacy of periurethral injections of bulking agent in women with urinary incontinence. Technology. 2021;11(1):85–9.
8. Hoe V, Haller B, Yao HH, O'Connell HE. Urethral bulking agents for the treatment of stress urinary incontinence in women: a systematic review. Neurourol Urodyn. 2021;40(6):1349–88.
9. Giammò A, Geretto P, Ammirati E, et al. Urethral bulking with Bulkamid: an analysis of efficacy, safety profile, and predictors of functional outcomes in a single-center cohort. Neurourol Urodyn. 2020;39(5):1523–8.
10. Itkonen Freitas A-M, Isaksson C, Rahkola-Soisalo P, Tulokas S, Mentula M, Mikkola TS. Tension-free vaginal tape and polyacrylamide hydrogel injection for primary stress urinary incontinence: 3-year followup from a randomized clinical trial. J Urol. 2022;208(3):658–67.
11. Brosche T, Kuhn A, Lobodasch K, Sokol ER. Seven-year efficacy and safety outcomes of Bulkamid for the treatment of stress urinary incontinence. Neurourol Urodyn. 2021;40(1):502–8.
12. Plotti F, Montera R, Terranova C, et al. Long-term follow-up of bulking agents for stress urinary incontinence in older patients. Menopause. 2018;25(6):663–7.
13. Braga A, Caccia G, Papadia A, et al. Urethral bulking agents for the treatment of recurrent stress urinary incontinence: a systematic review and meta-analysis. Maturitas. 2022;163:28–37.
14. Dobberfuhl AD. Evaluation and treatment of female stress urinary incontinence after pelvic radiotherapy. Neurourol Urodyn. 2019;38:S59–69.
15. Wilson S, Quek ML, Ginsberg DA. Transurethral injection of bulking agents for stress urinary incontinence following orthotopic neobladder reconstruction in women. J Urol. 2004;172(1):244–6.
16. Plotti F, Zullo MA, Palaia I, Angioli R, Panici PB. Urinary incontinence after radical vulvectomy treated with Macroplastique implantation. J Minim Invasive Gynecol. 2008;15(1):113–5.
17. Murless BC. The injection treatment of stress incontinence. BJOG Int J Obstet Gynaecol. 1938;45(1):67–73.

18. Kocjancic E, Mourad S, Acar Ö. Complications of urethral bulking therapy for female stress urinary incontinence. Neurourol Urodyn. 2019;38:S12–20.
19. Christensen LH. Host tissue interaction, fate, and risks of degradable and nondegradable gel fillers. Dermatologic Surg. 2009;35:1612–9.
20. Stenberg A, Larsson E, Läckgren G. Endoscopic treatment with dextranomer-hyaluronic acid for vesicoureteral reflux: histological findings. J Urol. 2003;169(3):1109–13.
21. Haab F, Zimmern PE, Leach GE. Urinary stress incontinence due to intrinsic sphincteric deficiency: experience with fat and collagen periurethral injections. J Urol. 1997;157(4):1283–6.
22. Hubmer MG, Hoffmann C, Popper H, Scharnagl E. Expanded polytetrafluoroethylene threads for lip augmentation induce foreign body granulomatous reaction. Plast Reconstr Surg. 1999;103(4):1277–9.
23. Hurtado EA, McCrery RJ, Appell RA. Complications of ethylene vinyl alcohol copolymer as an intraurethral bulking agent in men with stress urinary incontinence. Urology. 2008;71(4):662–5.
24. Sweat SD, Lightner DJ. Complications of sterile abscess formation and pulmonary embolism following periurethral bulking agents. J Urol. 1999;161(1):93–6.
25. Klapper-Goldstein H, Tamam S, Sade S, Weintraub AY. A systematic review of stem cell therapy treatment for women suffering from stress urinary incontinence. Int J Gynecol Obstet. 2022;157(1):19–30.
26. Aragona F, D'Urso L, Scremin E, Salmaso R, Glazel GP. Polytetrafluoroethylene giant granuloma and adenopathy: long-term complications following subureteral polytetrafluoroethylene injection for the treatment of vesicoureteral reflux in children. J Urol. 1997;158(4):1539–42.
27. Malizia AA, Reiman HM, Myers RP, et al. Migration and granulomatous reaction after periurethral injection of polytef (Teflon). JAMA. 1984;251(24):3277–81.
28. Toth G, Rubeiz H, Macdonald RL. Polytetrafluoroethylene-induced granuloma and brainstem cyst after microvascular decompression for trigeminal neuralgia: case report. Neurosurgery. 2007;61(4):E875–7.
29. Altomare D, La Torre F, Rinaldi M, Binda G, Pescatori M. Carbon-coated microbeads anal injection in outpatient treatment of minor fecal incontinence. Dis Colon Rectum. 2008;51:432–5.
30. Christensen LH, Breiting VB, Aasted A, Jørgensen A, Kebuladze I. Long-term effects of polyacrylamide hydrogel on human breast tissue. Plast Reconstr Surg. 2003;111(6):1883–90.
31. Zheng Y, Rovner E. Update on urethral bulking for stress urinary incontinence in women. Curr Urol Rep. 2022;23(10):203–9.
32. Siddiqui ZA, Abboudi H, Crawford R, Shah S. Intraurethral bulking agents for the management of female stress urinary incontinence: a systematic review. Int Urogynecol J. 2017;28:1275–84.
33. Capobianco G, Saderi L, Dessole F, et al. Efficacy and effectiveness of bulking agents in the treatment of stress and mixed urinary incontinence: a systematic review and meta-analysis. Maturitas. 2020;133:13–31.
34. de Vries AM, Wadhwa H, Huang J, Farag F, Heesakkers JP, Kocjancic E. Complications of urethral bulking agents for stress urinary incontinence: an extensive review including case reports. Urogynecology. 2018;24(6):392–8.
35. de Vries AM, van Breda HM, Fernandes JG, Venema PL, Heesakkers JP. Para-urethral injections with Urolastic® for treatment of female stress urinary incontinence: subjective improvement and safety. Urol Int. 2017;99(1):91–7.
36. Carlin BI, Klutke CG. Development of urethrovaginal fistula following periurethral collagen injection. J Urol. 2000;164(1):124.
37. Theofrastous J, Simpkins K. Urinary retention and intravesical hemorrhage following urethral collagen injections in women using warfarin. Int Urogynecol J. 2002;13:268–9.
38. Ramirez-Caban L, Malekzadeh M, Ossin DA, Hurtado EA. Clinical presentation and treatment of Macroplastique® urethral exposures: a retrospective case series. Int Urogynecol J. 2022;33(3):681–7.
39. Rodríguez D, Jaffer A, Hilmy M, Zimmern P. Bladder neck and urethral erosions after Macroplastique injections. LUTS. 2021;13(1):93–7.
40. Erekson EA, Sung VW, Rardin CR, Myers DL. Ethylene vinyl alcohol copolymer erosions after use as a urethral bulking agent. Obstet Gynecol. 2007;109(2 Part 2):490–2.
41. Berger MB, Morgan DM. Delayed presentation of pseudoabscess secondary to injection of pyrolitic carbon-coated beads bulking agent. Female Pelv Med Reconstr Surg. 2012;18(5):303.
42. Hilton P. Urethrovaginal fistula associated with 'sterile abscess' formation following periurethral injection of dextranomer/hyaluronic acid co-polymer (Zuidextrade) for the treatment of stress urinary incontinence-a case report. Bjog Int J Obstet Gynaecol. 2009;116(11):1527.
43. Patel S, Lazarowicz H, Hamm R. Long-term complications of bulking agents in the treatment of stress urinary incontinence: Results of a national survey. J Clin Urol. 2022:20514158221086405.
44. Pruthi RS, Petrus CD, Bundrick WS. New onset vesicovaginal fistula after transurethral collagen injection in women who underwent cystectomy and orthotopic neobladder creation: presentation and definitive treatment. J Urol. 2000;164(5):1638–9.
45. Bridges MD, Petrou SP, Lightner DJ. Urethral bulking agents: imaging review. Am J Roentgenol. 2005;185(1):257–64.
46. Gaines N, Gupta P, Khourdaji AS, et al. Radiographic misdiagnoses after periurethral bulking agents. Urogynecology. 2018;24(4):312–4.
47. Chulroek T, Wangcharoenrung D, Cattapan K, et al. Can magnetic resonance imaging differentiate among transurethral bulking agent, urethral diverticulum, and periurethral cyst? Abdom Radiol. 2019;44:2852–63.

48. Akinjise-Ferdinand O, Hubbard R, Osman NI, Chapple CR. A diagnostic conundrum: Is it a periurethral diverticulum/cyst or a bulking agent (Bulkamid)? Neurourol Urodyn. 2023;42(2):547–54.
49. Li H, Westney OL. Injection of urethral bulking agents. Urol Clin. 2019;46(1):1–15.
50. Vidart A, Zimmern PE. Migration of durasphere after transurethral injection for stress urinary incontinence. Urogynecology. 2004;10(1):39–40.

Sacral Neuromodulation

32

Hashim Hashim, Laura Thomas, and Steven W. Siegel

Introduction

Sacral Neuromodulation (SNM)/Sacral Nerve Stimulation (SNS) is a well-established treatment for several pelvic compartment conditions, most commonly the overactive bladder, voiding dysfunction and faecal incontinence. More recently, SNM has also been used to treat patients with other symptoms such as pelvic pain; however, this is currently not an approved indication despite evidence of its benefits in improving the quality of life in this group of patients [1].

It is theorised to work by stimulating the afferent sacral nerve roots S3 or S4, and final electrode placement is determined through the attainment of optimal motor or sensory patient response. Most patients undergo a test period before full system implantation. This test phase is performed via a percutaneous nerve evaluation (PNE), or an advanced tined lead test (ATL). If successful, then the patient progresses with an implantable pulse generator (IPG) attached to a lead containing four electrode contact points.

In recent years, there have been advances in technology, bringing rechargeable devices to the market, extending the battery life of the recharge-free options and enhancing the MRI status to facilitate full body MRIs. In addition to the changes in device technology, refinements have been made to the implantation techniques, facilitating less invasive surgical procedures, and improving patient outcomes.

Despite these developments, there are still known complications associated with SNM (Table 32.1) and this chapter aims to address some of the most frequently reported ones. It includes departmental insight into experienced complications and the learning that evolved from these. We discuss practical solutions to minimise the risk of complications through clear patient selection, ideal lead placement [2, 3] and good surgical practice.

H. Hashim (✉) · L. Thomas
Bristol Urological Institute, Southmead Hospital, Bristol, UK
e-mail: Laura.Thomas2@nbt.nhs.uk

S. W. Siegel
Centers for Continence Care and Female Urology, Metro Urology, Woodbury, MN, USA
e-mail: steven.siegel@neuspera.com

H. B. Goldman, J. Zillioux (eds.), *Complications of Urogynecology and Reconstructive Pelvic Surgery*, https://doi.org/10.1007/978-3-032-00339-3_32

Table 32.1 Insite trial adverse events [17, 18]

Adverse event	≤1 year $N = 272$	≤5 years $N = 272$	Adverse event	≤1 year $N = 272$	≤5 years $N = 272$
Undesirable change in stimulation	12%	22%	**Granuloma**	<1%	<1%
Implant site pain	7%	15%	**Hypersensitivity**	<1%	<1%
Implant site infection	3%	4%	**High impedance**	<1%	3%
Implant site erythema	1%	2%	**Implant site effusion**	<1%	1%
Lead fracture	1%	3%	**Implant site erosion**	<1%	<1%
Paresthesia	1%	5%	**Implant site pruritis**	<1%	<1%
Lead migration/dislodgment	1%	5%	**Incision site complication**	<1%	1%
Implant site irritation	<1%	1%	**Medical device complication (neurostimulator)**	<1%	<1%
Implant site reaction	<1%	<1%	**Muscle contracture**	<1%	<1%
Device malfunction (Lead)		1%	**Back pain**		1%
Migration of implant	<1%	1%	**Neurostimulator battery depletion**	<1%	<1%
Pollakiuria	<1%	3%	**Neurostimulator migration**	<1%	<1%
Sciatica	<1%	1%	**Pain**	<1%	<1%
Therapeutic product ineffective	<1%	13%	**Pain in extremity**	<1%	<1%
Arthralgia	<1%	<1%	**Post procedural complication**	<1%	<1%
Asthenia	<1%	<1%	**Pyrexia**	<1%	<1%
Cellulitis	<1%	<1%	**Radiculopathy**	<1%	<1%
Change in sensation of stimulation	<1%	1%	**Sacral pain**	<1%	<1%
Discomfort	<1%	<1%	**Sensory disturbance**	<1%	<1%
Dyskinesia	<1%	<1%	**Skin discoloration**	<1%	<1%
Fecal incontinence	<1%	<1%	**Urinary incontinence**	<1%	1%
Frequent bowel movements	<1%	<1%	**Total**	30%	57%

Complications Associated with Surgery

Infection

Infection is a disastrous outcome for any patient with an implanted device. Unmanaged infections result in device explantation and subsequently no therapeutic control for the patient. The rates of infection recorded in the literature vary from <1% to over 9% [4]. As such, every care should be taken to minimise infection during full system implants and tined lead, advanced tests. The rate of infections for PNE's is significantly lower, with none reported in our cohort of over 800 patients and <2% for full implants.

During the surgical procedure, every precaution should be taken. Masks should be worn to minimise infection risk, and the operating room/theatre should be clearly identified as one undertaking implants to reduce the through traffic of staff. A laminar flow OR is ideally used. It is advisable not to open each piece of kit until required by the operating surgeon, as this reduces both exposure time and the potential for wasted equipment should full implantation not be performed due to issues such as difficult lead placement.

There are also steps to be taken in regard to draping of the patient in theatre, which may decrease the infection rate. Most centres will tape the buttocks apart to observe the anus for motor responses.

If this is done, then a A 3M™ Ioban™ drape covering the area and pre-sacral area is adequate for visualisation and may improve sterility (Fig. 32.1).

During implantable pulse generator (IPG) placement, pocket size, depth and haemostasis are all issues that can impact infection rate and other local complications [5]. Make sure the device is about 2 cm beneath the skin, and creation of the pocket should use bipolar cautery and minimize blunt dissection to avoid bleeding. Adherence to protocol for patients on anticoagulants is therefore vital before surgical attendance.

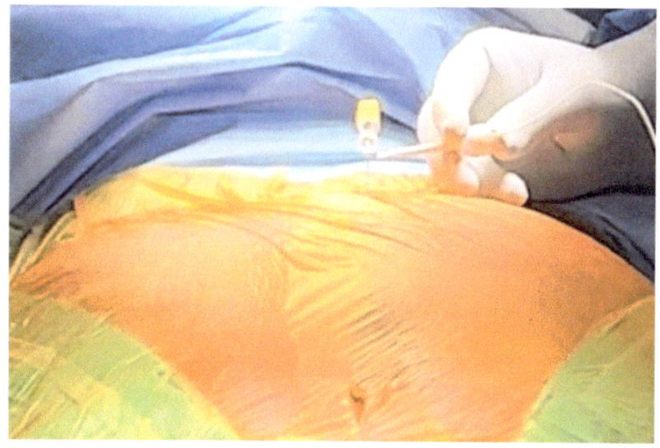

Fig. 32.1 A 3M™ Ioban™ drape to cover the anus and buttocks

The pocket should be parallel to the skin and appropriately sized for the device to prevent flipping or undue pressure on the incision. Research has shown that post-operative haematoma or a deep implant pocket of >3 cm are both significant risk factors for infection and subsequent explantation [6].

Consideration of pocket size is of greater importance when considering the IPG type being implanted. Rechargeable devices work optimally when the IPG lies flat within the patient; movement of the IPG may cause considerable problems extending the time required to both find the device and keep the charging unit connected. A rotated rechargeable IPG is problematic and may lead to further revision surgery (Fig. 32.2).

Consider marking the pocket site with patient cooperation in pre-op for any unusual body habitus or specific patient concern; this will aid inter-operative decision making. For rechargeable devices, patients can be made to wear the belt for recharging and ensuring that the recharging unit sits flat on the body (Fig. 32.3) and the site marked accordingly, especially in those who are wheelchair-bound.

Antibiotic impregnated materials, such as gentamycin-impregnated collagen, are utilised by some centres in an attempt to minimise infection [7]. Others use a gentamicin wash of the IPG pocket or wrap the IPG in a gentamicin-soaked swab prior to implantation. There is, however, minimal evidence showing the direct benefit

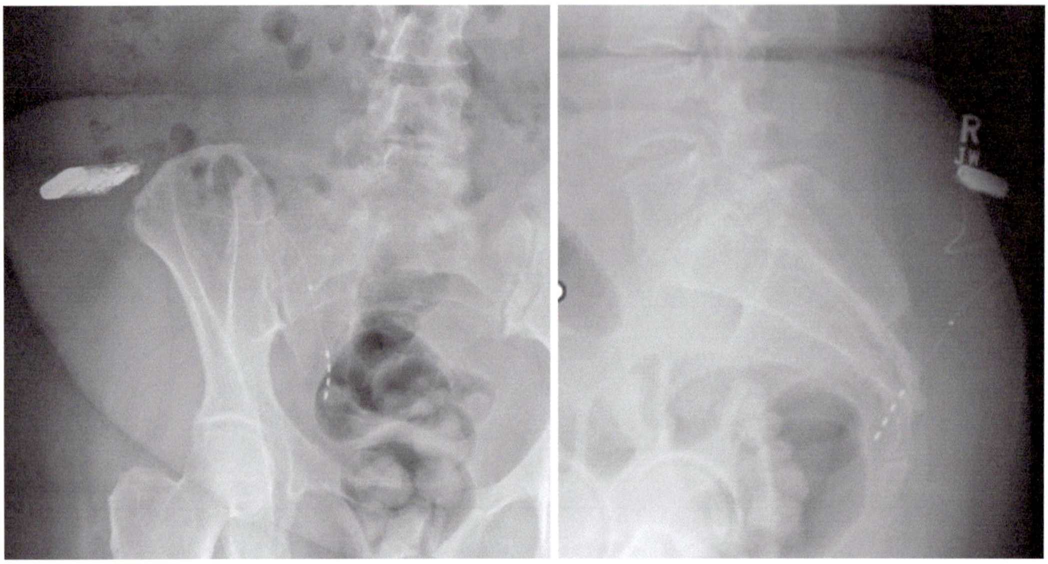

Fig. 32.2 Rotated rechargeable device making recharging difficult

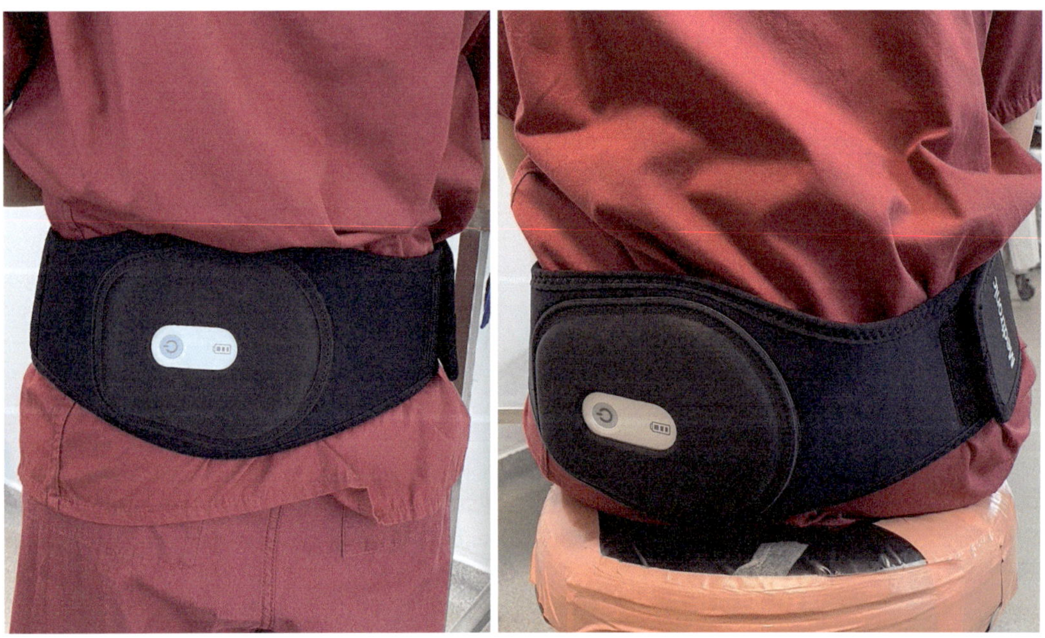

Fig. 32.3 Rechargeable device belt worn pre-op to check for optimal position of IPG and fitting of belt

of wrapping in a gentamicin-soaked swab, with concerns about fluid entering the lead connection port if devices are soaked prior to implantation.

For patients having an ATL or full implant, pre-operative intravenous broad-spectrum antibiotics, such as gentamicin and flucloxacillin or cephazolin, are given, and post-operatively, oral antibiotics are commonly given for 5 days following surgery, dependent on patient allergies and surgeon preference. It is our local practice to give a broad-spectrum antibiotic, such as co-amoxiclav, orally post-operatively. However, it is important to note that there is little data that supports the use of more than intraoperative gram-positive coverage. For the PNE, we do not give antibiotics.

If using a staged approach, it is also important to minimise the duration of time between surgical interventions. Ensuring sufficient trial time to determine device efficacy, whilst minimising time for potential infection of open incisions. A low threshold should be had for removing any infected device and a wait time of 3–6 months is advised for full healing to occur before re-implanting, and ideally on the contralateral side.

Management of infection post-implant often depends on the site of infection and whether it is localised to the device or more generalised, causing headaches and photophobia. Those with localised infection, such as skin redness, inflammation, and/or pain, can initially be treated with intravenous antibiotics based on microbiological advice to try to salvage the device. Bloods, including C-reactive protein (CRP) and white cell count, an ultrasound scan of the IPG and tined-lead to look for collections and oedema, need to be arranged. However, more often than not, an infected device needs extraction. It is frequently easy to extract due to the surrounding inflammation, and the entire device removal should be considered, rather than an attempt to salvage any component (Fig. 32.4). This can often be done in the office under purely local anesthesia.

If the infection is more generalised and especially in those with meningitis symptoms, it needs immediate extraction of the full implant.

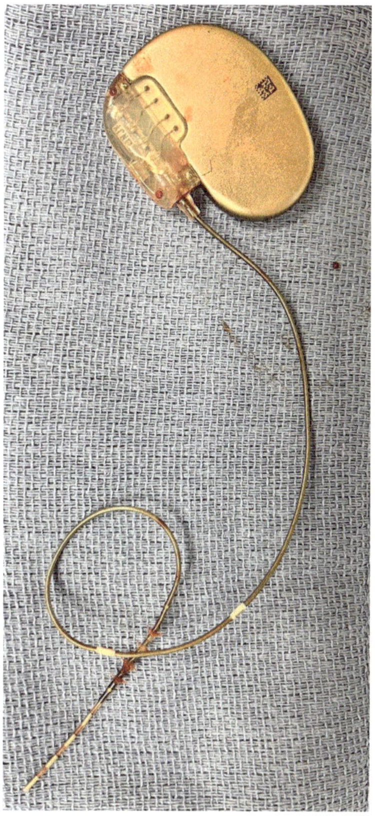

Fig. 32.4 Full removal of infected tined-lead and battery

Device Extraction

Tined lead extraction is frequently straightforward following a failed advanced test phase. This is not always the case once the lead has been in situ for a substantial period of time, and there is structural integrity of scar tissue surrounding the device. As such, it is not unusual for lead fractures to occur during explantation, and the remaining lead segments can be problematic, especially if the device is being removed for MRI purposes (pre-2020 tined leads). Research by Quirouet et al. [8] demonstrated that no significant heating was seen with lead fragments <5 cm when undergoing 1.5 M Tesla head MRI, however many newer devices are compatible with 3 M Tesla and therefore the impact of a 3 M Tesla MRI on fragments is unknown. The risk of lead fracture and possible fragment retention should be clearly discussed with patients prior to surgery, and a full discussion on patient preference noted.

While some have reported successful removal of the complete lead from the generator pocket even years after implantation [9], the more common method is to remove the lead by making a separate small 1–2 cm incision over the original pre-sacral point of insertion, and to dissect down along the lead until the tines may be seen.

Initially, the IPG is removed and gentle tugs on the lead from the battery pocket will help identify the insertion point or fluoroscopy can be used to identify the insertion point. It is often helpful to re-insert a stylet, which may have been used for placement of a new lead before extraction of the old. Care should be taken if electrocautery is used to dissect along the lead, since a breach in insulation can lead to stimulation of the nerve with electro-cautery. Others have described the use of a fascial or ureteral dilator in order to aid in dissection down the course of the lead. Dissection of scar tissue with McIndoe scissors has also been helpful. Once one of the tines is seen, the lead can be clamped with straight heavy grasping clips distally and slow, steady traction on the lead in the opposite direction of original insertion should be used. We also utilise the circular motion of the lead with slow and firm traction. Readjustment of the position of the clamp may be needed during the process. Even under these circumstances, the lead may fracture. If so, it is usually in a specific fashion due to how the lead was assembled. A "ghost" lead remains where no filament is left behind, and only the plastic housing with contacts remains (Fig. 32.5). In this circumstance, it may be difficult to remove the remaining portion of the lead without a sacral laminectomy, and the risk of nerve damage would seem to be less in leaving the lead in place. The filament is necessary to act as an antenna for MRI energy, so without it, it is unlikely the contacts will heat during MRI.

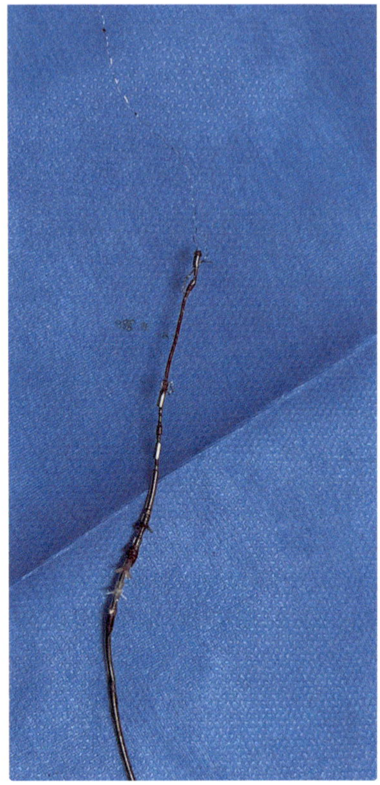

Fig. 32.5 Tined lead removed with fracture of the lead and retained electrode

Device-Related Complications

Allergic or Immune System Reactions to Implant

Currently, there is no formal guidance for the management of allergic reactions associated with sacral neuromodulators or their component parts. Iatrogenic allergic reactions can occur from the introduction of any foreign substances into a patient's body; however, there is a heightened risk of metals being the causative element. Nickel is the most commonly reactive material, with local dermatitis and pruritus being common symptoms. These can be difficult to distinguish from implant infection and care should be taken to explore all patient allergies before considering implantation. Treatment with antihistamines or local corticosteroid ointment may be possible for mild reactions; however, severe allergic reactions will likely require a full explanation. Before active management, it is essential to clearly distinguish whether the allergic reaction is in response to the implanted device or another element of the surgical procedure, such as the dressings. A thorough patient discussion before embarking on the SNM journey would help indicate the likelihood of patients experiencing these adverse effects and better inform the implant team.

Loss of Effective Symptom Control

Loss of effective symptom control is frequently cited in the literature. Carlton et al. [10] reviewed the FDA MAUDE database to assess the prevalence of reported complications and showed that loss or lack of efficacy was the most frequently reported complication. Desprez et al. [11] performed a 10-year follow-up study of 360 patients and noted a 23% loss of efficacy over that period. Although device explantation due to loss of efficacy has been reported to be lower [13], indicating that some benefit may still be achieved from the device, albeit not to the original level.

Determining the underlying cause for a loss of therapeutic benefit is complicated. It is important to differentiate between a device that never provided therapeutic benefit and one whose efficacy has declined. Regardless of ideal lead placement, a poor candidate with no true trial phase improvement will not experience the desired improvement, irrespective of intervention. Ensuring patients are carefully selected following national recommendations and objective benefits in relevant symptom categories is quantified through standardised diaries and questionnaires. Guidelines state that a 50% improvement is required prior to implantation, and the change in symptoms should be obvious and dramatic. Patients should never be persuaded into a full implant and expectation setting should be prudent. It is unlikely that a full system implant will give any greater benefit than the test phase, so careful counselling before implantation is important. Optimal lead placement and intra-operative response a good indicators of treatment success, but the only true predictor that we have is a successful trial outcome.

Lead migration can also be an explanation for declining efficacy. The lead has the potential to move in either direction, although more commonly it migrates inwards due to the tine design (Fig. 32.6). Outward migration may be contributed to by tension on the lead due to IPG positioning and patient size. Sometimes a knuckle/bulge is formed at the site of insertion of the lead. This can happen more in slim patients and can result in inward migration of the lead when the knuckle is pressed against a hard surface, such as a chair, before the lead has fully healed into place. In rare circumstances, patients themselves may "play" with the IPG and turn it, causing the lead to twist and be pulled out of the foramen [12]. Care must be taken to make a large enough incision to place a small retractor inside the incision and lift up on the retractor while tracking back towards the insertion site and deeply over to the IPG.

Placing the lead and the IPG on the same side may mitigate against this, although in slim patients, tunnelling across to the contralateral side may reduce slack on the lead and prevent an excess loop from forming at the pre-sacral site. Patients frequently report discomfort and dissatisfaction from these loops of the lead, and they may play a role in lead migration if they develop before scar tissue has had time to fully develop. The potential for lead migration can be reduced by clear patient guidance, warning of excessive or strenuous exercise for the initial 6–8 weeks post-implant.

Suboptimal lead placement causes problematic programming, often within the first 3–12 months. Intraoperative testing with motor responses at low amplitude levels is a good predictive factor for later device success. Lead migration is also more frequent within the first 6–8 weeks following implantation prior to scar tissue development. Persistence or recurrence of symptoms can often be mitigated by further reprogramming of the electrode. Optimal programming can ensure comfortable stimulation and delivery of therapy. The initial response to a loss of efficacy would be to utilise reprogramming before consideration of lead re-siting. Advances in technology allow patients to cycle between eleven programmes before requiring a face-to-face clinic appointment. Lead migration can be mitigated by appropriate programme selection and changes (Fig. 32.7), placing a focus on the electrode combination which appears closest to the nerve path.

Should changing the programme not deliver any improvement in symptoms remotely, then an impedance test should be a first-line check in the clinic to ensure any further programme changes

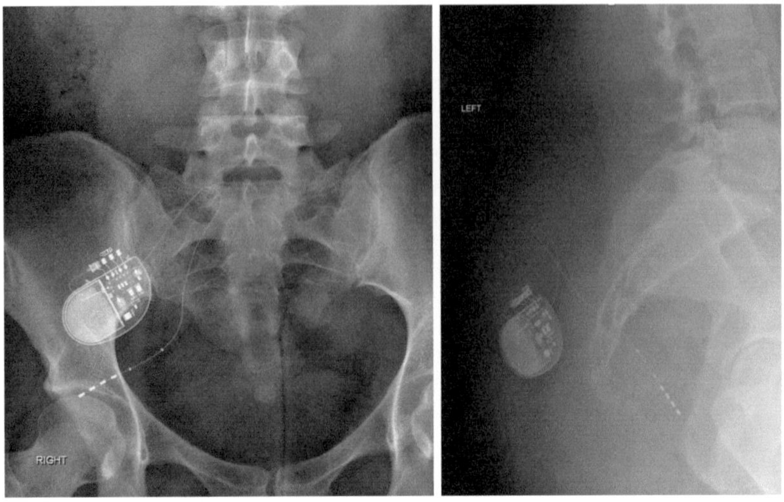

Fig. 32.6 Inward migration of tined lead

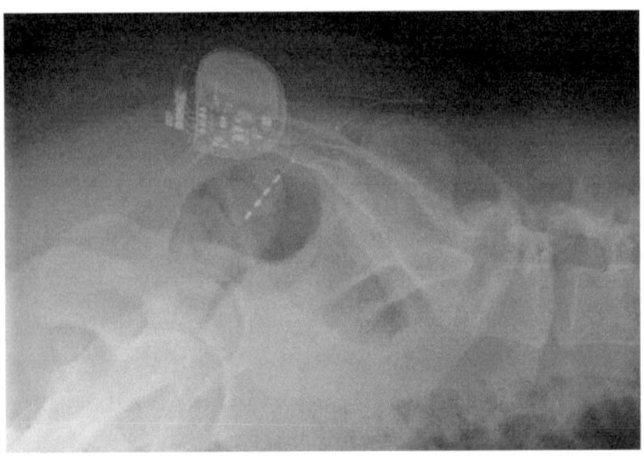

Fig. 32.7 Lead migration that was mitigated by change of programming

are viable. Impedance reports can be used as an indicator for appropriate electrode selection, avoiding ones with impedance readings outside of the recommended range. Tissue encapsulation around the electrodes can result in a higher electrical impedance, requiring higher stimulation amplitude to achieve therapeutic benefit. Increased impedance results indicate an open circuit break and low impedance results are indicative of a closed system break. Impedance results at either extreme are likely to prevent effective reprogramming if they appear on all electrode combinations and at this point, a lead replacement should be strongly considered.

If impedance results are acceptable, then expert opinion has shown some additional benefits from adjusting programme parameters. Increasing the stimulation frequency from the standard 14 Hz to 31 Hz has been demonstrated to optimise efficacy in a selection of patients and may be worth considering prior to lead re-siting [13].

Revision for Declining Efficacy

Once reprogramming options to improve efficacy have been exhausted, it is reasonable to consider lead revision. This is particularly true in cases where a prior peripheral nerve evaluation (PNE) demonstrated better symptomatic control than the permanent implant, which may indicate a poor permanent lead placement. Antero-posterior (AP) and lateral x-rays can be helpful in determining if there are obvious areas where lead position could be improved. Furthermore, if thresholds are high, it may suggest the lead is too inferior or lateral when entering the foramen. In the case of a successful PNE, with obvious problems identified with permanent lead placement, it is reasonable to correct the problems during revision and to connect to the IPG in a single-stage revision. If the response to the original trial is questionable in retrospect, it may be appropriate to perform a staged trial with the new lead, and to connect after bladder diaries confirm symptom control. If further improvement is not demonstrated, it may then be appropriate to remove all implanted devices.

Unwanted Sensation

Pain at IPG Site

Pain at the IPG site is another commonly reported complication with a variable prevalence rate. Chartier-Kastler et al. [14] performed a 5-year multicentre study of 291 patients, 6% of whom reported implant site pain. Understanding whether the pain is stimulation-oriented or mechanical is a first-line assessment. Some patients report 'pocket' pain associated with using the IPG as the anode when programming. Switching the device off and assessing discomfort will elicit whether this is causative, and if so, reprogramming will be required. Use of a bipolar setting may be more appropriate in these cases.

More commonly, however, site pain is mechanical and related to the position of the IPG. Careful placement and pocket sizing can prevent IPG movement, reducing the possibility of devices rotating, which in turn can pull the lead out of position. Also, the position of the IPG incision is important. It should be below the posterior superior iliac crest, usually by 8–10 cm, and lateral to the lateral sacral edge (upper outer part of the buttock). It should not be over either of these bony structures.

Conservative management of IPG site pain can include the use of ibuprofen gel, lidocaine plasters, Capsaicin 0.075% cream and in some cases injections of lidocaine, although the latter should be done with caution to avoid introducing infection. In persistent cases, re-positioning of the IPG is recommended. Once again, a full discussion with the patient is required to explore more ideal placement sites, and also to inform them of the risk of lead damage from surgical intervention. Erratic weight changes may influence IPG placement, and therefore, patient counselling before implantation is paramount.

Placement of the IPG on the opposite side may also be helpful for some situations, but the lead must be disconnected and re-tunnelled from the pre-sacral site to do so. In rare cases, the device can be placed in the abdomen (Fig. 32.8).

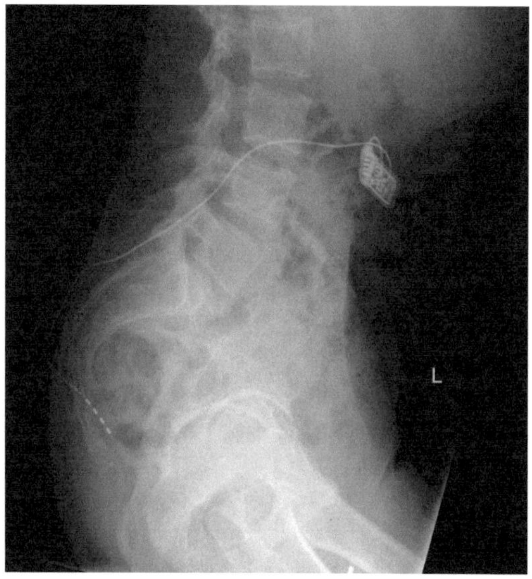

Fig. 32.8 Rechargeable Interstim Micro inserted into anterior abdominal wall do to lack of body fat in buttocks in patient with low BMI and previous extrusions of larger IPGs

This is an option for those who do not have sufficient buttock adipose to encapsulate the IPG fully (Fig. 32.9).

Referred Pain in Leg/Foot

In addition to site pain, some patients report discomfort radiating into their leg or foot. This is more frequently related to stimulation, be that the amplitude level of programme choice. In cases where leads have migrated inwards, avoidance of the more distal electrodes may mitigate against unwanted leg stimulation. Reprogramming of the standard pulse width parameter of 210 μsec has also been shown to affect nerve recruitment, with lower pulse widths being associated with a reduction in undesirable pain [13].

Prior to any reprogramming, patients should be advised to switch their devices off and monitor changes in discomfort. If the discomfort persists in the absence of stimulation, then it is unlikely that any device related changes will be of benefit and further exploration of pain is needed.

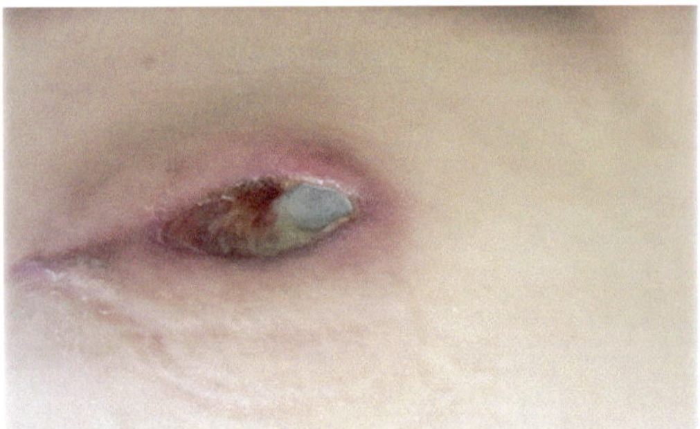

Fig. 32.9 Extruded Interstim II IPG in patient with low BMI

Suspected Nerve Damage

On rare occasions, patients report severe neuropathic pain or neurological symptoms post-implant. These patients are difficult to manage, especially if they are experiencing symptomatic benefit from their device. The cause of neuropathic pain is difficult to establish, and the case study below highlights an individual case experienced within our unit. Resolution of symptoms is not always achieved by device removal, and therefore, careful counselling of patients should include possible long-term pain.

Case Study

A 40-year-old male with refractory detrusor overactivity incontinence. Successful PNE trial phase with >50% improvement in symptoms. The patient experienced neurological pain immediately post-implant, describing pain radiating from the right buttock into the back of the right leg and calf, as far as the outer ankle and foot. He presented with weakness in the affected leg, preventing him from walking long distances or standing for prolonged periods of time.

Management through reprogramming was not beneficial. Removal of tined lead with IPG left in situ to allow potential lead re-implantation at a later date was also unsuccessful at reducing pain. Full system explanation was then performed and neurological pain and symptoms persisted. Mild symptom relief with Amitriptyline but unpleasant side effects.

Investigations included nerve conduction tests, which showed evidence of partial L5, S1/S2 radiculopathies. This indicates a possible nerve impingement due to IPG implantation.

Additional Possible Complications

Poor Candidate Selection

Whilst patient comorbidities are rarely an absolute contraindication, there are a number of patient factors which should be considered when selecting the most appropriate candidate. Research has shown that an elevated body mass index (BMI) has been linked to higher rates of explantation [15]. However, a better assessment may be to consider body habitus and associated weight distribution along with the likelihood of weight changes following implantation.

Additionally, Quirouet et al. [8] identified that diabetic men presented more difficult lead extraction cases. Diabetic patients have also been linked to higher rates of explantation due to infection [16]. The only true predictor of SNM success is the trial phase.

Careful lead placement with all 4 electrodes in an optimal position and eliciting correct nerve responses at low amplitude levels is critical to a successful implant. The device needs to be comfortable both in position and stimulation, as well as able to provide therapeutic benefits.

Pregnancy

There is limited evidence for the impact of SNM on pregnancy and due to the evident ethical considerations randomised control trial would raise, any research readily available is primarily extracted from case studies. A recent systematic review [16] demonstrated that SNM activation during pregnancy appears to be both safe and effective. This needs to be considered on an individual patient basis with open patient/clinician discussions about the possible risks and manufacturer recommendations. For those patients who are implanted to treat voiding dysfunctions or urinary retention, then the risk of SNM deactivation is a reoccurrence of these symptoms and a resulting need to catheterise. For many patients, catheterisation comes with an unacceptable risk of urinary tract infections and pyelonephritis, and therefore SNM activation should be carefully considered on a risk/reward basis.

Advice relating to the most ideal method of delivery is also scarce. Neither vaginal nor caesarean delivery can guarantee no damage to the IPG or electrode. Therefore, all implant information should be available to the obstetrician to guide their decision-making, including placement of epidural, use of surgical diathermy or patient positioning.

Post-delivery, patients who have had their devices deactivated may wish to reactivate them in the presence of a clinician. There is potential for device damage or electrode displacement during delivery or at some point throughout the pregnancy period. This, coupled with the extensive period of inactive time, may result in a loss of therapeutic effect or uncomfortable stimulation. Should either of these be the case, then it would be advisable to follow the relevant advice above.

Magnetic Resonance Imaging (MRI)

Advances in technology have meant that since August 2020, all implantable SNM devices have 1.5T and 3T full-body MR Conditional labelling. This positive development has opened up SNM as an appropriate treatment option for patients who require regular MRI scans. However, with advances in technology comes a greater need to understand the relevant safety considerations of fully body MRIs.

MR conditional labelling is dependent on the model of the device the patient has implanted. This information should be readily available on the patient's hospital records, but also on their personal handset or patient identification card. Whilst all new devices are MRI compatible, it is important to review all implant history. A new IPG connected to an existing pre-2020 lead creates a system that is still not MRI-compatible. An abandoned lead fragment from a previous implant may still act as an antenna and absorb radiofrequency signals present during the MRI.

MRI guidance can be obtained from the company and often this acts as the best resource for ensuring the safest possible MRI scan.

IPG Charging Difficulties

The advent of rechargeable devices has brought with it a new array of complications, most commonly ones that prevent an efficient connection between the implanted IPG and the charging unit. A poor connection results in a suboptimal charging experience for the patient, with the extended time needed to establish and maintain the connection to recharge. Problematic connections are most commonly due to a poor IPG position or equipment failure. Adaptations can be made to enhance connection through the application of pressure and direct skin contact; however, it is not uncommon for IPG re-siting to be required for acceptable charging.

Consideration of body habitus and technical ability should be high on the priority list when counselling patients on device choice. Pre-operative marking of IPG placement, along with charging belt sizing, is recommended to avoid early charging difficulties.

Unexpected Complications Associated with Percutaneous Nerve Evaluation (PNE)

Despite verbal and written instructions, there have been a number of leads cut by the patients during the course of the trial phase both terminat-

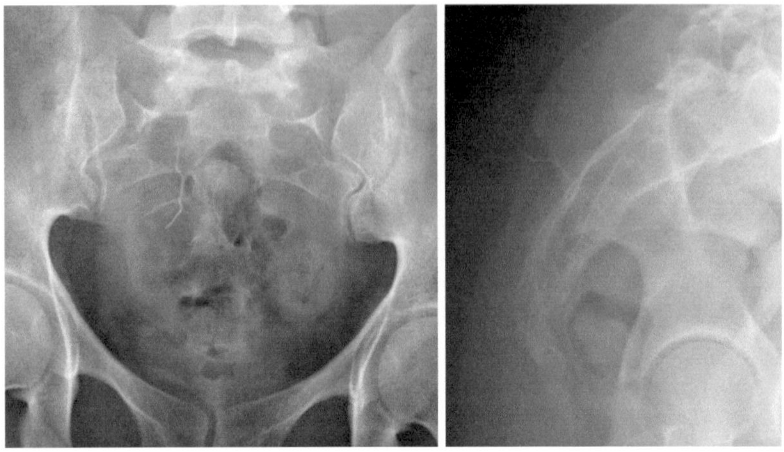

Fig. 32.10 Cut PNE lead that had to be removed surgically

ing the trial and also resulting in an untethered lead segment being left in the patient. Those cut flush to the skin have required urgent surgical intervention to extract the lead segment before inward migration (Fig. 32.10). Whilst difficult to mitigate against unexpected patient actions, secure dressings and use of gauze around the temporary lead may better protect against this, as well as writing on the dressings "Do Not Touch or Remove".

Conclusion

Sacral neuromodulation is a well-established modality for the treatment of lower urinary tract and pelvic floor dysfunction. Complications can happen from device implantation, leading to removal and/or revision. It is therefore important to be able to prevent these complications from happening, recognise them if they happen and manage them accordingly (Table 32.2).

Table 32.2 Summary of tips and tricks to manage and reduce complications

Complication	Management
Infection prevention	MRSA screening and urine culture pre-op Intravenous antibiotics (Flucloxacillin and Gentamicin or cephazolin) pre-op Masks Laminar flow OR Limit movement of personnel in the OR 2% Chlorhexidine skin prep Ioban Skin glue and dressing Changing of gloves at time of battery insertion Five days broad spectrum oral antibiotics post-op e.g. co-amoxiclav
Infection treatment	Intravenous antibiotics, removal of all device components, capsule removal, saline wash of the wound, VAC dressing (if poor wound healing)
Loss of symptom efficacy	Confirm any changes in medical history or medication Assess for any clear event associated with loss of efficacy, perform x-ray if any concerns about lead position or integrity Device check (impedance—open/closed break, battery—end of battery life) Replace or reprogramme if possible Change electrode configuration based on impedance check and X-ray (AP and lateral) Adjust device parameters, increase stimulation frequency In some cases cycling can be beneficial, especially in those patients who habituate or feel a benefit from the sensation
Pain in leg/ foot	Switch the device off and establish whether pain dissipates or is maintained If discomfort continues then unlikely that is it due to stimulation X-ray (AP and lateral) to determine lead position, assess for inward lead migration Change electrode configuration to target nerve Adjust device parameters, decrease pulse width
Pain at site of IPG	Switch the device off and confirm discomfort is maintained If discomfort reduces then consider reprogramming to avoid programmes using the Case as an anode Establish any cause (trauma, weight alterations etc) Basic pain relief guidance (tight clothing to minimise movement, ibuprofen gel, Capsaicin gel, lidocaine plasters) Surgical re-site or removal
MRI	Find suitable alternative. Leads prior to March 2020—Safe for head or extremity if 1.5T lateral bore magnet with send/receive coil. Extra concern about lead fragments. May be necessary to remove IPG and lead if no alternative. If lead post-2020, then MRI compatible up to 3T
Tined lead retention	Use 1–2 cm pre-sacral incision to remove in opposite direction of original placement. Can use stylet to stiffen. "Ghost lead" fragment with filament removed may be safe. May need to dissect onto fascia but avoid entering foramen without neurosurgical input
Pregnancy	Turn off before first trimester if possible. Consider bridging with BoNT before planned conception if has overactive bladder or commence intermittent catheterisation if voiding dysfunction. Some risks may increase by turning off e.g. UTI with voiding dysfunction. Shared decision making and discuss pros and cons of switching off with mother and obstetrician. Regarding caesareans, a single spinal injection may be safer than an epidural provided there is no chance of hitting the lead and electrodes

References

1. Greig J, Mak Q, Furrer MA, Sahai A, Raison N. Sacral neuromodulation in the management of chronic pelvic pain: a systematic review and meta-analysis. Neurourol Urodyn. 2023;42(4):822–36.
2. Hendrickson WK, Amundsen CL. Sacral neuromodulation: sacral anatomy and optimal lead placement. Int Urogynecol J. 2021;32(9):2545–7.
3. Matzel KE, Chartier-Kastler E, Knowles CH, Lehur PA, Muñoz-Duyos A, Ratto C, Rydningen MB, Sørensen M, van Kerrebroeck P, de Wachter S. Sacral neuromodulation: standardized electrode placement technique. Neuromodulation. 2017;20(8):816–24.
4. Agnello M, Brugnano S, Vottero M, Bertapelle P. Infection rate of a prolonged sacral Neuromodulation test: a large retrospective study. Neuromodulation. 2023;26(8):1845–50.
5. Myer ENB, Petrikovets A, Slocum PD, Lee TG, Carter-Brooks CM, Noor N, Carlos DM, Wu E, Van Eck K, Fashokun TB, Yurteri-Kaplan L, Chen CCG. Risk factors for explantation due to infection after sacral neuromodulation: a multicenter retrospective case-control study. Am J Obstet Gynecol. 2018;219(1):78.e1–9.
6. Myer EN, Petrikovets A, Slocum PD, Lee TG, Carter-Brooks CM, Noor N, Carlos DM, Wu E, Van Eck K, Fashokun TB, Yurteri-Kaplan L. Risk factors for explantation due to infection after sacral neuromodulation: a multicenter retrospective case-control study. Am J Obstet Gynecol. 2018;219(1):78–e1.
7. Simpson JAD, Peacock J, Maxwell-Armstrong C. Use of a gentamicin-impregnated collagen sheet (Collatamp(®)) following implantation of a sacral nerve stimulator for faecal incontinence. Color Dis. 2012;14(4):e200–2.
8. Quirouet A, Bhattacharyya PK, Dielubanza EJ, Gill BC, Jones SE, Goldman HB. Sacral neuromodulation device heating during lumbar and pelvic magnetic resonance imaging-a phantom study. Urology. 2017;107:61–6.
9. Martin S, Goldman HB. Removal of sacral Neuromodulation devices is an office procedure. Urology. 2023;177:65–8.
10. Carlton CE, Souders CP, Chertack NA, Goueli RS, Lemack GE, Anger JT, McClelland L, Carmel ME. Understanding a decade of safety reporting for sacral neuromodulation in the food and drug administration manufacturer and user facility device experience database. Neurourol Urodyn. 2023;42(8):1655–67.
11. Desprez C, Damon H, Meurette G, Mege D, Faucheron JL, Brochard C, Lambrescak E, Gourcerol G, Mion F, Wyart V, Sielezneff I, Siproudhis L, Etienney I, Ajamie N, Lehur PA, Duflot T, Bridoux V, Leroi AM. Club NEMO. Ten-year evaluation of a large retrospective cohort treated by sacral nerve modulation for fecal incontinence: results of a French multicenter study. Ann Surg. 2022;275(4):735–42.
12. Guzman-Negron JM, Derisavifard S, Goldman HB. Sacral neuromodulation lead twisting causes migration and loss of efficacy. Urogynecology. 2020;26(3):e13–5.
13. Dudding TC, Lehur PA, Sørensen M, Engelberg S, Bertapelle MP, Chartier-Kastler E, Everaert K, Van Kerrebroeck P, Knowles CH, Lundby L, Matzel KE. Reprogramming sacral neuromodulation for sub-optimal outcomes: evidence and recommendations for clinical practice. Neuromodulation Technol Neural Interface. 2021;24(7):1247–57.
14. Chartier-Kastler E, Le Normand L, Ruffion A, Saussine C, Braguet R, Rabut B, Ragni E, Perrouin-Verbe MA, Pierrevelcin J, Rousseau T, Gamé X, Tanneau Y, Dargent F, Biardeau X, Graziana JP, Stoica G, Brassart E, Fourmarier M, Yaghi N, Capon G, Ferchaud J, Berrogain N, Peyrat L, Pecoux F, Bryckaert PE, Karsenty G, Song S, Keller DUJ, Cornu JN. Five-year results from the prospective, multicenter, observational SOUNDS study of patients with overactive bladder treated with the InterStim system for sacral neuromodulation. Eur Urol Focus. 2023;9(5):765–72.
15. Feldkamp A, Amasyalı AS, Groegler J, Jellison F, Staack A. Evaluation of progression from first to second stage sacral neuromodulation and unplanned device removal. Turk J Urol. 2020;47(1):58–65.
16. Salehi-Pourmehr H, Atayi M, Mahdavi N, Aletaha R, Kashtkar M, Sharifimoghadam S, Hassanzadeh R, Hajebrahimi S. Is sacral neuromodulation effective and safe in pregnancy? A systematic review. Neurourol Urodyn. 2023;42(6):1329–43.
17. Noblett K, Benson K, Kreder K. Detailed analysis of adverse events and surgical interventions in a large prospective trial of sacral neuromodulation therapy for overactive bladder patients. Neurourol Urodyn. 2017;36(4):1136–9.
18. https://manuals.medtronic.com/content/dam/emanuals/neuro/MA12871A_a_009_view.pdf

Botulinum Toxin Injection

33

Melissa R. Kaufman and Elizabeth A. Rourke

Introduction

Few therapies have so galvanized the management of a urologic condition as that witnessed over the past decade regarding use of onabotulinumtoxinA (BoNT-A) for bladder dysfunction. The range of clinical applications in the urologic realm, coupled with relative ease of administration, has revolutionized therapeutic options for several prevalent conditions. Although injection of BoNT-A is generally considered low risk, there remain a number of critical considerations with regard to contraindications and adverse events which must be carefully weighed prior to including BoNT-A in a patient's treatment algorithm. Herein we discuss common urologic applications and the associated potential sequela of utilization of BoNT-A in the urinary tract.

M. R. Kaufman (✉)
Department of Urology, Vanderbilt University Medical Center, Nashville, TN, USA
e-mail: melissa.kaufman@vumc.org

E. A. Rourke
Department of Urologic Surgery, Louisiana State University Health Science Center, New Orleans, LA, USA
e-mail: erourk@lsuhsc.edu

History of Botulinum Toxin

Botulinum neurotoxin (BoNT) is produced by the gram-positive obligate anaerobe *Clostridium botulinum*, initially isolated in 1897 by van Ermengem [1]. Despite the weighty role of BoNT in the manifestations of food-borne botulism, decades of innovative research have exploited the toxin's properties, revealing a multitude of clinical applications that impact a variety of debilitating conditions. In addition to the urologic indications outlined below, BoNT is routinely employed for treatment of chronic migraines, pain, head and neck dystonia, hyperhidrosis, and anal fissures in addition to the commonly recognized cosmetic applications [2].

BoNT induces flaccid muscle paralysis by inhibiting release of the neurotransmitter acetylcholine from the presynaptic nerve terminal at the neuromuscular junction. In the lower urinary tract, effects are principally mediated at the parasympathetic presynaptic nerve terminal [3]. Generally considered the most potent neurotoxin recognized, and classified by the Centers for Disease Control and Prevention as a Category A bioweapons threat, it has been postulated that a mere 1 g of appropriately dispersed purified BoNT could be lethal to a million people [4, 5].

C. botulinum produces seven antigenically distinct serotypes of BoNT, each with multiple sub-types; however, only types A and B are cur-

H. B. Goldman, J. Zillioux (eds.), *Complications of Urogynecology and Reconstructive Pelvic Surgery*, https://doi.org/10.1007/978-3-032-00339-3_33

rently employed clinically [6]. Expansive discussion of the molecular mechanism of action and pharmacology of BoNT is outside the scope of this review and is extensively detailed in additional material [7]. However, several salient aspects are critical to understand applications, limitations, and complications for urologic utilization. The most commonly utilized serotype, type A, is a 150 kDa polypeptide with several domains imparting distinct functions. As mentioned above, end-organ lower urinary tract manifestations are mediated by BoNT-A at the parasympathetic presynaptic nerve terminal. BoNT-A directly cleaves synaptosomal-associated protein (SNAP-25), required for fusion of synaptic vesicles at the cellular membrane, thus specifically preventing release of neurotransmitters into the synaptic cleft [8]. However, despite our classic concepts of BoNT's impact on the neuromuscular junction, emerging robust data implicate a diversity of alternative mechanisms of action to account for the clinical effects demonstrated in the lower urinary tract [9]. BoNT-A inhibits the release of an assortment of neurotransmitters (acetylcholine, ATP, substance P), in addition to downregulating purinergic and capsaicin receptors on afferent neurons with potential culmination in a central desensitization [10]. Indeed, many of the alternative targets of BoNT-A have been previously implicated to contribute to the pathophysiology of detrusor overactivity and the overactive bladder (OAB) symptom complex. BoNT-A binds with high affinity to synaptic vesicle protein 2 (SV2), expressed predominantly in the parasympathetic fibers of the human bladder and additionally present in approximately half of the sensory fibers [11]. Clinical effect of BoNT-A likely integrates both efferent, parasympathetic pathways and afferent, nociceptive pathways. Sensory dysfunction can also be impacted by BoNT as a result of afferent neurotransmitter blockade, driving a reduction of bladder sensations (i.e., urinary urgency, frequency, and bladder pain) [10]. Also critical for understanding clinical utility and potential complications is that BoNT produces a reversible chemical denervation with recovery due to axonal sprouting and formation of novel synaptic connections [12]. Clinical results are not typically completely manifested for several weeks following injection, and the duration of response is variable depending on the indication, dosage, and patient symptomatology.

Clinical Applications in Urology

Use of BoNT in lower urinary tract disorders was pioneered by Dykstra and colleagues in 1988 for treatment of detrusor-external sphincter dyssynergia (DSD) [13]. Currently, BoNT-A is utilized predominantly for the Federal Drug Administration (FDA)-approved indications of neurogenic detrusor overactivity (NDO) and refractory overactive bladder (OAB) [14, 15]. Additional applications have been extensively investigated for benign prostatic hyperplasia (BPH), interstitial cystitis/bladder pain syndrome (IC/BPS), radiation cystitis, urethral stricture disease, detrusor underactivity, and myofascial pelvic pain with variable clinical results. Full synopsis of the current data regarding each of the urologic applications is outside the scope of this chapter and expertly detailed in several meta-analyses and reviews [16–18]. Potential complications associated with the commonly employed on-label usage are generally applicable to investigational applications. For the purposes of this discussion, adverse event (AE) is defined by the FDA as an "untoward medical occurrence associated with the use of a drug in humans, whether or not considered drug related" [19]. Overall, BoNT has demonstrated low adverse event rates, with the most common events being UTI and dysuria.

Hypersensitivities and Absolute Contraindications

Remarkably, there are few definitive contraindications to administration of BoNT-A for lower urinary tract applications. Several relative contraindications should be carefully weighed, but remain at the clinician's discretion. The primary absolute contraindications to BoNT-A administration include a known hypersensitivity to the toxin. Immediate hypersensitivity reactions have been reported, including anaphylaxis, serum sickness, urticaria, soft tissue edema, and dyspnea. A solitary fatal case of anaphylaxis was reported with lidocaine as the diluent, and thus the causal agent for the reaction remains unidentified [20]. Systemic spread is not well understood but postulated to be a combination of contributing factors, including dose, injection volume, and injection technique [21]. Systematic review of efficacy and safety for NDO revealed no reported anaphylactic reactions for detrusor injection in the neurogenic population in the published literature [22].

For bladder indications, a more consequential absolute contraindication includes the presence of active urinary infection at the time of injection. Clinical trials for both NDO and OAB indications excluded patients reporting more than 2 urinary tract infections (UTI) in the past 6 months or those taking chronic antibiotics for UTI treatment [14, 15]. Careful vigilance in assessing active infection must be undertaken by the treating physician, particularly for the neurogenic population, as atypical UTI symptoms may manifest. As will be discussed in a following section, UTI was the primary AE documented in multiple clinical trials. Therefore, embarking on detrusor injection in the setting of active infection significantly increases the global risk to the patient for adverse outcomes, including potential progression to urosepsis.

Special Populations

Although not an absolute contraindication, exceptional caution must be employed for patients with diagnoses of pre-existing peripheral motor neuron diseases, amyotrophic lateral sclerosis, or neuromuscular junction disorders such as myasthenia gravis or Lambert-Eaton syndrome. Such patients may demonstrate increased risk of generalized effects following BoNT injection, such as weakness, diplopia, ptosis, dysphonia, dysarthria, dysphagia, and respiratory compromise. Careful deliberation in collaboration with the treating neurologist should be undertaken prior to embarking on detrusor injections for this patient population as the risks often outweigh the potential benefits. Likewise, in spinal cord injury and MS patients with restrictive lung disease treated for NDO, at least a 15% reduction in forced vital capacity (FVC) was noted in BoNT-A treatment arms compared to placebo [20]. Therefore, exceptional caution and monitoring are mandated in patients with concomitant pulmonary pathology and neurologic disease in the periprocedural period.

Spinal cord injury patients additionally display elevated risk for autonomic dysreflexia (AD) with intradetrusor injection of BoNT-A as compared to placebo (1.5% versus 0.4%) [14]. These data suggest it may be prudent to forgo clinic injection and consider monitored anesthesia care for patients with known or potential issues with AD desiring BoNT-A injection.

BoNT-A is considered by the FDA as Pregnancy Category C, indicating there are no adequate and well-controlled studies conducted in pregnant women to determine safety [20]. In a 24-year retrospective review of the Allergen safety database, 232 eligible patients exposed to BoNT-A before/during pregnancy demonstrated comparable fetal defects to the general population. However, exposure to BoNT-A was most commonly seen before and during the first trimester, and the majority (40%) of the study population received <50 units [23]. In animal models, intramuscular injection resulted in reductions in fetal body weight and skeletal ossification. During the critical phases of organogenesis in rats and rabbits at doses which extrapolate to the maximum recommended human dose of 400 Units, daily injections revealed significant maternal toxicity, abortions, early deliveries, and even maternal death was observed. However, a single dose at three different periods resulted in no AEs on fetal development. Overall, it is recommended to only employ BoNT-A during pregnancy if the benefit significantly outweighs the risk. Likewise, it remains unknown if BoNT-A is secreted in breast milk, so caution should be exercised when administering to nursing mothers.

Note that the FDA-approved indications include only dosage regimens and applications for adults >18 years of age. Utilization of BoNT-A for bladder applications in the pediatric population, although widely investigated for decades and generally reported safe and effective, remains off-label.

For geriatric patients undergoing 100 Unit BoNT-A injections for OAB indications, AEs such as UTI and urinary retention were demonstrated to be markedly more common in patients 75 years of age or older compared to younger patients. Rates of UTI for patients ≥75 years receiving BoNT-A were 38% (placebo 19%) compared to 30% for patients 65–74 years old and 21% for patients ≤65 years of age [15]. In general, caution is recommended for dose selection in the geriatric population with preferential initiation at low dose ranges to accommodate for the amplified frequency of decreased hepatic, renal, or cardiac function in addition to concomitant diseases and pharmaceuticals.

Potential Drug Interactions

Significant possible drug interactions critical to consider include avoidance of co-administration of BoNT-A with aminoglycosides or curare-like compounds, which may interfere with neuromuscular transmission and potentiate toxin effects [24]. However, a more contemporary retrospective review of 220 OAB patients receiving a single dose of 160 mg IV Gentamicin prior to BoNT-A injection demonstrated no adverse extravesical neuromuscular side effects. Therefore, broadly employed periprocedural urologic antimicrobial medications such as gentamicin must be carefully considered in special circumstances (i.e., urine cultures susceptible to aminoglycosides alone) [25]. For patients treated for NDO or OAB, concurrent usage of anticholinergics may potentiate systemic antimuscarinic effects and the risk of urinary retention. Additionally, patients concurrently utilizing muscle relaxants may experience exaggeration of weakness following administration of BoNT-A.

Toxin Preparation Equivalence

Commercially available BoNT-A preparations in the United States include Botox® (onabotulinumtoxinA, Allergan Pharmaceuticals), Dysport® (abobotulinumtoxinA, Ipson Biopharm), and Xeomin® (incobotulinumtoxinA, Merz Pharmaceuticals). A single type B BoNT preparation is additionally available, Myobloc® (rimabotulinumtoxinB, Solstice Neurosciences, Inc.) Presently, only onabotulinumtoxin A and Dysport possess FDA approval for urinary tract indications. With substantial differences in dosing, efficacy, and safety profiles, these BoNT preparations should not be considered interchangeable. Indeed, significant inconsistencies were revealed between studies determining dose equivalency, and therefore no standardized data exists to provide robust clinical guidance for interchange of toxin preparations for intradetrusor applications [26].

Injection Technique and Local Complications

BoNT-A is administered via intradetrusor injection under local, regional or general anesthesia using a rigid or flexible cystoscope, frequently in a clinic setting. While no protocol regarding the location and number of injections is universally accepted, general best practices for injection have been previously described [27]. Prior to injection, 30 mL of 2% lidocaine are instilled into the bladder and allowed to dwell for 30–60 minutes to provide local anesthesia. For FDA-approved indications, 100 Units of BoNT-A is diluted in 10 mL preservative-free saline (OAB) or 200 Units is diluted in 30 mL preservative-free saline (NDO). If a 200-unit vial is being used, it is recommended to dilute this with 6 mL and then use 2 mL in a 10 mL syringe reconstituted with 8 mL of preservative free saline. Reconstitution techniques can vary but are geared to an injection concentration of 6.7–10 U/mL [28]. It is commonly injected in a grid pattern on the posterior bladder wall in 0.5 cc increments for OAB and 1 cc increments for NDO, separated by a distance of 1–1.5 cm. Dilution modification is commonly employed in clinical practice to provide 10 Units per cc, allowing reproducible 1 cc injection volumes for both indications. Injection depth is optimized at 2 mm, which, in most instances, allows spread of BoNT-A deep to the mucosal layers and directly into the detrusor and can be visualized as a rise in the bladder epithelium. If flexible cystoscopy is utilized, a 1 mL sterile normal saline injection should be performed at the end to ensure complete use of BoNT-A. Injections to the bladder dome are generally avoided to prevent perforation and extravesical injection. The trigone has previously been circumvented as an injection site due to a theoretical risk of vesicoureteral reflux, detailed in the following section.

Transient adverse events associated with the act of injection, rather than BoNT-A itself, include dysuria, pain, hematuria, bacteriuria, and elevation of post-void residual (PVR). Of note, most mild AEs occurred within the first week following injection. Occasionally, needle or anxiety-related events, such as vasovagal responses, may occur at the time of injection and should be treated per the clinician's standard of care. Additional AEs reported at low frequencies included nausea, depression, muscle spasm, constipation, de novo incontinence, generalized or localized muscle weakness, insomnia, dizziness, diarrhea, influenza, hypertension, headache, back pain, mycotic infection, multiple sclerosis (MS) relapse, pain, fever, and de novo autonomic dysreflexia.

Systemic Complications

As mentioned previously, BoNT is often considered the most potent biological toxin recognized; thus potential AEs from administration are theoretically profound [29]. Although generally considered a focal therapy on local peripheral nerves, a black box warning accompanies the prescribing information for BoNT-A, highlighting the prospect for systemic spread. Doses of BoNT-A are represented by mouse units (U), with one unit of toxin representing the dose necessary for mortality following intraperitoneal injection in 50% of a group of female mice. In humans, an extrapolated lethal dose of BoNT-A would range from 2000 to 3000 Units [30]. Although the incidence of such systemic events remains exceedingly rare, the clinician must employ a high index of suspicion for such sequela [31]. New onset symptoms such as focal or generalized muscle weakness, hoarseness or dysphonia, dysarthria, de novo or worsening urinary incontinence, difficulty with breathing or swallowing, and impaired vision are potential indications of regional or systemic toxin spread [32–34]. Reports of progression to respiratory depression and death have thus far been limited to children receiving elevated doses for skeletal muscle spasticity [35]. Meta-analysis of long-term efficacy and safety of 2309 patients encompassing 36 studies reported the overall risk of mild or moderate AEs in patients receiving BoNT-A to be 25% compared to 15% in controls [35]. The only AE occurring more significantly in the BoNT-A group was focal weakness, again highlighting the potential for infrequent, yet significant, AEs. Similar literature reviews for both OAB and NDO demonstrated the exceptional rarity of systemic events [22, 36, 37].

Urinary Tract Infection and Urinary Retention

The most prevalent AEs noted with BoNT-A injections for both OAB and NDO include urinary tract infection and urinary retention, complications which are frequently interrelated. Confounding analysis of these common sequela of BoNT-A injection is inconsistent application of definitions for urinary infection, retention, and thresholds for initiation of catheterization. Additionally, the duration and frequency of intermittent catheterization are not standardized or well documented in the available literature.

Meta-analysis of four randomized controlled trials (RCTs) for OAB encompassing 1263 patients reported rates of UTI in the BoNT-A treatment arm as 19.7% compared to 6% of controls [37]. Initial data for OAB indications demonstrated 18% rates of UTI with 100-unit injection [15]. For patients with diabetes, UTI rates were substantially elevated to 31% in the BoNT-A arm compared to 12% with placebo. When defined as symptomatic retention with PVR between 200 and 350 cc or PVR ≥350 cc, urinary retention in the BoNT-A group was reported at 6%. However, with more stringent criteria encompassing practical clinical scenarios, a well-designed trial utilized limits of 200 cc to define retention, and 43% of patients met criteria, with 75% of BoNT-A treatment arm patients requiring antibiotic therapy for UTI [38]. Retrospective analysis of a single institution's clinical practice revealed rates of urinary retention, defined as the need for catheterization, of 35% while the OAB registration trials demonstrated much lower rates at 5.4% [15, 39]. The comorbidity of infection and retention was demonstrated in the pivotal RCT, with UTI documented in patients experiencing PVR ≥200 cc at 44% compared to 23% in those with PVR ≤200 cc [15]. Meta-analysis of available RCTs reporting PVR demonstrates that injection of BoNT-A significantly increased PVR versus placebo (32.8% versus 2.0%), with initiation of intermittent catheterization of 8.4% in the treatment arms [37].

For NDO patients with either spinal cord injury (SCI) or MS, UTI was dramatically increased in the 200 Unit BoNT-A arm at 49% compared to 18% of controls [14]. Of patients who were spontaneously voiding prior to injection, 47% were initiated on catheterization during the course of the analysis for all causes, compared to 22% of placebo patients. No defined PVR for initiation of intermittent catheterization was employed in the protocol. MS patients demonstrated significant dose-dependent increases in PVR with retention rates at 200 Units BoNT-A of 29% compared to 5% of placebo controls, with concomitant large discrepancies in UTI reported at 50% in the treatment arm versus 28% of controls.

Overall, urinary retention remains a dominant driving force for patient selection for BoNT-A injection and a major clinical concern following the procedure. Appropriate counseling regarding a realistic risk for retention and the requirement for duration of intermittent catheterization is mandated for the physician performing BoNT-A injection for patients currently spontaneously voiding. Assessment of the patient's or caregiver's willingness and ability to perform intermittent catheterization is imperative prior to performing BoNT-A injection.

Likewise, ensuring the absence of active infection at the time of injection and closely monitoring for signs of infection following the BoNT-A procedure are critical. Many clinicians advocate preprocedural urine culture accompanied by pretreatment with culture-specific antibiotics for high-risk patients, such as those with chronic bacteriuria secondary to intermittent catheterization with UTI symptoms.

Hematuria

While primarily related to the act of detrusor injection, transient hematuria is common following BoNT-A injection. However, complications resulting from persistent bleeding may result in acute anemia, clot urinary retention, and the need for repeat anesthesia/procedures. Recent studies suggest that performing BoNT-A injection on patients on anticoagulation therapy does not pose an increased risk of postoperative bleeding, and therefore, the decision to stop anticoagulants may vary with physician practice preference or shared decision-making with the patient. A number of patients with neurogenic bladder may display significant fibrosis and even friable bladder mucosa. If greater than anticipated bleeding is encountered during the procedure, hemostasis should be obtained with electrocautery/fulguration, and consideration for placement of an indwelling catheter for several days, which would allow bladder irrigation, may be prudent. Indwelling catheter placement may be particularly beneficial for patients reliant on self-catheterization to reduce the risk of further mucosal trauma and clot retention, which are complex situations to manage with smaller caliber single-use catheters. Exceedingly infrequently is there a need to employ electrocautery for fulguration of active bleeding following BoNT-A injection.

Vesicoureteral Reflux

With collective evidence of BoNT-A's influence on sensory pathways, there has been a concomitant increased focus on trigonal and suburothelial injections. The trigone of the bladder is particularly rich in sensory receptors, which may enhance response to BoNT-A for a variety of indications. Injections to the trigone have traditionally been avoided out of concern for potential provocation of vesicoureteral reflux (VUR). Despite this apprehension, several studies have demonstrated trigonal injections to be safe and effective without evidence of resultant VUR [40, 41] Indeed, recent meta-analysis comparing trigonal and extratrigonal injection technique in patients with NDO and OAB revealed no significant differences with regard to adverse effects or short-term efficacy, suggesting that patient specific factors and dosing dominate response to BoNT-A rather than injection location [42]. Additionally, Jo et al. demonstrated significant improvement in dryness rates (41%), symptom scores (78%), and frequency of incontinence episodes (87%) in a 2018 meta-analysis of trigone injections versus trigone sparing [43].

Administration for Multiple Indications

Significant numbers of patients receive BoNT for multiple indications, most frequently in neurogenic patients for extremity spasticity in addition to detrusor overactivity. The maximum cumulative dose for treatment of adult patients is currently recommended to not exceed 400 Units in a 3-month interval [20]. These dosage limits were increased from 360 to 400 Units in January 2016. Such dosage restrictions are promoted due to the risk of seroconversion owing to BoNT-A antibody formation, rather than to address systemic toxicity, discussed at length in the following section. A retrospective cohort study of patients undergoing high-dose injections of BoNT-A for multiple indications demonstrated only transient adverse events, even with a median dose administration of 800 Units within the 3-month window [31]. As indications for BoNT-A injection are expanded, careful documentation regarding dosage utilization is critical and may often dictate a multi-disciplinary coordination of effort to accomplish the patient's goals for therapy.

Refractory Patients

Defining the cohort of patients who are initial or eventual non-responders for treatment is a multifaceted process, as the majority of studies only include patients who, by definition demonstrated a primary response to treatment [44]. For patients treated with repeat or high-dose injections, concerns exist regarding the immunogenicity of BoNT-A and eventual decrease in clinical response due to seroconversion and antibody formation. Early data with patients administered long-term therapy with BoNT-A identified non-responders who subsequently underwent antibody testing with a mouse protection assay (MPA) [45]. In this group, only 18% of patients tested positive for antibody formation. Notably, many of these patients began therapy as early as 1985 when the formulation for BoNT-A was composed with a higher protein content. Following a decrease in the protein content in 1997 from 25 to 5 ng/100 Units, the rate of antibody formation was reduced from 9.5% to 0% [46]. In a meta-analysis designed to assess for presence of neutralizing antibodies with the MPA, the highest rate demonstrated was 1.3% in patients treated for cervical dystonia [47]. Multiple modalities for antibody testing are available; however, these are not widely employed due to cost and logistical constraints. Recent analysis of long-term data for an extension trial of NDO patients included 240 patients followed for at least 4 years [48]. Rates of seroconversion as assessed by the MPA in the group receiving either 200 Units or 300 Units of BoNT-A were 2.1%, with the rate of those injected solely with 200 Units at only 1.5%. More critically, it remains unclear from several investigations if clinical response is consistently compromised in patients who develop neutralizing antibodies against BoNT-A for bladder applications [49].

Histologic Changes

Concern exists for potentiation of detrusor fibrosis following multiple applications of BoNT-A injection. Examination of the histological and ultrastructural impact of BoNT revealed minimal effect with regard to neuronal architecture and, in fact, demonstrated reduction in bladder wall fibrosis compared to untreated controls [50, 51]. Further analyses have confirmed that BoNT-A injections do not induce substantial inflammation, fibrosis, or dysplasia in the urothelium or suburothelium in patients treated for either NDO or OAB [52].

Conclusion

Overall, for FDA-approved bladder indications, BoNT-A is generally safe and well-tolerated with transient and self-limiting side effects. The substantial incidence of urinary retention and UTI mandates vigilance for identification of these complications and promotion of appropriate counseling such that patient outcomes closely match expectations. Potential concern for dosage limitations with BoNT-A treatment will amplify in the future as patients meet criteria for multiple indications due to continuously expanding applications. Clinicians should remain vigilant to reduce both the expected sequela of BoNT-A injections as well as potential systemic manifestations, despite the rarity of such severe events.

References

1. Van Ermengem E. Ueber einen neunen anaeroben Bacillus and seine Beziehungen zum Botulisms. Ztsch Hyg Infect. 1897;26(1):1.
2. Montecucco C, Molgo J. Botulinal neurotoxins: revival of an old killer. Curr Opin Pharmacol. 2005;5(3):274–9.
3. Simpson LL. Molecular pharmacology of botulinum toxin and tetanus toxin. Annu Rev Pharmacol Toxicol. 1986;26:427–53.
4. Arnon SS, Schechter R, Inglesby TV, Henderson DA, Bartlett JG, Ascher MS, et al. Botulinum toxin as a biological weapon: medical and public health management. JAMA. 2001;285(8):1059–70.
5. Pickett A. Botulinum toxin as a clinical product: manufacture and pharmacology. In: Foster KA, editor. Clinical applications of botulinum toxin. New York: Springer; 2014. p. 7–49.
6. Dressler D, Benecke R. Pharmacology of therapeutic botulinum toxin preparations. Disabil Rehabil. 2007;29(23):1761–8.
7. Foster KA. Molecular aspects of botulinum neurotoxin. New York: Springer; 2014.
8. Dolly O. Synaptic transmission: inhibition of neurotransmitter release by botulinum toxins. Headache. 2003;43 Suppl 1:S16–24.
9. Apostolidis A, Rahnama'i MS, Fry C, Dmochowski R, Sahai A. Do we understand how botulinum toxin works and have we optimized the way it is administered to the bladder? ICI-RS 2014. Neurourol Urodyn. 2016;35(2):293–8.
10. Apostolidis A, Dasgupta P, Fowler CJ. Proposed mechanism for the efficacy of injected botulinum toxin in the treatment of human detrusor overactivity. Eur Urol. 2006;49(4):644–50.
11. Dong M, Yeh F, Tepp WH, Dean C, Johnson EA, Janz R, et al. SV2 is the protein receptor for botulinum neurotoxin A. Science. 2006;312(5773):592–6.
12. Angaut-Petit D, Molgo J, Comella JX, Faille L, Tabti N. Terminal sprouting in mouse neuromuscular junctions poisoned with botulinum type A toxin: morphological and electrophysiological features. Neuroscience. 1990;37(3):799–808.
13. Dykstra DD, Sidi AA, Scott AB, Pagel JM, Goldish GD. Effects of botulinum A toxin on detrusor-sphincter dyssynergia in spinal cord injury patients. J Urol. 1988;139(5):919–22.
14. Ginsberg D, Gousse A, Keppenne V, Sievert KD, Thompson C, Lam W, et al. Phase 3 efficacy and tolerability study of onabotulinumtoxinA for urinary incontinence from neurogenic detrusor overactivity. J Urol. 2012;187(6):2131–9.
15. Nitti VW, Dmochowski R, Herschorn S, Sand P, Thompson C, Nardo C, et al. OnabotulinumtoxinA for the treatment of patients with overactive bladder and urinary incontinence: results of a phase 3, randomized, placebo controlled trial. J Urol. 2013;189(6):2186–93.
16. Chermansky CJ, Chancellor MB. Use of botulinum toxin in urologic diseases. Urology. 2016;91:21.
17. Mangera A, Apostolidis A, Andersson KE, Dasgupta P, Giannantoni A, Roehrborn C, et al. An updated systematic review and statistical comparison of standardised mean outcomes for the use of botulinum toxin in the management of lower urinary tract disorders. Eur Urol. 2014;65(5):981–90.
18. Chancellor MB, Elovic E, Esquenazi A, Naumann M, Segal KR, Schiavo G, et al. Evidence-based review and assessment of botulinum neurotoxin for the treatment of urologic conditions. Toxicon. 2013;67:129–40.
19. Code of Federal Regulations. Available from: http://www.accessdata.fda.gov/scripts/cdrh/cfdocs/cfcfr/CFRSearch.cfm?fr=312.32.

20. Allergan. Available from: http://www.allergan.com/assets/pdf/botox_pi.pdf.
21. De Laet K, Wyndaele JJ. Adverse events after botulinum a toxin injection for neurogenic voiding disorders. Spinal Cord. 2005;43(7):397–9.
22. Soljanik I. Efficacy and safety of botulinum toxin a intradetrusor injections in adults with neurogenic detrusor overactivity/neurogenic overactive bladder: a systematic review. Drugs. 2013;73(10):1055–66.
23. Brin MF, Kirby RS, Slavotinek A, Miller-Messana MA, Parker L, Yushmanova I, Yang H. Pregnancy outcomes following exposure to onabotulinumtoxinA. Pharmacoepidemiol Drug Saf. 2016;25(2):179–87.
24. Santos JI, Swensen P, Glasgow LA. Potentiation of Clostridium botulinum toxin aminoglycoside antibiotics: clinical and laboratory observations. Pediatrics. 1981;68(1):50–4.
25. Napier-Hemy TP, Feyisetan O, Stewart H, et al. Prophylactic intravenous gentamicin with sedation-free cystoscopic injection of BoNT-A: no demonstrable adverse extravesical neuromuscular effects in a pilot safety study of 220 idiopathic overactive bladder patients. J Clin Urol. 2023;16(2):91–5.
26. Fraint A, Vittal P, Comella C. Considerations on patient-related outcomes with the use of botulinum toxins: is switching products safe? Ther Clin Risk Manag. 2016;12:147–54.
27. Rovner E. Chapter 6: Practical aspects of administration of onabotulinumtoxinA. Neurourol Urodyn. 2014;33 Suppl 3:S32–7.
28. AUA Update Series Volume 43 Lesson 12.
29. Gill DM. Bacterial toxins: a table of lethal amounts. Microbiol Rev. 1982;46(1):86–94.
30. Smith CP, Chancellor MB. Emerging role of botulinum toxin in the management of voiding dysfunction. J Urol. 2004;171(6 Pt 1):2128–37.
31. Nuanthaisong U, Abraham N, Goldman HB. Incidence of adverse events after high doses of onabotulinumtoxinA for multiple indications. Urology. 2014;84(5):1044–8.
32. Nitti VW. Botulinum toxin for the treatment of idiopathic and neurogenic overactive bladder: state of the art. Rev Urol. 2006;8(4):198–208.
33. Wyndaele JJ, Van Dromme SA. Muscular weakness as side effect of botulinum toxin injection for neurogenic detrusor overactivity. Spinal Cord. 2002;40(11):599–600.
34. Bauer RM, Gratzke C, Roosen A, Hocaoglu Y, Mayer ME, Buchner A, et al. Patient-reported side effects of intradetrusor botulinum toxin type a for idiopathic overactive bladder syndrome. Urol Int. 2011;86(1):68–72.
35. Naumann M, Jankovic J. Safety of botulinum toxin type A: a systematic review and meta-analysis. Curr Med Res Opin. 2004;20(7):981–90.
36. Zhou X, Yan HL, Cui YS, Zong HT, Zhang Y. Efficacy and safety of onabotulinumtoxinA in treating neurogenic detrusor overactivity: a systematic review and meta-analysis. Chin Med J. 2015;128(7):963–8.
37. Cui Y, Zhou X, Zong H, Yan H, Zhang Y. The efficacy and safety of onabotulinumtoxinA in treating idiopathic OAB: a systematic review and meta-analysis. Neurourol Urodyn. 2015;34(5):413–9.
38. Brubaker L, Richter HE, Visco A, Mahajan S, Nygaard I, Braun TM, et al. Refractory idiopathic urge urinary incontinence and botulinum A injection. J Urol. 2008;180(1):217–22.
39. Osborn DJ, Kaufman MR, Mock S, Guan MJ, Dmochowski RR, Reynolds WS. Urinary retention rates after intravesical onabotulinumtoxinA injection for idiopathic overactive bladder in clinical practice and predictors of this outcome. Neurourol Urodyn. 2015;34(7):675–8.
40. Kuo HC. Comparison of effectiveness of detrusor, suburothelial and bladder base injections of botulinum toxin a for idiopathic detrusor overactivity. J Urol. 2007;178(4 Pt 1):1359–63.
41. Karsenty G, Elzayat E, Delapparent T, St-Denis B, Lemieux MC, Corcos J. Botulinum toxin type a injections into the trigone to treat idiopathic overactive bladder do not induce vesicoureteral reflux. J Urol. 2007;177(3):1011–4.
42. Davis NF, Burke JP, Redmond EJ, Elamin S, Brady CM, Flood HD. Trigonal versus extratrigonal botulinum toxin-A: a systematic review and meta-analysis of efficacy and adverse events. Int Urogyn J. 2015;26(3):313–9.
43. Jo JK, Kim KN, Kim DW, Kim YT, Kim JY, Kim JY. The effect of onabotulinumtoxinA according to site of injection in patients with overactive bladder: a systematic review and meta-analysis. World J Urol. 2018;36(2):305–17.
44. Dowson C, Khan MS, Dasgupta P, Sahai A. Repeat botulinum toxin-A injections for treatment of adult detrusor overactivity. Nat Rev Urol. 2010;7(12):661–7.
45. Mejia NI, Vuong KD, Jankovic J. Long-term botulinum toxin efficacy, safety, and immunogenicity. Mov Disord. 2005;20(5):592–7.
46. Jankovic J, Vuong KD, Ahsan J. Comparison of efficacy and immunogenicity of original versus current botulinum toxin in cervical dystonia. Neurology. 2003;60(7):1186–8.
47. Naumann M, Carruthers A, Carruthers J, Aurora SK, Zafonte R, Abu-Shakra S, et al. Meta-analysis of neutralizing antibody conversion with onabotulinumtoxinA (BOTOX(R)) across multiple indications. Mov Disord. 2010;25(13):2211–8.
48. Kennelly M, Dmochowski R, Schulte-Baukloh H, Ethans K, Del Popolo G, Moore C, et al. Efficacy and safety of onabotulinumtoxinA therapy are sustained over 4 years of treatment in patients with neurogenic detrusor overactivity: final results of a long-term extension study. Neurourol Urodyn. 2015;36:368.

49. Schulte-Baukloh H, Bigalke H, Miller K, Heine G, Pape D, Lehmann J, et al. Botulinum neurotoxin type A in urology: antibodies as a cause of therapy failure. Int J Urol. 2008;15(5):407–15.
50. Haferkamp A, Schurch B, Reitz A, Krengel U, Grosse J, Kramer G, et al. Lack of ultrastructural detrusor changes following endoscopic injection of botulinum toxin type a in overactive neurogenic bladder. Eur Urol. 2004;46(6):784–91.
51. Comperat E, Reitz A, Delcourt A, Capron F, Denys P, Chartier-Kastler E. Histologic features in the urinary bladder wall affected from neurogenic overactivity–a comparison of inflammation, oedema and fibrosis with and without injection of botulinum toxin type A. Eur Urol. 2006;50(5):1058–64.
52. Apostolidis A, Jacques TS, Freeman A, Kalsi V, Popat R, Gonzales G, et al. Histological changes in the urothelium and suburothelium of human overactive bladder following intradetrusor injections of botulinum neurotoxin type A for the treatment of neurogenic or idiopathic detrusor overactivity. Eur Urol. 2008;53(6):1245–53.

Pelvic Complications in Gender-Affirming Genital Surgery

34

Camryn Hawkins, Bethany Bandi, and Michele Fascelli

Introduction

With the increasing demand for gender-affirming care, urologists are encountering more patients who have undergone gender-affirming genital surgery (GGAS). This chapter will review the common complications of GGAS.

Feminizing Surgeries: Vaginoplasty and Vulvoplasty

Vaginoplasty is a surgical procedure to create a vagina for transgender women and non-binary individuals. There are several common approaches to feminizing GGAS, including penile inversion vaginoplasty, robotic peritoneal pull-through vaginoplasty, and intestinal interposition vaginoplasty [1]. As a portion of the vaginal canal is typically made of hair-bearing genital skin, permanent genital hair removal is required. For patients who cannot access hair removal or do not wish to maintain a vaginal canal postoperatively, a minimal depth vaginoplasty or vulvoplasty can be performed [2].

Regardless of technique, the surgical procedure commences with perineal dissection and deconstruction of the penile anatomy to make a clitoris, shortened and downward-oriented urethra, and removal of the testicles. Externally, portions of the penile shaft skin can be used to construct outer and inner labia. Creation of the vaginal canal requires meticulous dissection to separate the urethra, bladder, and prostate from the rectum, akin to a prostatectomy. For vaginal canal construction, the penile inversion method utilizes a combination of penile and scrotal skin to line the vaginal canal. Robotically, peritoneal tissue can be harvested from the posterior bladder and lateral to the rectum; these can then be advanced and surgically connected to any available inverted skin flaps. Robotic vaginoplasty may be performed as primary vaginoplasty or for recovery of lost vaginal depth. Use of intestinal interposition requires assessing which segment of bowel will reach through the pelvis and into the perineum. Intestinal interposition affords self-lubrication and may be a desired outcome.

Complications following vaginoplasty are associated with a range of potential complications that may occur intraoperatively or postoperatively. Rates of complication following penile

C. Hawkins
Northeast Ohio Medical University, Rootstown, OH, USA
e-mail: chawkins2@neomed.edu

B. Bandi · M. Fascelli (✉)
Department of Urology, Cleveland Clinic Foundation, Cleveland, OH, USA
e-mail: BANDIB@ccf.org; Fascelm2@ccf.org

H. B. Goldman, J. Zillioux (eds.), *Complications of Urogynecology and Reconstructive Pelvic Surgery*, https://doi.org/10.1007/978-3-032-00339-3_34

inversion vaginoplasty range from 20% to 70% with most complications occurring within the first 4 months following surgery [3, 4].

Bleeding

Bleeding and hematoma formation can be a significant acute complication, occurring in 3.2–12% of patients [4]. Bleeding represents the primary reason for early return to surgery [4]. The primary sources of hemorrhage are usually the corpus spongiosum surrounding the urethra or from the proximal stumps of the corpora cavernosa; it is critical to ensure adequate removal of the corporal tissue during penectomy and appropriate urethral and corporal closure [5]. An injection of epinephrine into the crus of the corpora cavernosa may help to control bleeding intraoperatively [6]. It is important to identify and treat hematomas as they can delay wound healing and increase the risk of infection or abscess formation. Application of a large bolster dressing to the perineal area and utilization of labial/vulvar drains may help to prevent hematoma formation [4, 6, 7].

Wound Healing and Graft Loss

Wound healing issues are common and most tend to be self-limiting [3, 4, 6]. Wound healing can present frequent challenges due to the complex nature of the surgical site, which often includes multiple incisions, flaps, and/or grafts. Wound dehiscence, which occurs in 5–33% of patients undergoing penile inversion vaginoplasty, most often occurs at sites of maximal tension [6], notably the posterior fourchette, due to the high tension placed on the penile skin. In the literature, it has been noted that as many as 75% of patients will experience some level of breakdown at the posterior fourchette due to the combination of tension, moisture, and mechanical dilation required while the tissue is healing [6]. Wound dehiscence will generally heal with local wound care without additional surgical intervention, but it is important to monitor as it may lead to infection, scarring, neovaginal stenosis, or necrosis. Granulation tissue, which is often a byproduct of wound dehiscence and the healing process, is reported as the most common complication following vaginoplasty [3]. Granulation tissue may cause pain, discharge, or bloody spotting from the vagina and can primarily be managed with silver nitrate applications or topical steroids. Additionally, vaginal necrosis and clitoral necrosis can affect 1–3% of patients. Due to the utilization of full or partial thickness skin grafts to line the vagina, the graft may be lost due to inadequate blood supply or perfusion. Treatment will often require antibiotics and a revision surgery to remove any necrotic tissue and regrafting of the vaginal canal [8]. It is important to perform preoperative counseling with patients about the importance of smoking cessation, diabetes control, and cardiovascular optimization to reduce the risks of graft loss and necrosis.

Vaginal Stenosis

Vaginal stenosis is often associated with inadequate vaginal dilation, poor graft integration, or incomplete dissection during the primary surgery. Stenosis occurs in about 9.8% of patients and can occur at the introitus or within the vaginal canal [9]. Stenosis at the introitus may often be the result of contraction due to wound dehiscence or granulation tissue formation. Prevention of vaginal stenosis is critically dependent on strict adherence to a dilation protocol to maintain vaginal patency (Fig. 34.1). Non-compliance with postoperative dilation protocol and post-surgical follow-up leads are cited sources for stenosis at the introitus and canal [4, 6]. Initial management of vaginal stenosis may include pelvic floor physical therapy with supervised or guided dilation, increased dilation frequency, and use of oil-based lubricants or steroids to help soften skin [4, 6, 10]. In cases where stenosis must be managed surgically, secondary repair will likely require augmentation with either buccal mucosa or skin grafts, where peritoneal tissue or intestinal segments can address stenosis and depth deficiencies.

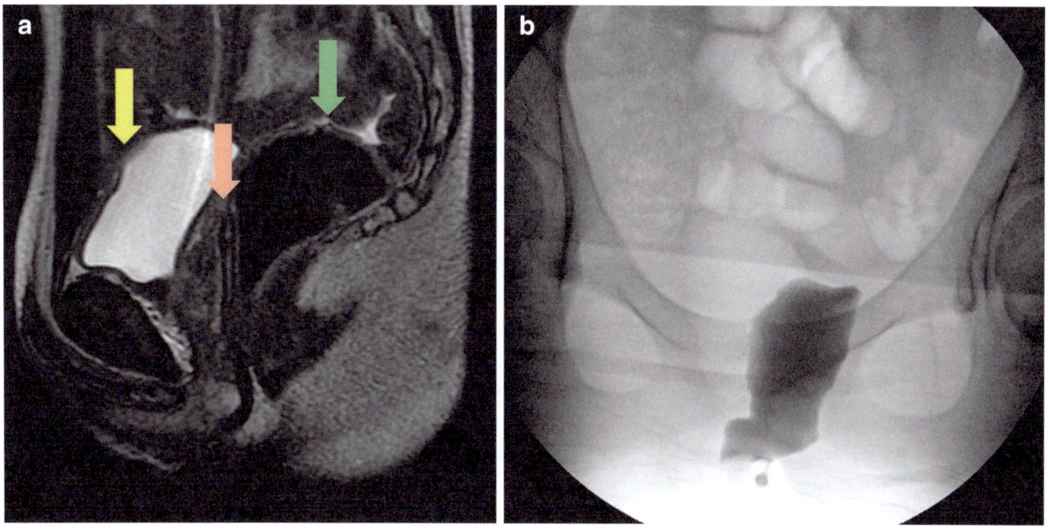

Fig. 34.1 A transgender female patient status post gender affirming vaginoplasty complicated by vaginal bleeding, pelvic pain, and immediate cessation of vaginal dilation due to granulation tissue, who presented with ongoing vaginal discharge from a pinpoint opening in the perineum. Office exam demonstrated pinpoint opening into an introital scar. MRI of the pelvis (panel **a**) demonstrated a vaginal lumen (orange arrow) without a visible fluid collection. The bladder (yellow arrow) and rectum (green arrow) were normal. A vaginogram (panel **b**) demonstrated proximal patency of approx. 8 cm above the introital stenosis

Colonic/Intestinal Vaginoplasty

Colonic vaginoplasty is an option as a secondary surgery for patients following failed primary penile inversion or robotic vaginoplasty [11]. Intestinal vaginoplasty can utilize portions of the small intestine, right colon, or sigmoid colon to create a vagina. Potential benefits of an intestinal vaginoplasty are the ability of the bowel interposition to self-lubricate and the potential for less lifelong dilation with persistent increased depth [3, 11]. Due to the intra-abdominal nature of the surgery, patients are at risk for bladder or bowel injury, anastomotic leak, abscess, fistula, postoperative ileus or potential small bowel obstruction, need for bowel diversion, and/or hemorrhage. Additionally, due to the length of the bowel interposition, some patients may experience prolapse of the vagina, requiring revision. Excessive discharge, which may contribute to malodor, has also been reported. The overall complication rate for intestinal or colonic vaginoplasty is between 6.4% and 8.3% [6, 11]. Patients who have a history of inflammatory bowel disease are not suitable candidates for this procedure.

Urologic Complications

Urologic complications following feminizing GGAS may include difficulty urinating, dysuria, urinary retention, hematuria, incontinence, or (recurrent) urinary tract infections. As many as 15 to 32% of patients reported a postoperative urinary complaint such as weak urinary stream, incomplete emptying, divergent stream, or incontinence [4, 8, 12]. Patients may present with deflected or slow stream, which may suggest an issue with the urethra, or may be a result of asymmetric labia, scarring, adhesions, or residual corporal tissue [4, 5]. Patients who present with a weak urinary stream or incomplete emptying should be evaluated to rule out urethral stricture/stenosis. Meatal or urethral stenosis has been found to occur in up to 14% of patients, with 21% of patients requiring a revision surgery [3, 5]. Pelvic floor physical therapy may be beneficial for patients who present with incontinence or dribbling issues early in the recovery period. Additionally, urethrovaginal fistulas may present with split or splayed streams, vaginal discharge with voiding, and fluid leakage [9]. Urethrovaginal fistulas can be repaired either transabdominally or transvaginally, depending on the location and surgeon's preference [9]. If the injury is recognized during the surgical dissection, a repair should be done to avoid further complications and is often challenging given the lack of robust interposition tissues available; if either of the bilateral bulbospongiosus muscles have yet to be removed at time of a urethral injury, these can be rotated into the vagina for interposition (Fig. 34.2).

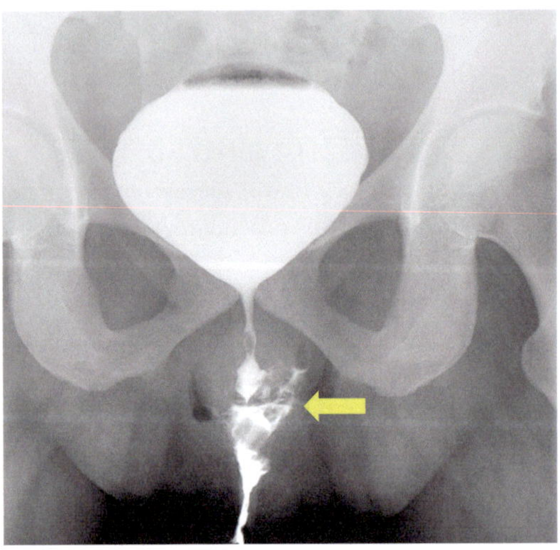

Fig. 34.2 A transgender female patient status post gender affirming vaginoplasty with intraoperative identification of left-sided bulbar urethral injury, with attempted repair utilizing bilateral bulbospongiosus muscles in a "pants-over-vest" interposition. Postoperative voiding cystourethrogram at 2 weeks demonstrated a small persistent leak of urine (yellow arrow) distal to the urinary sphincter. This was observed without an indwelling catheter, and the patient's cystoscopy at 6 weeks demonstrated a well-healed urethra

Rectal Injury

One of the most significant complications associated with feminizing GGAS is rectovaginal fistula, with an overall incidence reported between 0.8% and 1.7% [3]. Development of a rectovaginal fistula is strongly associated with rectal injury during the primary surgery (Fig. 34.3). One study found that approximately 17% of patients who had an identified rectal injury during surgery went on to develop a rectovaginal fistula [9]. In addition to injury during primary surgery, fistulas can also result from complications including abscesses, infection, hematoma, or a dilation injury. When a rectovaginal fistula is identified, conservative management, like a low -residue diet is unlikely to lead to resolution. More likely,

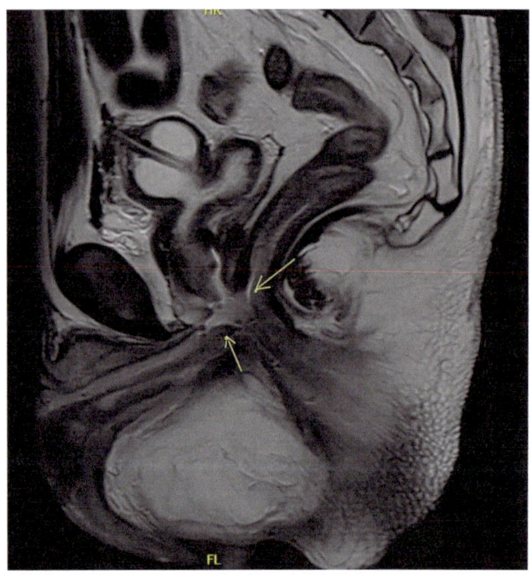

Fig. 34.3 A transgender female patient presented for consultation with a history of intraoperative rectal injury at the time of vaginoplasty repaired primarily. The patient developed a rectovaginal fistula despite an attempted repair. They underwent bowel diversion, and then, following a repeat endorectal advancement flap repair, the patient began having urine per rectum. A suprapubic tube was placed in the bladder and an MRI pelvis was performed demonstrating a prostatic urethra—vaginal—rectal fistula (two arrows)

these complex cases will necessitate surgical intervention, and it is critical to collaborate with a colorectal surgeon for repair [5, 9]. Dilation may need to be temporarily halted or augmented for patients with rectovaginal fistula to prevent worsening the condition, creating the possibility of vaginal depth loss [13].

Aesthetic/Cosmetic

If patients are not aesthetically satisfied, they may undergo revision surgery to improve the cosmetic appearance of the external genitalia. Revision rates range from 2% to 50%, with labiaplasty being cited as the most common revision surgery [3, 9]. Buried or recessed clitoris, which can affect clitoral sensation and visibility, was also a reason cited for revision for re-exposure or to minimize hypersensitivity [9].

Masculinizing Surgeries: Phalloplasty and Metoidioplasty

A phalloplasty is a complex reconstruction of a phallus utilizing a combination of free or pedicled flaps and skin grafts. Commonly, a radial forearm free flap or an anterolateral thigh flap (free or pedicled) is relocated to the prepubic location. Donor site is based on patient preference, anatomic suitability, and desired phallic goals (i.e., standing to void). The urethral reconstruction is factored into the donor sites' ability to be tubularized; the donor site must be of an appropriate thinness to allow for phallic bulk and creation of the urethra and shaft via tubularization. The length of the donor flap must allow for a urethral extension, which is typically set near the base of the clitoris. Microsurgical anastomoses of donor nerve and vasculature must be carefully performed and postoperatively monitored. At the second stage, the peri-urethral tissues—a combination of inner labia and anterior vaginal wall—are used to connect the native urethra to the phallic urethra (or pars pendulans). The newly created perineal portion of the urethra is also known as the pars fixa. Vaginectomy, clitoral burial, scrotoplasty (via rotational advancement of the outer labia), glansplasty, and perineal closure are part of the second-stage procedure. Pending return of sensation, the third stage of surgery is placement of penile and testicular prosthetics.

Metoidioplasty is the construction of a phallus based on a patient's existing genital tissue, primarily the now enlarged clitoris following a response to testosterone therapy. While erogenous sensation and erectile function are preserved, the length of a metoidioplasty is not typically sufficient for penetrative intercourse. For individuals seeking a metoidioplasty with urethral lengthening, a single-stage procedure can be performed. This begins with dorsal and ventral release of the clitoris to allow for maximal length. Release of the suspensory ligament can allow for ranges from 2 to 6 cm of additional length. The urethra is then created using the inner lining of the inner labia with or without buccal mucosa graft and an anterior vaginal wall flap. Vaginectomy and scrotoplasty are similarly performed at this stage. After appropriate healing, testicular prosthetics can be placed.

These masculinizing GGAS are accompanied by a wide range of surgical complications, which may influence both function and aesthetic outcomes of the surgery as well as the patient's overall quality of life. Urological complaints and issues collectively account for a large percentage of complications seen in these procedures and typically occur within the first several months following surgery, with nearly 75% of patients experiencing two or more complications [14]. Patients must cease nicotine use in preparation for reconstructive surgery as nicotine use remains a significant predictor for urethral complications [15].

Urethrocutaneous Fistula

Urethrocutaneous fistula is a common complication following both metoidioplasty and phalloplasty, with incidences ranging from 22% to 75% [14, 16]. These fistulae will most often develop at an anastomotic site and emerge along the ventral suture line [16, 17]. Fistula formation typically occurs in areas of poor vascularization, leading to inadequate vascular perfusion to the flap or graft, compromising tissue viability and healing (Fig. 34.4). One risk factor found to be associated with fistula formation is preservation of vaginal tissue at the time of surgery. One study found that fistulae occurred in up to 56% of patients who did not undergo vaginectomy compared to 14% of those who did have vaginectomy [14].

Patients who have developed a urethrocutaneous fistula will often present with urinary leakage from an ectopic site during voiding, possibly associated with a decreased force of urinary stream, incomplete bladder emptying, and post-void dribbling [16–18]. If a fistula is suspected,

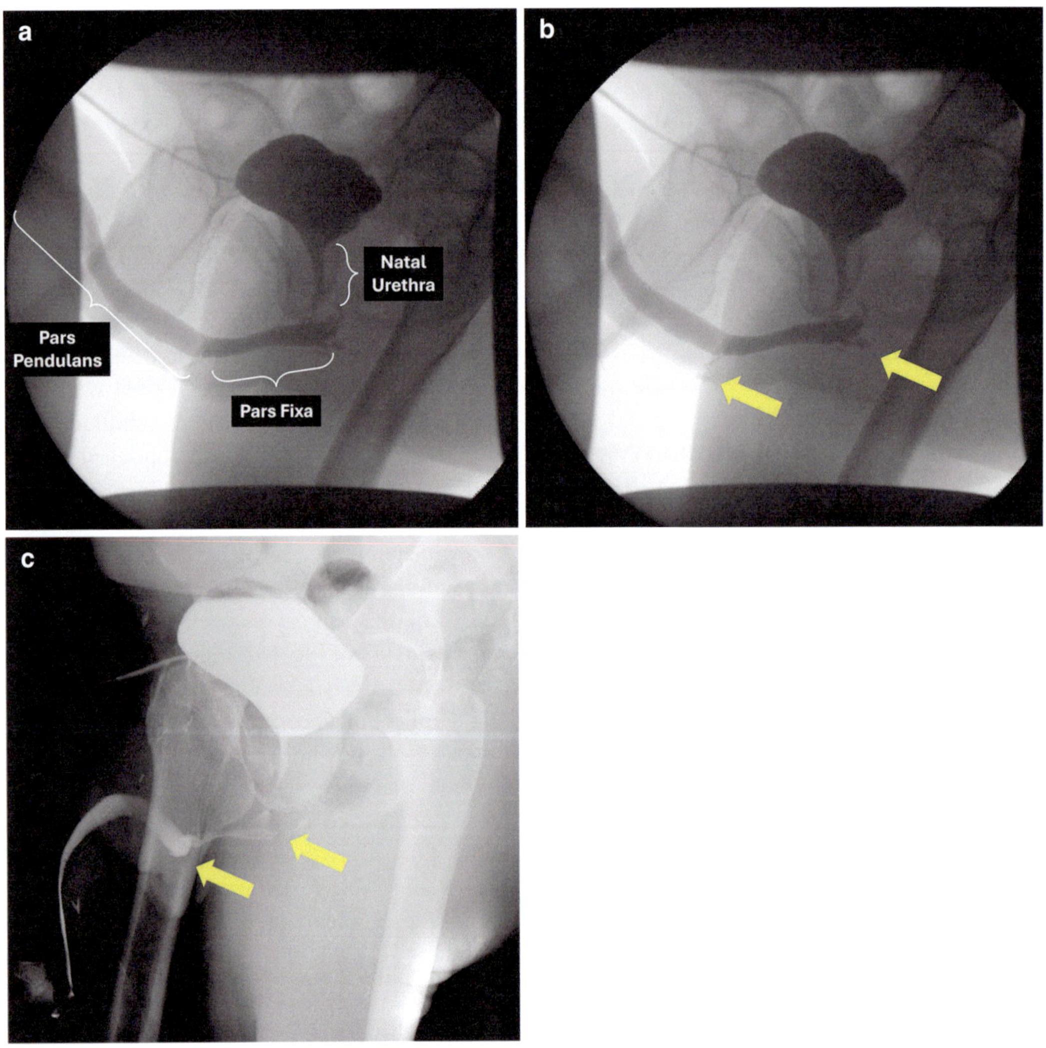

Fig. 34.4 A transgender male patient underwent voiding cystourethrogram via suprapubic tube following stage two of phalloplasty (urethral lengthening, vaginectomy, creation of scrotum and clitoral burial) after reporting perineal leakage. Panel **a** identifies the urethral segments. Two small urethrocutaneous fistulae are visualized (panel **b**) at the junction of the pars pendulans and pars fixa (left yellow arrow) and at the anastomosis of the pars fixa to the natal urethra (right yellow arrow). The suprapubic tube was maintained and a repeat voiding cystourethrogram demonstrated resolution of both fistulae (panel **c**)

concomitant stricture must also be assessed; a bladder scan may be helpful to assess for urinary retention. Flexible cystoscopy, retrograde urethrography, and/or a voiding cystourethrogram (VCUG) can be utilized to visualize the anatomy, location, and the extent of the fistula as well as assess for stricture concern. Management of a urethrocutaneous fistula will depend on the size, location, and persistence of the fistula [16, 18]. Spontaneous closure can occur for smaller fistulae typically within 2–3 months of diagnosis [14, 16, 17]. For larger or more persistent fistulae, surgical intervention is likely required and will often involve excision of the fistula tract with multilayer closure to ensure a durable repair [16, 18]. Some studies have suggested reducing fistula formation by utilizing vascularized tissue flaps, including bulbospongiosus muscles or gracilis muscle interposition at the time of urethral lengthening, providing additional urethral coverage and improved vascularity [14, 16]. However, this benefit in fistula reduction must be weighed against the increased surgical time and morbidity associated with grafting and transferring of flaps [16, 17] and eradicating a future interposition should need arise. Vaginectomy has been shown to decrease the incidence of urethrocutaneous fistula when performed at the urethral lengthening portion of the procedure [14].

Urethral Stricture

Urethral strictures, like fistulae, often present with urinary complaints and most commonly occur at sites of relative ischemia, poor vascular supply, or areas with scar tissue formation, making anastomotic junctions particularly susceptible [14, 16, 17]. In patients undergoing phalloplasty, strictures most frequently occur at the anastomotic junction between the pars fixa and the pars pendulans [17–19]; this has been reported to occur between pars fixa and pars pendulans (41%), in the phallic urethra (28%), in the meatus (15%), in the fixed urethra (13%), or may involve multiple segments (8%) [17–19].

Diagnosis requires flexible cystoscopy, retrograde urethrography, and/or VCUG [16, 17]. Management involves a wide range of interventions depending on severity. Temporary catheter dilation is a short-term measure that may provide some brief relief of symptoms [16, 17]. Endoscopic dilation (with or without steroid injection) and direct visualization internal urethrotomy (DVIU) provide direct visualization and treatment of short solitary strictures, but recurrence remains high [17]. For patients presenting with complex, multiple, or recurrent strictures, urethroplasty is the most definitive management strategy [16, 17]. Staged urethroplasty has been shown to provide the lowest recurrent rates at approximately 30% [16, 17, 19]. Despite these strategies, recurrence rates for masculinizing GGAS urethral strictures remain high, particularly among patients undergoing phalloplasty, whose stricture recurrence rates near 90% [16, 17]. This is attributed to the lack of vascular corpus spongiosum, underscoring the particular importance of conscientious surgical technique and postoperative management to prevent stricture formation and minimize risk of recurrence [17–19].

Persistent Vaginal Canal

Persistence of vaginal canal mucosa is a potential complication following vaginectomy (colpectomy) wherein the vaginal canal mucosa was incompletely ablated or excised [17] (Fig. 34.5). Performing vaginectomy has been shown to reduce the risk of urethral complications in patients undergoing trans masculine gender affirmation surgery [14, 17].

Patients with a persistent vaginal canal may present with high volume post-void dribbling, pelvic or perineal pain, fullness, or recurrent urinary tract infections [16, 17]. Urine or mucus may pool within the vaginal remnant, allowing it to remain patent and may lead to significant discomfort if not addressed [16]. This is best evaluated utilizing a pelvic MRI to identify remnant size and relationship to the surrounding anatomy [17]. Fluoroscopic evaluations can help assess the extent of the remnant and, when combined with cystoscopy, can facilitate identifying any

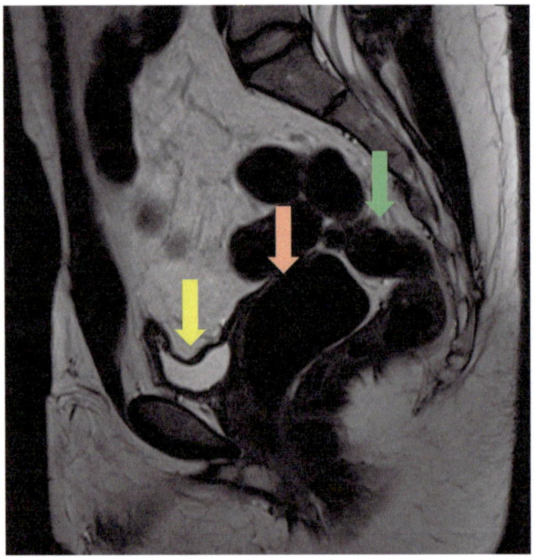

Fig. 34.5 A transgender male status post abdominal phalloplasty with vaginectomy and creation of scrotum presented with perineal pain. Operative reports described mucosal ablation of the vaginal canal. An MRI pelvis was performed and demonstrated a normal bladder (yellow arrow), a large, approximately 10 cm vaginal remnant/mucocele (orange arrow), and a normal rectum and colon (green arrow)

patent vaginal fistula that may have formed between the urethra and canal remnant [17]. Management of persistent vaginal canal requires surgical intervention with complete excision and obliteration of the remnant vaginal tissue.

Penile and Testicular Prostheses

Some patients undergoing phalloplasty may elect placement of penile or testicular prosthess. These are offered several months after initial surgery to allow for effective management of any surgical complications [14]. It is important to note that higher rates of infection and revision rates have occurred in TGD patients following prosthesis placement in comparison to cisgender males [14, 16]. Complications of penile prosethesis may include mechanical failure of the implant, malpositioning, extrusion, and implant instability due to the lack of corpora cavernosa within the phallus. The implant in TGD patients is anchored directly to the pubic bone to allow for greater stability and may result in prolonged pubic pain [14]. In the setting of infection, there is no standard of care or described salvage practice, though removal of infected prosthetics must be addressed promptly; antibiotic rescue may not be sufficient alone, though it is often attempted. Revisions for malfunction require understanding of the phallic vasculature as well as the increased risk to the shaft and erogenous sensation with each subsequent dissection near the previous nerve anastomoses.

Conclusion

Urologists play a vital role in the multidisciplinary care of TGD patients and are often involved in the initial evaluation and management of GGAS complications, including urethral strictures, fistulas, and voiding dysfunction. We are well-positioned to provide initial management and treatment for many complications with both feminizing and masculinizing GGAS and must continue to act as liaisons for appropriate referrals, educate providers, and advocate for system-wide culturally safe and inclusive healthcare environments.

References

1. Krakowsky Y, Shah G, Nguyen A-LV, Kavanagh AG, Potter E, Remondini T, Goldsher YW, Millman A. Gender-affirming care in urology: emergency care of the gender-affirming surgical patient—what the primary urologist needs to know. BJU Int. 2024;133:124–31. https://doi.org/10.1111/bju.16249.
2. Claeys W, Wolff DT, Zachou A, Hoebeke P, Lumen N, Spinoit AF. Variant genital gender-affirming surgery: a systematic review. BJU Int. 2025;135(1):40–53. https://doi.org/10.1111/bju.16513. Epub 2024 Aug 29
3. Gaither TW, Awad MA, Osterberg EC, Murphy GP, Romero A, Bowers ML, Breyer BN. Postoperative complications following primary penile inversion vaginoplasty among 330 male-to-female transgender patients. J Urol. 2018;199(3):760–5. https://doi.org/10.1016/j.juro.2017.10.013.
4. Hontscharuk R, Alba B, Hamidian Jahromi A, Schechter L. Penile inversion vaginoplasty outcomes: complications and satisfaction. Andrology. 2021;9(6):1732–43. https://doi.org/10.1111/andr.13030. Epub 2021 May 27

5. Schardein JN, Zhao LC, Nikolavsky D. Management of vaginoplasty and phalloplasty complications. Urol Clin North Am. 2019;46(4):605–18. https://doi.org/10.1016/j.ucl.2019.07.012.
6. Laungani A, Sapin-Leduc A, Belanger M, Brassard P. Strategies to prevent and mitigate common complications in gender affirming penile inversion vaginoplasty. Plast Aesthet Res. 2022;9:40. https://doi.org/10.20517/2347-9264.2021.110.
7. Das RK, Assi PE, Al Kassis S. Life-threatening bleeding following penile inversion vaginoplasty: case analysis and practice improvement. Eplasty. 2023;23:e72.
8. van der Sluis WB, de Haseth KB, Elfering L, Özer M, Smit JM, Budding AE, van Bodegraven AA, Buncamper ME, de Boer NKH, Mullender MG, Bouman MB. Neovaginal discharge in transgender women after vaginoplasty: a diagnostic and treatment algorithm. Int J Trans Health. 2020;21(4):367–72. https://doi.org/10.1080/26895269.2020.172571.
9. Mann RA, Kasabwala K, Kim N, Pariser JJ. The management of complications of feminizing gender affirming genital surgery. Urology. 2021;152:67–73. https://doi.org/10.1016/j.urology.2021.01.031.
10. Weinstein B, Schechter L. Wound healing complications in gender-affirming surgery. Neurourol Urodyn. 2023;42(5):990–5. https://doi-org.neomed.idm.oclc.org/10.1002/nau.25116
11. Hanley K, Wittenberg H, Gurjala D, Safir MH, Chen EH. Caring for transgender patients: complications of gender-affirming genital surgeries. Ann Emerg Med. 2021;78(3):409–15. https://doi.org/10.1016/j.annemergmed.2021.04.008.
12. Dy GW, Sun J, Granieri MA, Zhao LC. Reconstructive management pearls for the transgender patient. Curr Urol Rep. 2018;19(6):36. https://doi.org/10.1007/s11934-018-0795-y.
13. Stark T, Celtik K, Ting J, Purohit RS. Rectal injury during penile inversion vaginoplasty. Urology. 2024;192:141–5. https://doi.org/10.1016/j.urology.2024.05.043. Epub 2024 Jun 6
14. Jun MS, Crane CN, Santucci RA. What urologists need to know about female-to-male genital confirmation surgery (phalloplasty and metoidioplasty): techniques, complications, and how to deal with them. Minerva Urol Nefrol. 2020;72(1):38–48. https://doi.org/10.23736/S0393-2249.19.03611-7.
15. Esmonde N, Bluebond-Langner R, Berli JU. Phalloplasty flap-related complication. Clin Plast Surg. 2018;45(3):415–24. https://doi.org/10.1016/j.cps.2018.03.017.
16. Elyaguov J, Isakov R, Nikolavsky D. Evaluation and management of urologic complications following transmasculine genital reconstructive surgery. Neurourol Urodyn. 2023;42(5):979–89. https://doi.org/10.1002/nau.25100.
17. Fascelli M, Sajadi KP, Dugi DD, Dy GW. Urinary symptoms after genital gender-affirming penile construction, urethral lengthening and vaginectomy. Transl Androl Urol. 2023;12(5):932–43. https://doi.org/10.21037/tau-22-675.
18. Nikolavsky D, Hughes M, Zhao LC. Urologic complications after phalloplasty or metoidioplasty. Clin Plast Surg. 2018;45(3):425–35. https://doi.org/10.1016/j.cps.2018.03.013.
19. Santucci RA. Urethral complications after transgender phalloplasty: strategies to treat them and minimize their occurrence. Clin Anat. 2018;31(2):187–90. https://doi.org/10.1002/ca.23021.

Female Cystectomy: Pelvic Floor and Functional Perioperative Considerations

35

Shree Agrawal-Patel, Bahrom Ostad, Sandip P. Vasavada, and Jacqueline Zillioux

Introduction

Radical cystectomy with urinary diversion is considered the gold standard for muscle-invasive and certain non-muscle-invasive bladder cancers. In female patients, radical cystectomy traditionally includes removal of the bladder, uterus, fallopian tubes, bilateral ovaries, anterior vaginal wall, and partial or complete resection of the urethra. This extensive resection is considered standard for clinical T2 bladder cancer or greater to achieve optimal locoregional disease control [1].

This approach differs for non-oncologic cystectomy performed for conditions such as neurogenic bladder, poorly compliant bladder, or interstitial cystitis, where female reproductive organs are typically spared. Regardless of indication, cystectomy carries substantial potential implications for urinary function, sexual function, and quality of life [2–4]. This chapter reviews critical considerations for the perioperative care of female patients undergoing cystectomy, focusing on optimizing both oncologic and quality-of-life outcomes as well as addressing female-specific complications.

Anatomical Considerations

Understanding female cystectomy's anatomical impacts is crucial to optimizing functional outcomes and anticipating potential complications. Cystectomy with any form of urinary diversion—whether orthotopic neobladder, continent catheterizable reservoir, or urostomy—can significantly disrupt pelvic floor anatomy with several potential functional repercussions:

Structural:

- Anterior vaginal wall resection can translate to vaginal foreshortening and/or stenosis with subsequent dyspareunia.
- Clitoral devascularization during distal urethral dissection can lead to smooth muscle replacement by fibrous tissue [5]
- Hysterectomy and disruption of endopelvic fascia and lateral pelvic fascial support may predispose to pelvic organ prolapse and impact continence and/or voiding function in orthotopic urinary diversions [6]. These principles are explored in more detail in the pelvic organ prolapse prophylaxis section below.

S. Agrawal-Patel · S. P. Vasavada
Glickman Urological & Kidney Institute, Cleveland Clinic, Cleveland, OH, USA

B. Ostad · J. Zillioux (✉)
Department of Urology, University of Virginia Health, Charlottesville, VA, USA
e-mail: jmz7ga@uvahealth.org

H. B. Goldman, J. Zillioux (eds.), *Complications of Urogynecology and Reconstructive Pelvic Surgery*, https://doi.org/10.1007/978-3-032-00339-3_35

Neural:

- Sensation is carried by the pudendal, pelvic, and hypogastric nerves, which facilitate clitoral innervation and promote vaginal lubrication. Damage to these nerves during cystectomy can correlate to dyspareunia and decreased sexual stimulation [7–10].

Hormonal:

- Oophorectomy can result in early menopause, osteoporosis and/or increased cardiovascular risk [4, 11].

Patient Evaluation and Counseling

Preoperative Evaluation and Counseling

Preoperative counseling of female patients undergoing cystectomy should include a pelvic exam and extensive discussion about the perioperative risks, complications, and long-term outcomes. Initial evaluation should also include baseline sexual function and activity, urinary and bowel function, pelvic organ prolapse, and quality of life goals [12]. Further discussion should include the potential for organ-sparing and/or nerve-sparing approaches in addition to types of diversions and associated complications.

Often, additional time is necessary for comprehensive counseling; however, one survey-based study indicated many urologic oncology providers felt unable to provide this counseling to female patients in comparison with male patients [13]. Barriers to extensive counseling identified in this survey include: older patient age, inadequate clinic time, and poor understanding of patient's baseline sexual function. Perioperative counseling for sexual function remains low, with one study showing that only 13% of patients are counseled on sexual function [14]. Another study of 71 patients found that 27% wanted more information on the impact of cystectomy on personal sexual function and desired information for their partners [15]. Adequate counseling is likely critical for postoperative satisfaction, as suggested by one qualitative study in hysterectomy patients that found higher satisfaction among those counseled on potential postoperative sexual dysfunction compared to those not counseled, even among those who developed it [16].

Postoperative Evaluation

Postoperative pelvic examination and history are needed to assess pelvic floor-related complications or quality of life issues. Like preoperative baseline evaluation, questions should include assessment of urinary function, bowel function, sexual health concerns or dysfunction, and quality of life [4]. However, as with preoperative evaluation, current postoperative assessment patterns are inadequate: one group noted that just 10% of women were assessed for sexual dysfunction and 18% for pelvic organ prolapse after cystectomy [14].

There are a few validated questionnaires that can be utilized. The EORTC quality of life core questionnaire is a comprehensive 30-item questionnaire that has been proposed to capture patient survivorship issues, sexual function, bowel function, diversion issues, catheter use, and self-image [17]. Questionnaires can be given at each follow-up visit to monitor the progression of symptoms. In cases where reported symptoms or exam findings are concerning for a potential surgical pelvic complication, an MRI of the pelvis can be helpful.

The Female Sexual Function Index (FSFI) is a validated questionnaire that can be used to assess perioperative sexual function [18]. Its six domains evaluate desire, arousal, lubrication, orgasm, sexual satisfaction, and sex-related pain. The following factors can impact sexual function when counseling patients: choice of urinary diversion, cancer burden at the time of surgery, hormonal status, relationship status, pelvic organ prolapse, and other comorbid conditions. Patient factors associated with preserved sexual function include age younger than 60 years, cohabitation with a partner, and being sexually active [12].

Surgical Approaches and Prevention Strategies

This section focuses on surgical techniques to optimize sexual functional outcomes and reduce complication risk.

Organ- and Nerve-Sparing Techniques

Recent research has prompted a shift towards an organ- and nerve-sparing approach for radical cystectomy in select patients [1]. The benefits of an organ-sparing approach (a term broadly encompassing any of vaginal wall, ovarian, and uterine sparing approaches) include preservation of sexual function and maintaining pelvic floor support in preliminary studies [14, 19]. Nerve-sparing techniques are primarily employed to preserve sexual function postoperatively. Sexual dysfunction is related to neurovascular bundle damage, devascularization of the clitoris, total or partial urethrectomy, and/or anterior exenteration [4, 8, 20]. Organ-sparing approaches have demonstrated similar rates of cancer-specific survival, operative time, estimated blood loss, and recovery duration. Emerging data demonstrate similar rates of vaginal involvement in patients with clinical T3 disease compared to low-risk patients with or without neoadjuvant chemotherapy [21]. Performing vaginal-sparing radical cystectomy may portend similar oncologic outcomes.

Patient Selection

The current AUA guideline recommends organ-sparing approaches for organ-confined disease [1]. Relative contraindications include tumor involvement at the bladder neck or trigone and carcinoma in situ. Patients with concerning symptoms such as abnormal uterine bleeding or post-menopausal bleeding should undergo additional evaluation with gynecology, including cervical cancer screening, pelvic ultrasound, and potentially endometrial biopsy. However, there is limited data assessing the impact of organ-sparing approaches on disease progression in larger patient populations.

While ovarian-sparing approaches may preserve sexual function and libido, patient risk factors for potential ovarian cancer should be considered. Patients undergoing radical cystectomy may have germline mutations with recommendations for risk-reducing bilateral salpingoophorectomy. Known risk factors include BRCA1, BRCA2, BRIP1, ATM, RAD51C, MLH1, MSH2, MSH6, EPCAM [22]. At present, there is poor evidence to suggest a significant risk of bladder cancer metastatic spread to the ovaries necessitating prophylactic oophorectomy [23]. One study of over a thousand patients who underwent radical cystectomy over 40 years noted just a 0.05% incidence of ovarian involvement [24].

Technical considerations

Organ-Sparing

When performing an organ-sparing cystectomy, the peritoneal incision along the bladder and uterus junction must be more anterior near the bladder and less posterior near the rectum. The use of a vaginal probe with or without ultrasound may help to further define these planes and preserve innervation and vasculature [25]. A vaginal sparing approach and with neobladder diversion has been associated with sexual function recovery close to baseline function [3]. This approach maintains vaginal length to reduce dyspareunia and preserves the ability to continue penetrative intercourse. While traditional concerns regarding oncologic control in the setting of bladder cancer may promote a radical approach for cystectomy, emerging literature suggests organ-sparing radical cystectomy with or without orthotopic urinary diversion does not correlate to worse disease-free, cancer-specific, or overall survival [25–27]. In one report of 15 patients with T2bN0M0 or less bladder cancer who underwent genitalia, uterus, vaginal, and ovary-sparing cystectomy, three patients developed local recurrence and distant metastatic disease within 15 months, while 12 patients remained disease-free for a mean follow-up of 6 years [28].

Nerve-Sparing

The proposed technique is to preserve the nerves passing medially to the ureters as they cross the uterine and vaginal arteries and to preserve somatic nerve bundles as they course near the inferior bladder pedicles. Preserving the neurovascular bundle can preserve vaginal lubrication function and physiologic engorgement of the clitoris and the labia [5, 20].

Transecting the urethra can de-vascularize and impact the neurovascular supply to the clitoris, so careful dissection to preserve innervation is required [5, 27, 29, 30]. A modified approach includes meticulous dissection of the lateral vaginal walls, bladder neck, and proximal urethral to maintain the pudendal nerve flexus fibers to the clitoris [25, 31, 32]. In cases with bladder neck and trigone involvement of bladder cancer, urethral preservation is not indicated [33]. To avoid damage to the neurovascular bundles when dissecting the paraurethral structures, it is recommended to dissect from the 2 and 10 o'clock positions instead of the 4 and 8 o'clock positions [31]. There are also pelvic sensory fibers towards the vagina and cervix that are located around the anterior segment and fornix of the vagina. Some studies suggest using cold dissection to divide the tissue between the bladder and the anterior wall of the uterus and vagina to prevent thermal damage to the nerves [9, 34]. Endopelvic fascia should be preserved as it carries most of the autonomic fibers for continence and sexual function and may help prevent significant pelvic organ prolapse [4, 6].

In patients who undergo nerve-sparing approaches, especially in orthotopic diversion, there is no significant decline in FSFI scores reported in small cohort studies. At 1 year, 6 patients with nerve-sparing techniques are all sexually active without significant changes between the baseline and 1-year FSFI scores. Compared to a non-nerve-sparing cohort, 7 patients reported a significant decline in FSFI scores, on average 25 versus 11, with patient complaints including vaginal dryness, lack of arousal, dyspareunia, and notably, 6 patients discontinuing sexual intercourse. Stable FSFI scores are reported in other small cohorts of patients at 1 year following cystectomy [5, 35].

Reconstructive Considerations

Vaginal Reconstruction

Some studies suggest that if the anterior vaginal wall requires resection, reconstruction of the vaginal canal should be considered. Shortening or narrowing of the vaginal canal contributes to dyspareunia and can be prohibitive for vaginal intercourse. The commonly used clamshell reconstruction, wherein the posterior vaginal wall and cuff are mobilized and folded over to cover the anterior defect, can significantly shorten vaginal length. Restoring vaginal length can be done by re-tubularizing the posterior vaginal wall or use of bowel, rectus abdominis muscle, gracilis muscle, or skin grafts to reconfigure a neovagina adequate for penetrative intercourse [4, 36–40]. Creation of flaps or grafts for neovagina is also susceptible to complications and may compromise or occlude the introitus.

Split-thickness skin grafts can be harvested from the abdominal wall, thigh, and buttocks. If only a partial skin graft is needed, consider an anterior or posterior labial flap, or a thigh flap. If a more distal vaginal reconstruction needs to be performed, a thigh flap may be more appropriate. Once harvested, the graft is placed over a mold and then secured in the space of the native vagina to any vulvar tissue available [39].

If a more proximal vaginal defect requires reconstruction with tissue, a sigmoid or ileum colonic flap can be considered for an anastomosis to the remaining distal vaginal mucosal tissue. If there is a total vaginal defect, a combination of sigmoid colon and proximal thigh flaps can be utilized [41]. Postoperative complications following intestinal vaginoplasty include introital stenosis. In the gender-affirming literature, patients report high sexual satisfaction with intestinal vaginoplasty [37].

Pelvic Organ Prolapse Prophylaxis

Radical cystectomy compromises pelvic support in several ways that may increase risk of pelvic organ prolapse: hysterectomy affects cardinal-uterosacral ligament support, anterior vaginectomy and cystectomy disrupt paravaginal attachments to the arcus tendinous fascia, and anterior vaginectomy and urethrectomy impact endopelvic fascia and urogenital diaphragm support. These negative effects correspond to all three levels of pelvic organ support as described by De Lancey [42]. Vesicovaginal dissection with cystectomy may also negatively affect intrinsic vaginal tissue strength, and vaginal reconstruction following resection may alter vaginal lie and the vector forces thought to significantly contribute to pelvic organ support.

Multiple techniques have been explored to prevent pelvic organ prophylaxis after cystectomy, largely focused on orthotopic neobladders to prevent hypercontinence related to kinking of the neobladder neck with anterior wall prolapse. These techniques include:

- *Sacrocolpopexy*: concomitant mesh or fascia sacrocolpopexy techniques have been described in patients undergoing cystectomy with orthotopic neobladder [43–45]. One case series in 9 women reported a median 43 minutes added time with no hypercontinence postoperatively and no mesh complications or prolapse through nearly 5 years follow-up [43]. A 2015 small randomized controlled trial reported significantly improved objective and patient-reported urinary functional outcomes at 1 year in patients who underwent mesh sacrocolpopexy compared to controls [44]. From a technical perspective for these cases, the vagina is ideally spared, but if it requires resection, tubular reconstruction is preferred. We also note that peritoneum should be preserved to ensure adequate coverage to retroperitonealize the graft to avoid potential space for internal bowel herniation/obstruction [43, 45].
- *Mesh sacrospinous suspension*: one case report described concomitant laparoscopic mesh sacrospinous ligament suspension with no cystocele or mesh complications at 30-month follow-up [46].
- *Round ligament suspension*: A 2020 randomized trial involving 82 female patients with bladder cancer compared standard radical cystectomy with orthotopic neobladder to posterior neobladder suspension using preserved round ligaments. The study found a lower need for intermittent catheterization for retention at 2-year follow-up in the round ligament suspension group [47].
- *Other*: Other described techniques include paravaginal repair, vaginal-sparing technique with preservation of pubourethral ligaments, neobladder tacking to anterior rectus fascia, and omental flaps to provide posterior support [6, 48–51].

Pelvic Organ Prolapse Repair

While scant data exists on this topic, concomitant prolapse repair should be considered for patients with clinically significant baseline apical prolapse. We have previously utilized uterosacral ligament plication at the time of cystectomy due to minimal added time and morbidity, as well as the ability to avoid mesh-related complications [52]. Mesh sacrocolpopexy is also an option, although care should be taken to minimize urine spillage and preserve the peritoneum to facilitate retroperitonealization prior to bowel work.

Postoperative Functional Outcomes and Management

Sexual Function

Common issues after female cystectomy include dyspareunia, reduced libido, reduced vaginal lubrication, anorgasmia, and body image concerns related to urinary diversion. Approximately one-half of patients express postoperative dyspareunia and low libido with a significant decrease in vaginal lubrication [53]. Sexual function can also be altered by body image with different types of urinary diversions. Anorgasmia occurs in about half of patients postoperatively [15, 53, 54]. In a review of outcomes of patients undergoing cystectomy by Kessler et al., patients commonly experienced vasomotor symptoms in addition to sexual dysfunction symptoms [20]. Hormone therapy and symptomatic treatment with antidepressants, pain relievers, and anticholinergics can be provided [54].

Some therapeutic approaches to sexual dysfunction include the use of vaginal lubricant without topical irritants, vaginal estrogen treatment (vaginal DHEA, estriol, testosterone), and selective estrogen receptor modulators. Use of vaginal dilators to maintain vaginal patency can be considered. Trigger point injections or Botulinum toxin injections and pelvic floor physical therapy can assist in pelvic floor dysfunction and vaginal narrowing with symptomatic dyspareunia, although intravaginal work should only be utilized when pelvic exam confirms suture lines have healed well. Topical analgesia can also be used for penetrative intercourse. Sexual therapy and counseling should be recommended for patients with poor libido and anorgasmia to determine strategies such as enhanced partner communication, use of sex aids, and sensate focus to improve sexual satisfaction. Pharmacologic treatment with androgens, antidepressants, and flibanserin is also an option if symptoms persist [29].

Urinary Function

Patients who undergo orthotopic neobladder urinary diversion are at risk for daytime and/or nighttime incontinence as well as hypercontinence (urinary retention) [55].

Candidacy for orthotopic diversion is determined based on multiple factors such as disease burden, age, renal function, comorbidity burden, and prior pelvic radiation history [56]. Orthotopic neobladder is not contraindicated in patients with lymph node disease or extensive trigone involvement, but does require that the distal urethral margin is negative. There are also important functional considerations. First, as many patients are unable to empty completely postoperatively, patients should be willing and potentially able to perform intermittent catheterization. Second, women with intrinsic sphincter deficiency or foreshortened urethra are not ideal candidates, as incontinence would be likely to worsen postoperatively.

Many patients can spontaneously void with almost all achieving daytime continence and two-thirds preserving nighttime continence. Nighttime incontinence is thought to be related to reduced capacity and sphincter relaxation during sleep [55]. However, approximately half of all patients may require periodic intermittent self-catheterization after surgery. Voiding dysfunction is thought to be related to prolapse of the neobladder, causing kinking of the urethra and difficulty voiding (Fig. 35.1). Patients may also have pelvic floor dysfunction or excess sympathetic tone contributing to urinary retention. Hypercontinence and voiding dysfunction may

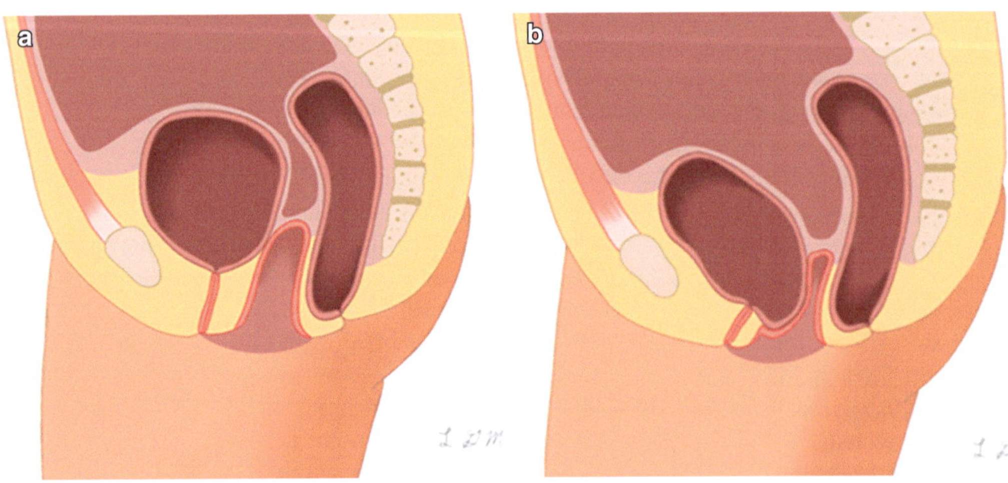

Fig. 35.1 Orthotopic neobladder hypercontinence related to prolapse. (**a**) Demonstrates orthotopic neobladder anatomy with normal support. (**b**) Neobladder prolapse during straining causes urethral kinking and bladder outlet obstruction. (Illustrations used with permission of Luis Gonzalez Miranda, MD, MPH)

also create a positive feedback cycle, where constant straining during voiding weakens the pelvic floor and leads to neocystocele formation [57].

Postoperative Pelvic Floor Complications and Management

Fistula

Fistulas can occur between neobladder and the vagina and likely result from inadvertent vaginal injury. The estimated incidence of neobladder vaginal fistula is 3–6% at higher volume centers, with fistulas typically occurring at the anterior vaginal wall near the neourethral anastomosis and presenting early postoperatively (weeks to months) [58]. They require a high index of suspicion to diagnose, as they can be mistaken for stress urinary incontinence, and pinpoint/smaller fistulas can be difficult to identify [59–61].

Apart from iatrogenic injury to the anterior vaginal wall, risk factors include prior radiation and local cancer recurrence. Overlapping suture lines may also predispose to fistula formation, so one proposed prevention technique is to transect the vagina with a longer anterior flap compared to the posterior vaginal flap so that the suture line can be away from the neobladder anastomosis [58, 62]. If a small entry is noted into the neobladder intraoperatively, it can be repaired primarily with an extended indwelling catheter period and cystography prior to removal to confirm no leak. Especially in patients with prior radiation treatment, interposition of an omental flap can be placed at the time of cystectomy [58, 59]. Other options include interposition of gracilis, peritoneal, or Martius flap, or vaginal reconstruction with autologous/cadaveric graft placement [58–60]. Rarely, patients may require conversion to an incontinent diversion such as an ileal conduit.

Repair of neobladder vaginal fistulas should follow the same tenets of vesicovaginal fistula repairs, with preference for transvaginal approach when feasible. Due to limited tissue mobility, lack of normal planes, and compromised tissue quality, an interposition graft/flap should be used. Additionally, care should be taken to avoid injury to the sphincter as there is a high risk of postoperative stress urinary incontinence [61]. Concomitant anti-incontinence procedures such as pubovaginal sling should be considered in patients with known stress urinary incontinence [63]. However, retropubic suspension may carry a higher risk of bowel perforation related to bowel adhesions deep in pelvis; approaches aimed at the obturator space or single incision approaches may be advisable, albeit with fascia or biologic substitution. Postoperatively, a larger bore catheter should be considered to accommodate neobladder mucous drainage [59].

Peritoneal vaginal fistulas are also possible in patients with non-orthotopic diversions. Patients may complain of continuous leakage or stress "urinary" incontinence. While many peritoneal fistulas represent delayed wound healing of vaginal cuff/repair and resolve spontaneously with time after cystectomy, those with persistent, bothersome leakage past 3 months should be offered surgical repair (Fig. 35.2). The urethrectomy or distal vagina overlying urethra is a common site. Repairs are challenging due to limited healthy tissue and loss of normal planes. If there is some vaginal redundancy available, a vaginal wall flap can be mobilized for coverage and Martius flap employed.

Pelvic Organ Prolapse

Pelvic organ prolapse (POP) following radical cystectomy is an uncommon but significant complication. While there is limited literature on its prevalence, a 2021 systematic review identified 5 retrospective cohort studies (mostly reflecting orthotopic neobladders) with postoperative POP incidences ranging from 0% to 23% [58]. The higher estimate comes from a cross-sectional survey-based study of women following radical cystectomy using the validated Pelvic Organ Prolapse Distress Index (POPDI-6) questionnaire, where 23% of the 35 respondents reported vaginal bulge symptoms at a mean 6-year follow-up [64]. Conversely, a more recent SEER Medicare 5% sample retrospective cohort study

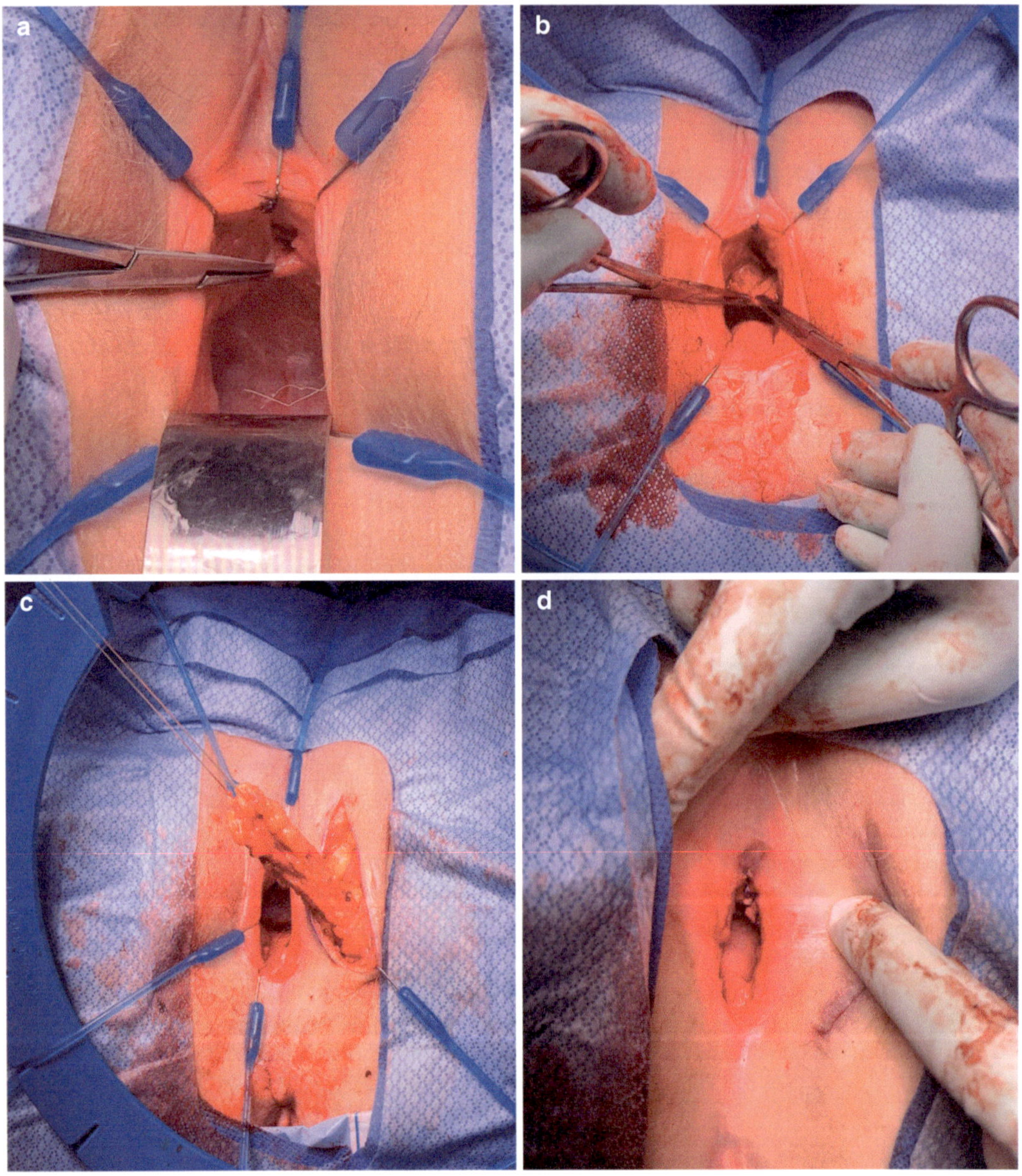

Fig. 35.2 Post-cystectomy peritoneal-vaginal fistula repair. This patient presented 1 year following radical cystectomy with ileal conduit for T4 muscle-invasive bladder cancer with bothersome leakage per vagina, worse with exercise and requiring several pads per day. (**a**) Exam revealed peritoneal vaginal fistula at site of urethrectomy, just 1 cm proximal from the old meatus site. (**b**) For the repair, an inverted U anterior vaginal wall flap was mobilized, although scarring restricted mobility. The fistula was debrided and repaired primarily with polyglactin sutures. (**c**) A modified Martius flap was developed and secured over the repair. (**d**) The vaginal wall flap was advanced for coverage and closure. The patient had durable resolution of symptoms at 9-month follow-up. (Photos courtesy of Dr. Jacqueline Zillioux)

estimated a 4.5% incidence of prolapse following radical cystectomy.

Surgical repair of POP following radical cystectomy presents numerous challenges. These may include poor vaginal tissue quality, with tissue overlying the prolapse often representing granulation tissue or peritoneum moreso than full thickness vaginal epithelium; loss of the "pubocervical fascia" anterior strength layer; limited vaginal length; bowel and/or neobladder adhesions to the vagina; significant intraabdominal adhesions and presence of urinary diversion; and (in the case of sacrocolpopexy following ileal conduit) proximity of longitudinal ligament of the sacrum to ureteroenteric anastomoses. These challenges are reflected by various case reports, several of which describe multiple repairs for recurrence [16, 57, 65–67]. Ultimately, each repair requires individualized surgical planning. Any intervention must balance the need for anatomical correction with the preservation of urinary function (ONB) and avoidance of complications such as graft infection, injury to the urinary diversion, and fistula formation.

Management Options

1. *Pessary*: Pessary use is generally not ideal in post-cystectomy patients due to the compromised integrity of the pelvic floor musculature and foreshortened vaginal vault, making pessary retention difficult and often ineffective [57]. Additionally, the often poor tissue quality raises concern for the risk of vaginal ulceration and dehiscence/evisceration for those with enteroceles [6]. There are no data regarding the efficacy of vaginal estrogen replacement for reducing this risk in this population, but common sense dictates it should be used when pessary management is attempted.
2. *Obliterative Surgery*: Colpocleisis is a good option for patients who do not wish to preserve future intravaginal sexual function. For patients with ONB, it is crucial to assess (occult) stress urinary incontinence preoperatively, as anti-incontinence surgeries (which are already challenging in this population) become even more challenging following colpocleisis. Additionally, anterior vaginal wall dissection in patients with ONB carries a risk of neobladder-vaginal fistula formation [57].
3. *Reconstructive Surgery*: Reconstructive options aim to restore pelvic support while maintaining vaginal function. The choice of approach is individualized based on factors such as vaginal length, anterior tissue quality, and the availability of supportive structures.
   - Transvaginal Repair: This approach is suitable for patients with a hostile abdomen with altered pelvic anatomy that makes abdominal access difficult. There are multiple approaches, including native tissue enterocele repair (Fig. 35.3). While mesh-based techniques have been described, the use of transvaginal mesh is controversial due to the risks of erosion and fistula formation [57, 68].
   - Abdominal Sacrocolpopexy: This approach, using either autologous fascia or synthetic mesh, provides a durable repair but is technically demanding due to adhesions and proximity to the urinary diversion [57]. Mesh is typically anchored to Cooper's ligament and the vaginal apex, sometimes requiring an "Eiffel Tower" shape for optimal fixation [43, 57, 66]. We have utilized a hybrid autologous and mesh technique, using autologous fascia lata graft for the anterior leaflet due to poor anterior tissue quality (Fig. 35.4).
   - Hybrid Techniques: Some cases may benefit from a combination of transvaginal and abdominal approaches, particularly when extensive reconstruction of support structures is needed [57].

Cuff Dehiscence/Vaginal Evisceration

Vaginal cuff dehiscence is a significant complication following cystectomy and, in the presence of bowel evisceration, is a surgical emergency. In a recent SEER study by Richter et al. it was identified as the most common vaginal complication [69]. Studies show this complication occurring in approximately 7–10% of cases [69, 70]. The median time to presentation was 25 days postop-

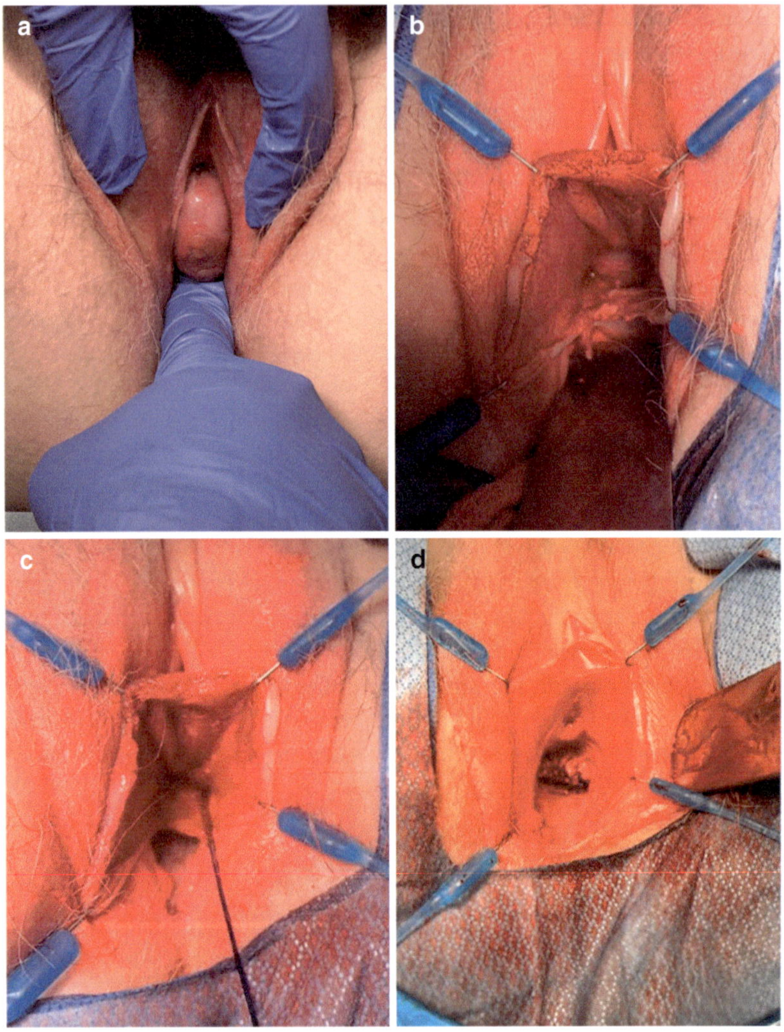

Fig. 35.3 Transvaginal enterocele repair for post-cystectomy prolapse. (**a**) This patient had a history of vaginal vault prolapse following robotic radical cystectomy status-post sacrocolpopexy (anterior leaflet autologous fascia lata with mesh posteriorly and apically, see Fig. 35.4). She presented 6 months later with recurrent symptomatic stage 3 anterior/apical vaginal vault prolapse. (**b–d**) Transvaginal enterocele repair was performed, closing the enterocele with purse string sutures using 0 polydioxanone (PDS). Of note, the recurrent prolapse appeared to occur between the distal edge of the autologous graft and the pubic bone. (Photos courtesy of Dr. Jacqueline Zillioux)

eratively, with most cases occurring within the first few months and almost all presenting within the first year after surgery [69].

The hallmark presentation of vaginal cuff dehiscence includes vaginal bleeding, pelvic pain, and a sensation of vaginal fullness or pressure. In severe cases, bowel evisceration can occur. The risk factors for dehiscence include previous hysterectomy and factors that compromise wound healing, such as radiation therapy, smoking, or advanced age with vaginal atrophy [69]. Patients should be closely monitored postoperatively for any signs of dehiscence, particularly in the early weeks following surgery. Figure 35.5 demonstrates an example of a patient 2 weeks status post radical cystectomy for muscle-invasive bladder cancer who presented with early prolapse and an area of concern for risk of cuff breakdown. This patient necessitated close monitoring, although dehiscence did not ultimately occur.

The management of vaginal cuff dehiscence depends on the severity of the condition and the presence of associated complications such as bowel evisceration. Limited cases without evisceration or infection may be managed conservatively with pelvic rest, vaginal estrogen therapy (for atrophic tissue), and close follow-up. However, non-operative management is rare, as most cases require surgical repair.

Dehiscence with bowel evisceration necessitates emergent surgery to reduce the risk of isch-

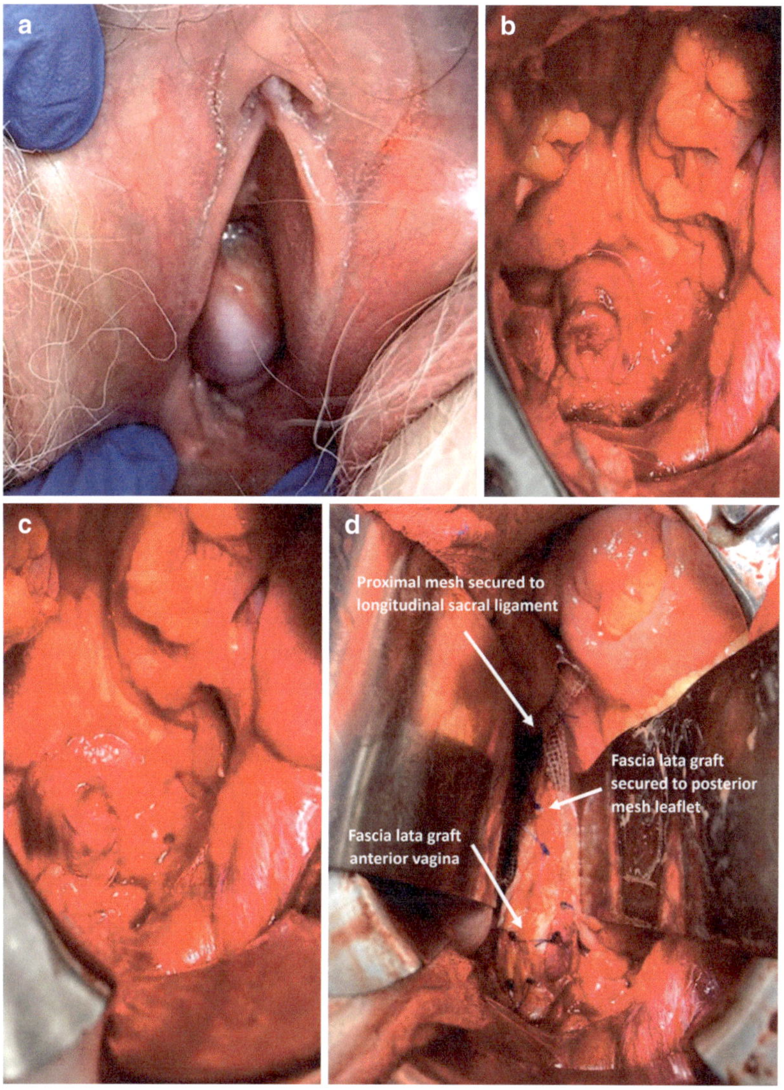

Fig. 35.4 Abdominal sacrocolpopexy using hybrid autologous and mesh graft for post-cystectomy prolapse. (**a**) This patient initially presented 1 year after radical cystectomy with ileal conduit for muscle-invasive bladder cancer with bothersome vaginal bulge (stage 2B anterior/apical). Anterior tissue was quite thin and poor quality. She elected abdominal sacrocolpopexy using autologous fascia lata graft for anterior leaflet affixed to mesh posteriorly and apically. (**b**) Intraoperatively, it became apparent that the clamshell flap from the time of her radical cystectomy had dehisced. Thin peritoneum/granulation tissue covered the defect/prolapse. (**c**) The vaginal mucosa was repaired with running 2-0 polyglactin suture. (**d**) A 4 × 8 cm autologous fascia lata graft was secured to a lightweight Y sacrocolpopexy mesh with polypropylene sutures, replacing the anterior leaflet of mesh with the autologous graft. The hybrid graft was affixed and tensioned in standard fashion to complete sacrocolpopexy. (Photos courtesy of Dr. Jacqueline Zillioux)

emia and peritonitis (Fig. 35.6). Surgical management can be performed trans-vaginally or trans-abdominally, depending on the emergent nature of the dehiscence, bowel viability, and the tissue quality [67]. Decision must then be made to attempt to repair the cuff with reconstruction of vaginal support or to perform colpocleisis, which can be challenging given inadequate tissue for mobilization to cover any exposed bowel. If the bowel is compromised, this must be addressed

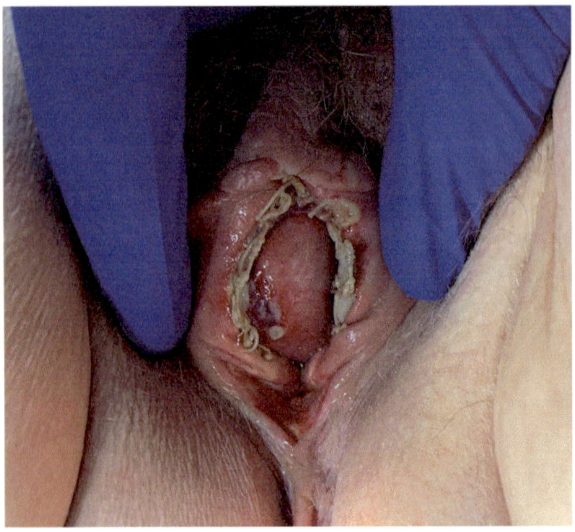

Fig. 35.5 Pelvic exam of a patient approximately two weeks status post radical cystectomy for muscle-invasive bladder cancer. She was noted to have stage 2 anterior/apical prolapse, which was placing some tension on the vaginal closure. Additionally, there was an area of concern for impending breakdown on the right aspect of the vaginal flap/cuff. This patient was advised to continue extended activity restrictions and was closely followed in the clinic. Dehiscence did not ultimately occur. (Photo courtesy of Dr. Jacqueline Zillioux)

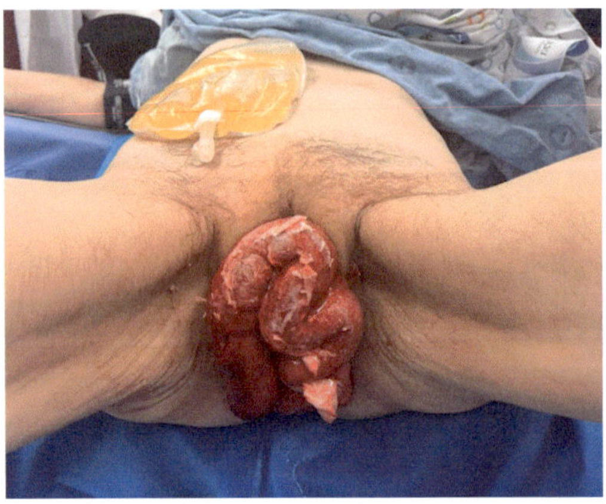

Fig. 35.6 Patient with bowel evisceration from vaginal cuff dehiscence after radical cystectomy with ileal conduit urinary diversion. (Photo courtesy of Dr. Sandip P. Vasavada)

with bowel resection and anastomosis or involvement of general surgery for further guidance. Colpususpension can be performed to prevent recurrent further prolapse, but enterocele repair with colpocleisis and levatormyorrhaphy is typically preferred in the emergent setting [67, 68]. If contributing factors such as poor tissue quality or excessive tension on the repair are identified, adjunct techniques like biological grafts or omental interposition may be utilized. Mesh-based repairs should only be used in select cases and with significant caution due to risks of erosion, infection, or bowel-related complication.

Conclusions

Cystectomy in women has numerous potential repercussions for sexual and pelvic floor function as well as quality of life; however, these outcomes remain understudied compared to male-specific outcomes. Patients require comprehensive counseling regarding sexual and pelvic floor risks and longitudinal follow-up that includes a focus on functional outcomes. Available data suggest that organ- and nerve-sparing approaches in appropriately selected patients can optimize functional outcomes. Urogynecology and Pelvic Reconstructive Surgery (URPS) collaboration is necessary for addressing pelvic floor complications when they do arise, as management is technically quite challenging and requires individualized approaches. Further study is necessary to determine prophylactic strategies to prevent complications and guide best practices for managing these complications.

References

1. Holzbeierlein J, Bixler BR, Buckley DI, et al. Treatment of non-metastatic muscle-invasive bladder cancer: AUA/ASCO/SUO Guideline (2017; Amended 2020, 2024). J Urol. 2024;212(1):3–10. https://doi.org/10.1097/JU.0000000000003981.
2. Westerman ME, Bree KK, Kokorovic A, et al. What women want: radical cystectomy and perioperative sexual function educational needs. Urology. 2021;157:181–7. https://doi.org/10.1016/j.urology.2021.06.012.
3. Clements MB, Atkinson TM, Dalbagni GM, et al. Health-related quality of life for patients undergoing radical cystectomy: results of a large prospective cohort. Eur Urol. 2022;81(3):294–304. https://doi.org/10.1016/j.eururo.2021.09.018.
4. Pederzoli F, Campbell JD, Matsui H, Sopko NA, Bivalacqua TJ. Surgical factors associated with male

and female sexual dysfunction after radical cystectomy: what do we know and how can we improve outcomes? Sex Med Rev. 2018;6(3):469–81. https://doi.org/10.1016/j.sxmr.2017.11.003.
5. Bhatt A, Nandipati K, Dhar N, et al. Neurovascular preservation in orthotopic cystectomy: impact on female sexual function. Urology. 2006;67(4):742–5. https://doi.org/10.1016/j.urology.2005.10.015.
6. Rapp DE, Zillioux J. Radical cystectomy in the female patient: the pelvic floor, sexual function, and patient/provider education. Urol Oncol Semin Orig Investig. 2024:S1078143924005465. https://doi.org/10.1016/j.urolonc.2024.07.007.
7. Graziottin A, Giraldi A. Anatomy and physiology of women's sexual function. In: Porst H, Buvat J, The Standards Committee Of The International Society For Sex, editors. Standard practice in sexual medicine. 1st ed. Wiley; 2006. p. 289–304. https://doi.org/10.1002/9780470755235.ch19.
8. Schoenberg M, Hortopan S, Schlossberg L, Marshall FF. Anatomical anterior exenteration with urethral and vaginal preservation: illustrated surgical method. J Urol. 1999;161(2):569–72.
9. Stenzl A, Colleselli K, Poisel S, Feichtinger H, Pontasch H, Bartsch G. Rationale and technique of nerve sparing radical cystectomy before an orthotopic neobladder procedure in women. J Urol. 1995;154(6):2044–9. https://doi.org/10.1016/S0022-5347(01)66688-6.
10. Park K, Goldstein I, Andry C, Siroky M, Krane R, Azadzoi K. Vasculogenic female sexual dysfunction: the hemodynamic basis for vaginal engorgement insufficiency and clitoral erectile insufficiency. Int J Impot Res. 1997;9(1):27–37. https://doi.org/10.1038/sj.ijir.3900258.
11. Hassan H, Allen I, Sofianopoulou E, et al. Long-term outcomes of hysterectomy with bilateral salpingo-oophorectomy: a systematic review and meta-analysis. Am J Obstet Gynecol. 2024;230(1):44–57. https://doi.org/10.1016/j.ajog.2023.06.043.
12. Davis L, Isali I, Prunty M, et al. Female sexual function following radical cystectomy in bladder cancer. Sex Med Rev. 2022;10(2):231–9. https://doi.org/10.1016/j.sxmr.2021.10.005.
13. Gupta N, Kucirka LM, Semerjian A, et al. Comparing provider-led sexual health counseling of male and female patients undergoing radical cystectomy. J Sex Med. 2020;17(5):949–56. https://doi.org/10.1016/j.jsxm.2020.01.025.
14. Voigt M, Hemal K, Matthews C. Influence of simple and radical cystectomy on sexual function and pelvic organ prolapse in female patients: a scoping review of the literature. Sex Med Rev. 2019;7(3):408–15. https://doi.org/10.1016/j.sxmr.2019.03.005.
15. Booth BB, Rasmussen A, Jensen JB. Evaluating sexual function in women after radical cystectomy as treatment for bladder cancer. Scand J Urol. 2015;49(6):463–7. https://doi.org/10.3109/21681805.2015.1055589.
16. Bradford A, Meston C. Sexual outcomes and satisfaction with hysterectomy: influence of patient education. J Sex Med. 2007;4(1):106–14. https://doi.org/10.1111/j.1743-6109.2006.00384.x.
17. Rammant E, Fox L, Beyer K, et al. The current use of the EORTC QLQ-NMIBC24 and QLQ-BLM30 questionnaires for the assessment of health-related quality of life in bladder cancer patients: a systematic review. Qual Life Res Int J Qual Life Asp Treat Care Rehabil. 2023;32(8):2127–35. https://doi.org/10.1007/s11136-022-03335-4.
18. Rosen C, Brown J, Heiman SL, R. The Female Sexual Function Index (FSFI): a multidimensional self-report instrument for the assessment of female sexual function. J Sex Marital Ther. 2000;26(2):191–208. https://doi.org/10.1080/009262300278597.
19. Laukhtina E, Deimling MV, Pradere B, et al. MP32-16 functional outcomes in female patients after traditional, organ- and nerve-sparing radical cystectomy and urinary diversion for bladder cancer: a systematic review and pooled analyses. J Urol. 2023;209 https://doi.org/10.1097/JU.0000000000003265.16.
20. Kessler TM, Burkhard FC, Studer UE. Clinical indications and outcomes with nerve-sparing cystectomy in patients with bladder cancer. Urol Clin North Am. 2005;32(2):165–75. https://doi.org/10.1016/j.ucl.2005.02.005.
21. Bree KK, Hensley PJ, Westerman ME, et al. Contemporary rates of gynecologic organ involvement in females with muscle invasive bladder cancer: a retrospective review of women undergoing radical cystectomy following neoadjuvant chemotherapy. J Urol. 2021;206(3):577–85. https://doi.org/10.1097/JU.0000000000001784.
22. National Cancer Institute. Genetics of breast and gynecologic cancers (PDQ®) – NCI; 2025. Accessed February 23, 2025. https://www.cancer.gov/types/breast/hp/breast-ovarian-genetics-pdq
23. Escott M, Avulova S, Bree KK, Westerman ME. Radical cystectomy and women's sexual health – can we do better? Curr Opin Urol. 2022;32(5):545–53. https://doi.org/10.1097/MOU.0000000000001026.
24. Avulova S, Benidir T, Cheville JC, et al. Prevalence, predictors, and oncologic outcomes of pelvic organ involvement in women undergoing radical cystectomy. Arch Pathol Lab Med. 2023;147(2):202–7. https://doi.org/10.5858/arpa.2021-0409-OA.
25. Menon M, Hemal AK, Tewari A, et al. Robot-assisted radical cystectomy and urinary diversion in female patients: technique with preservation of the uterus and vagina1. J Am Coll Surg. 2004;198(3):386–93. https://doi.org/10.1016/j.jamcollsurg.2003.11.010.
26. Miura H, Hatakeyama S, Tanaka T, et al. Oncological and functional outcomes of female reproductive organ-sparing radical cystectomy and ileal neobladder construction. Urol Oncol. 2023;41(5):254.e17–24. https://doi.org/10.1016/j.urolonc.2022.11.018.
27. Bhatta Dhar N, Kessler TM, Mills RD, Burkhard F, Studer UE. Nerve-sparing radical cystectomy and

orthotopic bladder replacement in female patients. Eur Urol. 2007;52(4):1006–14. https://doi.org/10.1016/j.eururo.2007.02.048.
28. Ali-El-Dein B, Mosbah A, Osman Y, et al. Preservation of the internal genital organs during radical cystectomy in selected women with bladder cancer: a report on 15 cases with long term follow-up. Eur J Surg Oncol EJSO. 2013;39(4):358–64. https://doi.org/10.1016/j.ejso.2013.02.004.
29. Kalampokis N, Grivas N, Ölschläger M, Hassan FN, Gakis G. Radical cystectomy in female patients – improving outcomes. Curr Urol Rep. 2019;20(12):83. https://doi.org/10.1007/s11934-019-0951-z.
30. Aboseif SR, Borirakchanyavat S, Lue TF, Carroll PR. Continence mechanism of the ileal neobladder in women: a urodynamics study. World J Urol. 1998;16(6):400–4. https://doi.org/10.1007/s003450050090.
31. Tuderti G, Mastroianni R, Flammia S, et al. Sex-sparing robot-assisted radical cystectomy with intracorporeal padua ileal neobladder in female: surgical technique, perioperative, oncologic and functional outcomes. J Clin Med. 2020;9(2):577. https://doi.org/10.3390/jcm9020577.
32. Pacchetti A, Pignot G, Le Quellec A, et al. Sexual-sparing robot assisted radical cystectomy in female: a step-by-step guide. Urology. 2021;156:322–3. https://doi.org/10.1016/j.urology.2021.06.002.
33. Coloby PJ, Kakizoe T, Tobisu KI, Sakamoto MI. Urethral involvement in female bladder cancer patients: mapping of 47 consecutive cysto-urethrectomy specimens. J Urol. 1994;152(5 Part 1):1438–42. https://doi.org/10.1016/S0022-5347(17)32440-0.
34. Stein JP, Stenzl A, Esrig D, et al. Lower urinary tract reconstruction following cystectomy in women using the kock ileal reservoir with bilateral ureteroileal urethrostomy: initial clinical experience. J Urol. 1994;152(5 Part 1):1404–8. https://doi.org/10.1016/S0022-5347(17)32431-X.
35. Nandipati KC, Bhat A, Zippe CD. Neurovascular preservation in female orthotopic radical cystectomy significantly improves sexual function. Urology. 2006;67(1):185–6. https://doi.org/10.1016/j.urology.2005.07.024.
36. Volkmer BG, Gschwend JE, Herkommer K, Simon J, Küfer R, Hautmann RE. Cystectomy and orthotopic ileal neobladder: the impact on female sexuality. J Urol. 2004;172(6 Part 1):2353–7. https://doi.org/10.1097/01.ju.0000145190.84531.66.
37. Bouman M, Van Zeijl MCT, Buncamper ME, Meijerink WJHJ, Van Bodegraven AA, Mullender MG. Intestinal vaginoplasty revisited: a review of surgical techniques, complications, and sexual function. J Sex Med. 2014;11(7):1835–47. https://doi.org/10.1111/jsm.12538.
38. Schove LR, Von Eschenbach AC. Sexual function and female radical cystectomy: a case series. J Urol. 1985;134(3):465–8. https://doi.org/10.1016/S0022-5347(17)47242-9.
39. Chen YBT, Cheng TJ, Lin HH, Yang YS. Spatial W-plasty full-thickness skin graft for neovaginal reconstruction. Plast Reconstr Surg. 1994;94(5):727–31. https://doi.org/10.1097/00006534-199410000-00027.
40. Mccraw JB, Massey FM, Shanklin KD, Horton CE. Vaginal reconstruction with gracilis myocutaneous flaps. Plast Reconstr Surg. 1976;58(2):176–83. https://doi.org/10.1097/00006534-197608000-00006.
41. Cordeiro PG, Pusic AL, Disa JJ. A classification system and reconstructive algorithm for acquired vaginal defects. Plast Reconstr Surg. 2002;110(4):1058–65. https://doi.org/10.1097/01.PRS.0000020988.13244.A0.
42. DeLancey JOL. What's new in the functional anatomy of pelvic organ prolapse? Curr Opin Obstet Gynecol. 2016;28(5):420–9. https://doi.org/10.1097/GCO.0000000000000312.
43. Stearns G, Donahue T, Fathollahi A, Dalbagni G, Sandhu J. Formal sacrocolpopexy reduces hypercontinence rates in female neobladder formation. Neurourol Urodyn. 2018;37(7):2281–5. https://doi.org/10.1002/nau.23584.
44. Życzkowski M, Muskała B, Kaletka Z, et al. Sacrocolpopexy with polypropylene tape as valuable surgical modification during cystectomy with orthotopic ileal bladder: functional results. Biomed Res Int. 2015;2015:1–4. https://doi.org/10.1155/2015/306191.
45. Truong H, Maxon V, Goh AC. Robotic female radical cystectomy. J Endourol. 2021;35(S2):S-106–15. https://doi.org/10.1089/end.2020.1190.
46. Törzsök P, Bauer S, Forstner R, Sievert KD, Janetschek G, Zimmermann R. Laparoscopic radical cystectomy and ileal neobladder for muscle invasive bladder cancer in combination with one stage prophylactic laparoscopic sacrospinal fixation to avoid future pelvic organ prolapse. J Endourol Case Rep. 2016;2(1):59–61. https://doi.org/10.1089/cren.2016.0029.
47. Zhou X, He P, Ji H, et al. Round ligament suspending treatment in orthotopic ileal-neobladder after radical cystectomy in women: a single-centre prospective randomised trial. BJU Int. 2021;128(2):187–95. https://doi.org/10.1111/bju.15306.
48. Zahran MH, Eldemerdash Y, Taha DE, Sheir K, Shaaban AA, Ali-El-Dein B. Chronic urinary retention after radical cystectomy and orthotopic neobladder in women: risk factors and relation to time. Urol Oncol. 2017;35(12):671.e11–6. https://doi.org/10.1016/j.urolonc.2017.07.032.
49. Littlejohn N, Cohn JA, Kowalik CG, Kaufman MR, Dmochowski RR, Reynolds WS. Treatment of pelvic floor disorders following neobladder. Curr Urol Rep. 2017;18(1):5. https://doi.org/10.1007/s11934-017-0652-4.
50. Finley DS, Lee U, McDonough D, Raz S, deKernion J. Urinary retention after orthotopic neobladder sub-

stitution in females. J Urol. 2011;186(4):1364–9. https://doi.org/10.1016/j.juro.2011.05.069.

51. Majdalany SE, Yaguchi G, Arora S, Ray C, Atiemo HO, Raza J. Genital sparing robot-assisted radical cystectomy with intracorporeal neobladder & paravaginal repair. Urology. 2023;179:202–3. https://doi.org/10.1016/j.urology.2023.05.031.
52. Zillioux J, Slopnick E, Almassi N, Vasavada S. V06-10 robotic uterosacral ligament plication at time of benign cystectomy. J Urol. 2022;207(Suppl 5) https://doi.org/10.1097/JU.0000000000002586.10.
53. Zippe CD, Raina R, Shah AD, et al. Female sexual dysfunction after radical cystectomy: a new outcome measure. Urology. 2004;63(6):1153–7. https://doi.org/10.1016/j.urology.2003.12.034.
54. Zahran MH, Fahmy O, El-Hefnawy AS, Ali-El-Dein B. Female sexual dysfunction post radical cystectomy and urinary diversion. Climacteric. 2016;19(6):546–50. https://doi.org/10.1080/13697137.2016.1225714.
55. Nseyo U, Ginsberg D. Functional outcomes of orthotopic neobladder in women. Curr Urol Rep. 2024;25(11):277–85. https://doi.org/10.1007/s11934-024-01223-7.
56. Stein JP, Penson DF, Lee C, Cai J, Miranda G, Skinner DG. Long-term oncological outcomes in women undergoing radical cystectomy and orthotopic diversion for bladder cancer. J Urol. 2009;181(5):2052–9. https://doi.org/10.1016/j.juro.2009.01.020.
57. Lee D, Zimmern P. Management of pelvic organ prolapse after radical cystectomy. Curr Urol Rep. 2019;20(11):71. https://doi.org/10.1007/s11934-019-0941-1.
58. Richter LA, Egan J, Alagha EC, Handa VL. Vaginal complications after radical cystectomy for bladder cancer: a systematic review. Urology. 2021;156:e20–9. https://doi.org/10.1016/j.urology.2021.07.001.
59. Kaufman MR. Neobladder-vaginal fistula: surgical management techniques. Curr Urol Rep. 2019;20(11):1–8. https://doi.org/10.1007/s11934-019-0934-0.
60. Gelber K, Bohrer J, Kim CO, Minaglia S. Vaginal repair of neobladder-vaginal fistula: a case report and review of the literature. Int Urogynecol J. 2013;24(1):175–8. https://doi.org/10.1007/s00192-011-1636-4.
61. Carmel ME, Goldman HB, Moore CK, Rackley RR, Vasavada SP. Transvaginal neobladder vaginal fistula repair after radical cystectomy with orthotopic urinary diversion in women. Neurourol Urodyn. 2016;35(1):90–4. https://doi.org/10.1002/nau.22687.
62. Flack CK, Monn MF, Kaimakliotis HZ, Koch MO. Functional and clinicopathologic outcomes using a modified vescica ileale padovana technique. Bladder Cancer Amst Neth. 2015;1(1):73–9. https://doi.org/10.3233/BLC-140002.
63. Bailey GC, Blackburne A, Ziegelmann MJ, Lightner DJ. Outcomes of surgical management in patients with stress urinary incontinence and/or neovesicovaginal fistula after orthotopic neobladder diversion. J Urol. 2016;196(5):1478–83. https://doi.org/10.1016/j.juro.2016.06.009.
64. Lipetskaia L, Lee TG, Li D, Meyer H, Doyle PJ, Messing E. Pelvic floor organ prolapse after radical cystectomy in patients with uroepithelial carcinoma. Female Pelvic Med Reconstr Surg. 2021;27(4):e501–4. https://doi.org/10.1097/SPV.0000000000000756.
65. Cruz AP, Chelluri R, Ramchandani P, Guzzo TJ, Smith AL. Post-cystectomy enterocele: a case series and review of the literature. Urology. 2021;150:180–7. https://doi.org/10.1016/j.urology.2020.03.063.
66. Zimmern PE, Wang CN. Abdominal sacrocolpopexy for repair of pelvic organ prolapse after radical cystectomy. Female Pelvic Med Reconstr Surg. 2019;25(3):218–21. https://doi.org/10.1097/SPV.0000000000000536.
67. Lin FC, Medendorp A, Van Kuiken M, Mills SA, Tarnay CM. Vaginal dehiscence and evisceration after robotic-assisted radical cystectomy: a case series and review of the literature. Urology. 2019;134:90–6. https://doi.org/10.1016/j.urology.2019.09.009.
68. Stav K, Dwyer PL, Rosamilia A, Lim YN, Alcalay M. Transvaginal pelvic organ prolapse repair of anterior enterocele following cystectomy in females. Int Urogynecol J Pelvic Floor Dysfunct. 2009;20(4):411–5. https://doi.org/10.1007/s00192-008-0786-5.
69. Richter LA, Osazuwa-Peters OL, Routh JC, Handa VL. Vaginal complications after cystectomy: results from a medicare sample. J Urol. 2022;207(4):789–96. https://doi.org/10.1097/JU.0000000000002336.
70. Kanno T, Ito K, Sawada A, et al. Complications and reoperations after laparoscopic radical cystectomy in a Japanese multicenter cohort. Int J Urol Off J Jpn Urol Assoc. 2019;26(4):493–8. https://doi.org/10.1111/iju.13917.

Index

H. B. Goldman, J. Zillioux (eds.), *Complications of Urogynecology and Reconstructive Pelvic Surgery*, https://doi.org/10.1007/978-3-032-00339-3

R

MIX
Papier aus verantwortungsvollen Quellen
Paper from responsible sources
FSC® C105338

If you have any concerns about our products,
you can contact us on
ProductSafety@springernature.com

In case Publisher is established outside the EU,
the EU authorized representative is:
Springer Nature Customer Service Center GmbH
Europaplatz 3, 69115 Heidelberg, Germany

Printed by Libri Plureos GmbH
in Hamburg, Germany